Handbook of
Liver Disease

FOURTH EDITION

Handbook of Liver Disease

LAWRENCE S. FRIEDMAN, MD
The Anton R. Fried, MD, Chair
Department of Medicine
Newton-Wellesley Hospital
Assistant Chief of Medicine
Massachusetts General Hospital
Professor of Medicine
Harvard Medical School
Professor of Medicine
Tufts University School of Medicine
Newton, Massachusetts

PAUL MARTIN, MD, FRCP, FRCPI
Professor of Medicine
Chief, Division of Gastroenterology and Hepatology
University of Miami Miller School of Medicine
Miami, Florida

ELSEVIER

ELSEVIER

1600 John F. Kennedy Blvd.
Ste 1800
Philadelphia, PA 19103-2899

HANDBOOK OF LIVER DISEASE, FOURTH EDITION   ISBN: 978-0-323-47874-8

Notices

Knowledge and best practice in this field are constantly changing. As new research and experience broaden our understanding, changes in research methods, professional practices, or medical treatment may become necessary.

Practitioners and researchers must always rely on their own experience and knowledge in evaluating and using any information, methods, compounds, or experiments described herein. In using such information or methods they should be mindful of their own safety and the safety of others, including parties for whom they have a professional responsibility.

With respect to any drug or pharmaceutical products identified, readers are advised to check the most current information provided (i) on procedures featured or (ii) by the manufacturer of each product to be administered, to verify the recommended dose or formula, the method and duration of administration, and contraindications. It is the responsibility of practitioners, relying on their own experience and knowledge of their patients, to make diagnoses, to determine dosages and the best treatment for each individual patient, and to take all appropriate safety precautions.

To the fullest extent of the law, neither the Publisher nor the authors, contributors, or editors, assume any liability for any injury and/or damage to persons or property as a matter of products liability, negligence or otherwise, or from any use or operation of any methods, products, instructions, or ideas contained in the material herein.

Previous editions copyrighted 2012, 2004, and 1998.

Library of Congress Cataloging-in-Publication Data

Names: Friedman, Lawrence S. (Lawrence Samuel), 1953- editor. | Martin, Paul, M.D., editor.
Title: Handbook of liver disease / [edited by] Lawrence S. Friedman, Paul Martin.
Description: Fourth edition. | Philadelphia, PA : Elsevier, [2018] | Includes bibliographical references and index.
Identifiers: LCCN 2017024152 | ISBN 9780323478748 (pbk. : alk. paper)
Subjects: | MESH: Liver Diseases | Handbooks
Classification: LCC RC845 | NLM WI 39 | DDC 616.3/62—dc23 LC record available at https://lccn.loc.gov/2017024152

Senior Content Strategist: Sarah Barth
Content Development Specialist: Meghan Andress
Publishing Services Manager: Patricia Tannian
Senior Project Manager: Claire Kramer
Design Direction: Amy Buxton

Printed in China.

Last digit is the print number: 9 8 7 6 5 4 3 2

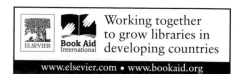

Working together to grow libraries in developing countries

www.elsevier.com • www.bookaid.org

In memory of Emmet B. Keeffe

CONTRIBUTORS

Sanath Allampati, MD
Assistant Professor
Department of Internal Medicine
West Virginia University
Morgantown, West Virginia

**Helen M. Ayles, MBBS, MRCP,
DTM&H, PhD**
Professor of Infectious Diseases and
    International Health
Clinical Research Department
London School of Hygiene and Tropical
    Medicine
London, England
Director of Research
ZAMBART Project
University of Zambia School of Medicine
Lusaka, Zambia

Bruce R. Bacon, MD
James F. King MD Endowed Chair in
    Gastroenterology
Professor of Internal Medicine
Division of Gastroenterology and
    Hepatology
Saint Louis University School of Medicine
St. Louis, Missouri

Sarah Lou Bailey, BSc, MBChB, MRCP
Clinical Research Fellow
Faculty of Infectious and Tropical Diseases
London School of Hygiene and Tropical
    Medicine
London, England

William F. Balistreri, MD
Director
Pediatric Liver Care Center
Department of Gastroenterology,
    Hepatology, and Nutrition
Children's Hospital Medical Center
Cincinnati, Ohio

Ji Young Bang, MBBS, MPH
Interventional Endoscopist
Center for Interventional Endoscopy
Florida Hospital
Orlando, Florida

Petros C. Benias, MD
Director of Endoscopic Surgery
Northwell Health System
Hofstra University
Manhassett, New York

Marina Berenguer, MD, PhD
Professor
Hepatology and Liver Transplantation Unit
La Fe University and Polytechnic Hospital
Valencia, Spain

Emily D. Bethea, MD
Fellow in Gastroenterology
Gastrointestinal Division
Massachusetts General Hospital
Chief Medical Resident
Department of Medicine
Brigham and Women's Hospital
Boston, Massachusetts

Kalyan Ram Bhamidimarri, MD, MPH
Assistant Professor of Clinical Medicine
Departments of Medicine and Hepatology
University of Miami
Miami, Florida

Christopher L. Bowlus, MD
Professor and Chief
Division of Gastroenterology and Hepatology
University of California, Davis
Sacramento, California

Andres Cardenas, MD, MMSc, PhD, AGAF, FAASLD
Consultant-Institute of Digestive Diseases
   and Metabolism
Institut de Investigacions Biomèdiques
   August Pi i Sunyer (IDIBAPS)
Hospital Clinic
University of Barcelona
Barcelona, Spain

Andres F. Carrion, MD
Direct of Hepatology
Assistant Professor of Medicine
Division of Gastroenterology and
   Hepatology
Texas Tech University Health Sciences
   Center
El Paso, Texas

Steve S. Choi, MD
Assistant Professor
Division of Gastroenterology
Department of Medicine
Duke University
Director, Hepatology
Department of Medicine
Durham Veterans Affairs Medical Center
Durham, North Carolina

Sanjiv Chopra, MBBS, MACP
Professor of Medicine
Harvard Medical School
Chief, James Tullis Internal Medicine Firm
Beth Israel Deaconess Medical Center
Editor-in-Chief, Hepatology Section,
   UpToDate
Boston, Massachusetts

Raymond T. Chung, MD
Director of Hepatology and Vice Chief
Division of Gastroenterology
Massachusetts General Hospital
Boston, Massachusetts

Jeremy F.L. Cobbold, PhD, MRCP
Clinical Lecturer in Hepatology
Imperial College London
London, England

Michael P. Curry, MD
Director of Hepatology
Department of Medicine
Beth Israel Deaconess Medical Center
Associate Professor of Medicine
Department of Medicine
Harvard Medical School
Boston, Massachusetts

Albert J. Czaja, MD, FACP, FACG, AGAF, FAASLD
Professor Emeritus of Medicine
Division of Gastroenterology and
   Hepatology
Mayo Clinic College of Medicine
Rochester, Minnesota

Teresita Gomez de Castro, MD
Pontifical Catholic University of Chile
Santiago, Chile

Andrew S. deLemos, MD
Clinical Assistant Professor of Medicine
University of North Carolina School of
   Medicine
Center for Liver Disease and Transplantation
Carolinas HealthCare System
Charlotte, North Carolina

Adrian M. Di Bisceglie, MD, FACP
Professor of Internal Medicine and
   Chairman
Department of Internal Medicine
Saint Louis University School of Medicine
St. Louis, Missouri

Anna Mae Diehl, MD
Professor of Medicine
Divison of Gastroenterology
Department of Medicine
Duke University
Durham, North Carolina

Robert J. Fontana, MD
Professor of Medicine
Department of Internal Medicine
University of Michigan
Ann Arbor, Michigan

Lawrence S. Friedman, MD
The Anton R. Fried, MD, Chair
Department of Medicine
Newton-Wellesley Hospital
Assistant Chief of Medicine
Massachusetts General Hospital
Professor of Medicine
Harvard Medical School
Professor of Medicine
Tufts University School of Medicine
Newton, Massachusetts

Pere Ginès, MD
Chairman
Liver Unit
Hospital Clinic
Professor
School of Medicine
University of Barcelona
Barcelona, Spain

Norman D. Grace, MD
Staff Physician
Division of Gastroenterology, Hepatology,
and Endoscopy
Department of Medicine
Brigham and Women's Hospital
Professor of Medicine
Tufts University School of Medicine
Lecturer on Medicine
Harvard Medical School
Boston, Massachusetts

Steven-Huy B. Han, MD, AGAF, FAASLD
Professor of Medicine and Surgery
David Geffen School of Medicine at
University of California, Los Angeles
Los Angeles, California

Gideon M. Hirschfield, MB BChir, PhD, FRCP
Professor of Autoimmune Liver Disease
Centre for Liver Research
National Institute for Health Research
Biomedical Research Unit
University of Birmingham
Birmingham, England

Michael G. House, MD, FACS
Associate Professor
Department of Surgery
Indiana University School of
Medicine
Indianapolis, Indiana

Christine E. Waasdorp Hurtado, MD, MSCS
Associate Professor of Pediatrics
Section of Pediatric Gastroenterology,
Hepatology, and Nutrition
Children's Hospital Colorado
University of Colorado School of Medicine
Colorado Springs, Colorado

Ira M. Jacobson, MD
Director of Hepatology
NYU Langone Medical Center
New York, New York

Kris V. Kowdley, MD, FACP
Director, Swedish/Providence Liver Care
Network
Swedish Liver Center and Organ Transplant
Seattle, Washington

Michelle Lai, MD, MPH
Assistant Professor
Department of Medicine
Harvard Medical School
Beth Israel Deaconess Medical Center
Boston, Massachusetts

Jay H. Lefkowitch, MD
Professor of Pathology and Cell Biology
Columbia University Medical Center
New York, New York

Chatmanee Lertudomphonwanit, MD
Division of Gastroenterology and
Hepatology
Department of Pediatrics
Faculty of Medicine
Ramathibodi Hospital
Mahidol University
Bangkok, Thailand

James H. Lewis, MD
Professor of Medicine and Director of
  Hepatology
Division of Gastroenterology
Georgetown University Medical Center
Washington, District of Columbia

Keith D. Lillemoe, MD, FACS
Chief of Surgery
Department of Surgery
Massachusetts General Hospital
W. Gerald Austen Professor of Surgery
Harvard Medical School
Boston, Massachusetts

Vincent Lo Re III, MD, MSCE
Associate Professor of Medicine and
  Epidemiology
Department of Medicine
Division of Infectious Diseases
Department of Biostatistics and
  Epidemiology
Perelman School of Medicine
University of Pennsylvania
Philadelphia, Pennsylvania

Hanisha Manickavasagan, MD
Department of Internal Medicine
Drexel University College of Medicine
Philadelphia, Pennsylvania

Paul Martin, MD, FRCP, FRCPI
Professor of Medicine
Chief, Division of Gastroenterology and
  Hepatology
University of Miami Miller School of
  Medicine
Miami, Florida

Marlyn J. Mayo, MD
Associate Professor
Department of Internal Medicine
University of Texas Southwestern Medical
  Center
Dallas, Texas

Mack C. Mitchell, MD
Professor
Department of Internal Medicine
University of Texas Southwestern Medical
  Center
Dallas, Texas

Kevin D. Mullen, MD, FRCPI, FAASLD
Professor of Medicine
Director of Digestive Diseases
West Virginia University
Morgantown, West Virignia

Santiago J. Muñoz, MD
Director of Hepatology
Medical Director, Liver Transplantation
Hahnemann University Hospital
Professor of Medicine
Drexel University College of Medicine
Philadelphia, Pennsylvania

Brent A. Neuschwander-Tetri, MD
Professor of Internal Medicine
Division of Gastroenterology and
  Hepatology
Saint Louis University School of Medicine
St. Louis, Missouri

Kelvin T. Nguyen, MD
Gastroenterology Fellow
Vatche and Tamar Manoukian Division of
  Digestive Diseases
David Geffen School of Medicine at
  University of California, Los Angeles
Los Angeles, California

Kavish R. Patidar, DO
Division of Gastroenterology, Hepatology,
  and Nutrition
Virginia Commonwealth University
Richmond, Virginia

Patricia Pringle, MD
Fellow
Divison of Gastroenterology
Department of Medicine
Massachusetts General Hospital
Boston, Massachusetts

Nicholas J. Procaccini, MD, JD, MS
Hepatologist
Swedish Liver Center and Organ
    Transplant
Gastroenterologist
Swedish Gastroenterology
Swedish Medical Center
Seattle, Washington

James Puleo, MD
Albany Gastroenterology Consultants
Albany, New York

K. Rajender Reddy, MD, FACP
Professor of Medicine
Division of Internal Medicine
University of Pennsylvania
Philadelphia, Pennsylvania

Hugo R. Rosen, MD, FACP
Waterman Endowed Chair in Liver Research
Professor of Medicine and Immunology
Division Head, Gastroenterology and
    Hepatology
University of Colorado School of Medicine
Aurora, Colorado

Arun J. Sanyal, MD
Division of Gastroenterology, Hepatology
    and Nutrition
Virginia Commonwealth University
Richmond, Virginia

Michael L. Schilsky, MD
Professor
Departments of Medicine and Surgery
Yale University School of Medicine
New Haven, Connecticut

Stuart Sherman, MD
Professor of Medicine and Radiology
Director of Endoscopic Retrograde
    Cholangiopancreatography
Department of Medicine
Indiana University School of Medicine
Indianapolis, Indiana

Ronald J. Sokol, MD
Professor and Vice Chair of Pediatrics
Arnold Silverman MD Chair in Digestive
    Health
Director of Colorado Clinical and
    Translational Sciences Institute
Chief, Section of Pediatric Gastroenterology,
    Hepatology, and Nutrition
Children's Hospital Colorado
University of Colorado School of Medicine
Aurora, Colorado

Erin Spengler, MD
Assistant Professor of Medicine
University of Wisconsin
Madison, Wisconsin

Elena M. Stoffel, MD
Assistant Professor of Medicine
Division of Gastroenterology
Department of Medicine
University of Michigan Health System
Ann Arbor, Michigan

**John A. Summerfield, MD, FRCP,
FAASLD**
Consultant in Gastroenterology
St. Mary's Hospital
London, England

Elliot B. Tapper, MD
Assistant Professor
Division of Gastroenterology and
    Hepatology
University of Michigan
Ann Arbor, Michigan

Tram T. Tran, MD
Medical Director, Liver Transplant
Professor of Medicine
Cedars Sinai Medical Center
David Geffen School of Medicine at
    University of California, Los Angeles
Los Angeles, California

Carmen Vinaixa, MD
Consultant
Digestive Medicine, Hepatology
La Fe University and Polytechnic Hospital
Valencia, Spain

Gwilym J. Webb, BM BCh, MA, MRCP
Clinical Research Fellow
National Institute for Health Research
   Birmingham Liver Biomedical Research
   Unit
University of Birmingham
Birmingham, England

Douglas M. Weine, MD
Gastroenterologist
Riverview Medical Center
Red Bank, New Jersey

Jacqueline L. Wolf, MD
Associate Professor
Department of Medicine
Harvard Medical School
Department of Gastroenterology/Medicine
Beth Israel Deaconess Medical Center
Boston, Massachusetts

**Florence S. Wong, MD, FRACP,
FRCP(C)**
Professor
Department of Medicine
Division of Gastroenterology
University of Toronto
Toronto, Ontario, Canada

Wei Zhang, MD, PhD
Internal Medicine Resident
Department of Internal Medicine
Saint Louis University School of Medicine
St Louis, Missouri

PREFACE

This fourth edition of *Handbook of Liver Disease* is the first for which Emmet B. Keeffe did not serve as a coeditor because of his untimely death as the third edition was published in 2012. A tribute to Emmet follows this Preface and the Acknowledgments. Succeeding Emmet as coeditor is Paul Martin, an accomplished editor and hepatologist in his own right.

The field of hepatology has continued to progress at a remarkable pace as the contents of the book illustrate. This is best exemplified by the paradigm-changing advances in the treatment of hepatitis C, which has been transformed from interferon-based therapy to the use of combinations of highly effective, direct-acting antiviral agents. Hepatitis C is now relatively easy to treat— and to cure—and the major challenge to eradication of the virus is the expense of the available drugs. The development of viral resistant mutations during treatment appears to be a less imposing obstacle. Reflecting the extraordinary pace of scientific developments in the field of viral hepatitis, the book now offers four, rather than two, chapters on the topic, with expanded attention to each virus.

Progress in other areas of hepatology has been no less impressive. Primary biliary cholangitis (formerly primary biliary cirrhosis) has a new name, more accurately reflecting the spectrum of disease, as well as a new treatment—obeticholic acid—for nonresponders or incomplete responders to ursodeoxycholic acid. Nonalcoholic fatty liver disease has emerged as the preeminent challenge, both epidemiologically and therapeutically, as hepatitis C is anticipated to come under control. There is much new information as well on autoimmune liver diseases, drug- and alcohol-induced liver disease, cirrhosis and portal hypertension, metabolic disorders of the liver, biliary disorders, and hepatobiliary neoplasms, among other topics, that is reflected in the fourth edition. Liver transplantation continues to have a central role in the practice of hepatology as advances proceed steadily toward new approaches to hepatic replacement and regeneration.

We are delighted to welcome a number of highly regarded new senior authors and their junior associates to the *Handbook*. The infusion of "new blood" ensures the vitality and currency of the book. Among the new authors are Erin Spengler and Robert J. Fontana (Acute Liver Failure), Kelvin T. Nguyen and Steven-Huy B. Han (Hepatitis A and Hepatitis E), Tram T. Tran (Hepatitis B and Hepatitis D), Elliot B. Tapper and Michael P. Curry (Hepatitis Caused by Other Viruses), James H. Lewis (Drug-Induced and Toxic Liver Disease), Kavish R. Patidar and Arun J. Sanyal (Ascites and Spontaneous Bacterial Peritonitis), Andres Cardenas and Pere Ginès (Hepatorenal Syndrome), Michael L. Schilsky (Wilson Disease and Related Disorders), Andres F. Carrion and Kalyan Ram Bhamidimarri (Liver Transplantation), and Ji Young Bang and Stuart Sherman (Cholelithiasis and Cholecystitis). We are equally grateful to our outstanding returning authors and coauthors.

As in the past, the goal of the *Handbook* is to provide a concise, accurate, up-to-date, and readily accessible (in print or online) reference for students of the liver and particularly for busy practitioners who need reliable information in "real time." We continue to use an outline format with many lists, tables, and color figures to convey information efficiently and effectively without compromising the depth and richness of the field. Our continued mission is to provide a resource that will be valuable to practicing gastroenterologists and hepatologists, as well as to internists, family practitioners, other specialists, and students and trainees in gastroenterology and hepatology or internal medicine.

—*Lawrence S. Friedman*
—*Paul Martin*

ACKNOWLEDGMENTS

We are grateful to all the authors for sharing their expertise and for staying true to the unique format of the book. We feel fortunate to be able to learn from the foremost authorities in the field of hepatology. We particularly appreciate the support, advice, and assistance of Suzanne Toppy and Sarah Barth, our acquisitions editors, Meghan Andress, our content development specialist, and Claire Kramer, our project manager, without whom this book would not have been possible. We thank our friend and esteemed colleague Bruce R. Bacon for his inspiring foreword. We are appreciative of our colleagues at Newton-Wellesley Hospital and the University of Miami School of Medicine for their support, and particularly our assistants, Alison Sholock and Maria del Rio, who provided invaluable and tireless editorial assistance. Finally, we are grateful to our families, especially our wives, Mary Jo Cappuccilli and Maria T. Abreu, for their steadfast support during the preparation of this fourth edition.

This book is dedicated to the memory of Emmet B. Keeffe, who cocreated the *Handbook of Liver Disease* and served as coeditor for the first three editions. Emmet worked tirelessly on the book, was a superb editor, and had a total mastery of the field of hepatology. He had a talent for clear, organized, and informative exposition, and an impressive feel for what was important to practitioners and to patients. He dealt with authors—and with his coeditor—in a direct yet respectful manner and delighted in discussing the ins and outs of liver disease and the finer points of English grammar. He was passionate about medicine and scholarship.

Emmet had a remarkably successful and productive academic career, but he is most remembered as a loving and devoted husband, father, and grandfather; a compassionate and effective physician; and a warm and generous friend who had no hint of pretense or formality. Emmet's professional life was a reflection of his love of people, dedication to the service of others, and devotion to the generation and communication of new knowledge.

A consummate "quadruple-threat"—an academician with strengths as a clinician, clinical investigator, educator, and administrator—Emmet's contributions spanned the breadth of gastroenterology and hepatology, from flexible sigmoidoscopy to liver transplantation, and he brought enlightenment to numerous areas. His particular interest was in the treatment and prevention of viral hepatitis. Emmet helped develop and lead three successful liver transplantations programs at Oregon Health and Science University, at California Pacific Medical Center, and at Stanford Medical Center. He held numerous leadership and editorial positions, including the presidencies of the American Society for Gastrointestinal Endoscopy from 1995 to 1996 and of the American Gastroenterological Association from 2004 to 2005. He also served as chair of the American Board of Internal Medicine (ABIM), Subspecialty of Gastroenterology and as a member of the ABIM Board of Directors in 2007. In addition to serving as coeditor of *Handbook of Liver Disease*, Emmet was editor-in-chief of the journal *Digestive Diseases and Sciences* at the time of his death.

Emmet had numerous friends around the world who admired his warmth, compassion, empathy, work ethic, integrity, grace, and wisdom. He was a natural leader who led by example and consensus building and was generous in his praise of others, yet always humble about his own accomplishments, which were prodigious. He was an international ambassador of gastroenterology and hepatology and truly beloved by all who knew him. The *Handbook of Liver Disease* is but one of his legacies.

CONTENTS

Handbook of
Liver Disease

FOREWORD

I am pleased and honored to have been asked to prepare a Foreword for the fourth edition of *Handbook of Liver Disease.* This handbook has become an incredibly valuable resource for all levels of medical providers who deal with patients who have liver disease. It is easy to use and not overly detailed; nonetheless, all the essentials are present. Reading through the forewords from previous editions of the book shows an interesting array of dramatic adjectives describing the progress that has been made in the field of hepatology. For example, the changes have been described as "astronomical" and "stunning." That seems still to be the case in light of continued new developments. For the young hepatologists in the field, it might be hard for them to consider a time when we as hepatologists could only identify problems but not do anything about them. Furthermore, I can remember when it was jokingly said that all we had in our armamentarium was furosemide and lactulose. Now, in 2017, the diagnostic and therapeutic advances have been phenomenal. One need only compare the exhibit area at the annual meeting of the American Association for the Study of Liver Diseases (AASLD) over the years. In 1977, there were only 11 exhibitors, whereas in 2017 in Washington, DC, there were 85 exhibitors. Indeed, hepatology has become a very successful growth area.

Perhaps the greatest developments in hepatology over the past 30 years have come in the field of viral hepatitis. In certain parts of the world, hepatitis B vaccination has significantly reduced the frequency of vertical transmission of the hepatitis B virus and in turn has reduced the risk of hepatocellular carcinoma (HCC) in young adults. In much of the United States, hepatitis D (delta) is rarely seen now, and identification of a case of hepatitis E is rare. However, the most dramatic example of progress in hepatology has been in the field of hepatitis C. The progress from the discovery of the hepatitis C virus (HCV) in the late 1980s to the ability to cure more than 90% to 95% of patients—and in some studies up to 100%—is truly remarkable. The new treatment regimens do not include interferon, are well tolerated, are safe, are highly effective, and usually require only 12 weeks of oral treatment. Unfortunately, the biggest current problem related to viral hepatitis, and particularly hepatitis C, is the increase in transmission of HCV associated with the opioid abuse problem in the United States. Also, the frequency of vertical transmission from mother to child is increasing slightly, and, unfortunately, the call for screening in baby boomers has not been vigorously received. Development of a hepatitis C vaccine has been slow, and some observers have opined that with treatment success approaching 100% with direct-acting antiviral agents, the need for a vaccine is not as great as once thought. At any rate, the availability of hepatitis C treatment regimens, with at least seven regimens by the end of 2017, has been a great achievement.

The explosion of successful therapies for hepatitis C has not been equaled for hepatitis B, but many of the scientists, clinicians, and investigators who had been working in hepatitis C are now working on treatments that will lead to cure of hepatitis B. Perhaps by the time the next edition of the *Handbook* has been prepared, we will have curative, direct-acting antiviral agents being tested for use in patients with hepatitis B.

The other major growth area in hepatology is nonalcoholic steatohepatitis (NASH). Although there may be three to five million Americans with hepatitis C and approximately two million with hepatitis B, it has been estimated that there may be as many as 25 million Americans with nonalcoholic fatty liver disease (NAFLD). Clinical trials are rapidly being initiated, and numerous new agents are being tested, some alone and some in combination. Most patients with NAFLD or NASH have insulin resistance, and it seems likely that two or more mechanisms for defining treatment may be necessary for success. It is also likely that the need for treatment may be long-term and perhaps lifelong. Therefore expense will be a major consideration for access to these treatments, and health care providers will have to be careful about this issue.

A significant number of patients who have elevated liver biochemical test levels are receiving medications known to cause liver dysfunction. The Drug-Induced Liver Injury Network (DILIN) has increased our attention to these disorders and has helped remind us of the need to focus on this area. Accordingly, all patients with abnormal liver enzyme levels must have their medication lists reviewed.

The autoimmune-mediated liver diseases include autoimmune hepatitis (AIH), primary biliary cholangitis (PBC), primary sclerosing cholangitis (PSC), and the overlap syndromes. The new findings in these disease states include recognition that overlap syndrome can develop in patients who initially present with AIH and progress to include PBC, or present with PBC and progress to include AIH. Occasionally, treatment needs to be adjusted. Also, the first new treatment in decades approved for patients with PBC is obeticholic acid, which is helpful in about one half of the patients who have had an inadequate or incomplete response to standard treatment with ursodeoxycholic acid. No new treatments have come about in AIH or in PSC, although trials of obeticholic acid in PSC are in progress.

In the area of inherited liver diseases, the changes and advances have not been as great in the past few years as they were in the 1990s, when new genes were being discovered. Most patients who have hereditary hemochromatosis with significant iron overload have two copies of a single mutation (C282Y). This is in stark contrast to the more than 600 disease-causing mutations found in the Wilson disease gene. This indicates that almost all patients with Wilson disease are compound heterozygotes.

Complications of chronic liver disease such as variceal bleeding, hepatic encephalopathy, fluid retention (ascites and edema), and hepatorenal syndrome are usually managed effectively and, when these problems occur, are often the precursors to liver transplantation. A dreaded complication of cirrhosis is the development of HCC, but current guidelines and recommendations for monitoring and standardized evaluation have led to outcomes that are acceptable. Most mid-to-large academic health centers now have teams of medical oncologists, hepatologists, transplant surgeons, pathologists, and interventional radiologists who meet regularly to discuss the management of patients with HCC. This multidisciplinary approach is necessary for successful outcomes in these complicated patients.

Therefore the developments in diagnosis and treatment for a variety of liver diseases have undergone tremendous advances since the publication of the previous edition of *Handbook of Liver Disease*. The changes that have developed in our field have led to improved care and better outcomes for our patients. We look with excitement to the future to see even greater changes that will further enhance the care that we provide.

Finally, I cannot resist adding a comment about Dr. Emmet B. Keeffe, to whom this edition of *Handbook of Liver Disease* is dedicated. I vividly remember several years ago visiting Emmet at Stanford. At the time, he was recovering from valvular heart surgery. It was mid-morning on a sunny day, and we sat outside enjoying a cup of coffee at a small shop. As if it were yesterday, I remember Emmet saying to me, "You know, Bruce, I found out with the recovery from this surgery that there is a life outside the hospital. Having some recovery time like this reminds me that we need to take time to take care of ourselves." This was vintage Emmet Keeffe and a valuable lesson for all of us as we go about our busy lives.

Congratulations to Drs. Friedman and Martin on an excellent fourth edition of the *Handbook of Liver Disease*.

—*Bruce R. Bacon*

CHAPTER 1

Assessment of Liver Function and Diagnostic Studies

Paul Martin, MD, FRCP, FRCPI ■ Lawrence S. Friedman, MD

KEY POINTS

1 Reflecting the liver's diverse functions, the colloquial term *liver function tests* (LFTs) includes true tests of hepatic synthetic function (e.g., serum albumin), tests of excretory function (e.g., serum bilirubin), and tests that reflect hepatic necroinflammatory activity (e.g., serum aminotransferases) or cholestasis (e.g., alkaline phosphatase [ALP]).

2 Abnormal liver biochemical test results are often the first clues to liver disease. The widespread inclusion of these tests in routine blood chemistry panels uncovers many patients with unrecognized hepatic dysfunction.

3 Normal or minimally abnormal liver biochemical test levels do not preclude significant liver disease, even cirrhosis.

4 Laboratory testing can assess the severity of liver disease and its prognosis; sequential testing may allow assessment of the effectiveness of therapy.

5 Although liver biopsy had been the gold standard for assessing the severity of liver disease, as well as for confirming the diagnosis for some causes, fibrosis is increasingly assessed by noninvasive means, most notably by ultrasound elastography, especially in chronic viral hepatitis.

6 Various imaging studies are useful in detecting focal hepatic defects, the presence of portal hypertension, and abnormalities of the biliary tract.

Routine Liver Biochemical Tests

SERUM BILIRUBIN

1. Jaundice
   - Often the first evidence of liver disease
   - Clinically apparent when serum bilirubin exceeds 3 mg/dL; patient may notice dark urine or pale stool before conjunctival icterus
2. Metabolism
   - Bilirubin is a breakdown product of hemoglobin and, to a lesser extent, heme-containing enzymes; 95% of bilirubin is derived from senescent red blood cells.
   - After red blood cell breakdown in the reticuloendothelial system, heme is degraded by the enzyme heme oxygenase in the endoplasmic reticulum.
   - Bilirubin is released into blood and tightly bound to albumin; free or unconjugated bilirubin is lipid soluble, is not filtered by the glomerulus, and does not appear in urine.

- **Unconjugated bilirubin** is taken up by the liver by a carrier-mediated process, attaches to intracellular storage proteins (ligands), and is **conjugated by the enzyme uridine diphosphate (UDP)–glucuronyl transferase** to form a diglucuronide and, to a lesser extent, a monoglucuronide.
- Conjugated bilirubin is water soluble and thus appears in urine.
- When serum levels of bilirubin glucuronides are elevated, some binding to albumin occurs *(delta bilirubin)*, leading to absence of bilirubinuria despite conjugated hyperbilirubinemia; this phenomenon explains delayed resolution of jaundice during recovery from acute liver disease until albumin-bound bilirubin is catabolized.
- Conjugated bilirubin is excreted by active transport across the canalicular membrane into bile.
- Bilirubin in bile enters the small intestine; in the distal ileum and colon, bilirubin is hydrolyzed by beta-glucuronidases to form unconjugated bilirubin, which is then reduced by intestinal bacteria to colorless urobilinogens; a small amount of urobilinogen is reabsorbed by the enterohepatic circulation and mostly excreted in the bile, with a smaller proportion undergoing urinary excretion.
- Urobilinogens or their colored derivatives urobilins are excreted in feces.

3. Measurement of serum bilirubin
   a. van den Bergh reaction
      - **Total serum bilirubin** represents all bilirubin that reacts with diazotized sulfanilic acid to form chromogenic pyrroles within 30 minutes in the presence of alcohol (an accelerating agent).
      - **Direct serum bilirubin** is the fraction that reacts with the diazo reagent in an aqueous medium within 1 minute and corresponds to **conjugated bilirubin.**
      - **Indirect serum bilirubin** represents **unconjugated bilirubin** and is determined by subtracting the direct reacting fraction from the total bilirubin level.
   b. More specific methods (e.g., high-pressure liquid chromatography) demonstrate that the van den Bergh reaction often overestimates the amount of conjugated bilirubin; however, the van den Bergh method remains the standard test.

4. Classification of hyperbilirubinemia
   a. **Unconjugated** (bilirubin nearly always <7 mg/dL)
      - Overproduction (presentation to liver of bilirubin load that exceeds hepatic capacity for uptake and conjugation): Hemolysis, ineffective erythropoiesis, resorption of hematoma
      - Defective uptake and storage of bilirubin: Gilbert syndrome (idiopathic unconjugated hyperbilirubinemia)
   b. **Conjugated**
      - Hereditary: Dubin-Johnson and Rotor syndromes, bile transport protein defects
      - Cholestasis (Bilirubin is not a sensitive test of hepatic dysfunction.)
        - Intrahepatic: Cirrhosis, hepatitis, primary biliary cholangitis, drug induced
        - Extrahepatic biliary obstruction: Choledocholithiasis, stricture, neoplasm, biliary atresia, sclerosing cholangitis
   c. **Very high bilirubin levels**
      - >30 mg/dL: Usually signifies hemolysis plus parenchymal liver disease or biliary obstruction; urinary excretion of conjugated bilirubin may help prevent even higher levels of hyperbilirubinemia; renal failure contributes to hyperbilirubinemia.
      - >60 mg/dL: Seen in patients with hemoglobinopathies (e.g., sickle cell disease) in whom obstructive jaundice or acute hepatitis develops.
   d. The diagnostic approach to the evaluation of an isolated serum bilirubin level is shown in Fig. 1.1.

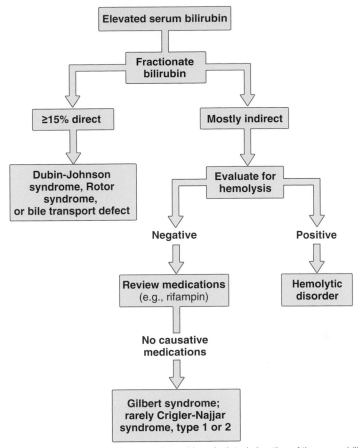

Fig. 1.1 Algorithm for the approach to a patient with an isolated elevation of the serum bilirubin level.

5. Urine bilirubin and urobilinogen
   - Bilirubinuria indicates an increase in serum conjugated (direct) bilirubin.
   - Urinary urobilinogen (rarely measured now) is found in patients with hemolysis (increased production of bilirubin), gastrointestinal hemorrhage, or hepatocellular disease (impaired removal of urobilinogen from blood).
   - Absence of urobilinogen from urine suggests interruption of the enterohepatic circulation of bile pigments, as in complete bile duct obstruction.
   - Urobilinogen detection and quantification add little diagnostic information to the evaluation of hepatic dysfunction.

SERUM AMINOTRANSFERASES (Table 1.1)

1. These intracellular enzymes are released from injured hepatocytes and are the most useful marker of hepatic injury (inflammation or cell necrosis).
   a. **Aspartate aminotransferase** (AST, serum glutamic oxaloacetic transaminase [SGOT])
      - Found in cytosol and mitochondria
      - Found in liver as well as skeletal muscle, heart, kidney, brain, and pancreas

TABLE 1.1 ■ **Causes of Elevated Serum Aminotransferase Levels**[a]

Mild Elevation (<5× normal)	**Marked Elevation (>15× normal)**
Hepatic: ALT predominant	Acute viral hepatitis (A–E, herpes)
Chronic viral hepatitis	DILI
Acute viral hepatitis (A–E, EBV, CMV)	Ischemic hepatitis
NAFLD	Autoimmune hepatitis
Hemochromatosis	Wilson disease
DILI	Acute bile duct obstruction
Autoimmune hepatitis	Acute Budd-Chiari syndrome
Alpha-1 antitrypsin deficiency	Hepatic artery ligation
Wilson disease	
Celiac disease	
Glycogenic hepatopathy	
Hepatic: AST predominant	
Alcohol-related liver injury (AST/ALT >2:1)	
Cirrhosis	
Nonhepatic	
Strenuous exercise	
Hemolysis	
Myopathy	
Thyroid disease	
Macro-AST	

[a]Almost any liver disease may be associated with ALT levels 5 times to 15 times normal.

ALT, Alanine aminotransferase; *AST,* aspartate aminotransferase; *CMV,* cytomegalovirus; *DILI,* drug-induced liver injury; *EBV,* Epstein-Barr virus; *NAFLD,* nonalcoholic fatty liver disease.

    b. Alanine aminotransferase (ALT, serum glutamic pyruvic transaminase [SGPT])
- Found in cytosol
- Highest concentration in liver (more sensitive and specific than AST for liver inflammation and hepatocyte necrosis)

2. Clinical usefulness
- **Normal levels of ALT are up to ~30 U/L in men and up to ~19 U/L in women.**
- Levels increase with body mass index (and particularly with trunk fat) and correlate with serum triglyceride, glucose, insulin, and leptin levels and possibly inversely with serum vitamin D levels. There is controversy as to whether levels correlate with the risk of coronary artery disease and mortality.
- Levels may rise acutely with a high caloric meal or ingestion of acetaminophen 4 g/day; coffee appears to lower levels.
- Aminotransferase elevations are often the first biochemical abnormalities detected in patients with viral, autoimmune, or drug-induced hepatitis; the degree of elevation may correlate with the extent of hepatic injury but is generally not of prognostic significance.
- In alcoholic hepatitis, the serum AST is usually no more than 2 to 10 times the upper limit of normal, and the ALT is normal or nearly normal, with an AST:ALT ratio >2; relatively low ALT levels may result from a deficiency of pyridoxal 5-phosphate, a necessary cofactor for hepatic synthesis of ALT. In contrast, in nonalcoholic fatty liver disease, ALT is typically higher than AST until cirrhosis develops.
- Aminotransferase levels may be higher than 3000 U/L in acute or chronic viral hepatitis or drug-induced liver injury; in acute liver failure or ischemic hepatitis (shock liver), even higher values (>5000 U/L) may be found.

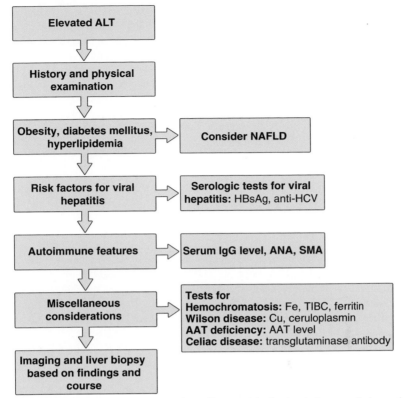

Fig. 1.2 Algorithm for the approach to a patient with a persistently elevated serum alanine aminotransferase level. *AAT*, Alpha-1 antitrypsin; *ANA*, antinuclear antibodies; *anti-HCV*, antibody to hepatitis C virus; *Cu,* copper; *Fe,* iron; *HBsAg*, hepatitis B surface antigen; *IgG*, immunoglobulin G; *NAFLD*, nonalcoholic fatty liver disease; *SMA*, smooth muscle antibodies; *TIBC*, total iron binding capacity.

- Mild-to-moderate elevations of aminotransferase levels are typical of chronic viral hepatitis, autoimmune hepatitis, hemochromatosis, alpha-1 antitrypsin deficiency, Wilson disease, and celiac disease.
- In obstructive jaundice, aminotransferase values are usually lower than 500 U/L; rarely, values may reach 1000 U/L in acute choledocholithiasis or 3000 U/L in acute cholecystitis, followed by a rapid decline to normal.

3. The approach to the patient with a persistently elevated ALT level is shown in Fig. 1.2.
4. Abnormally low aminotransferase levels have been associated with uremia and chronic hemodialysis; chronic viral hepatitis in this population may not result in aminotransferase elevation.

SERUM ALKALINE PHOSPHATASE

1. Hepatic ALP is one of several ALP isoenzymes found in humans and is bound to the hepatic canalicular membrane; various laboratory methods are available for its measurement, and comparison of results obtained by different techniques may be misleading.
2. **This test is sensitive for detection of biliary tract obstruction** (a normal value is highly unusual in significant biliary obstruction); interference with bile flow may be intrahepatic or extrahepatic.

- An increase in serum ALP results from increased hepatic synthesis of the enzyme, rather than leakage from bile duct cells or failure to clear circulating ALP; because it is synthesized in response to biliary obstruction, the ALP level may be normal early in the course of acute cholangitis when the serum aminotransferases are already elevated.
- Increased bile acid concentrations may promote the synthesis of ALP.
- Serum ALP has a half-life of 17 days; levels may remain elevated up to 1 week after relief of biliary obstruction and return of the serum bilirubin level to normal.

3. **Isolated elevation of alkaline phosphatase**
   - This may indicate infiltrative liver disease: Tumor, abscess, granulomas, or amyloidosis.
   - High levels are associated with biliary obstruction, sclerosing cholangitis, primary biliary cholangitis, immunoglobulin (Ig) G4–associated cholangitis, acquired immunodeficiency syndrome, cholestatic drug reactions, and other causes of vanishing bile duct syndrome; in critically ill patients with sepsis, high levels may result from secondary sclerosing cholangitis from ischemia with rapid progression to cirrhosis.
   - Nonhepatic sources of ALP are bone, intestine, kidney, and placenta (different isoenzymes); elevations are seen in Paget disease of the bone, osteoblastic bone metastases, small bowel obstruction, and normal pregnancy.
   - **A hepatic origin of an elevated ALP level is suggested by simultaneous elevation of either serum gamma-glutamyltranspeptidase (GGTP) or 5′-nucleotidase (5NT).**
   - Hepatic ALP is more heat stable than bone ALP. The degree of overlap makes this test less useful than GGTP or 5NT.
   - The diagnostic approach to an isolated elevated ALP level is shown in Fig. 1.3.
4. Mild elevations of serum ALP are often seen in hepatitis and cirrhosis.
5. Low serum levels of ALP may occur in hypothyroidism, pernicious anemia, zinc deficiency, congenital hypophosphatasia, and fulminant Wilson disease.

GAMMA-GLUTAMYLTRANSPEPTIDASE

1. Although present in many different organs, GGTP is found in particularly high concentrations in the epithelial cells lining biliary ductules.
2. It is a very sensitive indicator of hepatobiliary disease but is not specific. Levels are elevated in other conditions, including renal failure, myocardial infarction, pancreatic disease, and diabetes mellitus.
3. **GGTP is inducible, and thus levels may be elevated by ingestion of phenytoin or alcohol** in the absence of other clinical evidence of liver disease.
4. Because of its long half-life of 26 days, GGTP is limited as a marker of surreptitious alcohol consumption.
5. Its major clinical use is to exclude a bone source of an elevated serum ALP level.
6. Many patients with isolated serum GGTP elevation have no other evidence of liver disease; an extensive evaluation is usually not warranted. Patients should be retested after avoiding alcohol and other hepatotoxins for several weeks.

5'-NUCLEOTIDASE

1. 5NT is found in the liver in association with canalicular and sinusoidal plasma membranes.
2. Although 5NT is distributed in other organs, serum levels are believed to reflect hepatobiliary release by the detergent action of bile salts on plasma membranes.
3. Serum 5NT levels correlate well with serum ALP levels; **an elevated serum 5NT level in association with an elevated ALP level is specific for hepatobiliary dysfunction and is superior to GGTP in this regard.**

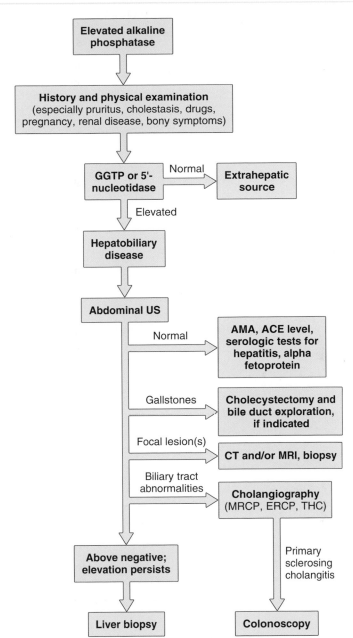

Fig. 1.3 Algorithm for the approach to a patient with isolated serum alkaline phosphatase elevation. *ACE,* Angiotensin-converting enzyme; *AMA,* antimitochondrial antibodies; *CT,* computed tomography; *ERCP,* endoscopic retrograde cholangiopancreatography; *GGTP,* gamma-glutamyltranspeptidase; *MRCP,* magnetic resonance cholangiopancreatography; *MRI,* magnetic resonance imaging; *THC,* transhepatic cholangiography; *US,* ultrasonography.

LACTATE DEHYDROGENASE

Measurement of lactate dehydrogenase (LDH) and the more specific isoenzyme LDH5 adds little to the evaluation of suspected hepatic dysfunction. High levels of LDH are seen in hepatocellular necrosis, ischemic hepatitis, cancer, and hemolysis. **The ALT/LDH ratio may help differentiate acute viral hepatitis (≥1.5) from ischemic hepatitis and acetaminophen toxicity (<1.5).**

SERUM PROTEINS

Most proteins circulating in plasma are produced by the liver and reflect its synthetic capacity.
1. Albumin
   - Albumin accounts for 75% of serum proteins.
   - Its half-life is approximately 3 weeks.
   - The concentration in blood depends on the albumin synthetic rate (normal, 12 g/day) and plasma volume.
   - **Hypoalbuminemia** may result from expanded plasma volume or decreased albumin synthesis. It is frequently associated with ascites and expansion of the extravascular albumin pool at the expense of the intravascular albumin pool. Hypoalbuminemia is common in chronic liver disease (an indicator of severity); it is less common in acute liver disease. It is not specific for liver disease and may also reflect glomerular or gastrointestinal losses.
2. Globulins
   a. Globulins are often increased nonspecifically in chronic liver disease.
   b. The pattern of elevation may suggest the cause of the underlying liver disease.
      - Elevated IgG: Autoimmune hepatitis
      - Elevated IgM: Primary biliary cholangitis
      - Elevated IgA: Alcoholic liver disease
3. Coagulation factors
   a. **Most coagulation factors are synthesized by the liver,** including factors I (fibrinogen), II (prothrombin), V, VII, IX, and X and have much shorter half-lives than that of albumin.
      - Factor VII decreases first in liver disease because of its shortest half-life, followed by factors X and IX.
      - Factor V is not vitamin K dependent, and its measurement can help distinguish vitamin K deficiency from hepatocellular dysfunction in a patient with prolonged prothrombin time. Serial measurement of factor V levels has been used to assess prognosis in acute liver failure; a value <20% of normal portends a poor outcome without liver transplantation.
      - Measurement of factor II (des-gamma-carboxyprothrombin) has also been used to assess liver function. Elevated levels are found in cirrhosis and hepatocellular carcinoma (HCC) and in patients taking warfarin, a vitamin K antagonist. Administration of vitamin K results in normalization of des-gamma-carboxyprothrombin in patients taking warfarin but not in those with cirrhosis.
   b. **The prothrombin time is useful in assessing the severity and prognosis of acute liver disease.** The one-stage prothrombin time described by Quick measures the rate of conversion of prothrombin to thrombin after activation of the extrinsic coagulation pathway in the presence of a tissue extract (thromboplastin) and calcium (Ca^{++}) ions. Deficiency of one or more of the liver-produced factors results in a prolonged prothrombin time.
   c. **Prolongation of the prothrombin time in cholestatic liver disease may result from vitamin K deficiency.**
      - Explanations for a prolonged prothrombin time apart from hepatocellular disease or vitamin K deficiency include consumptive coagulopathies, inherited deficiencies of a coagulation factor, or medications that antagonize the prothrombin complex.

- Vitamin K deficiency as the cause of a prolonged prothrombin time can be excluded by administration of vitamin K 10 mg; intravenous administration can cause severe reactions, and the oral route is preferable, if possible. (Subcutaneous administration is not recommended because of erratic absorption.) Correction or improvement of the prothrombin time by at least 30% within 24 hours implies that hepatic synthetic function is intact.
- The international normalized ratio (INR) is used to standardize prothrombin time determinations performed in different laboratories; however, the results are less consistent in patients with liver disease than in those taking warfarin unless liver-disease controls are used.
- The prothrombin time and INR correlate with the severity of liver disease but not with the risk of bleeding because of counterbalancing decreases in levels of anticoagulant factors (e.g., proteins C and S, antithrombin) and enhanced fibrinolysis in patients with liver disease.

Assessment of Hepatic Metabolic Capacity

Various drugs that undergo purely hepatic metabolism with predictable bioavailability have been used to assess hepatic metabolic capacity. Typically, a metabolite is measured in plasma, urine, or breath following intravenous or oral administration of the parent compound. These tests are not widely used in practice.

ANTIPYRINE CLEARANCE

1. Antipyrine is metabolized by cytochrome P-450 oxygenase with good absorption after oral administration and elimination entirely by the liver.
2. In chronic liver disease, good correlation exists between prolongation of the antipyrine half-life and disease severity as assessed by the Child-Turcotte-Pugh score (see Chapter 11).
3. Clearance of antipyrine is less impaired in acute liver disease and obstructive jaundice than in chronic liver disease.
4. Disadvantages of this test include its long half-life in serum, which requires multiple blood sampling, poor correlation with in vitro assessment of hepatic microsomal capacity, and alteration of antipyrine metabolism by increased age, diet, alcohol, smoking, and environmental exposure.

AMINOPYRINE BREATH TEST

1. This test is based on detection of $[^{14}C]O_2$ in breath 2 hours after an oral dose of $[^{14}C]$dimethyl aminoantipyrine (aminopyrine), which undergoes hepatic metabolism.
2. Excretion is diminished in patients with cirrhosis as well as those with acute liver disease.
3. The test has been used to assess prognosis in patients with alcoholic hepatitis and in cirrhotic patients who are undergoing surgery.
4. A limitation of the aminopyrine breath test is its lack of sensitivity in hepatic dysfunction resulting from cholestasis or extrahepatic obstruction.

CAFFEINE CLEARANCE

1. Caffeine clearance after oral ingestion can be assessed by measuring levels in either saliva or serum; the accuracy appears similar to the $[^{14}C]$aminopyrine breath test, without the need for a radioisotope.

2. Results are clearly abnormal in clinically severe liver disease, but the test is insensitive in mild hepatic dysfunction.
3. Caffeine clearance decreases with age or cimetidine use and increases with cigarette smoking.

GALACTOSE ELIMINATION CAPACITY

1. Galactose clearance from blood as a result of hepatic phosphorylation can be determined after either intravenous or oral administration; serial serum levels of galactose are obtained 20 to 50 minutes after an intravenous bolus, with correction for urinary galactose excretion.
2. At plasma concentrations >50 mg/dL, removal of galactose reflects hepatic functional mass, whereas at concentrations lower than this plasma level, clearance reflects hepatic blood flow.
3. [^{14}C]galactose is distributed in extracellular water and is affected by changes in volume.
4. Galactose clearance is impaired in acute and chronic liver disease as well as in patients with metastatic hepatic neoplasms but is typically unaffected in obstructive jaundice.
5. The oral galactose tolerance test incorporates [^{14}C]galactose with measurement of breath [^{14}C]O_2; the results of this breath test correlate with [^{14}C]aminopyrine testing.
6. [^{14}C]galactose testing is no more accurate than standard liver biochemical tests in assessing prognosis in patients with chronic liver disease.

LIDOCAINE METABOLITE

1. Monoethylglycinexylidide (MEGX), a product of hepatic lidocaine metabolism, is easily measured by a fluorescence polarization immune assay 15 minutes after administration of an intravenous dose of lidocaine.
2. The test may offer prognostic information about the likelihood of life-threatening complications in cirrhotic patients.
3. The test has also been used to assess the viability of donor liver allografts.
4. The test is easy to perform and has few adverse reactions, although it may be unsuitable for some cardiac patients. Test results may be affected by simultaneous use of certain drugs metabolized by cytochrome P-450 3A4 and high bilirubin levels; test results are affected by age and body mass index and are higher in men than in women.

Other Tests of Liver Function

SERUM BILE ACIDS

1. Bile acids are synthesized from cholesterol in the liver, conjugated to glycine or taurine, and excreted in the bile. Bile acids facilitate fat digestion and absorption within the small intestine. They recycle through the enterohepatic circulation; secondary bile acids form by the action of intestinal bacteria.
2. Detection of elevated serum bile acid levels is a sensitive marker of hepatobiliary dysfunction.
3. Various methods are available to assay individual and total bile acids; assaying an individual bile acid is probably as useful as measuring total bile acid concentration.
4. Numerous different bile acid tests have been described, including fasting and postprandial levels and determination of levels after a bile acid load, either oral or intravenous.
5. Normal bile acid levels in the presence of hyperbilirubinemia suggest hemolysis or Gilbert syndrome.

UREA SYNTHESIS

1. Hepatic metabolism of nitrogen from protein results in urea production. Urea is distributed in total body water and is excreted in urine or diffuses into the intestine, where urease-producing bacteria hydrolyze it to CO_2 and ammonia.
2. The rate of urea synthesis can be calculated from the urinary urea excretion and blood urea nitrogen after estimation of body water, with correction for gastrointestinal hydrolysis of urea.
3. The rate of urea synthesis is significantly reduced in cirrhosis and correlates with the Child-Turcotte-Pugh score, although it is insensitive for detection of well-compensated cirrhosis.

BROMSULPHALEIN

Clearance of bromsulphalein (BSP) after an intravenous bolus was formerly used to measure hepatic function. The most accurate information was obtained by the 45-minute retention test and initial fractional rate of disappearance. BSP testing fell out of favor because of reports of severe allergic reactions, lack of accuracy in distinguishing hepatocellular from obstructive jaundice, and the availability of simpler tests of liver function.

INDOCYANINE GREEN

This dye is removed by the liver after intravenous injection. A blood level can be obtained 20 minutes after administration, or levels can be determined by skin sensors. Compared with BSP, the hepatic clearance of indocyanine green is more efficient, and it is nontoxic. Its accuracy in assessing liver dysfunction is no better than standard Child-Turcotte-Pugh scoring. Its major role had been as a measure of hepatic blood flow.

NONINVASIVE SERUM MARKERS OF FIBROSIS

Various tests have been described to determine the extent of fibrosis in patients with chronic liver disease, thereby avoiding the need for liver biopsy.

Direct Markers
These markers include serum hyaluronate, procollagen III N-peptide, and matrix metalloproteinases. They are generally accurate in confirming cirrhosis and excluding severe liver disease in patients with minimal fibrosis.

Indirect Markers
Various formulas have been described that incorporate serum markers of fibrosis or routine laboratory tests, such as platelet count, INR, and serum aminotransferases.
- Examples include FibroSure, Fibrospect, and AST-to-platelet ratio index (APRI).
- **FibroSure is used most commonly in the United States** and includes α_2-macroglobulin, haptoglobin, apolipoprotein A1, bilirubin, and GGTP; it is most useful for excluding fibrosis (low score) or suggesting cirrhosis (high score); intermediate scores can reflect a varying degree of fibrosis.

Liver Biopsy

Despite advances in serologic testing and imaging, liver biopsy remains the definitive test in a number of settings: To confirm the diagnosis of specific liver diseases such as Wilson disease,

TABLE 1.2 ■ **Indications for Liver Biopsy**

Evaluation of abnormal liver biochemical test levels and hepatomegaly

Evaluation and staging of chronic hepatitis

Identification and staging of alcoholic liver disease

Recognition of systemic inflammatory or granulomatous disorders

Evaluation of fever of unknown origin

Evaluation of the pattern and extent of drug-induced liver injury

Identification and determination of the nature of intrahepatic masses

Diagnosis of multisystem infiltrative disorders

Evaluation and staging of cholestatic liver disease (primary biliary cholangitis, primary sclerosing cholangitis)

Screening of relatives of patients with familial diseases

Obtaining tissue to culture infectious agents (e.g., mycobacteria)

Evaluation of effectiveness of therapies for liver diseases (e.g., Wilson disease, hemochromatosis, autoimmune hepatitis, chronic viral hepatitis)

Evaluation of liver biochemical test abnormalities following transplantation

TABLE 1.3 ■ **Contraindications to Liver Biopsy**

Absolute	Relative
History of unexplained bleeding	Ascites
Prothrombin time >3–4 s over control	Infection in right pleural cavity
Platelets <60,000/mm³	Infection below right diaphragm
Prolonged bleeding time (>10 min)	Suspected echinococcal disease
Unavailability of blood transfusion support	Morbid obesity
Suspected hemangioma	
Uncooperative patient	

small-duct primary sclerosing cholangitis, and nonalcoholic fatty liver disease; to assess prognosis in most forms of parenchymal liver disease; and to evaluate allograft dysfunction in liver transplant recipients.

INDICATIONS

Indications for liver biopsy are shown in Table 1.2.

CONTRAINDICATIONS

Contraindications to liver biopsy are shown in Table 1.3. In patients with renal insufficiency, uremic platelet dysfunction should be corrected by infusion of arginine vasopressin (DDAVP), 0.3 μg/kg in 50 mL N saline intravenously, immediately before biopsy. Aspirin and nonsteroidal antiinflammatory drugs, which may also produce platelet dysfunction, are prohibited for 7 to 10 days before elective liver biopsy.

TECHNIQUE

1. Liver biopsy can be performed safely on an outpatient basis if none of the contraindications noted in Table 1.2 is present and the patient can be adequately observed for 2 to 3 hours after the procedure, with access to hospitalization if necessary (required in up to 5% of patients).
2. A local anesthetic is infiltrated subcutaneously and into the intercostal muscle and peritoneum. A short-acting sedative may be given to allay anxiety. Percussion identifies the point of maximal hepatic dullness.
3. The routine use of ultrasonography to mark the biopsy site or guide the biopsy needle has become standard. In diffuse liver disease, ultrasound-guided liver biopsy results in a higher yield and lower rate of complications than blind biopsy.
4. A transthoracic approach is standard; a subcostal approach should be attempted only with ultrasound guidance.
5. The biopsy is performed at end expiration; various needles (cutting [Tru-Cut, Vim-Silverman] or suction [Menghini, Klatskin, Jamshidi]) are used, including a biopsy "gun."
6. The biopsy site is tamponaded by having the patient lie on the right side.
7. When the standard approach is contraindicated (e.g., by coagulopathy or ascites), **transjugular biopsy** may be performed. This technique also allows determination of the hepatic venous wedge pressure gradient (see Chapter 11) to confirm portal hypertension, assess response to therapy with a beta-receptor antagonist, and determine prognosis.
8. Focal hepatic lesions are best sampled for biopsy under imaging guidance.
9. An adequate specimen for histologic interpretation should be at least 1.5 cm long and contains at least six portal triads.

COMPLICATIONS

1. Postbiopsy pain with or without radiation to the right shoulder occurs in up to one third of patients. Vasovagal reactions are also common. Serious complications are uncommon (<3%) and usually manifest within several hours of the biopsy. The fatality rate is 0.03% to 0.32%.
2. Intraperitoneal bleeding is the most serious complication. Increasing age, the presence of hepatic malignancy, and number of passes made are predictors of the likelihood of bleeding, as is the use of a cutting needle rather than a suction needle.
3. Patients who have clinical evidence of hemodynamically significant bleeding, persistent pain unrelieved by analgesia, or other evidence of a serious complication require hospital admission. Pneumothorax may require a chest tube, whereas serious bleeding may be controlled by selective embolization at angiography or, if necessary, surgical ligation of the right hepatic artery or hepatic resection.
4. Biopsy of a malignant neoplasm carries a 1% to 3% risk of seeding of the biopsy tract with tumor.

Hepatic Imaging

Several imaging modalities are available to assess the hepatic parenchyma, vasculature, and biliary tract. A logical sequence of initial and subsequent studies should be determined by the clinical circumstances (Table 1.4). The ready availability of abdominal imaging for unrelated complaints such as vague abdominal pain has led to the frequent detection of hepatic masses that are almost always benign and incidental to the patient's complaint but that require evaluation.

TABLE 1.4 ■ **Approach to Use of Imaging Studies**

Clinical Problem	Initial Imaging	Supplemental Imaging Studies (if necessary)
Jaundice	US	CT, if dilated ducts, an obstructing lesion, or suspicion of a mass in the pancreas or porta hepatis; MRCP to determine site and cause of dilated ducts
Hepatic parenchymal disease	US CT MRI	Doppler US, color Doppler US, or MRI with flow sequences if a vascular abnormality is suspected and in some instances of portal hypertension
Screening for liver mass	US	CT, MRI
Characterization of known liver mass	CT, MRI	MRI with liver-specific contrast media
Suspected malignancy	US- or CT-directed biopsy	Intraoperative US, CT portogram
Suspected benign lesion	US, CT, or MRI; nuclear medicine scan (e.g., ^{99m}Tc-labeled red blood cell scan) for suspected hemangioma	US- or CT-directed biopsy
Suspected abscess	US or CT US- or CT-directed aspiration	Nuclear medicine abscess scan (gallium or ^{111}In-labeled white blood cell scan)
Suspected biliary tract abnormalities	US to detect dilatation, biliary stones, or mass MRCP, ERCP, or THC to define ductal anatomy	CT or endoscopic US to detect stones or cause of extrinsic compression

CT, Computed tomography; *ERCP*, endoscopic retrograde cholangiopancreatography; *MRCP*, magnetic resonance cholangiopancreatography; *MRI*, magnetic resonance imaging; *THC*, transhepatic cholangiography; *US*, ultrasonography.

PLAIN ABDOMINAL X-RAY STUDIES AND BARIUM STUDIES

1. Plain abdominal x-ray studies add little to the evaluation of liver disease. On occasion, calcifications, usually resulting from gallstones, echinococcal cysts, or old lesions of tuberculosis or histoplasmosis, are detected. Tumors or vascular lesions may also be calcified.
2. A barium swallow is significantly less sensitive than endoscopy for detecting esophageal varices.
3. Wireless video capsule endoscopy has been used also to screen for esophageal varices.

ULTRASONOGRAPHY

1. Ultrasonography is the initial radiologic study of choice for many hepatobiliary disorders. It is relatively inexpensive, does not require ionizing radiation, and can be used at the bedside.
2. Ultrasound depicts interfaces in tissue of different acoustic properties. Contrast agents have been introduced to enhance the accuracy of ultrasonography; these include a microbubble technique for detection of discrete lesions and galactose-based contrast agents for assessment of vascularity.
3. Ultrasound cannot penetrate gas or bone, a characteristic that may preclude adequate examination of the viscera. Furthermore, increased resolution is generally at the expense of decreased tissue penetration.
4. "Real-time" ultrasonography demonstrates physiologic events such as arterial pulsation.

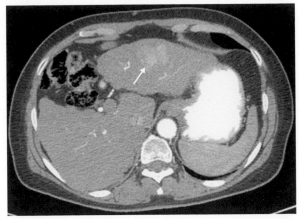

Fig. 1.4 Computed tomography scan showing a hepatocellular carcinoma (*arrow*).

5. Ultrasonography is better at detecting focal lesions than parenchymal disease and is the initial test of choice to detect biliary dilatation.
6. Hepatic masses as small as 1 cm may be detected by ultrasonography, and cystic lesions may be distinguished from solid ones.
7. Ultrasonography can also facilitate percutaneous biopsy of solid hepatic masses, drainage of hepatic abscesses, or paracentesis of loculated ascites.
8. Doppler ultrasonography is used to assess the patency of hepatic and portal vasculature in liver transplant candidates and recipients.

COMPUTED TOMOGRAPHY

1. Computed tomography (CT) is generally more accurate than ultrasonography in defining hepatic anatomy—normal and pathologic.
2. Oral contrast defines the bowel lumen, and intravenous contrast enhances vascular structures and increases anatomic definition.
3. Spiral, or helical, CT is a refinement that allows faster imaging at the peak of intravenous contrast enhancement. A more recent advance is multidetector CT, which permits imaging in a single breath-hold and three-dimensional reconstruction of the hepatic vasculature and biliary tract.
4. **CT with intravenous contrast is an excellent way to identify and characterize hepatic masses.** Cystic and solid masses can be distinguished, as can abscesses. Contrast enhancement after an intravenous bolus may be accurate enough to identify cavernous hemangiomas, which have a characteristic appearance. Neoplastic vascular invasion may also be identified. HCC exhibits arterial enhancement (Fig. 1.4), followed by rapid "washout."
5. CT can also suggest the presence of cirrhosis and portal hypertension, as well as changes consistent with fatty liver or hemochromatosis.
6. Limitations of CT are cost, radiation exposure, and lack of portability.

MAGNETIC RESONANCE IMAGING

1. Magnetic resonance imaging (MRI) can provide images in numerous planes and provides excellent resolution between tissues containing differing amounts of fat and water. Ultrafast sequencing obviates motion artifacts. Unlike CT, MRI does not require ionizing radiation, but there is a risk of nephrogenic systemic fibrosis in patients with impaired renal function after administration of gadolinium contrast.

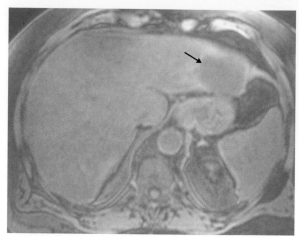

Fig. 1.5 Magnetic resonance imaging scan showing a hepatic hemangioma (*arrow*).

2. MRI is an excellent method for evaluating blood flow and can detect hepatic iron overload.
3. MRI is not portable, remains expensive, and has a slow imaging time, so physiologic events such as peristalsis can result in blurred images. The magnetic field used precludes imaging in patients with pacemakers or other metallic devices. Claustrophobic patients find the enclosed space in the scanner unpleasant, and many require sedation.
4. **MRI is the imaging study of choice in confirming the presence of vascular lesions, notably hemangiomas** (Fig. 1.5). **It is also useful in differentiating regenerative nodules from HCC;** on a T2-weighted image, the signal intensity of a regenerative nodule is equivalent to that of normal hepatic parenchyma, whereas that of a carcinoma is higher.
5. Use of liver-specific contrast media further enhances the accuracy of assessing hepatic mass characteristics by MRI.
6. Magnetic resonance cholangiopancreatography (MRCP) is a noninvasive alternative to diagnostic endoscopic cholangiopancreatography.
7. Magnetic resonance angiography, like CT angiography, is a useful method to assess the hepatic vasculature before hepatic resection.

RADIOISOTOPE SCANNING

1. Specific isotopes used are preferentially taken up by hepatocytes, Kupffer cells, or neoplastic or inflammatory cells. Radioisotope scanning is particularly helpful in the assessment of suspected acute cholecystitis, although for parenchymal and focal liver disease, ultrasonography and CT have largely superseded nuclear medicine studies.
2. Additional techniques include single-photon emission computed tomography (SPECT), which allows visualization of the cross-sectional distribution of a radioisotope, and positron emission tomography (PET) (see later), which provides information about blood flow and tissue metabolism.

POSITRON EMISSION TOMOGRAPHY

1. PET detects increased glucose metabolism characteristic of hepatic neoplasm.
2. Clinical applications include detection and staging of primary hepatic malignant diseases, evaluation of metastatic disease, and differentiation of benign from malignant hepatic tumors.

3. The accuracy of PET in HCC is limited by poor uptake of the most commonly used radiopharmaceutical (^{18}F-fluoro-2-deoxyglucose [FDG]) by well-differentiated tumors.

ULTRASOUND ELASTOGRAPHY

1. Ultrasound elastography incorporates an ultrasound transducer probe mounted on a vibrator to induce an elastic shear wave to measure hepatic stiffness, which reflects fibrosis. A commonly used technique is transient elastography, in which the results are expressed in kilopascals (kPa) and range from 2.5 to 75 kPa, with upper normal values approximately 5.5 kPa.
2. Ultrasound elastography is most accurate for excluding advanced fibrosis and cirrhosis and for suggesting cirrhosis; considerable overlap in results exists between when the fibrosis stage is intermediate.
3. The procedure is technically difficult in patients with obesity or ascites.
4. It may complement rather than replace liver biopsy.
5. Magnetic elastography is another emerging technique that uses magnetic resonance to measure liver stiffness.

FURTHER READING

Friedman LS. Controversies in liver biopsy: who, where, when, how, why? *Curr Gastroenterol Rep.* 2004;6:30–36.

Goessling W, Friedman LS. Increased liver chemistry in an asymptomatic patient. *Clin Gastroenterol Hepatol.* 2005;3:852–858.

Green RM, Flamm S. AGA technical review on the evaluation of liver chemistry tests. *Gastroenterology.* 2005;123:1367–1384.

Jang HJ, Yu H, Kim TK. Imaging of focal liver lesions. *Semin Roentgenol.* 2009;44:266–282.

Kechagias S, Ernersson A, Dahlqvist O, et al. Fast-food-based hyper-alimentation can induce rapid and profound elevation of serum alanine aminotransferase in healthy subjects. *Gut.* 2008;57:649–654.

Kim WR, Flamm SL, Di Bisceglie AM, et al. Serum activity of alanine aminotransferase (ALT) as an indicator of health and disease. *Hepatology.* 2008;47:1363–1370.

Kwo PY, Cohen SM, Lim JK. ACG clinical guideline: evaluation of abnormal liver chemistries. *Am J Gastroenterol.* 2017;112:18–35.

Lee TH, Kim WR, Poterucha JJ. Evaluation of elevated liver enzymes. *Clin Liver Dis.* 2012;16:183–198.

Marrero JA, Ahn J, Reddy KR. ACG clinical guideline: the diagnosis and management of focal liver lesions. *Am J Gastroenterol.* 2014;109:1328–1347.

Rockey DC, Caldwell SH, Goodman ZD, et al. Liver biopsy. *Hepatology.* 2009;49:1017–1044.

Ruhl CE, Everhart JE. Elevated serum alanine aminotransferase and γ-glutamyltransferase and mortality in the United States population. *Gastroenterology.* 2009;136:477–485.

Tapper EB, Castera L, Afdhal NH. FibroScan (vibration-controlled transient elastography): where does it stand in the United States practice. *Clin Gastroenterol Hepatol.* 2015;13:27–36.

Tripodi A, Mannucci PM. The coagulopathy of chronic liver disease. *N Engl J Med.* 2011;365:147–156.

Van Beers BE, Daire JL, Garteiser P. New imaging techniques for liver diseases. *J Hepatol.* 2015;62:690–700.

Watkins PB, Kaplowitz N, Slattery JT, et al. Aminotransferase elevations in healthy adults receiving 4 grams of acetaminophen daily: a randomized controlled trial. *JAMA.* 2006;296:87–93.

CHAPTER 2

Acute Liver Failure

Erin Spengler, MD ■ Robert J. Fontana, MD

KEY POINTS

1 Acute liver failure (ALF) is an uncommon but dramatic clinical syndrome that is associated with a high risk of mortality.

2 The defining features of ALF reflect mental status changes (i.e., hepatic encephalopathy [HE]) and coagulopathy in patients without preexisting liver disease.

3 Acetaminophen hepatotoxicity is the leading cause of ALF in the United States; nearly 50% of acetaminophen ALF cases reflect unintentional acetaminophen overdoses.

4 Treatment strategies for ALF include early transfer to a liver transplant center, disease-specific therapies in selected patients, and aggressive treatment of complications, including infection, renal failure, metabolic disorders, and cerebral edema, in an intensive care unit setting.

5 The etiology of ALF is the strongest predictor of spontaneous recovery; prognostic criteria are important in identifying patients with a low probability of survival without liver transplantation (LT).

6 LT is associated with a significant survival benefit in patients with ALF with a low probability of spontaneous recovery.

Overview

ALF is an uncommon but dramatic clinical syndrome characterized by a rapid decline in hepatic metabolic function and has a significant risk of mortality. ALF is defined by the onset of liver injury, HE, and coagulopathy (international normalized ratio [INR] >1.5) in patients with no antecedent history of liver disease. HE typically develops within 1 to 4 weeks of the onset of liver injury but may occur up to 12 to 24 weeks later (subacute liver failure). **Subacute liver failure** is associated with a lower likelihood of transplant-free survival (20% to 30%) and is more often seen with drug-induced liver injury (DILI) or idiopathic ALF.

1. There are approximately 2000 cases of ALF annually in the United States.
   a. ALF accounts for 31.2 hospitalizations and 3.5 deaths per million individuals each year.
   b. There are a variety of etiologies for ALF including drugs and toxins and metabolic, inflammatory, and viral diseases (Table 2.1).
2. ALF is associated with high short-term morbidity and mortality and accounts for approximately 5% of liver transplants.
3. Clinical outcomes and survival have improved significantly over the past 20 years in the United States despite similar disease severity and distribution of etiologies at presentation (see Table 2.1).
   a. Transplant-free survival (56% vs 45%), posttransplant survival (96% vs 88%), and overall survival (75% vs 67%) improved between 1998 and 2013.

TABLE 2.1 ■ **Causes of ALF and Disease-Specific Management**

Category	Cause	Evaluation and Diagnostic Testing	Treatment
Drugs and Toxins	Acetaminophen toxicity	Prescription and over-the-counter medication use, serum acetaminophen level, Rumack-Matthew nomogram, cysteine-acetaminophen adducts (if available)	N-acetylcysteine
	Idiosyncratic drug reaction	Medication history and timing, LiverTox website profile, dechallenge, liver biopsy	Withdrawal of suspect agent
	Amanita poisoning	History of mushroom ingestion	Penicillin G, silymarin, hemodialysis
Hepatotropic Viruses	Hepatitis A	IgM anti-HAV	—
	Hepatitis B	HBsAg, IgM anti-HBc, HBV DNA by PCR	Entecavir, tenofovir
	Hepatitis C	Anti-HCV, HCV RNA by PCR	
	Hepatitis D	HDAg, IgM anti-HDV, HDV RNA by PCR	Entecavir, tenofovir (for hepatitis B)
	Hepatitis E	IgM anti-HEV, IgG anti-HEV, HEV RNA by PCR (available at CDC)	—
Nonhepatotropic Viruses	Herpes simplex virus	HSV DNA by PCR, IgM anti-HSV, liver biopsy	Acyclovir
	Cytomegalovirus	CMV DNA by PCR, IgM anti-CMV, liver biopsy	Ganciclovir, valganciclovir
	Epstein-Barr virus	EBV DNA by PCR, serology, liver biopsy	Acyclovir, glucocorticoids
	Parvovirus B19	IgM anti-parvovirus, parvovirus DNA by PCR	—
	Adenovirus	ADV DNA by PCR	Cidofovir
Autoimmune Disease	Autoimmune hepatitis	ANA, SMA, anti-LKM, immunoglobulins, liver biopsy	Prednisone, azathioprine
Metabolic Diseases	Wilson disease	Ceruloplasmin, urinary and hepatic copper, slit-lamp examination, genetic testing	Oral chelators, zinc, plasmapheresis (?)
	Acute fatty liver of pregnancy	Clinical history, urine protein, DIC screen, ultrasonography, liver biopsy	Emergency delivery
	HELLP syndrome	Clinical history, urine protein, platelet count, hemolysis laboratory tests, ultrasonography, liver biopsy	Emergency delivery
	Preeclampsia or eclampsia	Clinical history, hypertension, proteinuria	Emergency delivery
Vascular Causes	Budd-Chiari syndrome	Doppler ultrasonography, CT, or MRI of liver, angiogram, evaluate for thrombophilia	IV heparin
	Sinusoidal obstruction syndrome	Clinical history, liver biopsy	Defibrotide
	Ischemic hepatitis	Clinical history, electrocardiogram, 2D echocardiogram with Doppler	Fluids, pressors, inotropes
Infiltrative Diseases	Metastatic malignancy	Imaging, liver biopsy	Chemotherapy
	Acute leukemia or lymphoma	Bone marrow aspiration, liver biopsy	Chemotherapy
	Systemic amyloidosis	Bone marrow aspiration, liver or other biopsy	Chemotherapy
Indeterminate Cause	Indeterminate ALF	Exclude other causes by laboratory testing and imaging	N-acetylcysteine (?)

2D, Two-dimensional; *ADV*, adenovirus; *ANA*, antinuclear antibodies; *anti-HBc*, antibody to hepatitis B core antigen; *anti-LKM*, antibodies to liver kidney microsome; *CDC*, Centers for Disease Control and Prevention; *CMV*, cytomegalovirus; *CT*, computed tomography; *DIC*, disseminated intravascular coagulation; *EBV*, Epstein-Barr virus; *HAV*, hepatitis A virus; *HBsAg*, hepatitis B surface antigen; *HBV*, hepatitis B virus; *HCV*, hepatitis C virus; *HDAg*, hepatitis D antigen; *HDV*, hepatitis D virus; *HELLP*, hemolysis, elevated liver enzymes, and low platelets; *HEV*, hepatitis E virus; *HSV*, herpes simplex virus; *Ig*, immunoglobulin; *IV*, intravenous; *MRI*, magnetic resonance imaging; *PCR*, polymerase chain reaction; *SMA*, smooth muscle antibodies.

TABLE 2.2 ■ **Stages of Hepatic Encephalopathy in Acute Liver Failure**

Stage	Spontaneous Survival Rate (%)	Mental Status
1	70	Mild changes in mood; mildly slurred speech; disorder of sleep rhythm, fluctuant, mild confusion
2	60	Accentuation of stage I encephalopathy; inappropriate behavior; mild somnolence
3	40	Somnolent, but arousable to verbal command; marked confusion, incoherent speech
4	20	Unarousable to painful stimuli (comatose)

   b. Reductions in blood product use, mechanical ventilation, and vasopressors may have led to improved outcomes, as has increased use of *N*-acetylcysteine (NAC) for nonacetaminophen ALF.

Pathophysiology

1. Most cases of ALF are characterized by massive hepatocyte necrosis resulting in liver failure; ALF without histologic evidence of hepatocellular necrosis can also be seen, as in acute fatty liver of pregnancy and Reye syndrome.
2. Hepatocyte necrosis and apoptosis may coexist in the setting of ALF. Hepatocyte necrosis occurs through adenosine triphosphate (ATP) depletion followed by cellular swelling and cell membrane disruption. Apoptosis is a process of programmed cell death triggered by extrinsic or intrinsic mechanisms and resulting in caspase activation, degradation of genetic material, and cell shrinkage.
3. The coagulopathy in ALF is due to reduced hepatic synthesis of clotting factors with a short half-life (e.g., factor V), increased consumption of clotting factors, and reduced thrombopoietin levels.
4. HE in ALF is due to reduced clearance of ammonia and other neurotoxins, portosystemic shunting, reduced integrity of the blood-brain barrier with astrocyte swelling, and increased intracranial blood flow (Table 2.2).
5. Reduced hepatic reticuloendothelial cell function leads to frequent bacterial and fungal infections.

Etiology

The most commonly identified causes of ALF are **acetaminophen overdose (50%), DILI (10% to 15%), and acute viral hepatitis (5% to 10%)**; a substantial proportion of cases remain indeterminate (12%) (Fig. 2.1).

ACETAMINOPHEN HEPATOTOXICITY

1. More than 60,000 acetaminophen overdose cases are reported annually in the United States with most being single-time-point suicide gestures; only approximately 1% of these patients have ALF.
2. Acetaminophen (see also Chapter 10) is a dose-dependent hepatotoxin and follows a typical pattern of injury (Table 2.3).
   a. A massive single-time-point ingestion of at least 6 to 10 g is required for ALF to occur, but 3 to 6 g per day over several days can also lead to hepatotoxicity.

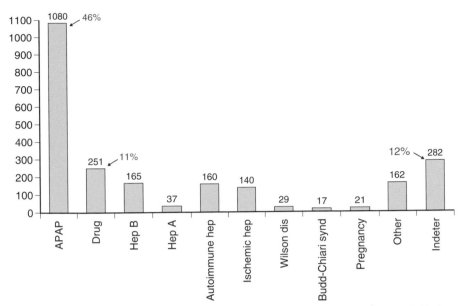

Fig. 2.1 Etiology of acute liver failure (ALF) in the United States. Among 2344 adult patients enrolled in the on-going Acute Liver Failure Study Group (ALFSG) registry, the leading cause of ALF remains acetaminophen (APAP) overdose (46%), followed by indeterminate ALF (12%), and idiosyncratic drug-induced liver failure (11%). *Dis*, disease; *hep*, hepatitis; *synd*, syndrome. (Data courtesy William M. Lee, University of Texas Southwestern, Dallas, TX.)

    b. Most patients present with serum aspartate aminotransferase (AST) and alanine aminotransferase (ALT) levels >1000 IU/L and minimally elevated total bilirubin (<3 g/dL) levels. Lactic acidosis and increases in serum creatinine levels are noted in 40% to 50% of cases.

    c. The serum acetaminophen level has diagnostic and prognostic utility in single-time-point ingestions; however, individuals with nonintentional overdose frequently have low or undetectable serum acetaminophen levels at presentation.

    d. Acetaminophen overdose is associated with a generally favorable prognosis (70% transplant-free survival). Patients with an acetaminophen-narcotic overdose frequently have a higher HE grade at presentation but a similar outcome.

3. Diagnostic testing: Serum acetaminophen level and clinical history of prescription narcotic-acetaminophen congeners and over-the-counter products; the acetaminophen Rumack-Matthew nomogram can help stratify hepatotoxicity risk after single-time-point ingestion (see Chapter 10, Fig. 10.2).

    a. A serum bilirubin >10 g/dL can lead to a false positive serum acetaminophen level (if a colorimetric assay is used).

    b. Serum cysteine-acetaminophen adducts are a promising diagnostic biomarker for acetaminophen hepatotoxicity.

4. Risk factors for increased susceptibility to acetaminophen-induced liver injury include alcohol use, barbiturate use, and poor nutritional status with fasting leading to intrahepatic glutathione depletion.

    a. Multiple acetaminophen-containing products are more frequently reported in nonintentional than intentional overdose ALF cases.

    b. The frequency of depression and alcohol use (40%) is similar in intentional and nonintentional cases.

    c. More than 400 over-the-counter products contain acetaminophen.

TABLE 2.3 ■ Management of Acetaminophen Overdose

Medical History

Review all prescription and over-the-counter medication use.
    Toxicity generally occurs with a total ingested dose >4 g
    Single-time-point ingestion: Use Rumack-Matthew nomogram at presentation and 4 hours later.
    Staggered/nonintentional overdose: Serum acetaminophen may be low or undetectable; give NAC
        whenever acetaminophen use is suspected.

Within 4 Hours of Ingestion

Ipecac syrup (15 mL once); repeat as needed.
    Gastric lavage of pill fragments
    Activated charcoal 1 g/kg orally or by nasogastric tube

N-acetylcysteine

Oral loading: 140 mg/kg followed by 70 mg/kg every 4 hours for 72 hours or until INR is <1.5
    To improve gastrointestinal tolerance, mix with carbonated beverage.
    Antiemetics: Prochlorperazine 10 mg, metoclopramide 10 mg, or ondansetron 4 mg by mouth or intrave-
        nously as needed
Consider IV NAC if severe nausea and vomiting.
    Intravenous dosing
        150 mg/kg in 250 mL of D5W over 1 hour
        50 mg/kg in 500 mL of D5W over 4 hours
        125 mg/kg in 1000 mL D5W over 19 hours
        100 mg/kg in 1000 mL D5W over 24 hours
    Monitoring: telemetry is recommended to identify arrhythmias and hypotension
        Anaphylactoid reactions (urticaria, wheezing, rash) should lead to cessation of the infusion and use of
            diphenhydramine and glucocorticoids.
        If hypotension and angioedema occur, stop the infusion and give fluids, glucocorticoids, and epinephrine.

Severity Assessment

Arterial pH, lactate, creatinine levels, and HE grade are of prognostic value.
    Serial INR, factor V, pH, and NH_3 levels every 12 hours
    Peak serum ALT level seen at 48–72 hours after presentation
    King's College criteria are better than the Model for End-stage Liver Disease score for assessing prognosis.

ALT, Alanine aminotransferase; *D5W*, dextrose 5% in water; *HE*, hepatic encephalopathy; *INR*, international normalized ratio; *IV*, intravenous; *NAC*, N-acetylcysteine; NH_3, ammonia.

5. Disease-specific treatment: **Oral or intravenous NAC started early and given for 48 to 72 hours** can diminish the likelihood of progression to LT and death (Table 2.3).
   a. Ipecac syrup, activated charcoal, and gastric lavage are recommended if intentional overdose occurred <4 hours earlier.
   b. Mixing NAC with a carbonated beverage or antiemetics improves gastrointestinal tolerability.

IDIOSYNCRATIC DILI AND TOXIN EXPOSURE

1. Idiosyncratic DILI is unpredictable liver injury and may reflect aberrant host metabolism and detoxification pathways. Latency from drug exposure to liver injury is usually <1 year. Most patients lack eosinophilia or other features of hypersensitivity on presentation.
   a. The most common agents implicated in ALF due to DILI are **antibiotics** (tetracycline, nitrofurantoin, trimethoprim-sulfamethoxazole), **antifungals** (ketoconazole),

antituberculosis drugs (isoniazid, pyrazinamide), and anticonvulsants (phenytoin, valproic acid, carbamazepine).

  b. Herbal and dietary supplements, including weight-loss products containing green tea extract, are an increasingly reported cause of severe DILI.

  c. Diagnostic testing: Exclude other specific causes of liver injury and obtain a medication history; medication discontinuation may not result in prompt improvement; liver biopsy findings can strengthen the diagnosis.

    ▪ The LiverTox website (http://livertox.nih.gov/) provides useful information on hepatotoxicity profiles and prior reports of DILI caused by individual drugs and herbal and dietary supplements.

    ▪ Assigning causality reflects the temporal association with clinical features and absence of other explanations.

  d. A specific antidote is generally not available. In addition to discontinuation of the culprit drug, other interventions include empiric use of NAC, which may improve transplant-free survival even in the absence of acetaminophen in patients with grade 1 or 2 HE.

  e. Glucocorticoids are of uncertain benefit but are frequently used if evidence of hypersensitivity or skin involvement is seen.

2. Toxin exposure secondary to ingestion of *Amanita* or *Galerina* species of mushrooms may lead to hepatic necrosis and, rarely, ALF, which may present with severe gastrointestinal symptoms, including diarrhea.

  a. Amatoxins are cyclic octapeptides that inhibit RNA polymerase II and lead to hepatocyte necrosis and renal tubular injury.

  b. Commercial testing for *Amanita* toxin is unavailable.

  c. Disease-specific treatment: Intravenous penicillin G, silymarin, and dialysis to reduce the circulating level of enterohepatically cleared amatoxins.

Viral Hepatitis (see also Chapters 3–6)

1. Hepatitis A virus (HAV) (see Chapter 3): Fecal-oral transmission; foodborne illness (preventable by vaccination)

  a. The incidence of acute symptomatic HAV in the United States is 1 in 100,000, with a case-fatality rate of 0.3%.

    ▪ The incidence of ALF in the United States due to HAV in adults has declined since 1995.

    ▪ Patients present with high serum AST and ALT levels, jaundice, and hepatitis symptoms.

  b. Persons at risk of ALF include those with underlying chronic liver disease, injection drug use, and advanced age.

  c. Diagnostic testing: Immunoglobulin M (IgM) antibody to HAV (anti-HAV)

  d. Disease-specific treatment: Supportive care; LT is needed in only 30% of HAV-related ALF.

2. Hepatitis B virus (HBV) (see Chapter 4): Parenteral, sexual, or perinatal transmission (preventable by vaccination)

  a. Most cases of acute hepatitis B in adults are asymptomatic; the incidence of reported acute hepatitis B in the United States is 1.5 per 100,000, with a case-fatality rate of 0.5% to 1.0%.

    ▪ Patients present with high serum AST and ALT levels, nausea, vomiting, and abdominal pain with jaundice.

  b. Diagnostic testing: Hepatitis B surface antigen (HBsAg) and IgM antibody to the hepatitis B core antigen (anti-HBc) may be present in serum in the setting of acute infection; detection of serum HBV DNA is the most reliable test in ALF.

   c. Risk factors for ALF include age >60 years, coinfection with hepatitis C virus (HCV), and coinfection with hepatitis D virus (HDV).
   d. Disease-specific therapy: Renally dosed oral nucleoside or nucleotide analogs (entecavir or tenofovir) are recommended in fulminant hepatitis B to improve the likelihood of recovery and reduce the viral load if LT is needed, but supporting data are limited.
   e. HBsAg-seropositive persons who receive chemotherapy or immunosuppressive therapy may develop reactivation of chronic HBV infection with a high viral load followed by fulminant hepatitis; therefore, antiviral prophylaxis is recommended in persons who receive immunosuppressants or chemotherapy.
      ■ Nearly 50% of fulminant hepatitis B in the United States appears to be due to HBV reactivation.
      ■ Rituximab, which depletes B cells, can lead to HBV reactivation in anti-HBc-positive patients who are HBsAg negative.
3. **HCV** (see Chapter 5): Parenteral, sexual transmission
   a. Acute hepatitis C is usually asymptomatic but can lead to icteric hepatitis and the need for hospitalization, but rarely ALF.
   b. Diagnostic testing: Serum HCV RNA (antibody to HCV may not yet be present)
   c. Disease-specific therapy: Data are limited regarding the efficacy and safety of direct-acting oral antiviral agents in acute HCV infection.
4. **HDV** (see Chapter 4): Parenteral and mucosal transmission (preventable by HBV vaccination)
   a. HDV is a defective virus that requires the presence of HBsAg for assembly of virions and infectivity.
   b. Infection may occur in the form of acute coinfection with HBV or as a superinfection in persons with chronic HBV infection, both of which are associated with an enhanced risk of ALF compared with HBV monoinfection.
   c. Diagnostic testing: Hepatitis D antigen (HDAg), HDV RNA by polymerase chain reaction (PCR) testing, anti-HDV (IgM and IgG); the availability of these tests is variable.
   d. Disease-specific therapy: Treatment is supportive; oral nucleoside and nucleotide analogs used for HBV infection have limited efficacy against HDV.
5. **Hepatitis E virus (HEV)** (see Chapter 3): Fecal-oral transmission, contaminated or undercooked pork, game animals (preventable by vaccination)
   a. Hepatitis E is a major cause of ALF in endemic regions of the world; sporadic acute HEV genotype 3 infection is rarely reported in Western patients, but 20% of the general U.S. population have detectable IgG anti-HEV in serum.
   b. Mortality is increased in pregnant women; the incidence of ALF with acute HEV infection has been reported to be as high as 70% in some populations, with mortality rates up to 20% in women infected during the third trimester.
   c. Diagnostic testing: IgM anti-HEV, IgG anti-HEV, HEV RNA by PCR from serum and stool (Centers for Disease Control and Prevention testing at http://www.cdc.gov/hepatitis/hev/labtestingrequests.htm)
   d. Disease-specific therapy: Treatment is supportive. Ribavirin is useful in chronic HEV infection.

NONHEPATOTROPIC VIRUSES (see Chapter 6)

1. **Herpes simplex virus (HSV)** and **varicella zoster virus (VZV)**
   a. Acute HSV or VZV infection can result in hepatitis and, rarely, ALF. HSV-associated ALF has a poor prognosis due in part to delayed diagnosis. HSV infection may be primary, without cutaneous or genital lesions, or due to reactivation.

- Immunocompromised patients are at increased risk of hepatitis and ALF.
- Cutaneous lesions and disseminated intravascular coagulation (DIC) are evident at presentation in approximately 50% of cases.

   b. Diagnostic testing: HSV DNA and VZV DNA by PCR; liver biopsy may be helpful in suspected cases (characteristic viral inclusions).
   c. Disease-specific therapy: Renally dosed intravenous acyclovir should be initiated immediately once the diagnosis is established or strongly suspected.

2. Cytomegalovirus (CMV)
   a. CMV infection is a major cause of morbidity in solid organ transplant recipients, although ALF is rare (see Chapter 33).
   b. The risk of severe hepatitis is greatest in CMV-seronegative transplant recipients of organs from CMV-seropositive donors.
   c. Diagnostic testing: CMV DNA by PCR, IgM and IgG anti-CMV; liver biopsy can be diagnostic.
   d. Disease-specific therapy: Immediate therapy with intravenous ganciclovir should be initiated if CMV hepatitis is suspected or confirmed.

3. Other viruses including parvovirus B19, Epstein-Barr virus (EBV), and adenovirus can rarely present as ALF in acute infection.
   a. **Parvovirus B19** infection is often associated with aplastic anemia.
   b. ALF is the leading cause of mortality in acute **EBV infection.** Some patients may have concomitant lymphoma or fever and severe adenopathy. Cholestatic ALF is also reported.
   c. Severe **adenovirus** hepatitis with ALF is more likely to occur in immunocompromised persons.
   d. Disease-specific therapy: Acyclovir and glucocorticoids may be tried in some cases.

AUTOIMMUNE HEPATITIS (see Chapter 7)

1. Autoimmune hepatitis (AIH) is more common in women (60%) than men, frequently presents as chronic hepatitis, and uncommonly presents with ALF or acute autoimmune hemolytic anemia with jaundice.
2. Diagnostic testing for autoimmune markers and liver biopsy should be performed when AIH is suspected.
   a. Serologic markers such as antinuclear antibodies (ANA), smooth muscle antibodies (SMA), and elevated immunoglobulin levels (especially IgG) are not always present in fulminant ALF.
   b. Liver biopsy specimens may show severe hepatocellular necrosis, interface hepatitis, plasma cell infiltration, pericentral venulitis, and hepatocyte rosettes.
   c. Drugs such as nitrofurantoin, minocycline, anti-PD-1 (programmed death-1) agents, and anti-CTLA-4 (cytotoxic T-lymphocyte-associated antigen 4) antibodies may induce AIH; discontinuation of the culprit drug and administration of glucocorticoids are recommended.
3. Disease-specific treatment: Glucocorticoid therapy (prednisone 40 to 60 mg/day) may be considered in fulminant AIH; some data suggest an increased rate of recovery.

VASCULAR OCCLUSION (see Chapter 21)

1. **Budd-Chiari syndrome** (acute hepatic vein thrombosis)
   a. Budd-Chiari syndrome typically presents with the acute onset of abdominal pain, ascites, and hepatomegaly due to hepatic venous outflow obstruction with engorgement.

    b. Diagnostic testing: Doppler ultrasonography, computed tomography (CT), or magnetic resonance venography; an underlying hypercoagulable disorder or myeloproliferative disease is found in 80% of cases; liver biopsy is used in selective cases to assess the severity of necrosis.

    c. Disease-specific treatment: All patients should be anticoagulated with intravenous heparin unless there is an overt contraindication. Thrombectomy, hepatic vein angioplasty, placement of a stent in the occluded vein, or transjugular intrahepatic portosystemic shunt (TIPS) placement may be considered. LT is considered for severe disease not responding to medical and radiologic interventions.

2. Sinusoidal obstruction syndrome (SOS)

    a. SOS (or veno-occlusive disease) may occur in patients who receive high-dose, induction chemotherapy before hematopoietic stem cell transplantation or after ingestion of large amounts of plant alkaloids (specific herbal teas).

    b. SOS presents with ascites, hepatomegaly, jaundice, and coagulopathy and is a rare cause of ALF.

    c. Diagnostic testing: Primarily through the patient's history, liver biopsy, and Doppler ultrasonography

    D. Disease-specific treatment: Primarily supportive; concomitant malignancy often precludes LT; defibrotide has been approved by the U.S. Food and Drug Administration for SOS.

ISCHEMIC HEPATITIS (see Chapter 22)

1. Ischemic hepatitis (hypoxic hepatitis, "shock liver") occurs most commonly after cardiac arrest, severe hypotension, or volume depletion or in the setting of cardiopulmonary collapse.

    a. ALF from ischemic hepatitis is rare; mortality is usually related to the precipitating event.

2. Cocaine or methamphetamine use may lead to drug-induced ischemic hepatitis.

3. Diagnostic testing: Compatible clinical history (hypotension, arrhythmia, cardiopulmonary disease); extremely high serum aminotransferase elevations; and acute kidney injury that improve with circulatory support

4. Disease-specific therapy: Volume resuscitation, vasopressors, inotropes, and treatment of the underlying cause

WILSON DISEASE (see Chapter 19)

1. Wilson disease is an autosomal recessive disease that presents most frequently in young adults.

    a. Patients may have neuropsychiatric manifestations at presentation (including depression).

    b. Kayser-Fleischer rings are identified with slit-lamp examination in only 50% of patients with hepatic disease.

    c. A mutation is identified in the *ATP7B* gene in 60% of white patients.

2. Diagnostic testing: Modest elevations in aminotransferase levels with an AST-to-ALT ratio of >2.2 and an alkaline phosphatase-to-bilirubin ratio of <4.

    a. A serum ceruloplasmin level is a useful screening test but is normal in 15% of affected patients.

    b. A 24-hour quantitative urine copper determination, liver biopsy with quantitative copper, and genetic testing may help confirm the diagnosis but should not delay a liver transplant evaluation and listing.

    c. Coombs-negative hemolytic anemia with jaundice and acute kidney injury occur frequently in patients with fulminant Wilson disease as a result of elevated free copper levels.

3. Disease-specific treatment: Albumin dialysis, plasmapheresis, or continuous hemofiltration to acutely lower serum copper can be attempted; however, interventions short of LT typically cannot arrest the course of ALF.

   a. Oral trientine (a chelating agent) and zinc therapy are frequently initiated.

   b. D-penicillamine may be associated with hypersensitivity and a worsening neurologic status.

   c. LT is needed in >95% of patients with fulminant Wilson disease.

MALIGNANT INFILTRATION (see Chapter 24)

1. Lymphomas, leukemias, and metastatic solid tumor infiltration of the liver (e.g., breast, lung) account for <1% of adult ALF cases.
   a. Clinical features of DIC may be present, and hepatic imaging may be abnormal.
   b. The diagnosis is frequently delayed; confirmation of isolated hepatic involvement may require transjugular or imaging-guided liver biopsy.
2. Disease-specific therapy: Prognosis is generally poor (<10% transplant-free survival), although some patients may benefit from salvage chemotherapy.

PREGNANCY-RELATED ALF (see Chapter 23)

1. Acute viral hepatitis; acute fatty liver of pregnancy; hemolysis, elevated liver enzymes, and low platelets (HELLP) syndrome; and preeclampsia and eclampsia may occur during pregnancy and result in ALF. The demographics and clinical presentation vary according to etiology.
2. Diagnostic testing: A serum beta-human chorionic gonadotropin level should be obtained in all women with ALF of childbearing age; all pregnant women with ALF should have a full workup for specific causes of ALF, especially acute viral hepatitis.
3. The mother should be closely monitored following delivery, since there is a risk of further hepatic decompensation after delivery.
4. Disease-specific treatment: Treatment varies according to the etiology of ALF; prompt delivery is often required.

ALF OF INDETERMINATE CAUSE

1. The etiology of ALF is unknown in 10% to 15% of cases in the United States despite extensive testing.
2. Serum acetaminophen-protein adducts in patients with ALF with high serum ALT and low serum bilirubin levels suggest that unsuspected acetaminophen hepatotoxicity may be responsible for up to 20% of indeterminate cases.
3. Disease-specific treatment: The rate of spontaneous recovery is low (30%), and LT is often required.

Treatment

INITIAL ASSESSMENT AND MANAGEMENT

1. **Rapidly determine the etiology of ALF** (Table 2.4).
   a. Directed history-taking may elicit potential causes of ALF including exposure risks, a history of depression or suicidal ideation, illicit drug or alcohol abuse, or ingestion of a hepatotoxic agent.
   b. Diagnostic studies should include toxicology screening, viral serologies, autoimmune markers, and hepatic imaging; abdominal ultrasonography may reveal hepatic surface nodularity associated with parenchymal collapse and regenerative nodule formation; a Doppler study may exclude Budd-Chiari syndrome.

TABLE 2.4 ■ Initial Clinical and Laboratory Assessment of ALF

Diagnostic Testing[a]

Medical and medication history, travel, exposures
Serum acetaminophen level, urine toxicity screen
Viral hepatitis: IgM anti-HAV, HBsAg, anti-HBc, anti-HCV, HCV RNA, IgM anti-HEV
Nonhepatotropic viruses: HSV DNA, EBV DNA, CMV DNA (all by PCR)
Wilson disease: Ceruloplasmin, urine copper, slit-lamp examination
Autoimmune hepatitis (AIH): ANA, SMA, quantitative immunoglobulin levels
Vascular disorders: Liver ultrasonography with Doppler
Ischemia: 2D echocardiogram with Doppler
Liver histology[b]: Only if malignancy, AIH, HSV suspected

Disease Severity

Serial laboratory testing every 12 hours
    Serum AST, ALT, bilirubin (total and direct), alkaline phosphatase
    INR, factor V, arterial blood gas, ammonia, lactate level
    Blood glucose, serum electrolytes, calcium, magnesium, phosphate
Encephalopathy grade, Glasgow coma score, presence of vital organ failure
    Head CT (if comma grade 2 or higher)
    ICP monitor if grade 4 HE or uninterpretable neurologic examination
Blood and urine cultures daily or infection suspected

Liver Transplantation Candidacy[c]

Medical and surgical assessment of prognosis and suitability
    Psychosocial assessment (substance abuse, compliance)
    Blood group determination
    HIV and other serologies
    Chest x-ray, ECG, and 2D echocardiogram
Contraindications: Sepsis, multiorgan failure, refractory hypotension, brain herniation

---

[a]Obtain initial diagnostic testing as soon as possible.

[b]Extent of necrosis on biopsy specimen is not associated with outcome.

[c]Complete within 24 hours of ICU admission and review periodically thereafter.

2D, Two-dimensional; *ALT*, alanine aminotransferase; *ANA*, antinuclear antibodies; *anti-HBc*, antibody to hepatitis B core antigen; *anti-HCV*, antibody to hepatitis C virus; *AST*, aspartate aminotransferase; *BUN*, blood urea nitrogen; *CMV*, cytomegalovirus; *CT*, computed tomography; *EBV*, Epstein-Barr virus; *ECG*, electrocardiogram; *HAV,* hepatitis A virus; *HBsAg*, hepatitis B surface antigen; *HE*, hepatic encephalopathy; *HEV,* hepatitis E virus; *HIV,* human immunodeficiency virus; *HSV*, herpes simplex virus; *ICP*, intracranial pressure; *ICU*, intensive care unit; *Ig*, immunoglobulin; *INR*, international normalized ratio; *IV*, intravenous; *PCR*, polymerase chain reaction; *SMA*, smooth muscle antibodies.

    c. Liver biopsy may be useful for prognostic purposes as well as to identify a specific etiology such as AIH, HSV hepatitis, or infiltration by malignant disease; if a liver biopsy is obtained, a transjugular approach is preferred due to coagulopathy.

2. Prompt transfer to an LT center is recommended.

3. Intensive care unit monitoring is critical to the prevention and management of complications such as shock, sepsis, acute kidney injury, and cerebral edema (Table 2.5).

4. Administer NAC in all patients with acetaminophen overdose. NAC can also provide survival benefit in adults with nonacetaminophen-associated ALF and grade 1 or 2 encephalopathy.

5. Assess the patient's probability of transplant-free survival.

    a. The etiology of ALF and severity of HE are the most important predictors of outcome; acetaminophen hepatotoxicity, acute hepatitis A, and ischemic hepatitis are associated with the most favorable rates of spontaneous recovery (60% to 70%).

TABLE 2.5 ■ **Management of Cerebral Edema**

General
Reduce external noise/stimuli (private room/ICU).
Elevate head of bed >30 degrees above horizontal at all times.
Mechanical intubation with sedation for grade 3 or 4 encephalopathy
Minimize endotracheal suctioning, movement, and Valsalva.
Propofol- or midazolam-based sedation

Specific
Consider placement of ICP monitor (epidural or parenchymal).
    Goal: ICP <25 mm Hg and CPP >50 mm Hg.
    Use vasopressors to maintain MAP >70 mm Hg.
Hyperventilation-induced hypocapnia to promote cerebral vasoconstriction
    Goal: PCO_2 of 28–30 mm Hg
Osmotherapy for ICP >25 mm Hg over 10 minutes
    Intravenous mannitol
        Bolus of 0.5 g/kg over 5 minutes (repeat every 2–6 hours)
        Maintain serum osmolarity <320 mOsm/L (with furosemide or dialysis).
        Caution: May cause pulmonary edema with acute kidney injury
    Intravenous hypertonic saline
        3% saline drip or 23% bolus infusion
        Goal: Serum sodium of 145–155 mEq/L
        Caution: Hyperchloremic, nongap acidosis
Barbiturate coma (for refractory cerebral edema)
    Intravenous pentobarbital
        Bolus of 100–150 mg over 15 minutes; continuous infusion of 1–3 mg/kg/hr
        Caution: Hypotension is common (use vasopressors if necessary)
    Excessive sedation: Monitor serum pentobarbital levels every 12 hours (target 20–35 mg/L).

CPP, Cerebral perfusion pressure; *ICP*, intracranial pressure; *ICU*, intensive care unit; *MAP*, mean arterial pressure; PCO_2, partial pressure of carbon dioxide.

TABLE 2.6 ■ **King's College Criteria for Adverse Outcomes in ALF[a]**

Acetaminophen Overdose	Nonacetaminophen ALF
Arterial lactate >3.5 mmol/L 4 hours after resuscitation	INR >6.5 (PT >100 seconds)
or	*or*
pH <7.30 or arterial lactate >3.0 mmol/L 12 hours after resuscitation	Three of the following:
	INR >3.5 (PT >50 seconds)
or	Age <10 or >40 years
INR >6.5 (PT >100 seconds)	Serum bilirubin >17.5 mg/dL
Serum creatinine >3.4 mg/dL	Duration of jaundice >7 days
Stage 3 or 4 encephalopathy	Etiology: Drug reaction

[a]Prognostic models should not be the sole criteria to determine appropriateness for liver transplant. Serial laboratory assessments (INR, factor V, NH_3) and detection of vital organ failure recommended (pressors, dialysis, intubation, infection).

INR, International normalized ratio; *PT*, prothrombin time.

    b. The most widely studied prognostic criteria for ALF are the **King's College criteria** (Table 2.6), which have a high specificity for mortality; however, failure to fulfill these criteria does not guarantee survival.

6. Assessment includes serial laboratory testing (INR, factor V, ammonia, and lactate levels) as well as organ system failure, HE grade, need for pressor support, mechanical intubation, and evidence of infection.

EVALUATION FOR LT (see Chapter 33)

1. All patients with ALF should be evaluated for possible LT.
2. Patients with ALF who fulfill listing criteria defined by the United Network for Organ Sharing (UNOS) may be assigned to category 1A and receive top priority for organ allocation (see Chapter 33).
   a. ABO-compatible whole LT is preferred; the waiting time for transplantation averages 1 to 10 days.
3. Contraindications to LT include extrahepatic malignancy, irreversible brain injury, severe cardiopulmonary disease, multiorgan failure, refractory hypotension, and sepsis.
4. Inadequate social support, active substance abuse, repeated suicide attempts, and severe comorbid psychiatric conditions may preclude LT candidacy.

MANAGEMENT OF COMPLICATIONS

1. HE and cerebral edema (see Table 2.5)
   a. **Encephalopathy is the defining feature of ALF and may progress rapidly and lead to increased risks of cerebral edema, intracranial hypertension, and death.**
      - Persons at higher risk of developing cerebral edema include those who present with a hyperacute course, have arterial ammonia levels >200 μmol/L, and develop grade 3 to 4 encephalopathy.
      - Cerebral edema develops in 35% and 75% of patients with grades 3 and 4 HE, respectively.
      - Hypoxia, systemic hypotension, decreased cerebral perfusion pressure (CPP), and swelling of astrocytes result from elevated blood ammonia levels and increased glutamine production within the brain.
      - Cerebral edema may ultimately lead to increased intracranial pressure (ICP), ischemic brain injury, and herniation.
      - Cerebral edema with intracranial hypertension is the most common cause of mortality in ALF.
   b. Monitoring cerebral edema and intracranial hypertension
      - Brain imaging and papilledema on funduscopy are not sensitive for intracranial hypertension; serial physical and neurologic examinations are recommended.
        - Abnormal pupillary reflexes, muscular rigidity, or decerebrate posturing may suggest the development of intracranial hypertension.
      - All sedatives and other medications that alter the sensorium should be strictly avoided.
        - Propofol and midazolam are preferred when needed due to short half-life.
      - CT of the head should be considered in patients with grade 2 to 4 HE to assess for cerebral edema or intracranial bleeding.
      - Placement of an ICP monitoring device may be considered in patients who are intubated and have grade 3 or 4 HE.
        - Administration of FFP and recombinant factor VIIa can facilitate safe placement of a pressure monitoring device.
   c. Management of cerebral edema and intracranial hypertension (see Table 2.5)
      - Measures should be taken to minimize elevations of ICP and maximize CPP.
        - The head of the bed should be elevated >30 degrees above horizontal.
      - Lactulose is not effective for the treatment of ALF.
      - Mannitol, hypertonic saline, hyperventilation, and a short-acting barbiturate may be considered once intracranial hypertension has been identified.
      - Therapeutic hypothermia to 32°C to 35°C with a cooling blanket is used in patients with refractory cerebral edema; the appropriate means of rewarming and impact on liver regeneration are uncertain.

2. Coagulopathy (Table 2.7)
    a. Coagulopathy is a key feature of ALF and an important prognostic indicator; although coagulopathy can be profound, serious bleeding events are uncommon (<10%).
    b. The platelet count, INR, and PT may be misleading in the setting of ALF and do not represent an accurate representation of a patient's coagulopathy and thrombophilia.
        ■ Serial factor V levels are useful as a prognostic marker in patients with ALF.
        ■ Thromboelastography or rotational thromboelastography may be a more accurate measure of coagulopathy.
        ■ Factor VIII levels are elevated in patients with hepatic necrosis and decreased in patients with DIC.
    c. Parenteral vitamin K (10 mg IV or PO) may be given if nutritional deficiency is suspected.

TABLE 2.7 ■ **Management of ALF Complications**

Major Complications	Pathogenesis	Management
Hypoglycemia	↓ Glucose synthesis	Blood glucose check every 1–2 hours Intravenous glucose supplementation (10% or 20% dextrose)
Encephalopathy	Cerebral edema	CT (if stage 3 or 4 HE) ICP monitoring (if stage 4) to determine CPP Elevation of head of bed >30 degrees above horizontal Consideration of osmotherapy (mannitol, hypertonic saline) or barbiturates Treatment of contributing factors (e.g., hypoglycemia, hypoxemia, fever) Avoidance of benzodiazepines/sedative medications
Infections	Reduced immune function Invasive procedures	Daily surveillance cultures of blood, urine, and sputum Preemptive broad-spectrum antibiotics (cephalosporin or fluoroquinolone and vancomycin)
Coagulopathy	Reduced clotting factor synthesis Thrombocytopenia, DIC	Monitor factor V, INR Vitamin K 10 mg intravenously or orally Platelet transfusions for bleeding or procedures if platelets <50,000/mm^3 Plasma infusions for bleeding or procedures if INR >1.5 Infusion of cryoprecipitate for bleeding or procedures if serum fibrinogen level <100 mg/dL Proton pump inhibitor for gastrointestinal bleeding prophylaxis
Hypotension	Hypovolemia Decreased vascular resistance	Hemodynamic monitoring of central pressures Volume repletion with blood or colloid Norepinephrine, vasopressin
Renal failure	Hypovolemia Hepatorenal syndrome Acute tubular necrosis	Volume repletion with blood or colloid Avoidance of nephrotoxins (e.g., aminoglycosides, contrast dye) CVVHD or hemodialysis
Respiratory failure	ARDS	Mechanical ventilation Propofol or midazolam for sedation Withdrawal of sedation every 12–24 hours

ARDS, Acute respiratory distress syndrome; *CPP,* cerebral perfusion pressure; *CT,* computed tomography; *CVVHD,* continuous venovenous hemodialysis; *DIC,* disseminated intravascular coagulation; *HE,* hepatic encephalopathy; *ICP,* intracranial pressure; *INR,* international normalized ratio.

   d. Platelet transfusions, plasma, and cryoprecipitate may reduce the bleeding risk associated with invasive procedures; correction of coagulopathy is otherwise NOT recommended unless clinically significant bleeding occurs.
      ■ Administration of recombinant factor VIIa may be considered after infusions of fresh frozen plasma for invasive procedures; thrombophilia, pregnancy, and cancer are contraindications.
   e. Proton pump inhibitors should be administered to all intubated patients because of the potential for gastrointestinal bleeding.
3. Renal failure
   a. May occur in up to 50% of patients with ALF
   b. Key early prognostic indicator, particularly in patients with acetaminophen hepatotoxicity, in which renal failure or the presence of acidosis is highly predictive of mortality
   c. The pathogenesis includes hypovolemia, acute tubular necrosis, or hepatorenal syndrome.
   d. Norepinephrine or dopamine infusion is used to mitigate circulatory dysfunction and severe hypotension.
   e. Renal replacement therapy with continuous venovenous hemodialysis is preferred over standard hemodialysis once renal or circulatory dysfunction develops.
4. Infection
   a. Surveillance cultures of blood, sputum, and urine are recommended in patients with ALF at presentation and when unexplained deterioration or systemic inflammatory response syndrome (SIRS) is evident.
      ■ 80% of patients with ALF develop a bacterial infection during hospitalization.
      ■ 20% develop a fungal infection (fever, hypotension on antibiotics).
   b. Empiric antimicrobial therapy should be initiated in any of the following circumstances.
      ■ Positive surveillance culture or fever
      ■ Grade 3 or 4 encephalopathy
      ■ Hemodynamic instability or the onset of SIRS
5. Metabolic disorders
   a. Hypoglycemia may result from decreased hepatic glycogen production and impaired gluconeogenesis. Blood glucose levels must be measured at frequent intervals, and continuous infusions of 10% to 20% glucose should be given if hypoglycemia is present.
   b. Hypophosphatemia may be seen in ALF as a result of ATP consumption in the setting of rapid hepatocyte regeneration as well as increased urinary loss. Life-threatening hypophosphatemia can occur, and phosphorus levels should be monitored frequently with prompt repletion.
   c. Electrolyte and metabolic derangements contribute to progressive HE and an increased risk of cerebral edema; therefore, they must be corrected promptly.
   d. Acidosis is an important predictor of mortality; a pH <7.3 is associated with a mortality rate of up to 95% in patients with acetaminophen overdose in the absence of LT.
   e. Alkalosis, reflecting hyperventilation, may be present in ALF.
   f. Hypoxemia may result from acute respiratory distress syndrome, aspiration, or pulmonary hemorrhage; patients with grade 3 or 4 encephalopathy should be intubated to protect the airway.

FUTURE THERAPIES

1. Extracorporeal hepatic assist devices such as albumin dialysis, auxiliary LT, and hepatocyte transplantation have been studied in an effort to improve clinical outcomes in ALF; although some improvements in physiologic parameters have been reported, no significant impact on survival has resulted to date.

2. Further study of bioartificial or nonbiological hepatic assist devices and the development of hepatocyte culture systems through tissue engineering may identify effective means of supporting patients with ALF through recovery or may provide a "bridge" to LT.

3. Medical therapies that stimulate hepatocyte regeneration and stem cell differentiation hold promise.

4. Medical therapies directed toward reducing hyperammonemia may reduce sequelae of cerebral edema.

FURTHER READING

Bari K, Fontana RJ. Acetaminophen overdose: what practitioners need to know. *Clin Liv Dis.* 2014;4:17–20.

Bernal W, Wendon J. Acute liver failure. *N Engl J Med.* 2013;369:2525–2534.

Fontana RJ, Ellerbe C, Durkalski VE, et al. Two-year outcomes in initial survivors with acute liver failure: results from a prospective, multicentre study. *Liver Int.* 2015;35:370–380.

Larsen FS, Wendon J. Prevention and management of brain edema in patients with acute liver failure. *Liver Transpl.* 2008;14(suppl 2):S90–S96.

Larson AM, Polson J, Fontana RJ, et al. Acetaminophen-induced acute liver failure: results of a United States multicenter, prospective study. *Hepatology.* 2005;42:1364–1372.

Lee WM, Hynan LS, Rossaro L, et al. Intravenous *N*-acetylcysteine improves transplant-free survival in early stage non-acetaminophen acute liver failure. *Gastroenterology.* 2009;137:856–864.

McPhail MJ, Farne H, Senvar N, et al. Ability of King's College criteria and model for end-stage liver disease scores to predict mortality of patients with acute liver failure: a meta-analysis. *Clin Gastroenterol Hepatol.* 2016;14:516–525.

O'Grady J. Timing and benefit of liver transplantation in acute liver failure. *J Hepatol.* 2014;60:663–670.

O'Grady JG, Alexander GJ, Hayllar KM, et al. Early indicators of prognosis in fulminant hepatic failure. *Gastroenterology.* 1989;97:439–445.

Ostapowicz G, Fontana RJ, Schiodt FV, et al. Results of a prospective study of acute liver failure at 17 tertiary care centers in the United States. *Ann Intern Med.* 2002;137:947–954.

Polson J, Lee W-M. AASLD position paper: the management of acute liver failure. *Hepatology.* 2005;41:1179–1197.

Reddy KR, Ellerbe C, Schilsky M, et al. Determinants of outcome among patients with acute liver failure listed for liver transplantation in the United States. *Liver Transpl.* 2016;22:505–515.

Reuben A, Tillman H, Fontana RJ, et al. Outcomes in adults with acute liver failure between 1998 and 2013: an observational cohort study. *Ann Intern Med.* Apr 5, 2016. [Epub ahead of print].

Rutherford A, Chung RT. Acute liver failure: mechanisms of hepatocyte injury and regeneration. *Semin Liver Dis.* 2008;28:167–174.

Stravitz RT, Kramer AH, Davern T, et al. Intensive care of patients with acute liver failure: recommendations of the U.S. Acute Liver Failure Study Group. *Crit Care Med.* 2007;35:2498–2508.

CHAPTER 3

Hepatitis A and Hepatitis E

Kelvin T. Nguyen, MD ■ Steven-Huy B. Han, MD, AGAF, FAASLD

KEY POINTS

1 Infection by the nonenveloped, enterically transmitted viruses, hepatitis A virus (HAV) and hepatitis E virus (HEV), generally causes self-limited infection, but severe hepatitis may develop in some cases; chronic hepatitis E has been recognized in immunosuppressed patients and can result in hepatic fibrosis and cirrhosis.

2 HEV genotypes 1 and 2, involved in acute HEV infection, are transmitted by the fecal-oral route, whereas HEV genotypes 3 and 4 have been implicated in chronic HEV infection and are transmitted by a zoonosis with domestic swine, wild boar, or wild deer as intermediates.

3 HAV vaccination is effective protection against infection. An effective HEV vaccine has been developed but is not approved for use in most countries.

4 In addition to immunocompromised patients, pregnant women and patients with preexisting liver disease are at increased risk for developing severe complications of hepatitis E.

5 Antiviral therapy for HAV is not available, in contrast to HEV, which responds to ribavirin, which is indicated in severe acute or chronic HEV infection.

Hepatitis A Virus

MOLECULAR BIOLOGY

1. Classified as a picornavirus, subclassified as the only member of the subclass hepatovirus
2. 27 to 28 nm in diameter with cubic symmetry
3. Positive single-stranded, linear RNA molecule, 7.5 kb in one open reading frame
4. One serotype in human beings; at least 6 genotypes
5. Although described as a nonenveloped virus, more recent evidence suggests that HAV may have enveloped and nonenveloped forms.
6. Contains a single immunodominant neutralization site
7. Contains four major virion polypeptides in a capsomere (Fig. 3.1)
8. Replication in cytoplasm of infected hepatocytes through an RNA-dependent RNA polymerase; no definitive evidence of persistent replication in the intestine
9. High degree of chemical and thermal resistance to inactivation, allowing HAV to persist in contaminated foods or fecal matter for weeks
10. Can survive exposure to bile and other detergents
11. Has been propagated in nonhuman primate and human cell lines
12. Does not result in prolonged viremia or an intestinal carrier state
13. Replicates in the liver and induces as yet unidentified immune responses

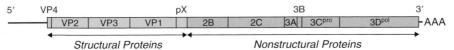

Fig. 3.1 Schematic showing organization of the 7.5-kb single-stranded, positive-sense RNA genome of hepatitis A virus. The 2227 amino acid residue polyprotein is composed of both structural and nonstructural proteins and is flanked by 5' and 3' untranslated RNA segments containing regulatory elements. *VP*, Virion protein. (Adapted from Walker C, Feng Z, Lemon S. Reassessing immune control of hepatitis A virus. *Curr Opin Virol.* 2015;11:7–13.)

EPIDEMIOLOGY AND RISK FACTORS

1. Incubation period: 15 to 50 days (average, 30 days)
2. **Worldwide distribution; annual global incidence is 1.5 million cases; hyperendemic in developing countries**
3. In developed countries with improved water and sanitation systems, the majority of the population reach adulthood without acquiring HAV infection and developing immunity. In developing countries where areas with socioeconomic development and hygienic improvement have led to a reduction in HAV transmission and a higher average age at the time of initial infection, there has been a paradoxical increase in the incidence of symptomatic HAV with more severe consequences, such as fulminant hepatitis and prolonged hospital stays and death, reflecting the increased severity of HAV infection acquired after childhood (Fig. 3.2).
4. HAV is excreted in the stools of infected persons for 1 to 2 weeks before and at least 1 week after the onset of illness, usually shortly after the serum alanine aminotransferase (ALT) level begins to increase.
5. Viremia is short lived, usually no longer than 3 weeks but occasionally up to 90 days in protracted or relapsing infection.
6. Prolonged fecal excretion (for months) is reported in infected neonates; the frequency, concentration of virus in stool, and epidemiologic importance remain uncertain.
7. Fulminant hepatitis A is increasingly uncommon since the advent of HAV vaccination.
8. Enteric (fecal-oral) transmission occurs predominantly by person-to-person household spread or an infected food handler; occasional outbreaks are linked to a common source:
   - Contaminated food
   - Bivalve mollusks
   - Water
9. Other risk factors for infection:
   - Daycare centers for infants, diapered children
   - Institutions for the developmentally disadvantaged
   - Travel to developing countries (the most common risk factor for Americans)
   - Oral-anal contact
   - Shared equipment or drugs in injection drug users
10. No evidence for maternal-neonatal transmission
11. The prevalence of HAV infection correlates with sanitary standards and larger households.
12. Transmission by blood transfusion or blood products is very rare.
13. No risk factors are identified in 30% to 40% of cases in the United States.
14. The overall seroprevalence of HAV infection in the United States is <30% and is declining rapidly with expanded use of the HAV vaccine.
15. Disease severity is increased in persons with preexisting liver disease or age ≥ 40 years.
16. HAV cellular receptor 1 (HAVcr1), a polymorphic variant, has been associated with an increased risk of severe hepatitis, possibly secondary to more avid binding of the virus to

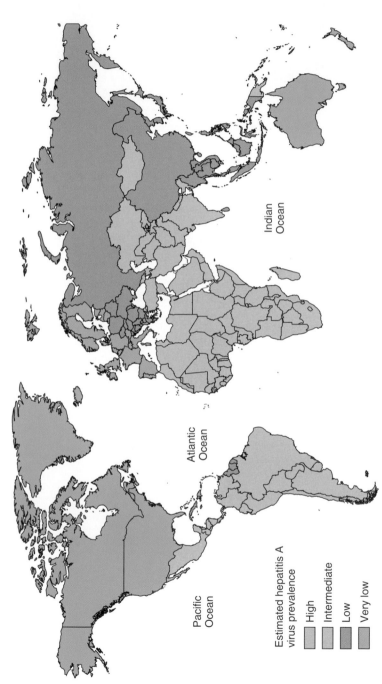

Fig. 3.2 Estimates of the prevalence of antibody to hepatitis A virus (anti-HAV), a marker of previous HAV infection, based on a systematic literature review conducted from 1990 to 2005. In addition, anti-HAV prevalence may vary within countries by subpopulation and locality. As used on this map, the terms "high," "medium," "low," and "very low" endemicity reflect available evidence of how widespread HAV infection is within each country, rather than precise quantitative assessments. (Adapted from Jacobsen KH, Wiersma ST. Hepatitis A virus seroprevalence by age and world region, 1990 and 2005. *Vaccine.* 2010;28:6653–6657.)

Estimated hepatitis A
virus prevalence

High

Intermediate

Low

Very low

Pacific
Ocean

Atlantic
Ocean

Indian
Ocean

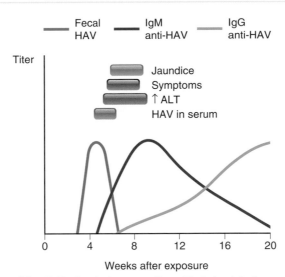

Fig. 3.3 Serologic course of hepatitis A virus infection.

hepatocytes, as well as a boost in the cytotoxicity of natural killer T cells against infected hepatocytes.

PATHOPHYSIOLOGY

After oral ingestion, HAV enters the portal circulation and reaches the liver after replication in intestinal cells. HAV enters hepatocytes, where further replication occurs resulting in a large amount of viral progeny released into the bile and intestinal lumen before being excreted in the feces Liver injury occurs via a host immune response.

CLINICAL FEATURES

Self-Limited Disease (Fig. 3.3)

1. **Disease severity ranges from asymptomatic infection to fatal acute liver failure; severity is increased in those with preexisting liver disease or age ≥40 years.**
   - The likelihood of symptomatic infection increases with age.
   - Children <6 years of age are typically asymptomatic.
   - Infectivity peaks between 2 weeks before and at least 1 week after symptoms begin.
   - **Some infected persons develop one or more relapses after an apparent initial partial or complete resolution of symptoms.** During relapse, there is ongoing viral replication, usually milder than the initial event, although prolonged cholestasis can occur, with eventual resolution (see discussion later in chapter).
2. Fever in acute viral hepatitis is generally uncommon, although it can occur in acute hepatitis A.
3. Prodromal symptoms abate or disappear with the onset of jaundice, although anorexia, malaise, and weakness may persist.
4. Jaundice is heralded by the appearance of dark urine and lightening of stool color; pruritus (usually mild and transient) may also occur.
5. Physical examination reveals mild hepatomegaly with tenderness.
6. Mild splenomegaly and posterior cervical lymphadenopathy are noted in 15% to 20% of patients.

Acute Liver Failure

See Chapter 2 for information about acute liver failure.

Cholestatic Hepatitis

1. Pruritus is prominent.
2. Persistent anorexia and diarrhea are present in a few patients.
3. Jaundice may persist for several months before eventual resolution.
4. The prognosis is excellent, usually with complete resolution without specific therapy.

Relapsing Hepatitis

1. Symptoms and liver biochemical test abnormalities recur weeks to months after apparent recovery.
2. Immunoglobulin (Ig)M antibody to HAV (anti-HAV) may remain positive, and HAV may once again be shed in stool.
3. Arthritis, vasculitis, and cryoglobulinemia may be observed.
4. Prognosis is excellent with complete recovery even after multiple relapses (particularly common in children).

EXTRAHEPATIC MANIFESTATIONS

Intracerebral hemorrhage has been reported as a complication of HAV infection, due mostly to aplastic anemia–induced thrombocytopenia. Other complications:

1. Acute kidney injury
2. Hemophagocytic lymphohistiocytosis
3. Pure red cell aplasia
4. Vasculitis with cutaneous manifestations
5. Arthritis
6. Autoimmune hemolytic anemia
7. Guillain-Barré syndrome
8. Pericarditis
9. Cryoglobulinemia
10. Myelopathy
11. Mononeuritis
12. Meningoencephalitis
13. Acute pancreatitis

LABORATORY FEATURES
Self-Limited Disease

1. Most prominent biochemical feature: Marked elevation of serum ALT and aspartate aminotransferase (AST) levels
2. Peak aminotransferase (ALT and AST) levels vary from 500 to 5000 U/L; ALT levels are generally higher than AST levels.
3. The serum bilirubin level is seldom >10 mg/dL, except in severe disease, acute liver failure, and cholestatic hepatitis.
4. Serum alkaline phosphatase levels are normal or mildly elevated.
5. The prothrombin time is normal or increased by 1 to 3 seconds.
6. The serum albumin level is normal or minimally depressed.
7. Peripheral blood counts are normal or mild leukopenia is present, with or without relative lymphocytosis.

Acute Liver Failure

See Chapter 2 for information about acute liver failure.

Cholestatic Disease

1. Serum bilirubin levels may exceed 20 mg/dL.
2. Serum aminotransferase levels are near normal despite cholestasis.
3. Variable elevation of serum alkaline phosphatase
4. Normal or nearly normal serum albumin
5. A prolonged prothrombin time, if present, is usually responsive to vitamin K administration.

Relapsing Hepatitis

1. After apparent normalization or near normalization of serum aminotransferase and bilirubin levels during convalescence, levels may rise again.
2. Infrequently, peak levels may exceed those of the initial bout.

HISTOLOGY

Liver biopsy is rarely performed in acute self-limited HAV infection.

Self-Limited Disease

1. Major hepatocyte injury
   - Focal hepatocyte necrosis
   - Loss of hepatocytes (cell dropout)
   - Ballooning degeneration
   - Apoptosis with Councilman-like bodies (mummified, hyalinized, necrotic hepatocytes extruded into a hepatic sinusoid)
2. Endophlebitis affecting the central vein
3. Diffuse mononuclear cell (CD8+ and natural killer cell) infiltrate
   - Within expanded portal tracts
   - Segmental erosion of the limiting plate
   - Within hepatic parenchyma
   - Kupffer cells are enlarged and hyperplastic and contain lipofuscin pigment and debris; remnants of injured hepatocytes are seen.

Cholestatic Disease

1. Hepatocyte degeneration and inflammation, as in self-limited hepatitis
2. Prominence of bile plugs in dilated biliary canaliculi and bilirubin staining of hepatocytes
3. Hepatocytes form multiple, scattered, ductlike structures (pseudoglandular transformation).

Relapsing Hepatitis

Changes are similar to those in self-limited disease.

DIAGNOSIS

For serologic diagnosis, see Table 3.1 and Fig. 3.3.
   - **IgM anti-HAV is detected during the acute phase and for 3 to 6 months thereafter, and rarely for as long as 24 months**.
   - The presence of IgG anti-HAV without IgM anti-HAV indicates past (resolved) infection or prior vaccination.

TABLE 3.1 ■ Serologic Patterns in the Diagnosis of Acute Hepatitis A and E

Agent	Acute Phase	Convalescence
HAV		
	Total anti-HAV positive	Development of IgG anti-HAV
	IgM anti-HAV positive	Disappearance of IgM anti-HAV
HEV		
	IgM anti-HEV positive and/or HEV RNA (in stool or serum)	Loss of HEV RNA; development of IgG anti-HEV
	IgG anti-HEV may be present	Loss of IgM anti-HEV

HAV, Hepatitis A virus; *HEV*, hepatitis E virus; *Ig*, immunoglobulin.

TREATMENT
Self-Limited Disease
1. **Supportive care in the outpatient setting is usually sufficient,** unless persistent vomiting or severe anorexia leads to dehydration and the need for inpatient admission.
2. Maintenance of adequate caloric and fluid intake is critical:
   - No specific dietary recommendations
   - Encourage a large breakfast, which is often the best tolerated meal in patients with acute hepatitis.
   - Prohibit use of alcohol during the acute phase.
3. Vigorous or prolonged physical activity should be avoided.
4. Limitation of daily activities and the need for rest periods are determined by the severity of the patient's fatigue and malaise.
5. All nonessential drugs should be discontinued.

Acute Liver Failure (see Chapter 2)
1. Intravenous *N*-acetylcysteine may be beneficial if given early after presentation; glucocorticoids are of no value.
2. Potential treatments for HAV infection require further investigation. Two categories are direct-acting antivirals (DAAs) and host-targeting agents (HTAs). There is a possible synergistic effect between the two drug classes. Potential drug targets in the HAV genomes include the following:
   - DAAs, such as protease inhibitors and internal ribosomal entry-site (IRES) inhibitors
   - HTAs, such as alpha interferon, gamma interferon, interferon-lambda 1, ribavirin, amantadine, and agents against key host enzymes or cellular factors

Cholestatic Hepatitis
1. The course may potentially be shortened by treatment with prednisone or ursodeoxycholic acid, but no clinical trials of efficacy are available to support this supposition.
2. Pruritus may be ameliorated by bile sequestrants such as cholestyramine.

Relapsing Hepatitis
Management is identical to that of self-limited HAV infection.

PREVENTION

Immunoprophylaxis is the cornerstone.

1. **Preexposure immunoprophylaxis**
   a. Inactivated HAV vaccine
      - Highly effective (efficacy rate, 95% to 100%); proven to be as effective as a live attenuated virus vaccine. One study has shown that one or two doses of inactivated vaccine achieve 93% to 100% seroprotection compared with 65% with one dose of the live attenuated HAV vaccine.
      - Highly immunogenic (nearly 100% in healthy subjects)
      - Protective antibodies induced in 15 days after first dose in 85% to 90% of recipients
      - Safe, well tolerated
      - Estimated duration of protection is 20 to 50 years, possibly lifelong.
      - Anti-HAV persists for 11 years after a single dose of inactivated HAV vaccine.
      - Injection site soreness is the major adverse event.
   b. **Inactivated HAV vaccine (HAVRIX and VAQTA) doses and schedules**
      - Adults 19 years of age or older: Two-dose (1440 ELISA U) regimen of HAVRIX (Glaxo-SmithKline), with the second dose 6 to 12 months after the first; or two-dose (50 U) regimen of VAQTA (Merck), with the second dose 6 to 18 months after the first
      - Children >12 months of age: Two-dose regimen of HAVRIX (720 ELISA U), with the second dose 6 to 12 months after the first; or two-dose (25 U) regimen of VAQTA, with the second dose 6 to 18 months after the first
   c. Indications for inactivated HAV vaccine
      - All children beginning at age 12 to 23 months
      - Travelers to high-risk areas (for those leaving immediately, immune globulin may be given simultaneously, at a different site, although the vaccine alone may be sufficient). Only 26.6% of travelers to countries with a high or intermediate prevalence of HAV currently receive HAV vaccination.
      - Homosexual, bisexual men, and adolescents
      - People who inject drugs
      - Native peoples of the Americas
      - Children and young adults in community-wide outbreaks
      - Children in regions, counties, and states with HAV attack rates higher than the national average
      - Patients with chronic liver disease
      - Patients with clotting disorders
      - Laboratory workers handling HAV
      - Food handlers when vaccination is deemed cost effective by local health officials
      - Household contacts of adoptees from endemic regions
      - Staff in daycare centers and waste water treatment workers
2. **Postexposure immunoprophylaxis**
   - HAV vaccine in the postexposure setting is as effective as immune globulin if given within 2 weeks of the onset of exposure for persons between 2 and 40 years of age; presumably, it is also effective in younger and older subjects, but it has not been studied in these groups.
   - Vaccine-induced immunity is longer lasting; therefore, vaccination is favored over administration of immune globulin.
   - The second vaccine dose should be administered 6 to 18 months later to provide extended protection.
   - The efficacy of immune globulin is well established, but availability is limited and it provides only short-term protection.

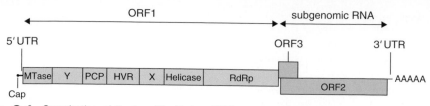

Fig. 3.4 Organization of the hepatitis E virus (HEV) genome. Nonstructural proteins are translated from ORF1 while the ORF2 and ORF3 structural proteins are translated from a single subgenomic RNA. *HVR,* Hypervariable region; *MTase,* methyltransferase; *ORF,* open reading frame; *PCP,* papain-like cysteine protease protease; *RdRp,* RNA-dependent polymerase; *UTR,* untranslated region; *X,* macro domain; *Y,* Y domain. (Adapted from Debing Y, Neyts J. Antivirals strategies for hepatitis E virus. *Antiviral Res.* 2014;102:106–118.)

- Immune globulin schedule and dose:
    - 0.02 mL/kg body weight, deltoid injection, as early as possible after exposure
    - Well tolerated; injection site soreness is major adverse effect
    - Indications: Household and intimate contacts of persons with acute HAV infection who refuse or cannot receive the HAV vaccine
3. In addition to vaccination, other general measures to protect against exposure to enteric viral hepatitis include heating foods to 85° C, use of household bleach for disinfection, handwashing, avoidance of uncooked or undercooked food, proper disposal of human waste, and ensuring the safety of the water supply.

Hepatitis E Virus

MOLECULAR BIOLOGY

1. Classified as Hepeviridae, subclassified as a hepevirus. The resulting illness was previously referred to as "enterically transmitted non-A, non-B hepatitis," now called hepatitis E owing to the alphabetical order of discovery of viral hepatitides; "e" also reflects "epidemic" and "endemic" disease. Hepeviridae, in addition to human HEV, includes viruses that infect pigs, rabbits, rats, deer, and mongoose and the more distant avian HEV. Human and swine HEV strains possess significant serologic cross reactivity.
2. 27 to 34 nm in diameter
3. Linear RNA molecule, 7.2 to 7.4 kb
4. RNA genome with three overlapping open reading frames encoding structural proteins and nonstructural proteins involved in HEV replication (Fig. 3.4)
   - RNA-dependent RNA polymerase (RNA replicase)
   - Helicase
   - Cysteine protease
   - Methyltransferase
   - Only one human serotype identified; four major genotypes
5. Immunodominant neutralization site on structural protein is encoded by a second open reading frame.
6. Can be propagated in transfected human hepatocellular carcinoma cell lines and in human embryo lung diploid cells
7. Can survive exposure to bile and other detergents
8. Shed in feces and transmitted through contaminated water and food
9. HEV can progress to chronic liver disease, albeit rarely.

10. Replicates in the liver and induces as yet unidentified immune responses
11. A third enterically transmitted hepatitis virus may exist that is transmissible to chimpanzees.

EPIDEMIOLOGY AND RISK FACTORS

1. First described in 1978 during an epidemic of hepatitis in Kashmir Valley, India. An estimated 52,000 cases of icteric hepatitis were been reported, resulting in 1700 deaths.
2. Incubation period: Approximately 40 days (range, 15 to 65 days)
3. **Widely distributed; seroprevalence data suggest that one-third of the world's population has been infected with HEV,** resulting in an approximate annual mortality of 70,000 persons; seroprevalence in the U.S. population is lower than in earlier reports.
4. HEV RNA is present in serum and stool during the acute phase. Fecal shedding of the virus occurs 1 to 2 weeks before and 2 to 4 weeks after the onset of symptoms.
5. **Most common form of sporadic hepatitis in young adults in the developing world**
6. **Largely waterborne outbreaks in Asia, Africa, and Central America**
7. Intrafamilial and secondary cases are uncommon.
8. Maternal-neonatal transmission is documented.
9. In the United States, cases have been reported in returning travelers and in recent immigrants from endemic regions; sporadic, rare cases of transmission from undercooked pork products, liver, and other organ meats, shellfish, and venison or by transfusion have been reported.
10. Prolonged viremia or fecal shedding is unusual; continued viral shedding is possible in rare cases in organ transplant recipients in whom chronic HEV infection is recognized.
11. Genotypes 1 and 2 have been isolated from sporadic human cases and waterborne outbreaks; genotypes 3 and 4 have been isolated from swine and other animals, including wild boar and deer, and apparently transmitted zoonotically to humans (Fig. 3.5).
12. Distinct epidemiologic patterns are observed in highly endemic regions such as tropical and subtropical countries in Asia, Africa, and Central America and nonendemic regions such as the United States, Western Europe, and developed countries of the Asia-Pacific region (Table 3.2).
13. In developed countries, risk factors for HEV infection include consumption of liver or meat more than once a month, male gender, non-Hispanic white ethnicity, residence in certain geographical areas, and keeping a pet.
14. Risk factors for chronic HEV infection are the consumption of game meat and therapeutic immunosuppression in organ transplant recipients. Dose reduction in immunosuppressive therapy can accelerate viral clearance.
15. Characteristics of each genotype are described in Table 3.3.
16. A case of transmission by an organ donor has been reported.

PATHOPHYSIOLOGY

1. After ingestion, HEV enters the portal circulation (similar to HAV). HEV RNA can be detected in serum, bile, and feces before the serum aminotransferase levels rise. HEV antigen can be demonstrated in hepatocytes 7 days after infection, with rapid spread to 70% to 90% of hepatocytes.
2. Hepatocyte injury is due to the host immune response. The increased mortality associated with pregnancy is thought to be due to an accentuated T-helper cell type 2 response.

CLINICAL FEATURES
Self-Limited Disease

1. In highly endemic regions, many patients do not recall initial acute hepatitis, suggesting HEV infection may be largely asymptomatic.

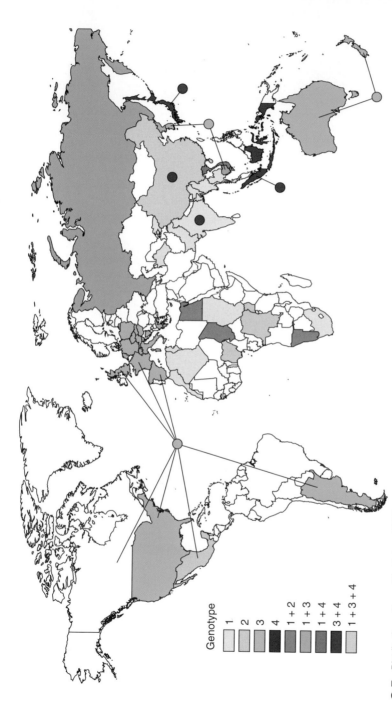

Fig. 3.5 Distribution of hepatitis E virus (HEV) genotypes in viral isolates obtained from humans and animals (predominantly pigs). The colors used for a country and the circle associated with it represent the predominant HEV genotypes of human and animal isolates, respectively, from that country. (Adapted from Aggarwal R, Jameel S. Hepatitis E. *Hepatology*. 2011;54:2218–2226.)

TABLE 3.2 ■ Features of Hepatitis E Virus Infection in Highly Endemic and Nonendemic Areas

Characteristic	Highly Endemic Areas	Nonendemic Areas
Human disease	Frequent; both sporadic and endemic cases	Infrequent sporadic cases
Reservoir	Primarily human; possibly environment	Suspected to be zoonotic (pigs, wild boars, and deer)
Primary routes of transmission	Fecal-oral; mainly through contaminated water	Ingestion of undercooked meat, possibly contact with animals
Characteristics of diseased persons	Young, healthy persons	Mostly elderly, with coexisting illnesses
Disease in pregnant women	High frequency of severe disease	Not reported
Prevalent genotypes[a]	1, 2, (4)	3, (4)
Chronic Infection	Not reported	May occur in immunosuppressed persons

[a]Numbers in parentheses indicate low frequency.

Adapted from Aggarwal R, Jameel S. Hepatitis E. *Hepatology*. 2011;54:2218–2226.

TABLE 3.3 ■ Hepatitis E Virus: Genotypes, Geographical Distribution, and Viral and Disease Characteristics

Genotype	Reservoir	Animal-to-Human Transmission	Waterborne Transmission	Geographic Distribution	Severity	Chronicity	Relation to Pregnancy	Epidemics
1	Human	No	Yes	South Asia, Central Asia, China, sub-Saharan Africa	Yes	No	Causes severe disease	Yes
2	Human	No	Yes	Mexico, Nigeria	Yes	No	NK	Yes
3	Swine	Yes	NK	Industrialized countries, United States, Europe, Japan	No	Yes	NK	No
4	Swine	Yes	Yes	Taiwan, Japan, China	No	NK	NK	No

NK, Not known.

Adapted from Shalimar S. Hepatitis E and acute liver failure in pregnancy. *J Clin Exp Hepatol*. 2013;3:213–224.

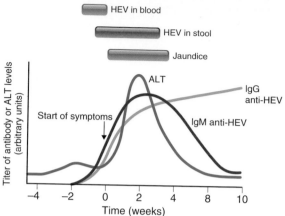

Fig. 3.6 Events during hepatitis E virus (HEV) infection. The course of a typical HEV infection is shown presymptoms and postsymptoms that include jaundice and liver damage (measured as ALT rise). The duration of viremia (HEV in blood), virus shedding (HEV in stool), and anti-HEV responses are shown. (Adapted from Aggarwal R, Jameel S. Hepatitis E. *Hepatology.* 2011;54:2218–2226.)

2. The serologic response is an initial IgM antibody to HEV (anti-HEV), followed by an IgG anti-HEV response. IgM anti-HEV titers wane in 4 to 6 months, although IgG anti-HEV persists for longer periods; the long-term protective efficacy of IgG anti-HEV seropositivity is unclear (Fig. 3.6).
3. Clinical syndromes caused by HEV are similar to those for other viral hepatitides, beginning with nonspecific constitutional and gastrointestinal symptoms:
   - Malaise, anorexia, nausea, and vomiting
   - Flulike symptoms including pharyngitis, cough, coryza, photophobia, headache, and myalgias
   - Loss of desire for alcohol or cigarette smoking
   - The onset of symptoms tends to be abrupt.
4. Fever, although uncommon, can occur. Prodromal symptoms abate or disappear with the onset of jaundice, although anorexia, malaise, and weakness may persist.
5. Jaundice is heralded by the appearance of dark urine and lightening of stool color; pruritus (usually mild and transient) may also occur. Physical examination reveals mild hepatomegaly with tenderness.
6. Mild splenomegaly and posterior cervical lymphadenopathy are noted in 15% to 20% of patients.
7. Extrahepatic manifestations may occur as for HAV infection (see earlier).

Acute Liver Failure (see Chapter 2)

1. **A high frequency, approaching 10% to 20%, is seen in pregnant women with HEV infection, particularly during the third trimester; high rates of maternal and fetal mortality result** (see upcoming discussion in chapter).
2. HEV may precipitate hepatic decompensation in patients with preexisting chronic liver disease.

HEPATITIS E AND PREGNANCY

1. HEV infection during pregnancy places mother and fetus at high risk of mortality and morbidity, including abortion, fetal demise, preterm labor, and maternal or neonatal death. Complications tend to occur during the second and third trimesters.

2. Maternal mortality is due to virus-induced acute liver failure.
3. Fetuses infected with HEV can develop icteric hepatitis, anicteric hepatitis, hyperbilirubinemia, prematurity, hypothermia, and hyperglycemia, with mortality rates approaching 50%.
4. The transmission rate from mother to fetus ranges from 33% to 100%.
5. Breastfeeding is considered safe in asymptomatic patients. However, if the mother has acute hepatitis E with a high viral load, substitution with formula is recommended due to the potential for transmission to the baby from infected breast milk or lesions on the mother's nipple.

CHRONIC HEPATITIS E

1. Recognized in HEV-infected immunosuppressed patients such as solid organ transplant recipients, patients with hematologic diseases, persons infected with human immunodeficiency virus, chemotherapy recipients, and patients on immunosuppressive treatment for rheumatologic disorders
2. Chronic HEV infection does not occur with genotypes 1 and 2, but mostly with genotype 3.
3. Pharmacologic drug effects on HEV replication are an area of ongoing investigation. Drugs that are known to cause inhibition of HEV replication include ribavirin and pegylated interferon alpha (both in vitro and in vivo), sofosbuvir, and mycophenolic acid (only in vitro, unknown in vivo). Drugs that are known to cause stimulation of HEV replication include mTOR (mechanistic target of rapamycin) inhibitors such as everolimus, rapamycin (both in vitro and in vivo), and calcineurin inhibitors such as cyclosporine and tacrolimus (only in vitro, unknown in vivo).

CHRONIC HEPATITIS E

1. Persistent increases in ALT and AST levels
2. Persistent evidence of HEV RNA in the serum and/or stool for at least 6 months

HISTOLOGY

Liver biopsy is rarely performed in acute self-limited viral hepatitis.

Self-Limited Disease
1. Major hepatocyte injury
   - Focal hepatocyte necrosis
   - Loss of hepatocytes (cell dropout)
   - Ballooning degeneration
   - Apoptosis with Councilman-like bodies (mummified, hyalinized, necrotic hepatocytes, extruded into a hepatic sinusoid)
2. Endophlebitis affecting the central vein
3. Diffuse mononuclear cell (CD8+ and natural killer cell) infiltrate
   - Within expanded portal tracts
   - Segmental erosion of the limiting plate
   - Within hepatic parenchyma
   - Kupffer cells enlarged and hyperplastic and containing lipofuscin pigment and debris; remnants of injured hepatocytes are seen.

Chronic Hepatitis E
1. Portal hepatitis with dense lymphocyte infiltration
2. Piecemeal necrosis (interface hepatitis)
3. Fibrosis with the possibility of progression to cirrhosis

DIAGNOSIS

For serologic diagnosis, see Table 3.1 and Fig. 3.6.

- Reference laboratories now offer serologic testing for HEV.
- IgM anti-HEV and IgG anti-HEV are detected early in infection.
- IgA anti-HEV may be useful for the diagnosis of acute HEV infection in patients who test negative for IgM anti-HEV.
- IgM anti-HEV may persist for at least 6 weeks after the peak of illness.
- IgG anti-HEV may remain detectable for as long as 20 months in self-limited infection.
- The presence of HEV RNA in stool or serum is confirmatory, but usually unnecessary unless chronic HEV is suspected during follow-up. Because IgM anti-HEV lacks specificity, HEV RNA may be useful to confirm acute HEV infection.
- A rapid HEV test can give results within 1 hour. Two rapid assays show a sensitivity of 93% to 96%, respectively, with a specificity of 100% for both. These tests can be useful in the clinic setting, particularly for patients with chronic liver disease or pregnant patients in whom quick testing is necessary to determine the need for urgent antiviral treatment.

TREATMENT
Self-Limited Disease

1. **Supportive care in the outpatient setting is usually sufficient,** unless persistent vomiting or severe anorexia leads to dehydration and the need for inpatient admission.
2. Maintenance of adequate caloric and fluid intake
   - No specific dietary recommendations
   - Encourage a large breakfast, which is often the best tolerated meal in patients with acute hepatitis.
   - Prohibit the use of alcohol during the acute phase.
3. Vigorous or prolonged physical activity should be avoided.
4. Limitation of daily activities and the need for rest periods are determined by the severity of the patient's fatigue and malaise.
5. All nonessential drugs should be discontinued.

Acute Liver Failure (see Chapter 2)

1. HEV-induced acute liver failure is uncommon except in pregnant women or patients with established cirrhosis. The incidence of acute liver failure is as high as 15% to 25%, with the highest mortality rate in pregnant women during the third trimester.
2. **Ribavirin (for at least 3 months) is the drug of choice for patients with or at high risk of acute liver failure.** There is a synergistic effect in vitro between ribavirin and pegylated interferon alpha. A significant side effect of ribavirin is severe anemia, whereas interferon can induce flulike symptoms, neuropsychiatric side effects, and acute rejection of solid organ allografts. **Both ribavirin and pegylated interferon are contraindicated in pregnant women due to teratogenicity.**
   - As of 2017, there is no approved treatment for acute hepatitis E, but ribavirin may provide benefit for patients with a poor prognosis or a high risk of acute liver failure, such as those with underlying chronic liver disease.
   - In chronic HEV infection, initial management includes a reduction of immunosuppressive medication, if possible; otherwise, ribavirin monotherapy or pegylated interferon alpha monotherapy for at least 3 months may be used. If the patient experiences breakthrough, relapse, or reinfection, the patient can be retreated for a longer duration.
   - Other potential HEV antiviral drugs include molecules that function as inhibitors of HEV

entry, RNA-dependent RNA polymerase inhibitors, methyltransferase inhibitors, which are involved in the capping of the viral RNA genome for infectivity, helicase inhibitors, which are involved in RNA unwinding during replication, and other molecules that target other viral proteins or host factors. These antivirals are under investigation.

PREVENTION

1. General measures to protect against exposure to enteric HEV infection include heating foods to 85° C, the use of household bleach for disinfection, handwashing, avoidance of uncooked or undercooked food, proper disposal of human waste, and ensuring safe sources of water.
2. IgG anti-HEV may be protective, but the efficacy of immune globulin containing anti-HEV is uncertain.
   - Two vaccines with proven efficacy have been developed and have undergone phase 3 clinical trial in China (HEV 239 vaccine) and Nepal (baculovirus-expressed 56-kD vaccine). The HEV 239 vaccine was licensed in China in 2012. It is based on a recombinant HEV genotype 1 antigen and has shown an efficacy rate of 94% to 100% in preventing acute symptomatic hepatitis E. The protection lasts up to 4.5 years. The vaccine is not globally licensed. Vaccines might be useful for travelers from developed countries to regions with high prevalence of hepatitis E and might be considered for high-risk persons, such as pregnant women, patients with chronic liver diseases, or immunosuppressed patients.
   - DNA vaccines are under investigation. Vaccination leads to synthesis of immunizing protein within host cells, which mimics natural infection and eventually leads to the induction of humoral and cellular responses.
   - Development of high-titer hyperimmune globulin is another possibility.
3. Transfusing an immunocompromised patient with blood products that have not been screened for HEV is associated with a risk of chronic HEV infection. Systemic screening of blood products for HEV should be considered in countries in which HEV is endemic.

FURTHER READING

Aggarwal R, Jameel S, Hepatitis E. *Hepatology*. 2011;54:2218–2226.

Blasco-Perrin H, Abravanel F, Blasco-Baque V, et al. Hepatitis E, the neglected one. *Liver Int*. 2016;36:130–134.

Chionne P, Madonna E, Pisani G, et al. Evaluation of rapid tests for diagnosis of acute hepatitis E. *J Clin Virol*. 2016;78:4–8.

Debing Y, Neyts J. Antivirals strategies for hepatitis E virus. *Antiviral Res*. 2014;102:106–118.

FitzSimons D, Hendrickx G, Vorsters A, Van Damme P. Hepatitis A and E: update on prevention and epidemiology. *Vaccine*. 2010;28:583–588.

Kamar N, Garrouste C, Haagsma E, et al. Factors associated with chronic hepatitis in patients with hepatitis E virus infection who have received solid organ transplants. *Gastroenterology*. 2011;140:1481–1489.

Kamar N, Izopet J, Tripon S, et al. Ribavirin for chronic hepatitis E virus infection in transplant recipients. *N Engl J Med*. 2014;370:1111–1120.

Kanda T, Nakamoto S, Wu S, et al. Direct-acting antivirals and host targeting agents against the hepatitis A virus. *J Clin Transl Hepatol*. 2015;3:205–210.

Lee GY, Poovorawan K, Intharasongkroh, et al. Hepatitis E virus infection: epidemiology and treatment implications. *World J Virol*. 2015;4:343–355.

Liu X, Chen H, Liao Z, et al. Comparison of immunogenicity between inactivated and live attenuated hepatitis A vaccines among young adults. A 3-year follow-up study. *J Infect Dis*. 2015;212:1232–1236.

Shalimar S. Hepatitis E and acute liver failure in pregnancy. *J Clin Exp Hepatol*. 2013;3:213–224.

Vaughan G, Rossi L, Forbi J, et al. Hepatitis A virus: host interactions, molecular epidemiology and evolution. *Infect Genet Evol*. 2014;21:227–243.

Victor JC, Monto AS, Surdina TY, et al. Hepatitis A vaccine versus immune globulin for post-exposure prophylaxis. *N Engl J Med.* 2007;357:1685–1694.

Zhang J, Zhang X, Huang S, et al. Long-term efficacy of a hepatitis E vaccine. *N Engl J Med.* 2015;372:914–922.

Zhu F, Zhang J, Zhang X, et al. Efficacy and safety of a recombinant hepatitis E vaccine in healthy adults: a large-scale, randomized, double-blind placebo-controlled, phase 3 trial. *Lancet.* 2010;376:895–902.

CHAPTER 4

Hepatitis B and Hepatitis D

Tram T. Tran, MD

KEY POINTS

1 Hepatitis B virus (HBV) infection is a major cause of acute liver failure, cirrhosis, and hepatocellular carcinoma (HCC).

2 HBV infection can be prevented by hepatitis B vaccination.

3 Acute HBV infection is most likely to resolve spontaneously in immunocompetent adults, especially if symptomatic. Progression to chronic infection is typical in children, the elderly, and immunocompromised persons, including hemodialysis patients.

4 HCC related to HBV infection can occur in a noncirrhotic liver.

5 Serum HBV DNA levels correlate with the risk of cirrhosis and HCC.

6 Indications for antiviral therapy are persistent viral replication with elevated serum aminotransferase levels.

7 Special populations such as pregnant patients with HBV infection and patients who are about to undergo immunosuppressive therapy should be considered for antiviral therapy even in the absence of standard indications.

8 Current first-line therapies for hepatitis B are entecavir, tenofovir, and pegylated interferon.

9 Long-term suppression of HBV with oral therapies has led to a reduction in the need for HBV-infected patients to undergo liver transplantation for decompensated cirrhosis. Regression of fibrosis and cirrhosis has been confirmed by serial liver biopsies with long-term therapy for HBV infection. A reduced frequency of HCC has also been observed with antiviral therapy for HBV.

10 Infection with hepatitis D virus (HDV) should be suspected in HBV-infected persons with clinically severe disease and low or absent HBV replication.

Hepatitis B Virus

VIROLOGY

1. Human-infecting member, the Hepadnaviridae family of hepatotropic DNA-containing viruses
2. Eight genotypes (A–H): Genotype C appears to be implicated in more severe chronic disease
3. 42-nm spherical particle with the following components:
   - A 27-nm-diameter, electron-dense, nucleocapsid core
   - A 7-nm-thick outer lipoprotein envelope
4. HBV core containing circular, **partially double-stranded DNA** (3.2 kb long) and the following components:
   - **DNA polymerase** protein with reverse transcriptase activity
   - **Hepatitis B core antigen (HBcAg)**, a structural protein of the nucleocapsid, which does not circulate in serum

- **Hepatitis B e antigen (HBeAg)**, a nonstructural, secretory protein that correlates imperfectly with active HBV replication
- **Hepatitis B X protein**, a transcriptional activator, which is linked to hepatocarcinogenesis

5. HBV outer lipoprotein envelope, which contains the following components:
   - **Hepatitis B surface antigen (HBsAg)**, with 3 envelope proteins: Major, large, and middle proteins
   - Minor lipid and carbohydrate components
   - HBsAg present in 22-nm spherical or tubular noninfectious particles, in excess of intact HBV particles
6. Variants
   a. One major serotype; many subtypes based on HBsAg protein diversity
   b. HBV mutant viruses emerge spontaneously as a consequence of poor proofreading ability of reverse transcriptase or emergence of antiviral resistance during therapy:
      - HBeAg-negative precore or core promoter mutants
      - HBV vaccine-induced escape mutants (rare)
      - Nucleos(t)ide-induced resistant mutants
7. Replication occurs through reverse transcription of pregenomic RNA.
8. The liver is the major, but not only, site of HBV replication.
9. Replication in vitro is limited in primary adult and fetal human hepatocytes.

EPIDEMIOLOGY

1. Incubation period: 15 to 180 days (average, 60 to 90 days)
2. HBV viremia lasts for weeks to months after acute infection.
3. **Chronic infection with persistent viremia develops in 1% to 5% of adults, 90% of infected neonates, and 50% of infants.**
4. Chronic infection is linked to chronic hepatitis, cirrhosis, HCC, and premature mortality.
5. Chronic infection can cause extrahepatic diseases: Vasculitis, lymphoma, membranous glomerulonephritis.
6. **Worldwide distribution: HBV carrier prevalence is <1% in the United States and 5% to 15% in Asia and sub-Saharan Africa; the incidence has declined in areas where HBV vaccine use has expanded.**
7. HBV is present in blood, semen, cervicovaginal secretions, saliva, and other body fluids.
8. **The risk of HBV transmission correlates with the serum HBV DNA level and presence of HBeAg.**
9. Modes of transmission
   a. **Blood-borne**
      - Transfusion of blood and blood products
      - Injection drug use
      - Hemodialysis
      - Exposure to blood in health care and other workers
   b. **Sexual**: Responsible for 50% of acute cases in the United States
   c. **Tissue penetration (percutaneous) or permucosal transfer**
      - Needlestick accidents
      - Muscosal exposure to body fluids
      - Reuse of contaminated medical equipment
      - Shared razor blades
      - Tattoos

- Acupuncture, body piercing
- Shared toothbrushes

d. **Maternal-neonatal and maternal-infant**
  - Perinatal transmission is associated with maternal serum HBV DNA levels >1,000,000 copies/mL (200,000 IU/mL).
  - Highest risk with maternal serum HBV DNA >10^8 copies/mL (2×10^7 IU/mL)

e. No evidence for fecal-oral spread

f. No identifiable risk factor in 25% of cases

ACUTE HEPATITIS B

Pathogenesis

1. Cell-mediated immune mechanisms are largely responsible for hepatocyte injury, including hepatocyte degeneration and apoptosis.
   - CD8+ and CD4+ T cell responses
   - Production of cytokines in the liver and systemically
2. Direct viral cytopathic effect
   - Postulated in immunosuppressed patients with exceedingly high levels of viral replication (evidence is indirect)

Clinical Features

1. **Disease severity ranges from asymptomatic (subclinical) hepatitis, to clinical acute symptomatic hepatitis, to acute liver failure** (Fig. 4.1); severity is increased in those with preexisting liver disease or age ≥40 years.
2. The initial clinical syndrome is similar to that for a general viral infection, with nonspecific constitutional and gastrointestinal symptoms.
   - Malaise, anorexia, nausea, and vomiting
   - Flulike symptoms, including pharyngitis, cough, coryza, photophobia, headache, and myalgias
3. The onset of symptoms is usually insidious.
4. Fever is uncommon.
5. A syndrome that is immune complex mediated and resembles serum sickness occurs in <10% of patients with HBV infection; it includes polyarthritis, polyarthralgias, angioedema,

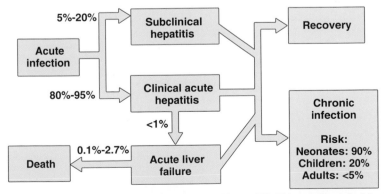

Fig. 4.1 Outcomes of acute hepatitis B. (Adapted from Hyams KC. Risks of chronicity following acute hepatitis B virus infection: a review. *Clin Infect Dis* 1995;20:992–1000; Liang TJ. Hepatitis B: the virus and disease. *Hepatology.* 2009;49:S13–S21.)

urticaria, maculopapular eruptions, purpura, petechiae, and, more rarely, hematuria and proteinuria or cutaneous or systemic vasculitis.

6. Prodromal symptoms abate or disappear with the onset of jaundice, although anorexia, malaise, and weakness may persist.
7. Jaundice (the icteric phase) is heralded by the appearance of dark urine and lightening of stool color; pruritus (usually mild and transient) may occur as jaundice increases.
8. The icteric phase lasts 1 to 3 weeks and is followed by a convalescent phase that may last for months and in which jaundice and symptoms abate and HBsAg, HBeAg, and HBV DNA disappear from serum.
9. Physical examination reveals mild enlargement and slight tenderness of the liver.
10. Mild splenomegaly and posterior cervical lymphadenopathy are noted in 15% to 20% of patients.

Laboratory Features

1. Most prominent biochemical feature: Marked elevation of serum alanine (ALT) and aspartate (AST) aminotransferase levels
2. Peak aminotransferase levels vary from 500 to 5000 U/L; ALT levels are generally higher than AST levels.
3. The serum bilirubin level is uncommonly higher than 10 mg/dL, except in severe disease, acute liver failure, and cholestatic hepatitis.
4. The serum alkaline phosphatase level is normal or mildly elevated.
5. The prothrombin time is normal or increased by 1 to 3 seconds.
6. The serum albumin level is normal or minimally depressed.
7. Peripheral blood counts: Normal or mild leukopenia with or without relative lymphocytosis
8. Serologic diagnosis is based on detection of HBsAg and immunoglobulin (Ig)M antibody to HBcAg (anti-HBc) in serum (Table 4.1).

Acute HBV Infection and Liver Failure

1. Acute liver failure is characterized by a striking coagulopathy with a prolonged prothrombin time (INR ≥1.5) (see Chapter 2).
2. Leukocytosis, hyponatremia, and hypokalemia are common.
3. Hypoglycemia
4. Marked elevations of serum bilirubin and aminotransferase levels, but the latter may decline toward normal despite disease progression.
5. Mild to moderate hypoalbuminemia

TABLE 4.1 ■ **Interpretation of HBV Serologic Markers**

HBsAg	IgG anti-HBc	IgM anti-HBc	Anti-HBs	Interpretation
−	−	−	−	Never infected and absence of immunity
+	+	−	−	Chronic infection
+	+	+	−	Acute infection or disease flare in chronic carrier
−	+	−	+	Recovered from past infection with immunity
−	−	−	+	Immunity from vaccination

Anti-HBc, Antibody to hepatitis B core antigen; *anti-HBs,* hepatitis B surface antibody; *HBsAg,* hepatitis B surface antigen; *HBV,* hepatitis B virus; *IgG,* immunoglobulin G; *IgM,* immunoglobulin M.

Treatment

1. **Outpatient observation is appropriate unless vomiting or severe anorexia persists and leads to dehydration, or features of acute liver failure develop.**
2. Caloric and fluid intake should be maintained.
   - No specific dietary recommendations
   - Prohibition of alcohol during the acute phase
3. Vigorous or prolonged physical activity should be avoided.
4. Daily activities should be limited, with rest periods determined by the severity of fatigue and malaise.
5. All nonessential medications should be discontinued.
6. Antiviral therapy
   - Not necessary because >95% of immunocompetent adults will recover spontaneously
   - Treatment with antiviral therapy has not shown to result in improvement in liver biochemical test levels or the rate of HBsAg loss.
   - If a patient has acute liver failure caused by HBV infection and may need liver transplantation, antiviral treatment is generally initiated and may reduce the likelihood of recurrent HBV infection posttransplantation.
   - Antiviral treatment should be considered in protracted cases of severe acute HBV infection (profound jaundice and a markedly prolonged prothrombin time); first-line treatment choices are entecavir and tenofovir (see discussion later in the chapter).

CHRONIC HEPATITIS B

Pathogenesis and Pathology

1. Most liver injury from HBV is caused by the host immune response with a cell-mediated response directed against HBcAg.
2. Cytotoxic T lymphocytes (CTLs) are the effector cells that mediate cell damage.
3. Non–antigen-specific immune responses, such as those mediated by inflammatory cytokines (tumor necrosis factor alpha, gamma interferon), may be more important for viral clearance than CTL-mediated mechanisms.
4. A hyperactive host response may lead to fulminant hepatitis, whereas a reduced host response increases the risk of chronic infection.
5. In patients who fail to clear virus, both the numbers of CD4+ and CD8+ T cells are markedly reduced.
6. Nonspecific histologic findings include a predominantly lymphocytic infiltrate, which may or may not be confined to the portal tracts.
7. Characteristic histologic findings of chronic hepatitis B include ground-glass hepatocytes in which the cytoplasm is stained pink with hematoxylin-eosin in response to massive production of HBsAg; HBcAg can be demonstrated in the hepatocyte nuclei, within the cytoplasm, and on the cell membrane.
8. Numerous systems are available for assessing the grade (severity of necroinflammation) and stage (severity of fibrosis); fibrosis stage is the most relevant histologic prognostic factor.

Clinical Features

1. Symptoms of chronic HBV range from none, to nonspecific complaints (fatigue, right upper quadrant pain), to complications of cirrhosis.
2. Extrahepatic manifestations occur in up to 20% of patients with chronic HBV infection and include arthralgias, polyarteritis nodosa, glomerulonephritis, mixed essential cryoglobulinemia, and other rare syndromes.

3. **The risk of chronicity depends on the age and immune function when a person is initially infected**, as follows:
   - **90% of infants** infected during the first year of life
   - **30% to 50% of children** infected between 1 and 4 years of age
   - **Approximately 5% of healthy adults**
   - **>50% of immunocompromised adults**
4. Approximately 25% of adults who become chronically infected during childhood will die of HBV-related cirrhosis or liver cancer.
5. **The four phases of serologic, virologic, and biochemical natural history of chronic HBV infection** are summarized in Fig. 4.2.
   - Progression from one stage to another and back (reversion) can occur.
6. The prevalence of HBeAg in persons with chronic hepatitis B declines with age, with spontaneous loss of HBeAg in 7% to 20% of patients per year.
7. Spontaneous loss of HBsAg in serum occurs infrequently (0.5% to 1% per year), with antibody to HBsAg (anti-HBs) developing in most persons who lose HBsAg.
8. The natural history and clinical outcomes of chronic hepatitis B are outlined in Fig. 4.3.
9. Factors associated with progression of chronic hepatitis B include older age (longer duration of infection), HBV genotype C, alcohol abuse, high serum levels of HBV DNA, concurrent infection with other viruses (human immunodeficiency virus [HIV], hepatitis C virus, HDV), environmental factors (smoking, aflatoxin), obesity, and diabetes mellitus.

Diagnosis
1. **The diagnosis of HBV infection relies initially on detection of HBsAg.**
2. When HBsAg is detectable, further laboratory testing to assess disease status and need for treatment is indicated (Fig. 4.4; see Fig. 4.2 and Table 4.1):
   - **Quantitative HBV DNA** by a sensitive assay
   - **Serum ALT level:** The ALT level should be measured every 3 to 6 months if the ALT is persistently normal and more often if it is elevated.

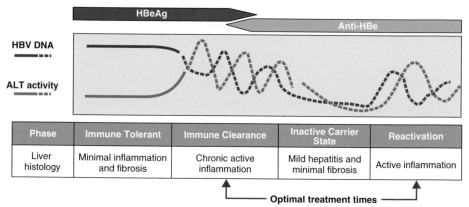

Phases of Chronic HBV Infection

Phase	Immune Tolerant	Immune Clearance	Inactive Carrier State	Reactivation
Liver histology	Minimal inflammation and fibrosis	Chronic active inflammation	Mild hepatitis and minimal fibrosis	Active inflammation

Optimal treatment times

Fig. 4.2 Phases of chronic hepatitis B virus (HBV) infection. *ALT*, Alanine aminotransferase; *anti-HBe*, antibody to hepatitis B e antigen; *HBeAg*, hepatitis B e antigen.

- **HBeAg and anti-HBe:** Define the type of chronic hepatitis B (i.e., HBeAg positive or HBeAg negative) and the end point of therapy (i.e., loss of HBeAg in HBeAg-positive patients).
- **Tests of liver disease severity:** Total bilirubin, serum albumin, and prothrombin time; international normalized ratio (INR); and platelet count (see Chapter 1)
- **Liver biopsy:** Optional in HBV infection but can determine the **histologic grade of inflammation and stage of fibrosis** and identify coexisting liver diseases such as steatohepatitis, iron overload, or autoimmune hepatitis. Ultrasound elastography or other noninvasive methods of staging fibrosis may be used in lieu of liver biopsy to aid in decisions about treatment. Liver biopsy may still be needed to determine the grade of inflammation (see Chapter 1).

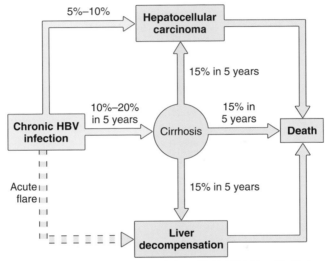

Fig. 4.3 Natural history of chronic hepatitis B. *HBV*, Hepatitis B virus.

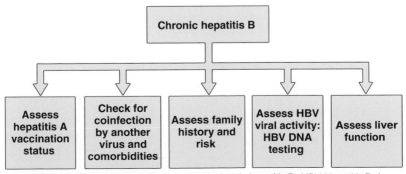

Fig. 4.4 Initial evaluation of the patient with chronic hepatitis B. *HBV*, Hepatitis B virus.

Treatment

1. Goals
   - Prevention of long-term complications (cirrhosis, HCC) and mortality by durable suppression of serum HBV DNA
   - **Primary treatment end point: Sustained decrease in serum HBV DNA to low or undetectable levels (<10 to 15 IU/mL)**
   - Secondary treatment end points: Decreased or normalized serum ALT level, improved liver histology, HBeAg loss with or without seroconversion to anti-HBe, HBsAg loss or seroconversion to anti-HBs and prevention of secondary spread of infection
2. Treatment criteria for chronic hepatitis B (Table 4.2)
   - Clinical and laboratory parameters do not show a consistent correlation with liver histology; management guidelines recommend liver biopsy in select patients based on age, serum HBV DNA levels, and HBeAg status.
3. Indications for HBV treatment (Table 4.3)
4. Therapeutic agents for treatment of chronic HBV (Table 4.4)
   - Oral agents: **First-line therapies are entecavir and tenofovir.**
     - Nucleos(t)ide analogs: Despite their high antiviral potency (greater than that of interferon), these drugs are not able to eradicate HBV from the liver, but they can maintain sustained suppression of replication.
     - Advantages: Potent; negligible adverse effects; oral administration; safe and effective for all age groups; suitable for cirrhotic and HIV-coinfected patients

TABLE 4.2 ■ Treatment Criteria for Chronic Hepatitis B

	HBeAg+		HBeAg−	
Guideline	HBV DNA IU/mL	ALT U/L	HBV DNA IU/mL	ALT U/L
NIH Consensus Conference 2009	>20,000	>2× ULN or + biopsy[a]	≥20,000	≥2× ULN or + biopsy
EASL 2012	>2,000	>ULN	>2,000	>ULN
United States Algorithm 2015	≥20,000	>ULN or + biopsy	≥2,000	>ULN or + biopsy
APASL 2012	≥20,000	>2× ULN	≥2,000	>2× ULN
AASLD 2009	>20,000	>2x ULN or + biopsy	>2,000	≥2× ULN or + biopsy

[a]Biopsy specimen indicates active hepatocellular inflammation.
AASLD, American Association for the Study of the Liver; *ALT*, alanine aminotransferase; *APASL*, Asian Pacific Association for the Study of the Liver; *EASL*, European Association for the Study of the Liver; *HBeAg,* hepatitis B e antigen; *HBV*, hepatitis B virus; *NIH*, National Institutes of Health, *ULN*, upper limit of normal.

TABLE 4.3 ■ Conditions in Which HBV Treatment Is and Is Not Indicated

Indicated	Not indicated
Chronic hepatitis B with elevated ALT levels and HBV DNA >2000 UI/mL	Acute hepatitis B
HBV DNA–positive cirrhotic patients	Immune tolerance phase
Decompensated cirrhotic patients	Inactive chronic carrier
Acute liver failure	
HBsAg-positive patient who is going to be immunosuppressed	

ALT, Alanine aminotransferase; *HBsAg*, hepatitis B surface antigen; *HBV*, hepatitis B virus.

- – Disadvantages: Lower rates of HBeAg and HBsAg seroconversion than with interferon; prolonged treatment required, which may lead to an increasing risk of antiviral drug resistance
- – **Entecavir** (nucleoside analog): Potent antiviral activity with a high genetic barrier to resistance and low rate of resistance; dose, 0.5 to 1 mg daily; adverse events include lactic acidosis (rare)
- – **Tenofovir** (nucleotide analog): Potent, with a high genetic barrier to resistance and low rate of resistance; less nephrotoxic than adefovir, another nucleotide analog; dose, 300 mg daily (tenofovir disoproxil fumarate) or 25 mg daily (tenofovir alafenamide); adverse events include Fanconi syndrome (rare) and decrease in bone density
  - ■ Parenteral agent: Pegylated interferon
    - – **Peginterferon alfa:** Consider in young, noncirrhotic patients with low HBV DNA levels, high serum ALT levels, and a favorable genotype (A > B > C > D). Treatment consists of 180 μg/week subcutaneously for 48 weeks.
    - – Advantages: Finite duration of treatment; absence of resistance; HBeAg seroconversion in up to 32% of HBeAg-positive patients at 48 weeks of treatment; clearance of HBsAg in 6% of patients
    - – Disadvantages: Many adverse effects; subcutaneous injections; frequent contraindications
  - ■ Avoid use of older agents—lamivudine, telbivudine, and adefovir— because of high resistance rates and/or low potency.
5. End points of therapy
   - ■ HBsAg seroconversion is the most desirable end point but it occurs at low rates.
   - ■ For HBeAg-positive patients: Treat until HBeAg seroconversion, and discontinue drug after consolidation period of 6 to 12 months after HBeAg seroconversion. Seroreversion is common, particularly in Asian patients.
   - ■ For HBeAg-negative patients: Treat indefinitely because relapse is common after cessation of therapy.
6. Resistance to antiviral drugs
   a. Diagnosis of resistance
      - ■ Viral rebound by at least 1.0 $\log_{10}$ compared with nadir; confirmed by repeat HBV DNA testing
      - ■ Exclusion of non–HBV-related causes of failure (i.e., poor adherence)

TABLE 4.4 ■ **FDA-Approved Therapies for HBV Infection**

Agent	Brand Name	Manufacturer	Year Approved
First-Line Therapy			
Entecavir	Baraclude	Bristol-Myers Squibb	2005
Tenofovir	Viread	Gilead Sciences	2008
Peginterferon alfa-2a	Pegasys	Roche Laboratories	2005
Second-Line Therapy			
Adefovir dipivoxil	Hepsera	Gilead Sciences	2002
Telbivudine	Tyzeka	Idenix and Novartis	2006
Third-Line Therapy			
Lamivudine	Epivir-HBV	GlaxoSmithKline	1998

FDA, Food and Drug Administration.

- Confirmation of genotypic resistance with HBV mutant detection, if available: HBV polymerase mutation(s) are associated with resistance.
- Confirmation of phenotypic resistance: Decreased in vitro susceptibility to an antiviral agent in patients adherent to therapy

b. The cumulative frequency of antiviral drug resistance is low (0% to 1%) for first-line oral therapies.

c. Monitoring for drug resistance:
- Repeated serum ALT and HBV DNA measurements
- Use of a sensitive HBV DNA assay and the same assay over time
- Frequency of assessments based on disease severity: For mild liver disease, at least every 6 months; for advanced disease or cirrhosis, every 3 months

Hepatitis B in Special Populations

PREGNANCY (Fig. 4.5)

1. For women of childbearing age who are chronically infected with HBV and are not currently on therapy and wish to become pregnant:
   a. Assess the severity of liver disease: If there is no evidence of advanced maternal liver disease (cirrhosis or advanced fibrosis), therapy can be deferred until the third trimester to reduce the risk of mother-child transmission.
   b. If there is clinical evidence of maternal advanced liver disease, start therapy with an oral antiviral agent to maintain clinical stability and prevent a flare or decompensation.
      - Tenofovir is the preferred option (Food and Drug Administration [FDA] category B).
2. For women of childbearing age who are already on medication and become pregnant:
   - Continue therapy as indicated for maternal disease status.
3. For women of childbearing age with active viral replication, consider therapy (see discussion earlier in the chapter).
4. Breastfeeding is considered safe with a low risk of HBV transmission.

REACTIVATION

Severe clinical reactivation of HBV can occur with immunosuppression in patients with evidence of HBV infection (HBsAg positivity) or evidence of prior infection (anti-HBc positivity).

1. **All patients who require immunosuppression should be screened for HBV infection (HBsAg, IgG anti-HBc)** (Fig. 4.6).
2. If the patient is positive for HBsAg, oral antiviral therapy should be initiated before the start of immunosuppressive therapy and continued for at least 6 to 12 months after immunosuppressive therapy is completed. Entecavir or tenofovir are first-line options because of their potency and low risk of resistance.
3. If the patient is negative for HBsAg but positive for anti-HBc, reactivation may still occur in the setting of high-risk immunosuppression (e.g., with rituximab). Reactivation in persons who are positive for anti-HBc can still occur even if they are also positive for anti-HBs.

PREVENTION

The cornerstone of immunoprophylaxis is the preexposure administration of HBV vaccine.

1. **Preexposure immunoprophylaxis with HBV vaccine**
   a. Recombinant yeast-derived vaccines
      - Contain HBsAg as the immunogen

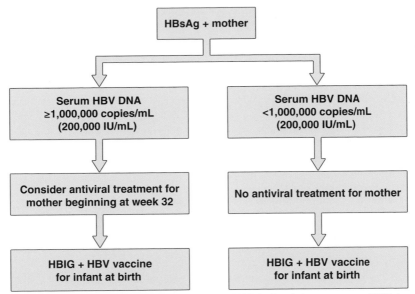

Fig. 4.5 Suggested management of hepatitis B virus (HBV) infection during pregnancy. *HBIG,* hepatitis B immune globulin; *HBsAg,* hepatitis B surface antigen.

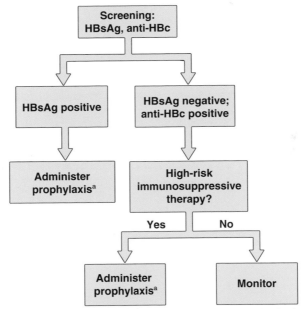

Fig. 4.6 Screening and prophylactic antiviral treatment for hepatitis B virus infection in patients undergoing chemotherapy or immunosuppressive therapy. Persons negative for hepatitis B viral markers do not require antiviral prophylactic treatment. [a]Options include lamivudine, telbivudine, and tenofovir. *Anti-HBc,* Antibody to hepatitis B core antigen; *HBsAg,* hepatitis B surface antigen.

- Highly immunogenic; induce protective levels of anti-HBs in >95% of healthy young (<40 years of age) recipients after all three doses
- It is 85% to 95% effective in preventing HBV infection or clinical hepatitis B.
- Principal side effects include the following:
  - Transient pain at the injection site in 10% to 25% of patients
  - Mild, short-lived fever in <3% of patients
- A booster dose of the vaccine may not be required even as long as 20 years after initial immunization (i.e., the vaccine may provide lifelong protection).
- A booster dose of the vaccine is indicated in immunocompromised persons if their anti-HBs titer is <10 mU/mL.
- HBV vaccination has no proven immunotherapeutic value in persons with established HBV infection.

  b. HBV vaccine doses and schedules
- Engerix-B (GlaxoSmithKline) is given by intramuscular (deltoid) injection in a dose of 20 μg of HBsAg protein for adults and 10 μg for infants and children through age 19 years, repeated 1 and 6 months later; for patients undergoing hemodialysis, a 40-μg dose (double dose of the 20-μg preparation) is given at 0, 1, 2, and 6 months.
- Recombivax HB (Merck) is given by intramuscular (deltoid) injection in a dose of 10 μg of HBsAg protein for adults and 5-μg doses for children up to age 19 years, repeated 1 and 6 months later; children between ages 11 and 15 years may receive 10 μg of Recombivax HB initially with a single booster at 4 to 6 months; for patients undergoing hemodialysis, a 40-μg 3-dose schedule is available.

  c. Indications
- Universal infant immunization is recommended shortly after birth.
- Catch-up vaccination of adolescents through 19 years of age (if not previously vaccinated) is recommended.
- Targeted high-risk groups:
  - Household and spouse contacts of HBV carriers
  - Native Alaskans, Pacific Islanders, and Native Americans
  - Health care workers and others exposed to blood (including first responders)
  - People who inject drugs
  - Men (including adolescents) who have sex with men, including bisexuals
  - Persons with multiple sexual partners
  - Workers in institutions for the developmentally disadvantaged
  - Recipients of high-risk blood products
  - Maintenance hemodialysis patients and staff
  - Incarcerated persons (in whom injection drug use and homosexual behavior may occur)
  - Household contacts of adoptees from endemic regions
  - Persons with preexisting liver disease (e.g., chronic hepatitis C)

2. **Postexposure immunoprophylaxis with HBV vaccine and hepatitis B immune globulin (HBIG),** a preparation of immune globulin containing high titers of anti-HBs

   a. Indications
- Susceptible sexual contacts of acutely HBV-infected persons
  - HBIG 0.04 to 0.07 mL/kg as early as possible after exposure
  - First of three HBV vaccine doses given at another site (deltoid) simultaneously or within a few days
  - Second and third vaccine doses given 1 and 6 months later
- Neonates of HBsAg-positive mothers identified during pregnancy
  - HBIG in a dose of 0.5 mL given within 12 hours of birth into the anterolateral muscle of the thigh

    – HBV vaccine in a dose of 5 to 10 μg given within 12 hours of birth (at another site in the anterolateral muscle), repeated at 1 and 6 months
    – Protective efficacy >95%

b. Prevention of maternal-child transmission

    ■ A high level of maternal viremia (1,000,000 copies/mL or >200,000 IU/mL) is associated with an increased risk of perinatal transmission (8% to 10%) even with appropriate vaccination of the infant.

    ■ See Fig. 4.5 for the suggested management strategy for women with HBV in pregnancy.

    ■ Infants born to mothers infected with HBV should receive standard vaccination and HBIG within 12 hours of birth (see previous discussion).

    ■ If antiviral therapy is initiated to reduce maternal-child transmission, it can be discontinued after birth, with monitoring of the mother for a subsequent flare; monitoring (serum ALT and HBV DNA) at least every 1 to 3 months for 6 months postpartum is suggested.

    ■ All women with HBV infection should be monitored for a flare throughout and after pregnancy because of the immunologic changes during pregnancy that may precipitate a flare.

Hepatitis D Virus

VIROLOGY

A defective RNA satellite virus (viroidlike) that requires the helper function of HBV for its expression and pathogenicity but not for its replication

1. Only 1 serotype recognized; 8 genotypes

2. 35-nm to 37-nm spherical particle, enveloped by the HBV lipoprotein coat (HBsAg)

3. 19-nm corelike structure containing an antigenic nuclear phosphoprotein (HDV antigen)
    ■ Binds RNA
    ■ Exists in two isoforms: Smaller 195 amino acid proteins and larger 214 amino acid proteins
    ■ Smaller HDV antigen transports RNA into the nucleus: Essential for HDV replication
    ■ Larger HDV antigen is prenylated: Inhibits HDV RNA replication and participates in HDV assembly

4. HDV RNA is 1.7 kb, single stranded, covalently closed, and circular.
    ■ HDV antigenome, a genome complement, and circular RNA are found in infected hepatocytes and, to a much lesser extent, in purified HDV particles.
    ■ HDV RNA is the smallest RNA genome among the animal viruses; HDV resembles plant satellite viruses.
    ■ The RNA genome can form an unbranched, rodlike structure by folding on itself through intramolecular base pairing.
    ■ Replication is limited to hepatocytes.

5. Primary chimpanzee, woodchuck, and human HCC cell lines have been transfected with HDV cDNA constructs expressing HDV RNA and HDV antigens.

PATHOGENESIS AND PATHOLOGY

1. HDV appears to be directly cytopathic; immune-mediated cell injury also occurs.

2. Necroinflammatory activity is often severe, but histologic features are not specific for chronic HDV infection.

3. HDV antigen (HDVAg) is readily demonstrated in nuclei and to a lesser extent in the cytoplasm of infected hepatocytes.

CLINICAL FEATURES AND NATURAL HISTORY

1. Incubation period: Estimated to be 4 to 7 weeks
2. Endemic in Mediterranean basin, Balkan peninsula, Central Europe, parts of Africa, Middle East, and Amazon basin
3. The incidence has declined with increasing use of the HBV vaccine.
4. HDV infection occurs in 2% to 5% of patients with chronic hepatitis B in the United States.
5. HDV viremia may be short lived (acute infection) or prolonged (chronic infection).
6. **HDV infections occur solely in persons at risk for HBV infection (coinfection or super-infection).**
7. Modes of transmission
   a. Blood-borne
      - Injection drug use is the predominant mode of spread in the United States.
      - Recipients of high-risk blood products
   b. Sexual
      - Men who have sex with men
      - Heterosexual transmission is inefficient.
   c. Maternal-neonatal, but frequency uncertain
8. Symptoms of HDV infection are nonspecific.
9. HDV infection should be suspected in the following settings:
   - Fulminant HBV infection
   - Acute HBV infection with initial improvement but subsequently relapse
   - Progressive chronic HBV infection in the absence of active HBV replication
10. **Coinfection** with HDV and HBV
    - Acute illness is generally more severe than in HBV monoinfection.
    - The risk of acute liver failure is increased.
    - The rate of chronicity is similar to that for acute HBV infection alone (<5%).
11. **Superinfection** with HDV in a patient with chronic HBV infection accelerates the natural history of chronic hepatitis B.
12. An association exists between HDV and the risk of HCC (mechanisms unknown).

SEROLOGIC AND VIROLOGIC TESTS

1. Both an enzyme immunoassay (EIA) and a radioimmunoassay (RIA) are available for the detection of total and IgM antibody to HDV (anti-HDV).
2. Persistence of IgM anti-HDV or an IgG anti-HDV titer >1:1000 correlates with the presence of ongoing viral replication.
3. An assay for HDV RNA is available only on a research basis, but it has utility in distinguishing ongoing from prior infection.
4. Coinfection and superinfection are distinguished by the presence or absence of IgM anti-HBc in serum.
5. Detection of HDVAg by immunohistochemical analysis of liver tissue is considered the gold standard for the diagnosis of persistent HDV infection; however, HDVAg staining is available only in research laboratories.

PREVENTION

1. Neither specific high-titer anti-HDV–containing immune globulin nor HDV vaccine is available.
2. HDV immunoprophylaxis depends on the prevention of HBV by use of HBV vaccine.

TREATMENT

1. Drugs
   - High-dose interferon alpha (9 MU three times a week) and peginterferon alfa, given for 1 year, have shown some efficacy in the treatment of chronic hepatitis D.
   - The efficacy of interferon alpha therapy should be assessed at 24 weeks by measuring HDV RNA levels.
   - More than 1 year of therapy may be necessary but is of unproven efficacy.
   - Some patients become HDV RNA negative and even HBsAg negative in serum, with accompanying improvement in histologic features.
   - Nucleos(t)ide analogs do not appear to affect HDV replication and related disease.
2. Liver transplantation (see Chapter 33)
   - Patients with chronic HDV infection are at lower risk for HBV recurrence than are those with chronic HBV infection alone.
   - HDV recurrence can be detected before signs of HBV reactivation.
   - Decreased recurrence rates and improved survival in patients with HDV cirrhosis compared with HBV cirrhosis may result from the inhibitory effects of HDV on HBV replication.
   - No specific treatment is available for preventing posttransplant recurrence of HDV infection, but it seems prudent to give combination therapy with an oral nucleot(s)ide and HBIG as for patients with posttransplant HBV infection.

FURTHER READING

Asselah T, Marcellin P, eds. Hepatitis B virus. *Clin Liver Dis.* 2013;17:375–506.

Fattovich G. Natural history and prognosis of hepatitis B. *Sem Liver Dis.* 2003;23:47–58.

Fung J, Lai CL, Tanaka Y, et al. The duration of lamivudine therapy for chronic hepatitis B: cessation vs. continuation of treatment after HBeAg seroconversion. *Am J Gastroenterol.* 2009;104:1940–1946.

Heller T, Rotman Y, Koh C, et al. Long-term therapy of chronic delta hepatitis with peginterferon alfa. *Aliment Pharmacol Ther.* 2014;40:93–104.

Iloeje UH, Yang HI, Su J, et al. Predicting cirrhosis risk based on the level of circulating hepatitis B viral load. *Gastroenterology.* 2006;130:678–686.

LeFevre ML. U.S. Preventive Services Task Force. Screening for hepatitis B virus infection in nonpregnant adolescents and adults: U.S. Preventive Services Task Force recommendation statement. *Ann Intern Med.* 2014;161:58–66.

Lok A, McMahon B, Brown R, et al. Antiviral therapy for chronic hepatitis B virus infection in adults: a systematic review and meta-analysis. *Hepatology.* 2015;63. 284–206.

McMahon BJ, Bulkow L, Simons B, et al. Relationship between level of hepatitis B virus DNA and liver disease: a population-based study of hepatitis B e antigen-negative persons with hepatitis B. *Clin Gastroenterol Hepatol.* 2014;12:701–706.

Romeo R, Del Ninno E, Rumi M, et al. A 28-year study of the course of hepatitis Delta infection: a risk factor for cirrhosis and hepatocellular carcinoma. *Gastroenterology.* 2009;136:1629–1638.

Terrault N, Bzowej N, Chang KM, et al. AASLD guidelines for treatment of chronic hepatitis B. *Hepatology.* 2016;63:261–283.

Wedemeyer H, Manns MP. Epidemiology, pathogenesis and management of hepatitis D: update and challenges ahead. *Nat Rev Gastroenterol Hepatol.* 2010;7:31–40.

Weinbaum C, Williams I, Mast E, et al. Recommendations for identification and public health management of persons with chronic hepatitis B virus infection. *MMWR Recomm Rep.* 2008;57:1–20.

WHO. *Guidelines for the prevention, care and treatment of persons with chronic hepatitis B infection.* Geneva, Switzerland: World Health Organization; May 12, 2015.

CHAPTER 5

Hepatitis C

Carmen Vinaixa, MD ■ Marina Berenguer, MD, PhD

KEY POINTS

1 Infection with the hepatitis C virus (HCV) is a major cause of chronic hepatitis, cirrhosis, and hepatocellular carcinoma (HCC), as well as the leading indication for liver transplantation in Western countries.

2 HCV infection is also implicated in a number of metabolic, immunologic, cardiovascular, and neuropsychiatric extrahepatic manifestations, including mixed cryoglobulinemia, cutaneous vasculitis, membranoproliferative glomerulonephritis, porphyria cutanea tarda, non-Hodgkin lymphoma, diabetes mellitus, insulin resistance, atherosclerosis, chronic fatigue, and cognitive impairment.

3 Screening for HCV has essentially eliminated transmission by transfusion, but new infections continue to occur as a result of spread by illicit drug use, sexual contact, and nosocomial exposures.

4 Effective and well-tolerated all-oral antiviral regimens afford the possibility of cure for the vast majority of chronically HCV-infected persons.

Overview

1. **Infection with HCV is a major cause of chronic liver disease with a substantial risk of progression to cirrhosis, which may be complicated by HCC.**
2. Risk factors for HCV acquisition include illicit drug use, sexual contact, including men who have sex with men, and health care interventions.
3. Acute HCV infection has a high rate of evolution to chronic infection. Icteric acute hepatitis C is more likely than subclinical infection to resolve spontaneously.
4. HCV-related liver disease is more severe in patients with concomitant hepatic insults, including alcohol abuse and nonalcoholic fatty liver disease. Coinfection with human immunodeficiency virus (HIV) and hepatitis B virus (HBV) also results in more severe liver disease.

Virology

1. A glycoprotein-enveloped, single-stranded RNA virus
2. 55- to 60-nm spherical particle; 33-nm nucleocapsid core
3. Classified among the Flaviviridae, in the *Hepacivirus* genus
4. The HCV genome is comprised of approximately 9.4 to 9.6 kb and encodes a large polyprotein of approximately 3,000 amino acid residues.
   - One third of the polyprotein consists of a series of structural proteins: An internal nucleocapsid, or core [C], protein and two glycosylated envelope proteins, termed E1 and E2, which are present in the lipid-containing envelope of the virus.

- The envelope proteins may generate neutralizing antibodies.
- A hypervariable region is localized in the E2 envelope protein.
■ The remaining two thirds of the polyprotein consists of nonstructural proteins (termed NS2, NS3, NS4A, NS4B, NS5A, and NS5B) involved in HCV replication: A zinc-dependent metalloproteinase in NS2/3, a nucleotide triphosphatase/helicase in NS3, a chymotrypsin-like serine protease in NS3/4A, an RNA-dependent RNA polymerase in NS5B, an interferon (IFN) sensitivity region in NS5A, and an ion channel, P7.

5. Only one HCV serotype has been identified. There are six major HCV genotypes (1–6) with multiple subtypes; the genotypes are distributed variably throughout the world.
6. Genotypes correlate with the likelihood of response of chronic HCV infection to antiviral treatment with IFN-based therapies. The genotype (and subtype) are also important in choosing a specific oral antiviral regimen (see discussion later in the chapter).

Epidemiology

1. Incubation period: 15 to 160 days
2. Wide geographic distribution
3. **Prolonged viremia and persistent infection are common, occurring in 55% to 85% of cases.** Persistent infection is linked etiologically to chronic hepatitis, cirrhosis, HCC, and premature death.
4. The seroprevalence of past and current HCV infection is 1.3% in the United States, close to 20% in some regions of Italy and Japan, and up to 40% in some villages in the Nile delta in Egypt.
5. Modes of transmission:
    ■ **Blood-borne transmission is the predominant mode:**
       - Injection drug use accounts for 85% of new cases in the United States.
       - Transfusion of blood and blood products (now exceedingly rare in the United States and other developed countries, with an estimated risk of <1 per 2,000,000 units transfused)
       - Hemodialysis
       - Tattoos; body piercing
       - Needlestick injury with a contaminated hollow-bore needle or blood splash to the eyes in a health care setting
       - Cocaine snorting
    ■ Sexual transmission: Low efficiency, low frequency. Sexual transmission in men who have sex with men is recognized increasingly as a risk factor.
    ■ Maternal-neonatal transmission: Low efficiency, low frequency. The efficiency of transmission is increased with HIV coinfection. Transplacental passage of maternal anti-HCV may be detectable in the infant for several months after delivery without actual transmission of the virus.
    ■ No evidence of fecal-oral transmission
    ■ Lack of identifiable risk factor in 10% of cases

Acute Hepatitis C

DIAGNOSIS (Fig. 5.1)

1. Antibodies to HCV (anti-HCV)
    ■ Antibodies to recombinant HCV antigens from structural and nonstructural regions are detectable in the serum of HCV-infected persons. Serologic diagnosis is based on detection of anti-HCV in serum.

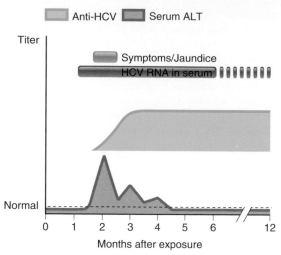

Fig. 5.1 Serologic course of acute hepatitis C virus (HCV) infection. *ALT,* Alanine aminotransferase.

- Anti-HCV is already detected in approximately 60% of patients during the acute phase of illness.
- Anti-HCV does not develop in <5% of infected persons and in a higher percentage of HIV-infected persons.
- Assays for immunoglobulin (Ig)M anti-HCV are under development.
- Anti-HCV generally persists for prolonged periods following acute infection in both self-limited and chronic HCV infections.

2. HCV RNA
    - **The earliest marker in the serum of persons with acute HCV infection**
    - Appears within a few weeks of infection
    - Testing for HCV RNA is used to detect viremia in seropositive persons and to exclude infection in seronegative persons.

NATURAL HISTORY

1. Infection is self-limited in 15% to 45% of acutely infected persons (and a higher percentage of acutely infected children); spontaneous resolution of HCV infection is more frequent in symptomatic cases and in persons with the interleukin-28B (IL28B; IFN lambda 3 [IFNL3]) genotype CC than in those with IL28B genotypes CT and TT.
2. Acute hepatitis C is rarely associated with acute liver failure.
3. HCV infection with prolonged viremia and elevated, fluctuating, or normal serum aminotransferase levels persist in the remainder of patients with acute hepatitis C and may ultimately result in cirrhosis and its complications (see discussion later in the chapter).

TREATMENT AND PREVENTION

1. **Antiviral therapy is highly effective in acute HCV infection. Therapy should be delayed for a minimum of 3 to 4 months to allow for the possibility of spontaneous resolution.** If viremia persists beyond 3 to 4 months, the treatment regimen should be based on the HCV genotype, as for chronic HCV infection (see discussion later in the chapter).
2. Immunoprophylaxis of HCV infection is not available, although neutralizing antibodies have been identified; development of an HCV vaccine is in progress.

3. Anti-HCV screening and nucleic acid testing of blood for HCV RNA have reduced the risk of transfusion-associated hepatitis C dramatically in the United States (<1 per 2,000,000 units transfused).
4. Safe sexual practice for contacts of HCV-infected persons with more than one partner may be appropriate.
5. Needle-exchange programs reduce HCV transmission in people who inject drugs.

Chronic Hepatitis C

PATHOGENESIS AND PATHOLOGY

1. Three mechanisms of pathogenesis of HCV-related liver injury have been proposed: Direct cytopathic damage, immune-directed hepatocyte destruction, and viral-induced autoimmunity; the weight of evidence suggests that immune-mediated mechanisms predominate, with destruction of hepatocytes by sensitized T cells.
2. Pathologic features range from minimal periportal lymphocytic inflammation to active hepatitis with bridging fibrosis, hepatocyte necrosis, and cirrhosis; steatosis, lymphoid aggregates, and bile duct damage are frequent; these findings are common with other viral and nonviral causes of liver disease.
3. Noninvasive approaches to the assessment of the extent of liver fibrosis have been developed. Several noninvasive tests are based on direct or indirect markers of liver fibrosis (alone or in combination). Ultrasound elastography (specifically, transient elastography) is the most widely used and validated technique; it measures liver stiffness and predicts advanced fibrosis and cirrhosis accurately and has been used increasingly instead of liver biopsy to monitor fibrosis progression and the need for antiviral treatment (see Chapter 1).
4. Role of liver biopsy:
    - Assessment of the severity of liver damage (grade of hepatic necroinflammation and stage of fibrosis); increasingly reserved for patients in whom the results of noninvasive tests are inconclusive
    - Detection of other concomitant diseases such as hemochromatosis, alcohol-induced injury, and nonalcoholic steatohepatitis (NASH)
    - Determination of the rate of disease progression in patients with a known date of infection or prior liver biopsy results

CLINICAL FEATURES AND NATURAL HISTORY

1. Most patients with chronic HCV infection have persistent or intermittent elevations of serum alanine aminotransferase (ALT) levels, although serum ALT levels remain normal in one third of cases.
2. Most patients are asymptomatic; when symptoms are present, the most common is fatigue. Other symptoms include musculoskeletal pain, pruritus, sicca syndrome, depression, anorexia, abdominal discomfort, impaired concentration, and a reduced quality of life. The intensity of symptoms is not related to the severity of liver disease.
3. Once cirrhosis is established, patients are predisposed to complications of portal hypertension; jaundice is rare until hepatic decompensation occurs (see Chapter 11).
4. **Extrahepatic manifestations:** 40% to 74% of patients develop at least one extrahepatic manifestation during the course of their disease; rheumatologic and cutaneous manifestations are the most common. HCV-induced cryoglobulinemia should be excluded. Chronically HCV-infected patients are at increased risk of insulin-resistance, diabetes mellitus, renal disease, cardiovascular events, and malignant lymphoma (Table 5.1).

TABLE 5.1 ■ **Extrahepatic Manifestations of Hepatitis C Viral Infection**

Metabolic
Insulin resistance
Diabetes mellitus

Cardiovascular
Atherosclerosis
Cardiac and cerebrovascular events/mortality

Neuropsychiatric
Fatigue
Cognitive impairment

Immunologic
Rheumatoid arthritis

Hematologic
Mixed cryoglobulinemia
Non-Hodgkin lymphoma

5. Natural history (Fig. 5.2)
   ■ Disease progression is typically silent.
   ■ Only a few patients have severe outcomes during the first 2 decades of infection; **at least 20 to 30 years of infection are required to develop clinically significant disease.**
     – Once cirrhosis develops, actuarial survival is 83% to 91% at 5 years and 79% after 10 years in the absence of clinical decompensation.
     – Survival decreases to 50% at 5 years among those in whom clinical decompensation occurs; the cumulative probability of developing an episode of decompensation is 4% to 5% at 1 year and increases to 30% at 10 years.
   ■ **The risk of developing HCC is 1% to 4% per year once cirrhosis is established.**
   ■ Factors associated with progression of chronic hepatitis C include male gender, infection after 40 years of age, alcohol consumption >50 g/day, immunosuppression, elevated serum ALT levels, significant necroinflammation and fibrosis on biopsy, and insulin resistance with obesity or diabetes mellitus.

DIAGNOSIS

1. **Anti-HCV**
   ■ Serologic testing with anti-HCV does not confirm active infection because anti-HCV persists indefinitely after spontaneous or treatment-induced resolution (see discussion earlier in chapter).
   ■ The sensitivity of anti-HCV is 97% to 100%; the positive predictive value is 50% to 95%; false-negative results are more likely in immunosuppressed patients including those who are HIV positive.
2. **HCV RNA:** Used to confirm active infection
   ■ HCV RNA testing should be performed in the following patients:
     – Those with a positive anti-HCV result
     – Those in whom antiviral treatment is being considered (a quantitative assay should be used)

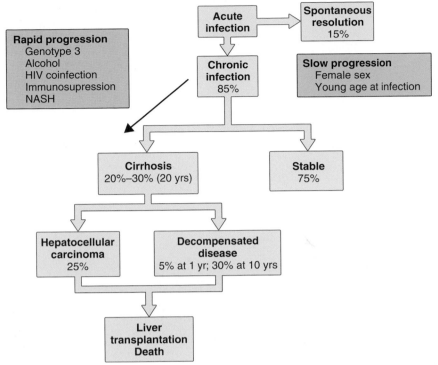

Fig. 5.2 Natural history of chronic hepatitis C. *HIV,* Human immunodeficiency virus; *NASH,* nonalcoholic steatohepatitis.

  - Those with unexplained liver disease and a negative anti-HCV result if they are immunocompromised or suspected of having acute HCV infection
- Real-time polymerase chain reaction (PCR)–based HCV RNA assays have wide linear ranges for the quantification of HCV and sensitivity similar to that of qualitative tests; these tests are preferred to assess the significance of a positive anti-HCV result and to monitor the response to antiviral treatment (see discussion later in chapter).

SCREENING AND COUNSELING

1. Universal testing of the population is not currently recommended.
2. **In the United States, screening is recommended for people born between 1945 and 1965, reflecting the high prevalence of HCV infection in the "baby boomer" cohort.**
3. Screening for risk factors involves identifying persons who are at the highest risk of HCV infection (see discussion earlier in chapter).
4. Once a patient is determined to be at risk, HCV testing should be performed.
5. Persons infected with HCV should be counseled on how to decrease the risk of HCV transmission:
   - Avoid sharing dental or shaving equipment.
   - Cover bleeding wounds to prevent contact with others.
   - Discontinue illicit injection drugs.
   - Do not donate blood, organs, tissue, or semen.
   - Be aware that barrier protection is not needed in monogamous relationships.
   - Avoid excessive alcohol use.
   - For susceptible persons, undergo hepatitis A and B vaccination.

TREATMENT

Treatment can interrupt disease progression and reduce complications of HCV-related cirrhosis.

1. Goals of therapy
   a. **The primary goal of therapy is to eradicate infection early enough in the course to prevent progression to end-stage liver disease and HCC. Sustained virologic response, defined as absence of viremia 12 weeks (SVR12) following completion of antiviral therapy, indicates cure of HCV infection.**
   b. Histologic improvement, often with regression of fibrosis, results in improved outcomes, including a reduction in morbidity and probably mortality.
   c. Additional benefits include prevention of HCV transmission.
2. Indications
   a. **All viremic patients with chronic HCV infection are candidates for antiviral therapy.**
   b. **Patients with advanced fibrosis or cirrhosis and other patients with clinically significant manifestations of HCV infection are at high priority for treatment.**
   c. Other high-priority groups include those with the following:
      - HIV and/or HBV coinfection
      - A liver transplant
      - Clinically significant extrahepatic manifestations: Symptomatic vasculitis associated with HCV-related mixed cryoglobulinemia, HCV immune complex-related nephropathy, and non-Hodgkin B cell lymphoma
      - Debilitating fatigue (regardless of fibrosis stage)
      - A high risk of transmitting HCV:
        - Active injection drug users
        - Men who have sex with men with high-risk sexual practices
        - Women of childbearing age who wish to become pregnant
        - Patients undergoing hemodialysis
        - Incarcerated persons
3. Available drugs
   a. Peginterferon (Peg-IFN) alfa-2a and alfa-2b
   b. Ribavirin (RBV)
   c. **Direct-acting antivirals (DAAs)** (Table 5.2):
      - **NS3-4 protease inhibitors:** Active against genotypes 1 and 4
        - First generation: Boceprevir, telaprevir (both now withdrawn from market), only in combination with Peg-IFN and RBV
        - Second generation: Simeprevir, asunaprevir (not approved in the United States), paritaprevir, grazoprevir
      - **NS5B polymerase inhibitors:** Pangenotypic (i.e., active against all HCV genotypes)
        - Nucleotide analog: Sofosbuvir
        - Nonnucleoside analog: Dasabuvir
      - **NS5A replication complex inhibitors:**
        - Pangenotypic: Daclatasvir, velpatasvir
        - Genotypes 1 and 4: Ledipasvir, ombitasvir, elbasvir
4. Treatment regimens (approved drugs): IFN-free regimens, composed of different combinations of DAAs, are the standard of care (where available) and are highly effective and well tolerated (Table 5.3).
5. Definitions of response to treatment
   - **Rapid virologic response (RVR):** HCV RNA undetectable by week 4
     - RVR does not predict SVR with IFN-free regimens.
   - **End of treatment (EOT) response:** Undetectable HCV RNA at the end of treatment

TABLE 5.2 ■ Direct-Acting Antiviral Agents Approved by the FDA as of 2017

	Potency	Barrier to Resistance	Side Effects	Drug Interaction Potential	Drugs
NS3/4A protease inhibitors	High, variable among genotypes	Low-medium	Rash, anemia, bilirubin elevation	High	Boceprevir[a] Telaprevir[a] Simeprevir Paritaprevir Grazoprevir Glecaprevir[b] Voxilaprevir[c]
NS5A inhibitors	High	Low	Variable	Low-moderate	Daclatasvir Ledipasvir Ombitasvir Elbasvir Velpatasvir Pibrentasvir[b]
NS5B polymerase nonnucleoside inhibitors	Variable	Low	Variable	Variable	Dasabuvir
NS5B polymerase nucleos(t)ide inhibitors	Moderate-high	High	Mitochondrial toxicity; drug-drug interactions (e.g., with ART)	Low	Sofosbuvir

[a]Withdrawn from market with advent of better agents.

[b]Approval pending in 2017.

[c]Approval pending in 2017; used in combination with sofosbuvir and velpatasvir.

ART, Antiretroviral therapy; *FDA,* Food and Drug Administration.

TABLE 5.3 ■ Treatment Regimens and Their Efficacies by Genotype, Prior Treatment, and Presence or Absence of Cirrhosis

Genotype (gt)	Treatment Regimen	Duration (weeks)	Efficacy (%)[a]
1 **No cirrhosis**			
Treatment-naïve patients	Sofosbuvir + simeprevir (+ribavirin if gt 1a)	12	87–97
	Sofosbuvir + ledipasvir	8–12	95–100
	Sofosbuvir + daclatasvir	12	95–100
	Paritaprevir/ritonavir-boosted + ombitasvir + dasabuvir (+ribavirin if gt 1a)	12	96 (gt 1a) 100 (gt 1b)
	Sofosbuvir + velpatasvir	12	98–99
Treatment-experienced patients	Sofosbuvir + simeprevir +/− ribavirin	12	79–97
	Sofosbuvir + ledipasvir	12	95
	Sofosbuvir + daclatasvir	12	95–100
	Paritaprevir/ritonavir-boosted + ombitasvir + dasabuvir + ribavirin	12	96
	Sofosbuvir + velpatasvir	12	98–99
Cirrhosis			
Treatment-naïve or treatment-experienced patients	Sofosbuvir + ledipasvir	12 (naïve) 24 (experienced)	96 98
	Sofosbuvir + ledipasvir + ribavirin	12	96–98

Continued

TABLE 5.3 ■ Treatment Regimens and Their Efficacies by Genotype, Prior Treatment, and Presence or Absence of Cirrhosis—cont'd

Genotype (gt)	Treatment Regimen	Duration (weeks)	Efficacy (%)[a]
Treatment-experienced patients and negative predictors of response (e.g., platelets <75,000/mm^3)	Sofosbuvir + ledipasvir + ribavirin	24	100
Treatment-naïve or treatment-experienced patients	Sofosbuvir + daclatasvir	24	95–100
	Sofosbuvir + daclatasvir + ribavirin	12	95–100
	Paritaprevir/ritonavir-boosted + ombitasvir + dasabuvir (+ribavirin if gt 1a)	24 (gt 1a) 12 (gt 1b)	95 100
	Sofosbuvir + velpatasvir	12	94
2			
Treatment-naïve patients with or without cirrhosis	Sofosbuvir + ribavirin	12	85–100
Treatment-experienced patients with cirrhosis	Sofosbuvir + ribavirin	16–24	87 (16 weeks) 100 (24 weeks)
Treatment-experienced or ribavirin-intolerant patients	Sofosbuvir + daclatasvir	12	80–92
	Sofosbuvir + velpatasvir	12	99–100
3 **No cirrhosis**			
Treatment-naïve or treatment-experienced patients	Sofosbuvir + daclatasvir	12	96
Cirrhosis			
Treatment-naïve or treatment-experienced patients	Sofosbuvir + daclatasvir + ribavirin	24	88
4			
Treatment-naïve or treatment-experienced patients	Sofosbuvir + simeprevir	12	N/A
	Sofosbuvir + daclatasvir	12	N/A
	Sofosbuvir + ledipasvir	12	93–95
	Paritaprevir/ritonavir-boosted + ombitasvir + ribavirin	12	100
	Grazoprevir + elbasvir	12	87–97
	Sofosbuvir + velpatasvir	12	100
5 and 6			
Treatment-naïve or treatment-experienced patients	Sofosbuvir + ledipasvir	12	95 (gt 5) 95–96 (gt 6)
	Grazoprevir + elbasvir +/– ribavirin	12	25–100 (gt 5) 75–100 (gt 6)
	Sofosbuvir + velpatasvir	12	97 (gt 5) 100 (gt 6)

[a]Sustained virologic response at 12 weeks.

N/A, Not available.

- **Sustained virologic response (SVR):** Undetectable HCV RNA at 12 (SVR12) or 24 (SVR24) weeks after the end of treatment. SVR12 is currently considered to be equivalent to SVR24 as a measure of efficacy.
- **Nonresponse:** Failure to achieve undetectable HCV RNA at any time point during therapy
- **Relapse:** An EOT response followed by return of HCV RNA in serum after treatment discontinuation

6. Factors associated with SVR
   - Current DAA combinations achieve excellent efficacy results (SVR rates >90% in most cases), with durations of 12 weeks and without the need to add IFN or RBV, even in the presence of classic predictors of nonresponse: High body mass index (BMI), HIV coinfection, gender, African American race, prior treatment failure, advanced liver disease, and prior liver transplantation
   - Factors associated with reduced SVR rates with IFN-free regimens include the following:
     - The presence of cirrhosis, especially if decompensated
     - Previous treatment failure (nonresponse to IFN-based therapy)
     - Infection with HCV genotype 3, which has replaced genotype 1 as the most challenging genotype in the IFN-free era
   - In general, the strategies used in the presence of these factors are one or both of the following:
     - Extending treatment to 24 weeks
     - Adding RBV

7. Adverse effects of treatment:
Adverse events occur in approximately 25% of patients treated with IFN-free regimens and are generally mild. The most frequent adverse events include asthenia, headache, anemia (especially with RBV-containing regimens), and insomnia.

8. Special considerations:
   - **Drug-drug interactions**
   Numerous and complex drug-drug interactions are possible with DAAs, especially when the combination contains a protease inhibitor (metabolized by cytochrome-P450 3A4). Recommendations can be found at www.hep-druginteractions.org.
   - **Resistant-associated substitutions** (RASs)
     - NS3/4A: RASs related to protease inhibitors disappear after approximately 1 year, permitting retreatment with same family of drug after this time period.
     - NS5A: RASs associated with NS5A inhibitors persist for long periods of time after treatment, possibly limiting the efficacy of subsequent retreatment with the same drug.
     - Routine testing for RASs before treatment is not recommended because RASs are not associated with reduced SVR rates, unless therapy with elbasvir or grazoprevir is planned.

9. Long-term follow-up
   - Noncirrhotic patients with other risk factors for liver disease (alcohol consumption, NASH, coinfections) who achieve an SVR should undergo serum ALT levels and noninvasive liver fibrosis assessment at yearly intervals.
   - Annual HCV RNA testing is recommended for persons who inject drugs and for HIV-seropositive men who have unprotected sex with men. Periodic testing should also be offered to other persons at ongoing risk of reexposure to HCV.
   - Cirrhotic patients who achieve an SVR should undergo testing with a complete blood count, liver biochemical tests, and hepatic ultrasonography (with or without alpha fetoprotein testing) every 6 months to survey for HCC (see Chapter 29). The risk of HCC

remains 1% to 3% per year in patients with cirrhosis. The risk depends on the severity of liver disease, age of the patient, and presence of diabetes mellitus.

- Patients without an SVR should undergo laboratory testing and noninvasive liver fibrosis assessment at yearly intervals if cirrhosis is absent and every 6 months, with ultrasonography, if cirrhosis is present. Consider retreatment with another regimen.

10. **Liver transplantation** (see Chapter 33)
    - **Cirrhosis due to HCV is the most common indication for liver transplantation in the Western world.**
    - **Posttransplant recurrence of HCV infection after liver transplantation is universal.**
    - Progression of HCV is accelerated in the posttransplant setting.
    - Histologic evidence of liver injury is present in approximately 50% of patients 1 year after transplantation, and the rate increases with follow-up.
    - Histologic findings typical of posttransplant HCV infection of the liver graft include hepatic steatosis, portal and parenchymal mononuclear infiltrates, and hepatocyte swelling and necrosis.
    - Short-term survival is similar to that observed in patients who undergo liver transplantation for nonviral liver disease, but long-term survival is reduced by HCV recurrence.
    - IFN-based therapy with and without RBV was used in the past to treat posttransplant HCV recurrence; transient reductions in serum HCV RNA levels were observed, but sustained biochemical and virologic responses was uncommon (around 33% with Peg-IFN plus RBV and around 60% with triple therapy containing Peg-IFN, RBV, and a first-generation protease inhibitor [telaprevir or boceprevir]).
    - Results of treatment with IFN-free regimens in the transplant setting are excellent. Therefore, **all liver transplant recipients with HCV infection should receive antiviral treatment with DAAs.**
    - IFN-free regimens can be administered either before transplantation to prevent HCV graft infection and, in some instances, avoid liver transplantation if significant improvement in liver function and portal hypertension is achieved or after transplantation to treat recurrent HCV infection. Excellent SVR rates are achieved with both strategies when sofosbuvir-based regimens are used. Caution is advised when treating patients with severe liver impairment (Model for End-stage Liver Disease [MELD] score >20 [see Chapter 33]), given the lack of data and cases of potential hepatotoxicity reported in the literature.

FURTHER READING

Buti M, Riveiro-Barciela M, Esteban R. Management of direct-acting antiviral agent failures. *J Hepatol.* 2015;63:1511–1522.

Castera L, Sebastiani G, Le Bail B, et al. Prospective comparison of two algorithms combining non-invasive methods for staging liver fibrosis in chronic hepatitis C. *J Hepatol.* 2010;52:191–198.

Centers for Disease Control and Prevention. Testing for HCV infection: an update of guidance for clinicians and laboratorians. *MMWR Morb Mortal Wkly Rep.* 2013;62:362–365.

Dick TB, Lindberg LS, Ramirez DD, et al. A clinician's guide to drug-drug interactions with direct-acting antiviral agents for the treatment of hepatitis C viral infection. *Hepatology.* 2016;63:634–643.

European Association for the Study of the Liver. EASL Clinical Practice Guidelines: EASL recommendations on treatment of hepatitis C 2015. *J Hepatol.* 2015;63:199–236.

Feld JJ, Jacobson IM, Hézode C, et al. Sofosbuvir and velpatasvir for HCV genotype 1, 2, 4, 5, and 6 Infection. *N Engl J Med.* 2015;373:2599–2607.

Felmlee DJ, Coilly A, Chung RT, et al. New perspectives for preventing hepatitis C virus liver graft infection. *Lancet Infect Dis.* 2016;16:735–745.

Goodman ZD. Grading and staging systems for inflammation and fibrosis in chronic liver diseases. *J Hepatol.* 2007;47:598–607.

Hepatitis C guidance. AASLD-IDSA recommendations for testing, managing, and treating adults infected with hepatitis C virus. *Hepatology.* 2015;62:932–954.

Naggie S, Cooper C, Saag M, et al. Ledipasvir and sofosbuvir for HCV in patients coinfected with HIV-1. *N Engl J Med.* 2015;373:705–713.

Negro F, Forton D, Craxi A, et al. Extrahepatic morbidity and mortality of chronic hepatitis C. *Gastroenterology.* 2015;149:1345–1360.

Pawlotsky JM. Hepatitis C virus resistance to direct-acting antiviral drugs in interferon-free regimens. *Gastroenterology.* 2016;151:70–86.

Petta S, Maida M, Macaluso FS, et al. Hepatitis C virus infection is associated with increased cardiovascular mortality: a meta-analysis of observational studies. *Gastroenterology.* 2016;150:145–155.

van der Meer AJ, Veldt BJ, Feld JJ, et al. Association between sustained virological response and all-cause mortality among patients with chronic hepatitis C and advanced hepatic fibrosis. *JAMA.* 2012;308:2584–2593.

CHAPTER 6

Hepatitis Caused by Other Viruses

Elliot B. Tapper, MD ■ Michael P. Curry, MD

KEY POINTS

1 Systemic viral infections can cause liver injury that ranges from mild asymptomatic and transient elevation of serum aminotransferase levels to acute icteric hepatitis or rarely severe hepatitis with acute liver failure (ALF).

2 The clinical presentation may be indistinguishable from liver injury caused by the principal hepatotropic viruses.

3 Mild liver enzyme elevations are a common feature of many systemic viral infections and can occur as a bystander effect.

4 In general, specific antiviral therapy is not available.

Overview

1. Hepatic dysfunction is frequently encountered in systemic, nonhepatotropic viral infections and may reflect the host immune response rather than direct viral injury.
2. Hepatic involvement in systemic viral infections does not result in chronic liver injury.
3. Although most systemic nonhepatospecific viral infections cause mild hepatocellular dysfunction, more severe liver disease may occur.
4. These nonhepatotropic viruses include cytomegalovirus (CMV), herpes simplex virus (HSV), Epstein-Barr virus (EBV), varicella-zoster virus (VZV), human herpesvirus 6 (HHV-6), and nonherpes viruses including adenovirus, Dengue virus, Chikungunya virus, Ebola virus, and influenza virus (Table 6.1).
5. Serologic testing is available for most viruses that have the potential to cause liver injury.

Viruses with Frequent Hepatic Involvement

CYTOMEGALOVIRUS

1. CMV has a seroprevalence rate of 30% to 70% in the general population, reflecting prior infection.
2. Primary infection of immunocompetent hosts is usually clinically indistinguishable from infectious mononucleosis caused by EBV. Symptoms include fever, myalgia, cervical lymphadenopathy, and, in >75% of patients, mild elevations in the liver enzymes.
3. Recovery from a primary infection results in lifelong latent infection with the possibility of replication and reactivation if the host immune response becomes compromised.
4. CMV infection in an immunocompromised host can occur because of reactivation of latent infection or as a primary infection after first exposure.
5. CMV-induced liver injury can be more severe in the immunocompromised host. Symptoms and signs may include tender hepatomegaly and jaundice. Hepatic involvement by CMV is

TABLE 6.1 ■ **Viral Infections that May Involve the Liver**

Virus	Histology	Severity	Treatment
Viruses with Frequent Hepatic Involvement			
Cytomegalovirus	Lobular microabscesses, often surrounding hepatocytes with nuclear and/or cytoplasmic inclusions	Usually mild, rarely severe	Valganciclovir (if mild), ganciclovir (severe); cidofovir (refractory)
Epstein-Barr virus (EBV)	Diffuse sinusoidal lymphocytic infiltration, EBV-encoded RNA (EBER)–positive tissue staining	Usually mild, rarely severe	Case reports suggest ganciclovir
Viruses with Less Frequent Hepatic Involvement			
Herpes simplex virus	Hepatocyte necrosis, pauciinflammatory infiltrates, Cowdry type A inclusion bodies, and multinucleated hepatocytes	Always severe	Acyclovir
Varicella zoster virus	–	Usually mild, rarely severe	Acyclovir
Adenovirus	Staining for adenoviral antigens; randomly scattered punched-out lesions, large nuclei with inclusions consisting of waxy-appearing dense material with unstained clear zones	Usually mild, rarely severe	Case reports suggest cidofovir
Influenza virus	Inflammatory infiltrate without direct infection of hepatocytes	Always mild	Supportive care
Viruses Uncommon in the United States but with Frequent Hepatic Involvement			
Chikungunya	–	Always mild	Supportive care
Dengue virus	–	Usually mild	Supportive care
Ebola virus	Widespread necrosis with periportal mononuclear cells and Kupffer cell hypertrophy	Usually severe	Supportive care

frequently accompanied by gastrointestinal tract injury and symptoms (ulcers, nausea, vomiting) and pneumonia.

6. Severe CMV-induced liver injury is characterized histologically by small collections (microabscesses) of inflammatory cells (mainly neutrophils) throughout the hepatic lobule, often surrounding hepatocytes with nuclear and/or cytoplasmic inclusions, so-called "owl's eye" inclusions.

7. CMV is a common infection in patients with acquired immunodeficiency syndrome (AIDS) and has been associated with papillary stenosis and sclerosing cholangitis (AIDS cholangiopathy) (see Chapter 27).

8. The diagnosis is made in the appropriate clinical context with polymerase chain reaction (PCR) testing or histologic evidence of infection.

9. Infection is usually defined as *primary* if the patient has no evidence of prior exposure (i.e., negative immunoglobulin [Ig]G anti-CMV) or *recurrent* if the patient has detectable IgG anti-CMV.

10. Treatment of CMV infection is not always indicated in immunocompetent patients, unless the infection is severe or life threatening.

11. Many immunocompromised patients at risk for CMV are routinely tested by a PCR assay or treated prophylactically with an antiviral agent. Treatment of viremia before the onset of symptoms is considered preemptive.

12. Drugs approved for the treatment of CMV infection include oral ganciclovir, valganciclovir, intravenous ganciclovir, intravenous foscarnet, and intravenous cidofovir.

13. Ganciclovir-resistant strains of CMV are emerging.
14. The choice and duration of treatment are dependent on the severity of disease and the immune status of the patient. Repeated assessments for CMV viremia should be made.
15. Organ transplantation recipients at risk of CMV reactivation usually receive 3 to 6 months of prophylactic therapy after transplantation.

EPSTEIN-BARR VIRUS

1. Of the world's population, 90% have serologic evidence of prior EBV infection.
2. Primary infection typically manifests as infectious mononucleosis (fever, lymphadenopathy, and mild elevations in liver enzyme levels).
3. Of patients with EBV mononucleosis, 90% have mild elevations in serum aminotransferase levels.
4. Cholestasis with jaundice is reported in 45% of patients with primary EBV infection, with a 5% case-fatality rate reported in both immunocompetent and immunocompromised patients.
5. Half of the deaths from mononucleosis, while rare, are attributable to ALF. Less than 1% of all cases of ALF, however, are attributable to EBV. EBV-associated ALF carries with it a 25% transplant-free survival.
6. The monospot test, which detects heterophile antibodies, is sensitive but not specific.
7. Liver injury attributable to EBV mononucleosis can be diagnosed clinically by the combination of symptoms with consistent serology (IgM directed against the viral capsid antigens [IgM anti-EBV VCA]).
8. Definite severe EBV infection is confirmed by the combination of serologic evidence of virus (by a PCR assay) and evidence of EBV-associated hepatopathology on light microscopy (diffuse sinusoidal lymphocytic infiltration) with or without EBV-encoded RNA (EBER)–positive tissue staining.
9. Treatments with demonstrated efficacy in clinical trials are lacking. Acyclovir inhibits EBV in vitro and reduces viral shedding in the oropharynx but has little to no effect on symptoms. Ganciclovir use has been supported by a study of two children with EBV hepatitis.

Viruses with Less Frequent Hepatic Involvement

HERPES SIMPLEX VIRUS

1. The two types of HSV (HSV-1 and HSV-2) have seroprevalence rates of 57.7% and 17.0%, respectively, in the general population.
2. HSV infections typically manifest as orolabial or genital lesions. Rare presentations include meningitis, encephalitis, and hepatitis.
3. HSV hepatitis usually occurs in neonates, pregnant women, and immunocompromised patients.
4. Only 50% of patients have associated mucocutaneous involvement.
5. Mild asymptomatic elevations in serum aminotransferase levels are seen in 14% of patients with acute HSV genital infection.
6. HSV hepatitis is rare. Approximately 137 cases have been reported, and the frequency of HSV hepatitis in a cohort of patients with ALF is 0.3%. Patients present with fever, leukopenia, and elevated serum aminotransferase levels.
7. The prognosis of HSV hepatitis is poor, with a transplant-free survival rate of 24.8%.
8. Liver biopsy findings consistent with HSV infection include extensive hepatocyte necrosis with adjacent congestion, pauciinflammatory infiltrates, Cowdry type A inclusion bodies (purple nuclear inclusions with a clear halo), and multinucleated hepatocytes.

9. The diagnosis of primary infection complicated by hepatitis is made by the combination of viremia (detected by a PCR assay) and consistent histology, whereas reactivation hepatitis occurs when there is serologic evidence of prior infection (IgG anti-HSV-1 or anti-HSV-2).

10. Although prospective trials are lacking, treatment with intravenous acyclovir (10 mg/kg 3 times a day) may be effective.

11. Liver transplantation should be considered for patients who meet criteria for ALF that does not reverse with antiviral therapy.

OTHER VIRUSES

1. **Varicella zoster virus (VZV):** Disseminated varicella infection typically presents as pneumonia with infrequent, mildly elevated liver enzyme levels. Up to 25% of children with primary varicella infection have elevated liver enzymes. There are a few reports of ALF attributable to VZV in patients with a confluence of vesicular rash, positive VZV by a PCR assay, and severe liver injury. Primary varicella infection in organ transplant recipients has been associated with ALF. Treatment is the same as for HSV: Intravenous acyclovir, 10 mg/kg three times a day for 7 to 10 days.

2. **Adenovirus** is a double-stranded DNA virus that is frequently implicated in upper respiratory tract and ocular infections. Confirmation of adenoviral hepatitis requires evidence of systemic infection (positive PCR assay, antigenemia, or viral blood culture) and liver biopsy specimens consistent with a viral infection—either stains for adenoviral antigens or diagnostic morphology (randomly scattered punched-out lesions, large nuclei with inclusions consisting of waxy-appearing dense material with unstained clear zones). Most reported cases have been in organ transplant recipients. Severe adenoviral hepatitis has a poor prognosis with a low rate of spontaneous recovery. Treatment may be attempted with cidofovir.

3. **Influenza** is an RNA virus associated with pandemic infections and a predominance of respiratory symptoms. Mild asymptomatic elevations of liver enzyme levels are common. However, influenza does not directly infect hepatocytes. Influenza infection induces the expansion of CD8+ T cells, which cause "collateral damage" to the liver while interacting with Kupffer cells.

4. **Human herpesvirus 6** is a rare cause of liver injury, lymphadenopathy, and a nonspecific rash. A detectable viral load (positive PCR assay) or serology (IgM anti-HHV-6) in the absence of other potential causes for the symptoms is considered diagnostic. One study suggested that HHV-6 may be responsible for non-A–E–associated ALF; HHV-6 antigens were isolated in the liver tissue by immunohistochemistry in 12 of the 15 cases.

Viruses Uncommon in the Unites States but with Frequent Hepatic Involvement

1. **Chikungunya** is an RNA virus associated with an epidemic fever marked by flulike symptoms and arthralgia. In the early phase of infection (<14 days), serum aminotransferase levels range from 49 to 311 U/L without evidence of severe liver injury (i.e., coagulopathy or jaundice).

2. **Dengue** virus, the most common mosquito-borne RNA virus worldwide, is highly prevalent in tropical climates. Over 80% of patients with Dengue fever, including 84.4% of patients with hemorrhagic-type fever, present with elevated serum alanine aminotransferase (ALT) levels without severe liver injury. The mechanism of injury is not defined. The mortality rate associated with severe hepatitis associated with Dengue fever is 2.7% in affected adults and over 50% in the pediatric population.

3. **Ebola** virus is an epidemic RNA virus associated with hemorrhagic shock syndrome. Independent of shock, 77% of patients present with elevated liver enzyme levels, and 100%

develop liver injury during the index hospitalization. Serum aspartate aminotransferase (AST) and ALT levels rise to about 200 U/L, with an AST > ALT. Jaundice develops in over 50% of patients during the course of infection. A marked elevation in the alkaline phosphatase level (to 900 U/L) was noted in American patients treated in 2014. Fatalities were more frequent in patients with an AST level of 900 U/L during the Sudan Ebola virus epidemic in Uganda in 2000. Histology in this series showed widespread necrosis with periportal mononuclear cells and Kupffer cell hypertrophy, without prominent bile duct damage.

4. Liver injury was prominent in **severe acute respiratory syndrome** (SARS) caused by a coronavirus, with elevation of the serum aminotransferase levels, and may have reflected direct hepatic injury by the virus. After an outbreak of SARS in Asia in 2002, no further cases have been identified.

VIRUSES OF UNCLEAR PATHOGENICITY

1. **Transfusion transmitted (TT) virus** is a single-stranded, circular, hepatotropic DNA virus spread by both blood-borne and enteric transmission routes. Although it is prevalent in patients with specific risk factors (transfusions, intravenous drug use, and sex workers), TT virus is also found in the serum of some patients with ALF, cirrhosis, and liver cancer but has not been consistently implicated in liver injury.

2. **SEN virus** is a single-stranded, circular, hepatotropic DNA virus detected in 1.8% of American blood donors. In Japan, it was identified in 22% of healthy subjects and 38% of patients undergoing hemodialysis. It appears to be transmitted by transfusion. In a study of 12 patients with non-A-E-transfusion–related hepatitis, 11 (92%) had serologic evidence of SEN viremia; however, in a follow-up case-control study, no etiologic role for SEN in the cause of cryptogenic hepatitis could be established, nor was it associated with more severe hepatitis.

3. **Hepatitis G virus** (or GB virus C) is an RNA virus in the same family as hepatitis C virus (Flaviviridae). Although it was originally thought to cause transfusion-related hepatitis, no etiologic role has been established. Hepatitis G may be associated with favorable outcomes in patients with human immunodeficiency virus infection.

FURTHER READING

Adams DH, Hubscher SG. Systemic viral infections and collateral damage in the liver. *Am J Pathol.* 2006;168:1057–1059.

Adams LA, Deboer B, Jeffrey G, et al. Ganciclovir and the treatment of Epstein-Barr virus hepatitis. *J Gastroenterol Hepatol.* 2006;21:1758–1760.

Bradley H, Markowitz LE, Gibson T, et al. Seroprevalence of herpes simplex virus types 1 and 2—United States, 1999-2010. *J Infect Dis.* 2014;209:325–333.

Drebber U, Kasper HU, Krupacz J, et al. The role of Epstein-Barr virus in acute and chronic hepatitis. *J Hepatol.* 2006;44:879–885.

Gandhi MK, Khanna R. Human cytomegalovirus: clinical aspects, immune regulation, and emerging treatments. *Lancet Infect Dis.* 2004;4:725–738.

Härmä M, Höckerstedt K, Lautenschlager I. Human herpesvirus-6 and acute liver failure. *Transplantation.* 2003;76:536–539.

Kew M. Hepatitis viruses (other than hepatitis B and C viruses) as causes of hepatocellular carcinoma: an update. *J Viral Hepat.* 2013;20:149–157.

Khan E, Kisat M, Khan N, et al. Demographic and clinical features of Dengue fever in Pakistan from 2003-2007: a retrospective cross-sectional study. *PloS One.* 2010;5:e12505.

Lyon GM, Mehta AK, Varkey JB, et al. Clinical care of two patients with Ebola virus disease in the United States. *N Engl J Med.* 2014;371:2402–2409.

Mellinger JL, Rossaro L, Naugler WE, et al. Epstein-Barr virus (EBV) related acute liver failure: a case series from the US Acute Liver Failure Study Group. *Dig Dis Sci.* 2014;59:1630–1637.

Norvell JP, Blei AT, Jovanovic BD, et al. Herpes simplex virus hepatitis: an analysis of the published literature and institutional cases. *Liver Transpl.* 2007;13:1428–1434.

Papic N, Pangercic A, Vargovic M, et al. Liver involvement during influenza infection: perspective on the 2009 influenza pandemic. *Influenza Other Respir Viruses.* 2012;6:e2–e5.

Ronan B, Agrwal N, Carey EJ, et al. Fulminant hepatitis due to human adenovirus. *Infection.* 2014;42: 105–111.

Taubitz W, Cramer JP, Kapaun A, et al. Chikungunya fever in travelers: clinical presentation and course. *Clin Infect Dis.* 2007;45:e1–e4.

Uyeki TM, Mehta AK, Davey Jr RT, et al. Clinical management of Ebola virus disease in the United States and Europe. *N Engl J Med.* 2016;374:636–646.

CHAPTER 7

Autoimmune Hepatitis

Albert J. Czaja, MD, FACP, FACG, AGAF, FAASLD

KEY POINTS

1. Criteria for the diagnosis of autoimmune hepatitis have been codified with development of two diagnostic scoring systems that can support clinical judgment in the diagnosis of difficult cases.

2. Presentations range from acute severe (fulminant) to asymptomatic and mild.

3. Genetic factors within (DRB1*0301, DRB1*0401, DRB1*1301, DQB1*0201, DRB1*07) and outside (diverse polymorphisms) the major histocompatibility complex (MHC) may affect occurrence, clinical phenotype, severity, and outcome.

4. Budesonide in combination with azathioprine is an alternative regimen especially for treatment-naïve noncirrhotic patients with mild, uncomplicated disease or risk for severe glucocorticoid-induced complications (vertebral collapse, diabetes mellitus, hypertension, psychosis).

5. Overlapping features with primary biliary cholangitis (PBC) or primary sclerosing cholangitis (PSC) commonly require therapy with prednisone or prednisolone in combination with low-dose ursodeoxycholic acid.

6. Calcineurin inhibitors and mycophenolate mofetil may be effective in patients with refractory disease or intolerance to the primary medications.

Definition

1. Self-perpetuating hepatic inflammation of unknown cause characterized by interface hepatitis, hypergammaglobulinemia, and autoantibodies

2. Other diseases that have similar features have been excluded, including Wilson disease, chronic viral hepatitis, drug-induced liver disease (most commonly, minocycline or nitrofurantoin), celiac disease, nonalcoholic steatohepatitis, PBC, and PSC.

NOMENCLATURE

1. The designation autoimmune hepatitis, or idiopathic autoimmune hepatitis, indicates that the disease does not have a recognized etiologic agent and must be distinguished from diseases of similar phenotype that have well-defined causes.

2. Type 1 and type 2 autoimmune hepatitis are clinical descriptors that distinguish patients with antinuclear (ANA) and/or smooth muscle (SMA) antibodies from those with antibodies to liver kidney microsome type 1 (anti-LKM1), respectively.

Diagnosis

1. Codified criteria for *definite* and *probable* diagnoses have been established by an international panel (Table 7.1).

TABLE 7.1 ■ **International Criteria for Definite or Probable Diagnosis of Autoimmune Hepatitis**

Diagnostic Features	Definite Diagnosis	Probable Diagnosis
Exclusion of other diseases	Alcohol intake <25 g/day No hepatotoxic drugs Normal α-1 AT phenotype Normal ceruloplasmin level Normal iron and ferritin levels No active hepatitis A, B, or C	Alcohol intake <50 g/day No hepatotoxic drugs Heterozygous α-1 AT phenotype Abnormal copper or ceruloplasmin level (Wilson disease excluded) Nonspecific iron or ferritin abnormalities No active hepatitis A, B, or C
Inflammatory indices	Predominant serum AST and ALT abnormalities Serum AP normal or ≤2-fold ULN	Predominant serum AST and ALT abnormalities Serum AP >2-fold ULN
Autoantibodies	ANA, SMA, or anti-LKM1 >1:80 in adults and >1:20 in children No AMA	ANA, SMA, or anti-LKM1 >1:40 in adults or any titer/level in children No AMA Absent ANA, SMA and anti-LKM1 but positive for atypical pANCA, anti-SLA, anti-LC1, or anti-ASGPR
Immunoglobulins	Globulin, γ-globulin, or IgG level >1.5-fold ULN	Hypergammaglobulinemia
Histologic findings	Interface hepatitis (moderate–severe) No biliary lesions, granulomas, or prominent changes suggestive of another disease	Interface hepatitis (moderate–severe) No biliary lesions, granulomas, or prominent changes suggestive of another disease

ALT, Alanine aminotransferase; *AMA,* antimitochondrial antibodies; *ANA,* antinuclear antibodies; *AP,* alkaline phosphatase; *ASGPR,* asialoglycoprotein receptor; *AST,* aspartate aminotransferase; *AT,* antitrypsin; *IgG,* immunoglobulin G; *LC1,* liver cytosol type 1; *LKM1,* liver kidney microsome type 1; *pANCA,* perinuclear antineutrophil cytoplasmic antibodies; *SLA,* soluble liver antigen; *SMA,* smooth muscle antibodies; *ULN,* upper limit of normal ranges.

Adapted from Alvarez F, Berg PA, Bianchi FB, et al. *J Hepatol.* 1999;31:929–938, with permission of Elsevier BV and the European Association for the Study of the Liver.

2. Two scoring systems developed by the International Autoimmune Hepatitis Group (IAIHG) can support clinical judgment in the diagnosis of difficult cases, but neither has been validated by prospective studies. For both scoring systems antibody levels are determined by indirect immunofluorescence and expressed in titers.
   a. Revised original scoring system (Table 7.2)
      ■ Developed as research tool to ensure comparable patient populations in clinical studies; subsequently used as diagnostic aid in clinical practice
      ■ Comprehensive template that evaluates 13 clinical categories, renders 27 grades, including response to glucocorticoid treatment, and yields a total score that supports a "definite" or "probable" diagnosis
      ■ Sensitivity, 100%; specificity, 73%; and accuracy, 82% using retrospective clinical experiences as the gold standard
      ■ Major value: Enables comprehensive clinical evaluation of all pertinent disease features before or after treatment and supports clinical judgment in difficult cases
   b. Simplified scoring system (Table 7.3)
      ■ Developed to ease application at bedside
      ■ Evaluates four clinical categories; renders nine possible grades; and yields a total score that supports a "definite" or "probable" diagnosis

TABLE 7.2 ■ **Revised Original International Scoring System for the Diagnosis of Autoimmune Hepatitis**

Variable	Finding	Score	Variable	Score
Gender	Female	+2	Alcohol use <25 g/day	+2
AP:AST or ALT ratio	>3	−2	>60 g/day	−2
	<1.5	+2	HLA DRB1*03 or DRB1*04	+1
γ-globulin or IgG levels	>2-fold ULN	+3	Concurrent immune disease	+2
	1.5–2-fold ULN	+2	Other liver-related markers	+2
	1–1.4-fold ULN	+1	Interface hepatitis	+3
ANA, SMA, or anti-LKM1	>1:80	+3	Plasmacytic infiltrate	+1
	1:80	+2	Hepatocyte rosettes	+1
	1:40	+1	No characteristic features	−5
	<1:40	0	Biliary changes	−3
AMA	Positive	−4	Fat, granulomas, other	−3
Viral markers	Positive	−3	Complete treatment response	+2
	Negative	+3	Relapse after treatment	+3
Hepatotoxic drugs	Yes	−4		
	No	+1		

Pretreatment score:	**Posttreatment score:**
Definite diagnosis **>15**	Definite diagnosis **>17**
Probable diagnosis **10–15**	Probable diagnosis **12–17**

AMA, Antimitochondrial antibodies; *ANA*, antinuclear antibodies; *AP*, alkaline phosphatase; *ALT*, alanine aminotransferase; *AST*, aspartate aminotransferase; *HLA*, human leukocyte antigen; *IgG*, immunoglobulin G; *LKM1*, liver kidney microsome type 1; *SMA*, smooth muscle antibodies; *ULN*, upper limit of normal range.

Adapted from Alvarez F, Berg PA, Bianchi FB, et al. *J Hepatol.* 1999;31:929–938, with permission of Elsevier BV and the European Association for the Study of the Liver.

- Does not grade treatment response
- Sensitivity, 95%; specificity, 90%; and accuracy, 92% using retrospective clinical experiences as the gold standard
- Major value: Ease of application and support of clinical judgment in difficult cases

Pathogenesis

1. Molecular mimicry between foreign and self-antigens induces loss of immune tolerance to self-antigens.
2. Imprecise (promiscuous) targeting by activated lymphocytes extends the immune response to homologous antigens (epitope spread).
3. The receptor-mediated (extrinsic) apoptotic pathway is activated by liver-infiltrating CD8+ lymphocytes especially around portal tracts (interface hepatitis).
4. Apoptotic bodies become neoantigens, and their inadequate clearance stimulates the production of autoantibodies and the adaptive immune response in a self-amplification loop.
5. Apoptotic bodies stimulate Kupffer cells to release chemokines and reactive oxygen species that increase the apoptosis of hepatocytes and activate hepatic stellate cells to transform into myofibroblasts.

TABLE 7.3 ■ **Simplified International Scoring System for the Diagnosis of Autoimmune Hepatitis**

Variable	Finding	Score
Autoantibodies		
ANA or SMA	1:40	+1
	≥1:80	+2
Anti-LKM1	≥1:40	+2
Anti-SLA	Positive	+2
Serum Immunoglobulin Level		
Immunoglobulin G	>ULN	+1
	>1.1-fold ULN	+2
Histologic Findings		
Interface hepatitis, no incompatible findings	Compatible with AIH	+1
Interface hepatitis, lymphoplasmacytic infiltration	Typical of AIH	+2
Viral Markers		
Hepatitis A, B, and C markers	Negative	+2
Aggregate score:		
Definite diagnosis		**≥7**
Probable diagnosis		**6**

AIH, Autoimmune hepatitis; *ANA*, antinuclear antibodies; *LKM1*, liver kidney microsome type 1; *SLA*, soluble liver antigen; *SMA*, smooth muscle antibodies; *ULN*, upper limit of normal range.

Adapted from Hennes EM, Zeniya M, Czaja AJ, et al. *Hepatology*. 2008;48:169–176, with permission of John Wiley & Sons, Inc. and the American Association for the Study of Liver Disease.

6. Activated Kupffer cells and hepatic stellate cells generate reactive oxygen species.
7. Reactive oxygen species increase permeability of the inner membrane of hepatocyte mitochondria (intrinsic apoptotic pathway), which allows release of cytochrome c into the cytoplasm, formation of a macromolecular complex (apoptosome), and activation of a caspase cascade that enhances the apoptosis of hepatocytes.
8. Proinflammatory and immune cells bearing ligands for specific chemokines migrate to sites of liver injury attracted by the chemokines (especially CXCL9 and CXCL10).
9. Regulatory T cells with antiinflammatory and immunosuppressive actions are attracted to the sites of tissue injury and counterregulate the proinflammatory response.
10. Deficiencies in the number and function of the regulatory T cells, possibly aided by a perturbed (galectan 9–mediated) ligation pathway, may favor the proinflammatory response and impair the apoptosis of type 1 T helper (Th1) lymphocytes and dendritic cells.
11. The release of proinflammatory cytokines (interleukin [IL]-1, IL-12, tumor necrosis factor-alpha, interferon-gamma) by cells of the innate and adaptive immune response increase the differentiation and proliferation of antigen-sensitized liver-infiltrating CD8[+] lymphocytes and support a cell-mediated form of cytotoxicity.
12. The release of the antiinflammatory cytokines (IL-4, IL-5, IL-10, and IL-13) counterregulate the proinflammatory response and promote the differentiation of B lymphocytes into plasma cells that produce antibodies and support an antibody-dependent form of cytotoxicity mediated by natural killer cells.

13. Genetic factors within (*DRB1*0301, DRB1*0401, DRB1*1301, DQB1*0201, DRB*07*) and outside (polymorphisms of *CTLA-4, Fas, TNFA, VDR, STAT4, TGF-β1, SH2B3,* and *CARD10*) the MHC vary in different ethnic populations and age groups, and they can affect occurrence, clinical phenotype, severity, and outcome.

14. Natural killer T (NKT) cells and gamma delta lymphocytes have both stimulatory and inhibitory immune actions and may be key regulators of the proinflammatory response.

15. The role of regulatory T cells has been challenged by findings that cells defined by the phenotype, CD4⁺CD25⁺CD127⁺(low)Foxp3⁺, are increased in number in the peripheral blood and liver tissue of patients with autoimmune hepatitis and have unimpaired immunosuppressive function.

16. Cytochrome P450 2D6 (CYP2D6) and formiminotransferase cyclodeaminase (FTCD) are the principal target antigens in autoimmune hepatitis characterized by the presence of anti-LKM1.

Classification

1. **Type 1 autoimmune hepatitis**
   a. Characterized by SMA and/or ANA
   b. Atypical perinuclear antineutrophil cytoplasmic antibodies (pANCA) are present in 50% to 92%, and antibodies to soluble liver antigen (anti-SLA) are present in 15%.
   c. **Most common type and affects all ages**
   d. Female-to-male ratio is 3.6 to 1.
   e. Concurrent extrahepatic immune diseases in 38%, including the following:
      - Autoimmune thyroiditis (12%)
      - Graves disease (6%)
      - Ulcerative colitis (6%)
      - Celiac disease (1% to 3%)
      - Rheumatoid arthritis (1%)
      - Pernicious anemia (1%)
      - Systemic sclerosis (1%)
      - Coombs-positive hemolytic anemia (1%)
      - Idiopathic thrombocytopenic purpura (1%)
      - Leukocytoclastic vasculitis (1%)
      - Nephritis (1%)
      - Erythema nodosum (1%)
      - Fibrosing alveolitis (1%)
   f. Acute onset in 40% and acute severe (fulminant) presentation in 3% to 6%
   g. **Associated with *DRB1*0301* (North America and northern Europe), *DRB1*0401* (North America and northern Europe), *DRB1*0404* (Mexico), *DRB1*0405* (Japan), *DRB*1301* (South America)**
   h. Principal autoantigen unknown
   i. Cirrhosis at presentation in 25%
2. **Type 2 autoimmune hepatitis**
   a. Characterized by anti-LKM1
   b. Antibodies to liver cytosol type 1 (anti-LC1) in 32%
   c. Atypical pANCA absent
   d. Affects mainly children (age range, 2 to 14 years)
   e. Only 4% of North American adults with autoimmune hepatitis have anti-LKM1.
   f. Commonly associated with concurrent immune diseases, including vitiligo, insulin-dependent diabetes mellitus, and autoimmune thyroiditis

g. Frequent organ-specific autoantibodies (antibodies to parietal cells, thyroid, or islets of Langerhans)

h. Acute or acute severe (fulminant) presentation possible

i. **DQB1∗0201 is the principal genetic risk factor in strong linkage disequilibrium with DRB1∗07 and DRB1∗03.**

j. **CYP2D6 is the principal target antigen.**

k. **FTCD is targeted by anti-LC1.**

l. Five antigenic sites are located within recombinant CYP2D6, and amino acid sequence between positions 193 and 212 is main epitope of anti-LKM1.

m. Homologies exist between recombinant CYP2D6 and the genomes of hepatitis C virus, cytomegalovirus, and herpes simplex virus type 1 providing an opportunity for cross-reactive immune responses.

n. Anti-LKM1 in 10% of patients with chronic hepatitis C in Europe, but rarely in the United States

o. **Similarities in clinical phenotype, genetic factors, treatment strategies, and outcome between type 1 and type 2 autoimmune hepatitis have challenged the need for the classifications, especially in adults, and the IAIHG has not endorsed typing.**

p. Typing has greatest value in research studies to maintain homogeneity of patient populations and experimental models.

Epidemiology

1. The mean annual incidence of type 1 autoimmune hepatitis is 1 to 1.9 cases per 100,000 per year in ethnically similar populations of Western Europe, and the point prevalence is 11 to 16.9 per 100,000.

2. Type 2 autoimmune hepatitis is rare, with an estimated prevalence of 3 cases per 1,000,000 and an annual incidence of 0.16 per 1,000,000.

3. Autoimmune hepatitis accounts for 11% to 23% of cases of chronic hepatitis and affects 100,000 to 200,000 persons in the United States.

4. Autoimmune hepatitis results in 2.6% of liver transplants in Europe and 5.9% in the United States.

5. Its prevalence is highest in white populations of northern Europe, North America, and Australia and may relate to their high frequency of human leukocyte antigen (HLA) DRB1∗03 and DRB1∗04.

6. **Autoimmune hepatitis occurs in diverse ethnic groups and all age ranges worldwide.**

Presentation (Table 7.4)

1. **Chronic hepatitis**
   a. Typically indolent liver inflammation associated with fatigue and arthralgia
   b. Jaundice may be present.
   c. Cirrhosis at presentation in 25% suggests chronic aggressive subclinical phase.

2. **Acute or acute severe (fulminant) hepatitis**
   a. Acute onset in 25% to 75% of patients
   b. Acute severe (fulminant) presentation characterized by hepatic encephalopathy within 26 weeks of disease discovery in 3% to 6% of North American and European patients
   c. Classic features may be absent or less pronounced in acute severe (fulminant) disease:
      ▪ ANA absent or weakly positive in 29% to 39%
      ▪ Serum immunoglobulin G (IgG) level normal in 25% to 39%
      ▪ Centrilobular hemorrhagic necrosis and massive or submassive liver necrosis in 86%
      ▪ Disease-specific heterogeneous hypoattenuated regions within the liver by unenhanced computed tomography (CT) in 65%

TABLE 7.4 ■ **Presentations of Autoimmune Hepatitis**

Presentation	Features
Chronic hepatitis	Fatigue and arthralgia common symptoms Jaundice frequent basis for medical evaluation Cirrhosis present in 25%
Acute hepatitis	Symptoms and manifestations develop abruptly coincident with the onset or discovery of autoimmune hepatitis May resemble acute viral or drug-induced hepatitis May reflect spontaneous exacerbation of chronic disease Occurs in 25%–75% of patients
Acute severe (fulminant)	Hepatic encephalopathy develops within 26 weeks of disease discovery ANA absent or weakly positive in 29%–39% Serum IgG level normal in 25%–39% Centrilobular hemorrhagic necrosis and massive or submassive liver necrosis in 86% Heterogeneous hypoattenuated regions within the liver by unenhanced CT in 65% Occurs in 3%–6% of North American and European patients
Asymptomatic	Occurs in 25%–34% Symptoms develop in 26%–70% Histologic findings similar to symptomatic patients
Antibody negative	Typical findings except negative for ANA, SMA, LKM1 Comprehensive scoring system diagnostic in 19%–34% Anti-SLA, atypical pANCA or other markers may support diagnosis IgA antibodies to tissue transglutaminase or endomysium may implicate celiac disease
Graft dysfunction after liver transplantation	Recurrent AIH in 8%–12% after 1 year and 36%–68% after 5 years De novo AIH in 1%–7% up to 9 years (mainly children)
AIH-PBC overlap syndrome	Predominant features of AIH, AMA, and histologic features of bile duct injury or loss
AIH-PSC overlap syndrome	Predominant features of AIH, absent AMA, histologic features of bile duct injury or loss, and cholangiographic changes of focal biliary strictures and dilatations
AIH-cholestasis overlap syndrome	Predominant features of AIH, absent AMA, histologic features of bile duct injury or loss, and normal cholangiography May include AMA-negative PBC and small duct PSC

AIH, Autoimmune hepatitis; *AMA,* antimitochondrial antibodies; *ANA,* antinuclear antibodies; *CT,* computed tomography; *IgA,* immunoglobulin A; *IgG,* immunoglobulin G; *LKM1,* liver kidney microsome type 1; *pANCA,* perinuclear antineutrophil cytoplasmic antibodies; *PBC,* primary biliary cholangitis; *PSC,* primary sclerosing cholangitis; *SLA,* soluble liver antigen; *SMA,* smooth muscle antibodies.

3. **Asymptomatic presentation**
   a. No symptoms in 25% to 34% at time of newly discovered liver biochemical test abnormalities
   b. Symptoms develop in 26% to 70% within 2 to 120 months (mean interval, 32 months).
   c. Histologic findings are similar between asymptomatic and symptomatic patients at presentation, including moderate to severe interface hepatitis (87% versus 93%), periportal fibrosis (41% versus 41%), and bridging fibrosis (39% versus 48%).
   d. Untreated patients improve spontaneously less frequently (12% versus 63%) and less completely than treated patients with severe symptomatic disease, and they have a lower 10-year survival rate (67% versus 98%).
   e. The asymptomatic state does not preclude the need for treatment.

4. **Antibody-negative (cryptogenic) hepatitis**
   a. Clinical and laboratory findings are typical of autoimmune hepatitis, but ANA, SMA, and anti-LKM1 are absent.
   b. Diagnostic scoring system of the IAIHG or clinical judgment reclassifies 19% to 34% of patients with cryptogenic hepatitis as autoimmune hepatitis.
   c. Implicated as etiology of acute liver failure in 7% of British patients and 24% of Japanese patients
   d. ANA and SMA may emerge later in the course of the disease.
   e. Testing for nonstandard antibodies may direct the diagnosis:
      - Antibodies to soluble liver antigen (anti-SLA) occur in 14% to 20% of seronegative patients and have high specificity for autoimmune hepatitis.
      - Atypical pANCA can support the diagnosis in some patients.
      - Immunoglobulin A (IgA) antibodies to tissue transglutaminase or endomysium may implicate celiac disease as a mimic of autoimmune hepatitis.
   f. Autoantibody-negative patients respond as well to glucocorticoid therapy as autoantibody-positive patients with disease of similar severity.
   g. **Autoimmune hepatitis should be considered in all patients with unexplained acute or chronic hepatitis.**
5. **Graft dysfunction after liver transplantation**
   a. Autoimmune hepatitis recurs after liver transplantation in 8% to 12% after 1 year and 36% to 68% after 5 years (range, 2 months to 12 years).
   b. Hypergammaglobulinemia, increased serum levels of IgG, conventional autoantibodies, and interface hepatitis with or without portal plasma cell infiltration characterize recurrence.
   c. Autoimmune hepatitis can develop de novo in 1% to 7% of patients (mainly children) 1 month to 9 years after transplantation for nonautoimmune liver disease.
   d. **Autoimmune hepatitis must be considered in all patients with graft dysfunction after liver transplantation.**
6. **Overlap syndrome with PBC**
   a. Definition: Features of autoimmune hepatitis coexist with antimitochondrial antibodies (AMA) and histologic findings of bile duct injury or loss.
   b. "Paris criteria" provide objective basis for the diagnosis:
      - Two of three features associated with autoimmune hepatitis, including serum alanine aminotransferase (ALT) level ≥5-fold the upper limit of the normal range (ULN), IgG level ≥2-fold ULN or the presence of SMA, and interface hepatitis on histologic examination
      - Two of three features associated with PBC, including serum alkaline phosphatase level ≥2-fold ULN or gamma-glutamyltranspeptidase (GGTP) level ≥5-fold ULN, AMA, and florid duct lesions or destructive cholangitis on histologic examination
      - The sensitivity and specificity of the Paris criteria are 92% and 97%, respectively, using clinical judgment as the gold standard.
      - The Paris criteria have been endorsed by the European Association for the Study of the Liver (EASL) with the recommendation that diagnosis of this syndrome requires the presence of interface hepatitis.
   c. The predominant disease component influences the initial treatment strategy.
      - Patients with classic features of autoimmune hepatitis and background features of PBC manifested mainly by a serum alkaline phosphatase level ≤2-fold ULN (outside Paris criteria) can respond to conventional glucocorticoid therapy, entering remission in 81% and failing to respond in 14%.
      - Patients with predominately PBC and background features of autoimmune hepatitis can respond to conventional therapy with ursodeoxycholic acid (13 to 15 mg/kg daily).

- Patients with PBC and marked features of autoimmune hepatitis that satisfy the Paris criteria have higher frequencies of esophageal varices, gastrointestinal bleeding, ascites, and death from hepatic failure or requirement for liver transplantation than patients with classic PBC who receive similar therapy with ursodeoxycholic acid.
- Combination therapy with glucocorticoids and ursodeoxycholic acid (13 to 15 mg/kg daily) has been endorsed by EASL for all patients satisfying the Paris criteria despite the lack of strong clinical evidence.
- Limited experience using combined budesonide, azathioprine, and ursodeoxycholic acid has not favored this regimen.

7. **Overlap syndrome with PSC**
   a. Definition: Features of autoimmune hepatitis, cholestatic laboratory findings, histologic evidence of cholestasis including bile duct injury or loss, and focal biliary strictures and dilations by magnetic resonance cholangiography (MRC) or endoscopic retrograde cholangiography (ERC)
   b. Histologic features of bile duct injury, portal edema, and/or ductopenia and normal cholangiogram compatible with small duct PSC
   c. Clues to diagnosis: Inflammatory bowel disease, suboptimal response to glucocorticoid therapy, and/or rising serum alkaline phosphatase level
   d. Variably responsive to glucocorticoids alone or in combination with ursodeoxycholic acid (20% to 100% response in small studies); limited experience with calcineurin inhibitors; and mycophenolate mofetil ineffective in children
   e. Therapy with prednisone or prednisolone and ursodeoxycholic acid (13 to 15 mg/kg daily) is endorsed by EASL and the American Association for the Study of Liver Diseases (AASLD) despite a lack of strong clinical evidence.
   f. Biliary changes suggestive of PSC in 8% of adults with classic autoimmune hepatitis assessed by MRC, but similar frequency of these changes in nonautoimmune liver diseases and hepatic fibrosis rather than PSC is the probable basis for this diagnostic confusion.

8. **Overlap syndrome with undefined cholestasis**
   a. Definition: Features of autoimmune hepatitis with cholestatic laboratory and histologic features, normal cholangiography, and no AMA
   b. Heterogeneous syndrome that probably includes patients with AMA-negative PBC or small duct PSC
   c. Poor response to glucocorticoid regimen, and variable response to ursodeoxycholic acid alone or in combination with glucocorticoids
   d. No regimen has been preferred or endorsed by a liver society
   e. Treatment is individualized to predominant manifestations and commonly includes low-dose ursodeoxycholic acid (13 to 15 mg/kg daily) alone or in combination with a glucocorticoid (10 mg daily).
   f. Clinical and laboratory improvements may not be accompanied by histologic improvements.

Clinical and Laboratory Features

1. Easy fatigability is the most common symptom (85%), whereas weight loss is unusual and intense pruritus precludes the diagnosis.
2. Hepatomegaly (78%) and jaundice (69%) are the most common physical findings of severe or advanced disease, and thrombocytopenia is indicative of cirrhosis.
3. **Serum aspartate aminotransferase (AST) or ALT levels ≥10-fold ULN or ≥5-fold ULN in conjunction with serum γ-globulin level ≥2-fold ULN indicate severe disease and compel the prompt institution of therapy (3-year mortality of 50% and 10-year mortality of 90% if untreated).**

4. Hyperbilirubinemia is present in 83%, and the serum level is ≤3-fold ULN in 54%.
5. **Serum alkaline phosphatase level is increased in 81%, but it is ≤2-fold ULN in 67%; levels >4-fold ULN occur in only 10% and suggest another disease or an overlap syndrome.**
6. Polyclonal hypergammaglobulinemia is typical, and an increased serum IgG level is a hallmark of the disease.
7. Concurrent ulcerative colitis indicates the need for MRC cholangiography or ERC to exclude PSC.

HISTOLOGIC FEATURES

1. Interface hepatitis (Fig. 7.1) is required for the diagnosis, but lobular (panacinar) hepatitis (Fig. 7.2) in conjunction with interface hepatitis is within the histologic spectrum.
2. Plasma cell infiltration (Fig. 7.3) is characteristic but not specific or essential for the diagnosis (present in 66%).
3. Centrilobular (zone 3) necrosis may be an early or severe histologic stage, coexists with interface hepatitis in 78%, and can accompany cirrhosis.

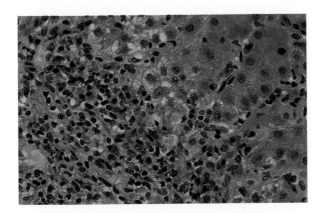

Fig. 7.1 Histopathology of interface hepatitis in autoimmune hepatitis. Disruption of the limiting plate of the portal tract by mononuclear inflammatory infiltrate that extends into the acinus is shown (hematoxylin and eosin, ×400).

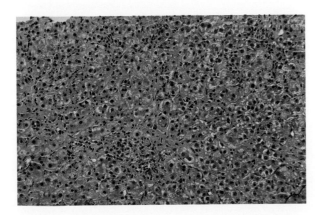

Fig. 7.2 Histopathology of panacinar hepatitis in autoimmune hepatitis. Mononuclear inflammatory cells line the sinusoidal spaces in association with liver cell degenerative and regenerative changes (hematoxylin and eosin, ×100).

4. **Prominent cholestatic changes (bile duct destruction, ductopenia) or histologic features suggestive of another disease (e.g., steatosis, granulomas, copper, or iron) suggest an alternative diagnosis.**
5. Cirrhosis is present in 25% of patients at diagnosis.

AUTOANTIBODIES

1. Standard autoantibodies (Table 7.5)
   a. **ANA**
      - Present in 80% of patients with autoimmune hepatitis
      - Lack both organ and disease specificity, occurring in 21% of patients with chronic alcoholic liver disease, 32% with nonalcoholic fatty liver disease, 28% with chronic viral hepatitis, and 39% with PBC or PSC
      - Specificity only 76%, and diagnostic accuracy only 56% if isolated finding

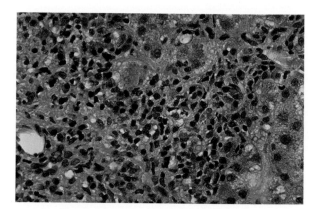

Fig. 7.3 Histopathology of plasma cell infiltration in autoimmune hepatitis. Plasma cells typified by perinuclear cytoplasmic haloes contribute to the mononuclear inflammatory infiltrate within the portal tract (hematoxylin and eosin, ×400).

TABLE 7.5 ■ **Standard and Nonstandard Antibodies in Autoimmune Hepatitis**

Standard Antibodies

Type	Features
ANA	Present in 80% of AIH Specificity, 76%; accuracy, 56% as single marker Supports diagnosis of type 1 AIH
SMA	Present in 63% of AIH; concurrent with ANA in 43% Specificity, 96%; accuracy, 61% as single marker Specificity, 99%; accuracy, 74% when concurrent with ANA Supports a diagnosis of type 1 AIH
LKM1	Present in 3%–4% of North American adults and 14%–38% of British children Coexists with ANA or SMA in 1%–3% Concurrent with anti-LC1 in 24%–32% Supports a diagnosis of type 2 AIH Directed against CYP2D6

TABLE 7.5 ■ **Standard and Nonstandard Antibodies in Autoimmune Hepatitis—cont'd**

Standard Antibodies

Type	Features
Atypical pANCA	Present in 50%–92% of type 1 AIH; absent in type 2 AIH Detected in chronic ulcerative colitis, PSC, PBC, chronic hepatitis C, and minocycline-induced autoimmune disease May be the sole marker of AIH in cryptogenic chronic hepatitis Reactive against nuclear membrane (not cytoplasm) of human neutrophils Directed against β-tubulin isotype 5 in 88% of seropositive patients
SLA	Present in 7%–22% with AIH (15% in the United States) Specificity for AIH, 99% Associated with severity, relapse, mortality, liver transplantation, DRB1*0301 Directed against Sep (O-phosphoserine) tRNA:Sec (selenocysteine) tRNA synthase
Actin	Present in 74% with type 1 AIH and 86% of patients with SMA Occurs in immune-mediated nonliver diseases Concurrent with anti-α-actinin in 66% of patients with AIH Concurrence with anti-α-actinin associated with severity and acute onset Directed against polymerized filamentous actin (F-actin)
LC1	Coexists with anti-LKM1 in 24%–32% of type 2 AIH Mainly detected in European children and young adults aged ≤20 years May be the sole marker in otherwise seronegative patients Directed against formiminotransferase cyclodeaminase
ASGPR	Present in 67%–88% of AIH and frequent in other acute and chronic liver diseases Associated with liver inflammation and disappear with successful therapy Failure to disappear during therapy is associated with relapse May be useful in assessing cryptogenic chronic hepatitis, monitoring treatment response, and determining the end point of treatment Directed against lectins on the hepatocyte surface that bind glycoproteins that lack sialic acid (asialoglycoproteins)

AIH, Autoimmune hepatitis; *ANA,* antinuclear antibodies; *ASGPR,* antibodies to asialoglycoprotein receptor; *CYP2D6,* cytochrome P450 2D6; *LC1,* antibodies to liver cytosol type 1; *LKM1,* antibodies to liver kidney microsome type 1; *pANCA,* perinuclear antineutrophil cytoplasmic antibodies; *PBC,* primary biliary cholangitis; *PSC,* primary sclerosing cholangitis; *SLA,* antibodies to soluble liver antigen; *SMA,* smooth muscle antibodies.

b. **SMA**
- Present in 63% of patients with autoimmune hepatitis
- Lack both organ and disease specificity, occurring in 7% of patients with chronic hepatitis C, 4% with alcoholic liver disease, 6% with PBC, and 16% with PSC
- Specificity is 96% and diagnostic accuracy is 61% if isolated finding.
- **Concurrent with ANA in 43% of patients with autoimmune hepatitis, and the diagnostic specificity of concurrent markers is 99% with a diagnostic accuracy of 74%.**

c. **Anti-LKM1**
- Present in only 3% to 4% of North American adults with autoimmune hepatitis
- Low sensitivity counterbalanced by high specificity (99%)
- Detected in 14% to 38% of British children with autoimmune hepatitis
- Coexist with ANA or SMA in only 1% to 3% of North American adults with autoimmune hepatitis; this exclusivity has justified the designation of two types of autoimmune hepatitis.
- Anti-LC1 coexist with anti-LKM1 in 24% to 32% of patients and may be the sole marker of type 2 autoimmune hepatitis.

2. Nonstandard autoantibodies (see Table 7.5)
  a. Atypical pANCA
    ■ Reactivity against nuclear membrane (not cytoplasm) of human neutrophils warrants the designation "atypical."
    ■ β-tubulin isotype 5, a 50-kDa protein on the inner side of the nuclear envelope, is the target antigen in 88%.
    ■ Atypical pANCA cross-react with an evolutionary precursor bacterial protein, and intestinal microorganisms may trigger the immune response.
    ■ Detected in 50% to 92% of patients with type 1 autoimmune hepatitis
    ■ Absent in type 2 autoimmune hepatitis
    ■ Occur in chronic ulcerative colitis, PSC, PBC, chronic hepatitis C, and minocycline-induced autoimmune disease
    ■ May be sole marker of autoimmune hepatitis and useful in reclassifying patients who are otherwise seronegative or cryptogenic
  b. Anti-SLA
    ■ Present in 7% to 22% of patients, and frequency varies among ethnic groups (occurrence in the United States, 15%; Germany, 19% to 22%, and Japan, 7%).
    ■ Specificity for autoimmune hepatitis, 99%
    ■ Target antigen is a transfer ribonucleic acid (RNA)–protein complex designated as SEPSECS [Sep (O-phosphoserine) tRNA:Sec (selenocysteine) tRNA synthase].
    ■ Detected in 14% to 20% of patients who would otherwise have been classified as seronegative or cryptogenic chronic hepatitis
    ■ Associated with HLA DRB1*0301, severe clinical and histologic findings, long treatment requirement, relapse after drug withdrawal, death from liver failure, and need for liver transplantation
    ■ Antibodies to ribonucleoprotein/Sjögren syndrome A antigen (anti-Ro/SSA) also present in 96% of patients with anti-SLA
  c. Antibodies to actin (anti-actin)
    ■ Directed against polymerized filamentous actin (F-actin)
    ■ Present in 74% with type 1 autoimmune hepatitis and 86% of patients with SMA
    ■ Detected in diverse immune mediated diseases, including systemic lupus erythematosus, Sjögren syndrome, rheumatoid arthritis, celiac disease, diabetes mellitus, autoimmune thyroiditis, and Crohn disease
    ■ Associated with α-actinins, which are cross-linking proteins that bind to actin
    ■ Antibodies to α-actinin (anti-α-actinin) are present in 66% of patients with autoimmune hepatitis and anti-F actin, and the combination of antibodies is specific for the diagnosis.
    ■ Double reactivities for actin and anti-α-actinin have been associated with clinical and histologic severity and an acute onset of disease.
    ■ The baseline serum level of anti-α-actinin may be an independent predictor of treatment response (low levels, treatment response; high levels, incomplete response or relapse after drug withdrawal).
    ■ Assay for anti-actin has not been standardized, and the assay for anti-α-actinin is investigational and not generally available.
  d. Anti-LC1
    ■ Coexist with anti-LKM1 in 24% to 32% of patients with type 2 autoimmune hepatitis
    ■ Present in 12% to 33% of patients with chronic hepatitis C and anti-LKM1 and rarely in patients with ANA or SMA
    ■ Directed against the cytosolic enzyme FTCD
    ■ Mainly detected in European children and young adults aged ≤20 years; rare in white North American adults
    ■ Serum levels fluctuate with disease activity and response to treatment.

- May be the sole marker of autoimmune hepatitis in patients seronegative for SMA, ANA, and anti-LKM1
- Assay not generally available in the United States
  e. Antibodies to asialoglycoprotein receptor (anti-ASGPR)
  - Present in 67% to 88% of patients with autoimmune hepatitis
  - Detected in 57% of patients with acute hepatitis A, 35% with acute hepatitis B, 14% to 100% with PBC, 14% with chronic hepatitis C, 8% with alcoholic liver disease, and 7% with chronic hepatitis B
  - Directed against lectins (ASGPR) on the hepatocyte surface that can bind glycoproteins from which sialic acid has been removed (asialoglycoproteins)
  - Associated with laboratory and histologic features of inflammatory activity and disappear during successful glucocorticoid therapy
  - Failure to induce disappearance during treatment associated with relapse after drug withdrawal
  - Potential clinical uses: Assessment of patients seronegative for other markers, monitor treatment response, determine end point of treatment
  - Assay has not been standardized and is not generally available.

Treatment

REGIMENS

1. **Prednisone or prednisolone, in combination with azathioprine,** is the preferred regimen except in patients with severe cytopenia (leukocyte count, $<2.5 \times 10^9/L$; platelet count, $<50 \times 10^9/L$), absent thiopurine methyltransferase (TPMT) activity, or concerns about the effects of azathioprine on pregnancy (Table 7.6).
   a. **All patients warrant treatment regardless of symptom status or laboratory findings because autoimmune hepatitis is a progressive, self-perpetuating, inflammatory liver disease of indefinite duration and fluctuating severity.**
   b. Standard dose regimen: 4-week induction phase followed by maintenance phase using lower doses of the same medications and continued until end point
   c. Weight-based regimen: Used mainly in Europe where prednisolone is preferred over prednisone; doses of prednisolone (1 mg/kg daily) and azathioprine (1 to 2 mg/kg daily)
   d. Azathioprine is a category D drug for pregnancy, and an alternative equally effective regimen using higher doses of prednisone or prednisolone alone should be used during pregnancy.
   e. TPMT activity has not been predictive of azathioprine toxicity in autoimmune hepatitis, but its absence has been associated with bone marrow failure; TPMT activity is appropriate to assess before therapy, especially in cytopenic patients.
   f. **Determinations of leukocyte and platelet counts should be performed at regular intervals (every 1 to 3 months) throughout the treatment period to monitor for myelosuppression (regardless of TMPT activity).**
   g. Continue therapy until normalization of serum AST, ALT, bilirubin, and γ-globulin levels and all histologic manifestations of disease activity have disappeared before considering drug withdrawal.
2. Prednisone or prednisolone alone is an effective alternative regimen to combination therapy; higher doses of glucocorticoid are a substitute for azathioprine (see Table 7.6).
   a. Preferred in patients with severe cytopenia, absent TMPT activity, or pregnancy
   b. Standard dose regimen: 4-week induction phase followed by maintenance phase using a lower dose of the same medication
   c. Associated with higher frequency of glucocorticoid-induced side effects than the combination regimen with azathioprine (44% versus 10%)

TABLE 7.6 ■ Standard Treatment Regimens for Autoimmune Hepatitis

Regimen	Doses		Relative contraindications
Prednisone or prednisolone plus azathioprine	Glucocorticoid: 30 mg × 1 week 20 mg × 1 week 15 mg × 2 weeks 10-mg maintenance until end point	Azathioprine: 50-mg maintenance until end point	Severe cytopenia TPMT deficiency Pregnancy
	Weight-based schedule: 1 mg/kg daily	Weight-based schedule: 1–2 mg/kg daily	
Prednisone or prednisolone monotherapy	60 mg × 1 week 40 mg × 1 week 30 mg × 2 weeks 20-mg maintenance	None	Obesity Osteopenia Emotional instability Brittle diabetes mellitus Labile hypertension Postmenopausal state Acne
Budesonide plus azathioprine	Budesonide: 3 mg × 2–3 times daily (6–9 mg daily)	Azathioprine: 1–2 mg/kg daily	Cirrhosis Severe disease Rescue therapy Concurrent immune-mediated diseases Severe cytopenia TPMT deficiency Pregnancy

TPMT, Thiopurine methyltransferase.

    d. Continue therapy until normalization of serum AST, ALT, bilirubin, and γ-globulin levels and all histologic manifestations of disease activity have disappeared before considering drug withdrawal.
3. Budesonide in combination with azathioprine (see Table 7.6)
    a. Glucocorticoid with high first-pass hepatic clearance (>90%) and metabolites devoid of glucocorticoid activity
    b. Budesonide (3 mg two to three times daily) in combination with azathioprine (1 to 2 mg/kg daily) normalized serum AST and ALT levels more frequently (47% versus 18%) and with fewer side effects (28% versus 53%) than conventional combination therapy with prednisone (40 mg daily tapered to 10 mg daily) and azathioprine (1 to 2 mg/kg daily) when administered for 6 months in a large randomized clinical trial.
    c. Management option, especially in treatment-naïve noncirrhotic patients with mild uncomplicated disease or individuals at risk for glucocorticoid-related complications
    d. Frequency of histologic resolution and durability of response uncertain
    e. Autoimmune hepatitis can "break through" during therapy.
    f. Ineffective as salvage or rescue regimen
    g. Major advantage in pediatric patients is less weight gain.

DRUG-RELATED SIDE EFFECTS

1. Glucocorticoid-induced complications
    a. Cosmetic changes include facial rounding, dorsal hump formation, striae, weight gain, acne, alopecia, and facial hirsutism.

b. Metabolic effects include diabetes mellitus, obesity, hyperlipidemia, and hypertension.

c. Skeletal changes include osteopenia and vertebral compression.

d. Psychiatric effects include emotional instability and psychosis.

e. Somatic effects include cataract formation, pancreatitis, opportunistic infection, and malignancy.

f. Cosmetic changes most common and develop in 80% after 2 years of therapy with glucocorticoid alone or in combination with azathioprine

g. Severe side effects (intolerable obesity, severe cosmetic changes, osteopenia, vertebral compression) compel discontinuation of treatment in 13% and usually develop during treatment with glucocorticoid monotherapy (20 mg daily) for ≥18 months.

h. Preemptive adjunctive management for all patients, especially postmenopausal women, should include:
- Regular weight-bearing exercise
- Calcium and vitamin D_3 supplements
- Periodic bone densitometry if protracted treatment
- Bisphosphonates as indicated for progressive osteopenia
- Vaccination for hepatitis A and hepatitis B if uninfected and seronegative for viral antibodies

2. Azathioprine-induced complications

a. Nausea, vomiting, rash, pancreatitis, opportunistic infection

b. Cholestatic hepatotoxicity (can be mistaken for refractory disease)

c. Cytopenia in 46%, most commonly associated with underlying cirrhosis; warrants discontinuation of the drug in 6%

d. Bone marrow failure, rare

e. Category D drug for pregnancy based on animal studies (congenital defects not observed in clinical experiences with inflammatory bowel disease or transplantation)

f. Extrahepatic malignancy (risk is 1.4-fold that in age- and sex-matched normal population and no cell type predominates)

g. Preemptive adjunctive management should include:
- Determination of TPMT activity pretreatment
- Assessment of leukocyte and platelet counts at 1- to 3-month intervals
- Dose reduction for profound cytopenia (can reverse or stabilize the decline)
- Avoid drug in pregnancy since nonessential in management
- Uncertain value of determining blood thioguanine levels

3. Budesonide-induced complications

a. Typical glucocorticoid-induced side effects mainly in treated patients with cirrhosis presumably because of increased systemic bioavailability of the drug

b. Withdrawal symptoms when replacing prednisone or prednisolone with budesonide presumably because of decreased systemic bioavailability of the drug

c. Concurrent extrahepatic immune-mediated diseases (arthritis, vasculitis) may be exacerbated.

FACTORS THAT AFFECT INITIAL OUTCOME (Table 7.7)

1. Prognostic models

a. Model of End-stage Liver Disease (MELD) score ≥12 points at presentation has sensitivity of 97% and specificity of 68% for treatment failure.

b. Failure of the United Kingdom End-stage Liver Disease (UKELD) score to decrease by at least 2 points within 7 days of treatment has a sensitivity of 85% and specificity of 68% for death from hepatic failure, need for emergency transplantation, or requirement for second-line immunosuppressive medication in patients with icteric autoimmune hepatitis.

TABLE 7.7 ■ **Factors Affecting the Immediate Outcome of Autoimmune Hepatitis**

Factor	Implications
Mathematical models	MELD score ≥12 points at presentation Sensitivity, 97%; specificity, 68% for treatment failure Failure of UKELD score to decrease by ≥2 points within 7 days of treatment in icteric patients Sensitivity, 85%; specificity, 68% for liver-related death, transplantation, or need for next line of drug therapy

Rapidity of treatment response	Inability to normalize or prevent worsening of at least one liver biochemical test (especially serum bilirubin level) within 2 weeks of treatment in patients with multilobular necrosis and associated with:
	    Death from hepatic failure within 4 months
	    Need for liver transplantation evaluation
	Improvement to normal or near-normal liver biochemical test levels and liver tissue within 12 months of treatment compared with ≥36 months and associated with:
	    Lower frequency of cirrhosis, 18% vs. 54%
	    Lower frequency of liver transplantation, 2% vs. 15%

Age	≤30 years:
	    Fail conventional glucocorticoid therapy more commonly than patients ≥60 years old (24% vs. 5%) and have HLA DRB1*03 more often (58% vs. 23%)
	≥60 years:
	    Have cirrhosis more commonly (33% vs. 10%), fail treatment less frequently, and have HLA DRB1*04 more often (47% vs. 13%) than patients aged ≤30 years

HLA phenotype	HLA DRB1*0301:
	    Associated with early age onset, severe disease, slow or nonresponse to treatment, relapse after drug withdrawal, and need for liver transplantation in white North American and British adults
	HLA DRB1*0401:
	    Associated with complete remission, low frequency of progression to cirrhosis or need for liver transplantation in northern European patients

Concurrent immune-mediated diseases	Concurrent inflammatory bowel disease associated with PSC in 41% and poor response to glucocorticoids ASC in 50% of children with AIH and associated with a shortened transplant-free survival
Serologic markers	Anti-SLA associated with HLA DRB1*0301, relapse, and reduced overall and transplant-free survival Anti-actin and anti-α-actinin associated with clinical, laboratory, and histologic severity

AIH, Autoimmune hepatitis; *anti-SLA,* antibodies to soluble liver antigen; *ASC,* autoimmune sclerosing cholangitis; *HLA,* human leukocyte antigen; *MELD,* Model for End-stage Liver Disease; *PSC,* primary sclerosing cholangitis; *UKELD,* United Kingdom End-stage Liver Disease.

2. Rapidity of treatment response
   a. Multilobular necrosis on histologic examination and inability to normalize or prevent worsening of at least one liver biochemical test abnormality within 2 weeks of glucocorticoid treatment (especially failure of hyperbilirubinemia to improve) associated with death from hepatic failure within 4 months and justify liver transplantation evaluation
   b. Improvement to normal or near-normal liver biochemical test levels and liver histology within 12 months of conventional glucocorticoid treatment associated with lower frequency of progression to cirrhosis (18% versus 54%) and liver transplantation (2% versus 15%) than patients who require continuous therapy for ≥36 months to achieve the same response
3. Clinical phenotype at presentation
   a. Individuals who are ≤30 years old fail conventional glucocorticoid therapy more commonly than individuals ≥60 years old (24% versus 5%), and they have HLA DRB1*03 more often (58% versus 23%).

TABLE 7.8 ■ **Treatment Outcomes in Autoimmune Hepatitis**

Outcome	Definition	Frequency
Remission	Normal liver biochemical tests and liver tissue	Normal liver tests in 66%–91% ≤2 years Normal liver tissue in 22% ≤2 years Near-normal liver tissue in 45% ≤2 years
Treatment-free state	Sustained remission after treatment	Achievable in 19%–40%
Relapse	Recurrent symptoms, increase in serum AST or ALT ≥3-fold ULN, and hypergammaglobulinemia	Occurs in 50% within 6 months and as many as 86% within 3 years Can progress to cirrhosis in 10% or liver failure in 3%
Incomplete response	Improvement but no remission after 3 years	Occurs in 13% Increasing risk of drug-related side effects
Treatment failure	Worsening of liver biochemical tests and/or histologic findings despite compliance with therapy	Occurs in 9%

ALT, Alanine aminotransferase; *AST*, aspartate aminotransferase; *ULN*, upper limit of normal.

b. Individuals who are ≥60 years old have cirrhosis more commonly at presentation (33% versus 10%), fail conventional glucocorticoid treatment less frequently, and have HLA DRB1*04 more often (47% versus 13%) than adults aged ≤30 years.

c. HLA DRB1*0301 is associated with early age onset disease, severe inflammatory activity, slow or nonresponse to treatment, relapse after drug withdrawal, and need for liver transplantation in white North American and British adults.

d. Treatment failure is uncommon in patients with HLA DRB1*04, and HLA DRB1*0401 and is associated with a high frequency of complete remissions and lower frequencies of cirrhosis and need for liver transplantation in northern European patients.

e. Cirrhosis at presentation has been associated with poor survival and the requirement for liver transplantation in some studies.

f. Concurrent inflammatory bowel disease is associated with cholangiographic changes of PSC in 41% and poor response to glucocorticoids.

g. Autoimmune sclerosing cholangitis is present in 50% of children with autoimmune hepatitis and associated with a shortened transplant-free survival.

h. Gender does not influence the frequency of treatment response or long-term outcome unless men with HLA DRB1*03 are compared with women with HLA DRB1*04.

4. Serologic markers

a. Anti-SLA are associated with reduced overall and liver-transplant-free survival.

b. Anti-SLA are present in 53% to 100% of patients who relapse after glucocorticoid withdrawal, and 83% of patients with these antibodies have HLA DRB1*0301.

c. Antibodies to both actin and α-actinin are associated with clinical (91% versus 52%) and histologic activity (91% versus 50%) more frequently and with higher serum AST levels at presentation (328±760 U/L versus 125±219 U/L) than untreated patients without these antibodies.

TREATMENT OUTCOMES (Table 7.8)

1. **Remission** (Fig. 7.4)

a. Normal liver biochemical test levels in 66% to 91% of patients within 2 years

b. Normal liver histology in 22% and near-normal liver tissue in 45%

c. Nonprogression or reversal of hepatic fibrosis in 79%

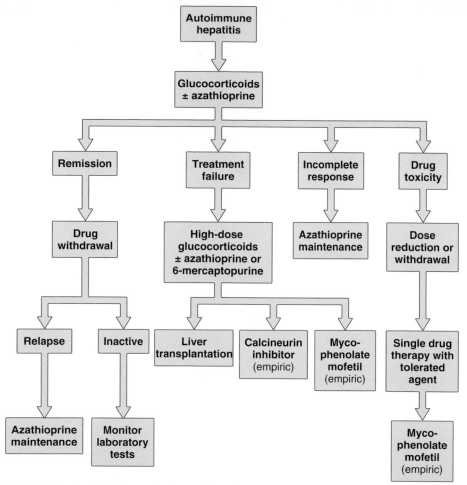

Fig. 7.4 Treatment algorithm and outcomes for autoimmune hepatitis. The diagnosis of autoimmune hepatitis justifies treatment with prednisone alone or a lower dose in combination with azathioprine (glucocorticoids
with or without azathioprine). Treatment is continued until remission, treatment failure, incomplete response,
or drug toxicity. Depending on treatment response, additional treatment may be necessary, including the
empiric use of nonstandard salvage therapies for treatment failure or drug toxicity (calcineurin inhibitors or mycophenolate mofetil). Mycophenolate mofetil has been effective for patients with azathioprine intolerance. Liver
transplantation is the most effective salvage therapy and should not be deferred in decompensated patients.

    d. Average treatment duration until normal liver tests and normal or near-normal liver his-
       tology, 22 months in the United States and 24 months in Europe
    e. Remission within 12 months is associated with a lower frequency of progression to cirrhosis
       (18% versus 54%) and need for liver transplantation (2% versus 15%) than remission after
       ≥3 years of treatment.
  2. **Incomplete response** (see Fig. 7.4)
    a. Connotes improvement insufficient to satisfy remission criteria after 3 years of treatment
    b. Occurs in 13%
    c. The frequency of side effects exceeds the frequency of achieving remission if standard
       therapy is extended beyond 3 years.

3. **Treatment failure** (see Fig. 7.4)
   a. Connotes worsening of liver biochemical tests and/or histologic findings despite compliance with treatment strategy
   b. Occurs in 9%
   c. **Requires reconfirmation of original diagnosis, laboratory tests, and liver tissue examination to exclude viral hepatitis, overlap syndrome, nonalcoholic (glucocorticoid-induced) fatty liver disease, and azathioprine- or other drug-induced liver injury**
4. **Drug toxicity** (see Fig. 7.4)
   a. Severe glucocorticoid side effects (mainly cosmetic changes) occur in 13% of patients, and severe azathioprine intolerance (mainly nausea, vomiting, and cytopenia) develop in <10%.
   b. The incriminated drug must be reduced in dose or discontinued and the tolerated medication increased in dose to stabilize laboratory tests.
   c. Dose reduction or withdrawal ameliorates or reverses most side effects, especially nausea, vomiting, rash, and cytopenia.
   d. Mycophenolate mofetil (1 to 2 g daily) has been effective in 58% of azathioprine-intolerant patients, but therapy is associated with side effects (in 3% to 34%) that may resemble those of azathioprine, especially cytopenia, and is contraindicated in pregnancy.

MANAGEMENT AFTER REMISSION

1. Treatment withdrawal
   a. **Treatment withdrawal should only be considered when there has been complete resolution of symptoms, normalization of serum AST, ALT, bilirubin, and γ-globulin levels, and reversion of hepatic architecture to normal.**
   b. Liver tissue examination before drug withdrawal optimizes the opportunity for a treatment-free state since histologic changes are present in 55% of patients with normal laboratory tests.
   c. Histologic resolution lags behind clinical and laboratory resolution by 3 to 6 months, and the liver tissue examination should be performed no sooner than 3 months after normal liver biochemical test levels are achieved.
   d. Withdrawal should be gradual and well monitored over a 6-week period (Table 7.9). Serum AST, ALT, bilirubin, and γ-globulin levels should be performed every 3 weeks during and after discontinuation of the drugs to monitor for relapse for at least 3 months. Tests should then be performed every 6 months for 1 year and then at annual intervals indefinitely if remission is sustained.
   e. The decision to terminate therapy must be individualized and modified by the completeness of the disease response and estimates of long-term tolerance of the medication.
2. Treatment-free state (see Table 7.8)
   a. Connotes a clinically inactive, nonprogressive state during the period of observation after drug withdrawal
   b. Frequency of success and duration of inactivity are variable.
   c. Achievable in 19% to 40% of patients in follow-up studies of at least 3 years' duration
   d. Remissions sustained for at least 1 year after withdrawal have a low frequency of subsequent relapse (≤10%), and durations of inactivity have ranged from 68 to 198 months (mean, 130±7 months).
   e. **Complete laboratory and histologic resolution before drug withdrawal is the main factor associated with a sustained treatment-free state.** Of the 22% of patients who achieve normal liver tissue, 72% maintain normal laboratory tests for 71±11 months after drug withdrawal, including 62% for >5 years (range, 5.4 to 11.5 years).

TABLE 7.9 ■ **Withdrawal Schedule after Remission in Autoimmune Hepatitis**

| Weeks after remission | Combination Regimen | | Monotherapy |
	Prednisone or prednisolone (mg/day)	Azathioprine (mg/day)	Prednisone or prednisolone (mg/day)
1	7.5	50	15
2	7.5	50	10
3	5	50	5
4	5	25	5
5	2.5	25	2.5
6	2.5	25	2.5
Thereafter	None	None	None

Indefinite monitoring for relapse: Serum AST, ALT, and γ-globulin levels at 3-week intervals during and after drug withdrawal for at least 3 months, then at 6-month intervals for 1 year, then at annual intervals lifelong

ALT, Alanine aminotransferase; *AST*, aspartate aminotransferase.

   f. Histologic resolution implies the absence of plasma cells (<5% to 10% of the portal cell population).
   g. Age and ethnicity, fibrotic stage during therapy, rapidity of the treatment response, concurrent immune diseases, presence of anti-SLA, and HLA phenotype (DRB1*0301) may also influence occurrence of a treatment-free state, but none has been recognized across studies.
3. Relapse after drug withdrawal (see Table 7.8)
   a. Occurs in 50% within 6 months and as many as 86% within 3 years
   b. Defined by increase in serum AST or ALT level ≥3-fold ULN and hypergammaglobulinemia
   c. Liver tissue examination is not necessary if laboratory findings are consistent with relapse, with no other diagnostic considerations.
   d. Reinstitution of the original treatment regimen induces laboratory resolution in 94% after 4±1 months and improvement to normal or near-normal liver tissue in 59% after 8±2 months.
   e. Relapse can progress to cirrhosis in 10% or liver failure in 3%, and the early detection of relapse and prompt reinstitution of therapy are essential in minimizing these risks.
   f. Serum AST, ALT, and γ-globulin levels should be monitored at 3-week intervals during and after drug withdrawal for at least 3 months, then at 6-month intervals for 1 year, then at lifelong annual intervals (longest interval before relapse, 22 years).
   g. The frequency of relapse increases with each previous relapse, and the consequences of repeated relapses include drug-induced side effects (>70%), progression to cirrhosis (38%), and death from liver failure or requirement for liver transplantation (20%).
   h. **Long-term maintenance therapy with azathioprine (2 mg/kg daily) is preferred after the first relapse and following restoration of normal laboratory tests during retreatment with the original regimen.**
   i. Indefinite low-dose prednisone or prednisolone (up to 10 mg daily; median dose, 7.5 mg daily) can be used after the first relapse and restoration of normal laboratory tests if azathioprine intolerance is suspected.
   j. Long-term maintenance regimens with azathioprine may require the periodic addition of a glucocorticoid if laboratory instability emerges.

4. Indefinite treatment without an attempt at immediate drug withdrawal
    a. Treatment can be maintained indefinitely usually in a reduced dose guided by patient tolerance and laboratory changes without a commitment to drug withdrawal.
    b. Risks of relapse and retreatment can be avoided, but treatment may be lifelong and include patients who potentially could be treatment-free (19% to 40%).
    c. **Long-term low-dose maintenance regimens with prednisone or prednisolone (<10 mg daily) in combination with azathioprine (25 to 50 mg daily) or azathioprine alone (2 mg/kg daily) to maintain stable liver biochemical test levels are usually well tolerated and do not preclude the opportunity to become treatment-free after a protracted interval of disease inactivity.**
    d. Well-monitored periodic efforts at dose reduction and drug withdrawal are warranted in patients committed to indefinite treatment who have stable inactive disease.
    e. A treatment-free state is ultimately achievable in 12% after low-dose maintenance therapy for 69±8 months (range, 5 to 264 months).
    f. **The main management misstep is to preclude the possibility of a treatment-free state from the outset and implement indefinite therapy without flexibility or individualization.**
    g. The decision between immediate drug withdrawal after remission or indefinite therapy with the possible late opportunity for drug withdrawal must counterbalance patient tolerance of the medication against the low but possible risks of relapse and retreatment.

MANAGEMENT AFTER A SUBOPTIMAL TREATMENT OUTCOME (Table 7.10)

1. Treatment failure
    a. Institute high-dose prednisone or prednisolone (30 mg daily) in conjunction with azathioprine (150 mg daily) or prednisone or prednisolone alone (60 mg daily) if cytopenia or intolerance of azathioprine is present.
    b. Continue the high-dose regimen for at least 1 month and then taper the dose after each month of laboratory improvement until conventional maintenance doses are achieved.
    c. **A high-dose regimen induces clinical and biochemical improvement in 70% within 2 years but histologic resolution in only 20%.**
    d. Indefinite therapy is frequently necessary, with the risk of side effects and liver failure.
    e. Calcineurin inhibitors have been used as rescue agents in multiple small single-center studies, and potential benefits must be counterbalanced against the risk of toxicity.
        ■ **Cyclosporine** (Neoral, 2 to 5 mg/kg daily, with dose adjustments to achieve trough levels of 100 to 300 ng/mL) has led to improvement in 93% of patients in a composite of 10 studies involving 133 patients, including 32 patients with glucocorticoid intolerance or refractory disease. No response, noncompliance, or drug intolerance in 7%
        ■ **Tacrolimus** (0.5 to 1 mg daily adjusted according to tolerance to a maintenance level of 1 to 3 mg daily to achieve a serum level of 3 ng/mL [range, 1.7 to 10.7 ng/mL]) has improved 98% of patients with refractory disease in a composite of 3 studies involving 41 patients. No response or treatment-ending drug intolerance in 2%
        ■ Caveats: Possibility of serious side effects, including neurotoxicity; mainly immunosuppressive rather than antiinflammatory actions; probable indefinite treatment; expensive; ineffective in preventing recurrent or de novo autoimmune hepatitis after liver transplantation; possible paradoxic effect of enhancing autoreactivity; requires experience in administering and monitoring the drug
    f. **Mycophenolate mofetil** (1.5 to 2 g daily) is an alternative rescue agent that has led to improvement in 23% of refractory patients in a composite of 11 small clinical experiences.
        ■ Caveats: Side effects develop in 3% to 34%, most commonly nausea and leukopenia; serious congenital malformations if given during pregnancy, including microtia or anotia,

TABLE 7.10 ■ **Management of Adverse Outcomes in Autoimmune Hepatitis**

Adverse Outcome	Regimen

Relapse after drug withdrawal	Preferred:
	  Original glucocorticoid regimen until normalization of laboratory tests
	  Azathioprine, 2 mg/kg daily, with tapered withdrawal of glucocorticoid
	Alternative (azathioprine intolerant):
	  Original glucocorticoid regimen until normalization of laboratory tests
	  Gradual reduction of glucocorticoid dose to lowest level possible to maintain normal tests (≤10 mg daily; median dose, 7.5 mg daily)

Incomplete response (after 36 months of treatment)	Indefinite individualized combination regimen:
	  Prednisone or prednisolone, <10 mg daily, plus azathioprine, 25–50 mg daily
	Indefinite fixed-dose azathioprine regimen:
	  Azathioprine, 2 mg/kg daily
	Multiple adjustments may be necessary to maintain stable, near-normal liver tests

Treatment failure	Preferred regimen:
	  High-dose prednisone or prednisolone, 30 mg daily, plus azathioprine, 150 mg daily, or prednisone or prednisolone alone, 60 mg daily, if cytopenia or azathioprine intolerance
	  Continue at fixed dose for 1 month
	  Reduce glucocorticoid by 10 mg and azathioprine by 25 mg each month of laboratory improvement
	  Return to conventional maintenance doses
	Alternative regimens:
	  Cyclosporine (Neoral, 2–5 mg/kg daily, trough levels of 100–300 ng/mL): Improvement, 93%; side effects, ≤7%
	  Tacrolimus (0.5–1 mg daily; adjusted to 1–3 mg daily; serum level, 3 ng/mL [range, 1.7–10.7 ng/ml]): Improvement, 98%; side effects, ≤2%
	  Mycophenolate mofetil (1.5–2 g daily): Improvement, 23%; side effects, 3%–24%
	Liver transplantation: 5-year patient and graft survivals, 83%–92%; recurrence, 8%–12% at 1 year and 36%–68% at 5 years; retransplantation, 8%–23%

external auditory canal atresia, orofacial clefts, coloboma, hypertelorism, micrognathia, and congenital heart defects (mitral atresia, double outlet right ventricle, pulmonic stenosis, and anomalous pulmonary venous return)

   g. Liver transplantation is justified at the first sign of decompensation (usually ascites).

2. Incomplete response

   a. Long-term empirical management with low-dose prednisone (up to 10 mg daily) and azathioprine (50 to 75 mg daily) or azathioprine alone (2 mg/kg daily) to maintain serum AST and ALT levels <3-fold ULN and no interface hepatitis

3. Liver transplantation

   a. Consider in all patients with a MELD score >16 points, acute decompensation, intractable symptoms, treatment intolerance, or liver cancer (see Chapter 33)

   b. 5-year patient and graft survivals, 83% to 92%; actuarial 10-year survival, 75%

   c. Recurrent autoimmune hepatitis in 8% to 12% at 1 year and 36% to 68% at 5 years

   d. Recurrence is associated with progression to cirrhosis, graft failure, or retransplantation in 8% to 23% of adults and 50% of children.

   e. Asymptomatic histologic recurrence may precede clinical recurrence by 1 to 5 years.

   f. Mainstay treatment for recurrence is prednisone or prednisolone alone or in combination with azathioprine (not antirejection regimens).

   g. Alternative immunosuppressive agents can be considered for refractory recurrence (mycophenolate mofetil, rapamycin, or switching calcineurin inhibitor).

    h. Retransplantation may be complicated by recurrence in the new graft.

    i. Graft and patient survival rates after recurrence have been 78% to 87% and 89% to 100%, respectively, and graft and patient survival rates have been similar to those of patients transplanted for other liver diseases.

    j. The frequency of acute (81% versus 47%), glucocorticoid-resistant (38% versus 13%), and chronic (11% versus 2%) graft rejection is higher in autoimmune hepatitis than in nonautoimmune (alcoholic) liver disease.

    k. Gradual withdrawal of glucocorticoids is possible in 68% after transplantation (commonly attempted after the first year), and complications of hypercholesterolemia, hypertension, and diabetes mellitus are decreased.

Long-Term Outcomes

1. Survival

    a. The 10-year survival rates from liver-related death or requirement for liver transplantation in treated patients with and without cirrhosis at presentation is 89% and 90%, respectively, and the 20-year survival rate is 70%.

    b. Survival from all causes of death or liver transplantation is 82% and 48% at 10 years and 20 years, respectively.

    c. The standardized mortality ratio is 1.63 for all causes of death (95% confidence interval, 1.25 to 2.02) and 1.86 for liver-related death or need for liver transplantation (95% confidence interval, 1.49 to 2.26).

2. Hepatocellular carcinoma

    a. The frequency in cirrhosis is 1% to 9%, and the annual rate of occurrence in cirrhosis is 1.1% to 1.9%.

    b. The standardized incidence ratio is 23.3 (95% confidence interval, 7.5 to 54.3) in Sweden, and the standardized mortality ratio is 42.3 (95% confidence interval, 20.3 to 77.9) in New Zealand.

    c. **The principal risk factor is long-standing cirrhosis, and patients at risk are characterized mainly by cirrhosis for ≥10 years, manifestations of portal hypertension, persistent liver inflammation, and immunosuppressive therapy for ≥3 years.**

    d. Surveillance has not been formally endorsed by the American Association for the Study of Liver Diseases because the annual rate of occurrence may be below threshold for surveillance, but hepatic ultrasonography every 6 months in patients with cirrhosis is a reasonable clinical decision, especially with cirrhosis for ≥10 years.

3. Extrahepatic malignancy

    a. Extrahepatic malignancies occur in 5%; incidence, 1 case per 194 patient-years

    b. Standardized incidence ratio, 2.7 (95% confidence interval, 1.8 to 3.9) in New Zealand

    c. Nonmelanoma skin cancers are most common, and neoplasms of the bladder, blood, breast, cervix, lymphatic tissue, soft tissue, and stomach are possible.

    d. Hematologic and lymphoproliferative diseases do not predominate as in patients receiving chronic immunosuppressive therapy after organ transplantation.

    e. Malignancies typically develop after 18 to 164 months (mean interval, 116±23 months).

    f. Patients are not distinguished from tumor-free patients by age, gender, cumulative duration of immunosuppressive therapy (42±9 months versus 60±4 months, $P = .7$), or individual features of liver disease, including the presence of cirrhosis.

    g. Treatment and outcomes are related to the nature and stage of the tumor at diagnosis.

    h. Survival is >70% during a mean follow-up of 48±25 months.

    i. Standard cancer surveillance recommendations should be maintained, including complete skin examination, mammography, gynecologic evaluation, and colonoscopy.

FURTHER READING

Czaja AJ. Performance parameters of the diagnostic scoring systems for autoimmune hepatitis. *Hepatology.* 2008;48:1540–1548.

Czaja AJ. Autoantibody-negative autoimmune hepatitis. *Dig Dis Sci.* 2012;57:610–624.

Czaja AJ. Drug choices in autoimmune hepatitis: part A—steroids. *Expert Rev Gastroenterol Hepatol.* 2012;6:603–615.

Czaja AJ. Drug choices in autoimmune hepatitis: part B—non-steroids. *Expert Rev Gastroenterol Hepatol.* 2012;6:617–635.

Czaja AJ. Rapidity of treatment response and outcome in type 1 autoimmune hepatitis. *J Hepatol.* 2009;51:161–167.

Czaja AJ. Special clinical challenges in autoimmune hepatitis: the elderly, males, pregnancy, mild disease, fulminant onset, and nonwhite patients. *Semin Liver Dis.* 2009;29:315–330.

Czaja AJ. Acute and acute severe (fulminant) autoimmune hepatitis. *Dig Dis Sci.* 2013;58:897–914.

Czaja AJ. Review article: the management of autoimmune hepatitis beyond consensus guidelines. *Aliment Pharmacol Ther.* 2013;38:343–364.

Czaja AJ. Cholestatic phenotypes of autoimmune hepatitis. *Clin Gastroenterol Hepatol.* 2014;12:1430–1438.

Czaja AJ. Current and prospective pharmacotherapy for autoimmune hepatitis. *Expert Opin Pharmacother.* 2014;15:1715–1736.

Czaja AJ. Review article: permanent drug withdrawal is desirable and achievable for autoimmune hepatitis. *Aliment Pharmacol Ther.* 2014;39:1043–1058.

Czaja AJ. Transitioning from idiopathic to explainable autoimmune hepatitis. *Dig Dis Sci.* 2015;60:2881–2900.

Gleeson D, Heneghan MA. British Society of Gastroenterology (BSG) guidelines for management of autoimmune hepatitis. *Gut.* 2011;60:1611–1629.

Manns MP, Czaja AJ, Gorham JD, et al. Practice guidelines of the American Association for the Study of Liver Diseases: diagnosis and management of autoimmune hepatitis. *Hepatology.* 2010;51:2193–2213.

Vierling JM. Autoimmune hepatitis and overlap syndromes: diagnosis and management. *Clin Gastroenterol Hepatol.* 2015;13:2088–2108.

CHAPTER 8

Alcoholic Liver Disease

Steve S. Choi, MD ■ Anna Mae Diehl, MD

Overview

1. Alcohol is used by nearly 75% of Americans. Consequently, alcohol abuse and dependence are common, with 12-month and lifetime prevalence rates of 13.9% and 29.1%, respectively.
2. ALD is one of the most serious medical consequences of long-term alcohol abuse and is the **most common cause of cirrhosis in the Western world.** ALD accounted for approximately 50% of deaths from cirrhosis in the United States in 2013.
3. Alcohol abuse and dependence rates are higher for men (18%) than for women (10%) and for white than for black persons; however, the black population is more prone to develop progression of liver disease to cirrhosis.
4. The prevalence of alcohol abuse and dependence is typically inversely related to age, with younger age groups most likely to have an alcohol disorder; however, the prevalence of alcohol abuse and dependence has risen in adults age 60 years and over.

DIAGNOSIS OF ALCOHOL DEPENDENCE AND ABUSE

1. **Alcohol dependence** (three items required):
   ■ Alcoholic beverages often taken in larger amounts or over a longer period than intended
   ■ Persistent desire for alcohol or one or more unsuccessful attempts to cut down or control use

- A great deal of time spent in obtaining alcohol, drinking it, or recovering from its effects
- Recurrent use at times when alcohol use is physically hazardous (e.g., driving while intoxicated) or frequent intoxication or withdrawal symptoms despite major obligations at work, school, or home
- Social, occupational, or recreational activities discontinued or reduced because of alcohol use
- Continued alcohol use despite knowledge of having persistent or recurrent social, psychological, or physical problems that are caused or exacerbated by alcohol use
- Marked tolerance: Need for markedly increased amounts of alcohol (at least a 50% increase) to achieve intoxication or desired effect or a markedly diminished effect with continued use of the same amount
- Characteristic withdrawal symptoms
- Alcohol taken to relieve or avoid withdrawal symptoms

2. **Alcohol abuse** (one item required):
   - Continued use despite knowledge of having a persistent or recurrent social, occupational, psychological, or physical problem that is caused or exacerbated by the use of the substance
   - Recurrent use in situations in which its use is physically hazardous

SCREENING FOR ALCOHOL PROBLEMS

CAGE Questionnaire:
a. Have you ever felt you ought to **cut down** on your drinking?
b. Have people **annoyed** you by criticizing your drinking?
c. Have you ever felt bad or **guilty** about your drinking?
d. Have you ever had a drink first thing in the morning (**eye opener**) to steady your nerves or get rid of a hangover?

Two or more positive responses imply the presence of an alcohol disorder.

Alcohol Use Disorders Identification Test

Developed by the World Health Organization (WHO), the Alcohol Use Disorders Identification Test (AUDIT) is a simple method of screening for excessive drinking that can be administered as an interview or written questionnaire (Table 8.1). By standardizing alcohol content, the AUDIT can assess alcohol consumption, drinking behaviors, and alcohol-related problems.

TABLE 8.1 ■ **AUDIT Questionnaire (Self-Report Version)**

Questions	Points				
	0	1	2	3	4
1. How often do you drink alcohol?	Never	Monthly or less	2–4 times a month	2–3 times a week	4 or more times a week
2. How many drinks containing alcohol do you have on a typical day when you are drinking?	1 or 2	3 or 4	5 or 6	7–9	10 or more
3. How often do you have 6 or more drinks on one occasion?	Never	Less than monthly	Monthly	Weekly	Daily or almost daily
4. How often during the past year have you found that you were not able to stop drinking once you started?	Never	Less than monthly	Monthly	Weekly	Daily or almost daily

TABLE 8.1 ■ **AUDIT Questionnaire (Self-Report Version)—cont'd**

	Points				
Questions	0	1	2	3	4
5. How often during the past year have you failed to do what was normally expected of you because of drinking?	Never	Less than monthly	Monthly	Weekly	Daily or almost daily
6. How often during the past year have you needed a first drink in the morning to get yourself going after a heavy drinking session?	Never	Less than monthly	Monthly	Weekly	Daily or almost daily
7. How often during the past year have you had a feeling of guilt or remorse after drinking?	Never	Less than monthly	Monthly	Weekly	Daily or almost daily
8. How often during the past year have you been unable to remember what happened the night before because of your drinking?	Never	Less than monthly	Monthly	Weekly	Daily or almost daily
9. Have you or someone else been injured because of your drinking?	Never	Less than monthly	Monthly	Weekly	Daily or almost daily
10. Has a relative, friend, doctor, or other health care worker been concerned about your drinking or suggested you cut down?	No	—	Yes, but not in the last year	—	Yes, during the past year

Total Score[a] (sum of points for each question)

[a]For total scores between 8 and 15, simple advice focused on the reduction of hazardous drinking is recommended. For scores between 16 and 19, brief counseling and continued monitoring are recommended. For scores of 20 or above, further diagnostic evaluation for alcohol dependence is recommended.

Risk Factors for Alcoholic Liver Disease

1. In all societies studied, a positive correlation exists between average per capita consumption of alcohol and the frequency of cirrhosis.
2. The amount ingested and the duration of intake correlate with the incidence of alcohol-related liver disease.
3. Above a **threshold** level of daily alcohol consumption (estimated to be **60 to 80 g/day for men** and **20 g/day for women**), the risk of hepatotoxicity increases dramatically.
4. Despite consistently high daily consumption of alcohol, progression of chronic ALD to cirrhosis is uncommon. Fewer than 20% of men consuming more than two 6-packs of beer per day for 10 years become cirrhotic.
5. Several advisory committees have recommended that alcohol consumption be limited to no more than two drinks per day for healthy men and no more than 1 drink per day for healthy nonpregnant women.

SPECIFIC RISK FACTORS

1. **Gender:** The toxic effects of alcohol per dose are greater in women than men; however, this difference cannot be explained solely by differences in body composition or alcohol distribution. Gastric mucosal alcohol dehydrogenase activity is lower in women than in men, thereby leading to greater hepatic metabolism of ingested alcohol in women.

2. **Genetic variability in alcohol-metabolizing enzymes:** Polymorphisms of the **alcohol dehydrogenase** and **aldehyde dehydrogenase** enzymes seem to protect certain persons from ethanol toxicity. Persons of Asian descent frequently inherit a "slow" aldehyde dehydrogenase isoenzyme, thereby increasing serum levels of acetaldehyde. The resulting flushing, nausea, and dysphoria (disulfiram-like reaction) may explain why habitual alcohol use and ALD are less common in Asians.

3. **Nutrition:** Ethanol interferes with intestinal absorption and storage of nutrients and reduces appetite for nonalcoholic sources of calories and can result in protein, vitamin, and mineral deficiencies.

4. **Presence of an infection with a hepatotropic virus or another chronic liver disease:** Acute and chronic hepatitis B or C accelerate the progression of ALD. Fatty liver disease related to obesity and insulin resistance (i.e., nonalcoholic fatty liver disease) can also coexist with ALD, and the combined effects of both diseases may promote more serious liver damage than would occur if either disease was present alone.

5. **Concurrent exposure to drugs or toxins:** Long-term consumption of alcohol induces the activity of microsomal enzymes and thus potentiates the metabolism of drugs, solvents, and xenobiotics. For example, therapeutic doses of acetaminophen can cause more severe hepatic damage in ALD. Similarly, treatment with or prolonged exposure to tolbutamide, isoniazid, and industrial solvents accelerate ALD.

6. **Immunologic derangements:** ALD is modulated by alterations in the cellular immune system, including increased reactivity of T and B cells and increased expression of major histocompatibility complex (MHC) class I and class II DR antigens. Increased levels of the immune modulatory cytokines tumor necrosis factor (TNF), interleukin (IL)-1, and IL-6 are common in ALD. Alterations of the humoral immune system include increased levels of circulating immunoglobulins, the presence of autoantibodies (against nuclear, smooth muscle, liver cell membrane, liver-specific protein, and alcoholic hyaline antigens), and the development of antibodies against neoantigens, proteins altered by reaction to acetaldehyde, malondialdehyde, and various radicals.

7. **Alterations in intestinal microbiota:** Alcohol dependency alters the intestinal microbiota. The resulting derangement in the microbiome promotes increased intestinal permeability. This process is mediated by interactions of lipopolysaccharide (LPS) and peptidoglycans with toll-like receptor (TLR)-4, thereby increasing levels of proinflammatory cytokines such as IL-1.

8. **Continued alcohol ingestion:** Patients with alcoholic liver injury who persistently consume alcohol have a greater risk of progression to cirrhosis. Conversely, abstinence almost guarantees clinical improvement and, in many cases, regression of histologic injury.

Clinical Features

HISTORY

1. Eliciting a history of habitual alcohol consumption is essential in implicating alcohol as the cause of liver disease.

2. The type of alcoholic beverage consumed does not influence the likelihood of developing hepatotoxicity. The amount of ethanol (in grams) consumed in spirits, wine, or beer can be estimated by multiplying the volume of the beverage in milliliters by the percentage of that beverage that is pure ethanol (spirits = 40%, wine = 12%, beer = 5%) times the specific gravity (0.8) of ethanol.

3. The AUDIT questionnaire can screen for alcohol dependency and assess alcohol consumption and drinking behaviors (see Table 8.1).

4. Accelerated disease progression is likely when alcohol abuse is accompanied by one or more of the following: Viral hepatitis, acetaminophen intake, obesity, exposure to solvents, a family history of ALD, hemochromatosis, Wilson disease, or alpha-1 antitrypsin deficiency.

TABLE 8.2 ■ **Laboratory Abnormalities in Alcoholic Liver Disease**

Laboratory Test	Result
Serum AST/ALT ratio	>2 and both generally <300 U/L
Serum alkaline phosphatase	Elevated
Serum bilirubin	Varying degree of elevation often with indirect hyperbilirubinemia due to hemolysis
Prothrombin time	Normal to prolonged
Serum albumin	Normal to decreased
Hematocrit value	Typically mild macrocytic anemia; may be normal
White blood cell count	May be elevated in acute alcoholic hepatitis due to leukemoid reaction
Platelet count	Normal to decreased
Serum triglycerides	Typically increased, especially in active drinkers
Serum potassium, phosphate, magnesium	Often deficient in active drinkers
Serum glucose	Hyperglycemia common

ALT, Alanine aminotransferase; *AST*, aspartate aminotransferase.

SYMPTOMS AND SIGNS

1. The clinical features of ALD are variable, ranging from a complete absence of symptoms to florid features of advanced liver failure and complications of portal hypertension. Because portal hypertension may occur in alcoholic hepatitis even in the absence of established cirrhosis, alcoholic hepatitis can be difficult to distinguish from alcoholic cirrhosis unless a liver biopsy is performed.
2. Patients may have one or more of the following: Fever, weakness, anorexia, nausea and vomiting, malaise, confusion, sleep-wake cycle alterations, hepatomegaly, splenomegaly, cachexia, jaundice, spider telangiectasias, Dupuytren contractures, gynecomastia, testicular atrophy, parotid/lacrimal gland enlargement, asterixis, Muercke lines, white nails, and decreased libido; however, none of these features is specific or pathognomonic for ALD.
3. Other sequelae of excess alcohol may be present, including alcoholic cardiomyopathy, pancreatitis and pancreatic insufficiency, and neurotoxicity.

LABORATORY FEATURES (Table 8.2)

Diagnosis

1. The diagnosis of ALD is typically established in patients with evidence of liver disease and a history of significant alcohol use. Given the dearth of pathognomonic symptoms and signs of ALD, the elimination of other potential causes of liver injury is mandatory.
2. Imaging is not typically helpful in implicating alcohol as the cause of liver disease, although surveillance for hepatocellular carcinoma in the setting of alcoholic cirrhosis is recommended.
3. Liver biopsy is not essential for the diagnosis of ALD, but it may be helpful in staging fibrosis and in ascertaining the presence and impact of other chronic liver diseases.

Histology and Spectrum of Disease

FATTY LIVER (STEATOSIS)

This disorder is a consequence of alcohol oxidation. Fatty liver results when the intracellular redox potential and redox-sensitive nutrient metabolism are disturbed. An excessive accumulation of reducing equivalents favors metabolic pathways that lead to the accumulation of intracellular lipid (Fig. 8.1). The excess lipid is stored in large droplets within individual hepatocytes. With abstinence, the normal redox potential is restored, the lipid is mobilized, and fatty liver resolves completely. Although reports have noted fatal outcomes and progression to cirrhosis, **fatty liver is generally considered a benign, reversible condition.**

ALCOHOLIC HEPATITIS

1. This disease is characterized by **steatosis, hepatocellular necrosis, and acute inflammation** (Fig. 8.2). The steatosis is most pronounced in zone 3 of the hepatic acinus. Characteristic eosinophilic fibrillar material (Mallory hyaline, or Mallory-Denk bodies) may be seen in swollen (ballooned) hepatocytes. These condensations of cytoskeletal intermediary filaments result from the formation of acetaldehyde-tubulin adducts. Although characteristic of alcoholic hepatitis, they are not specific and are also seen in other forms of hepatitis. Focally intense lobular infiltration of polymorphonuclear leukocytes distinguishes alcoholic hepatitis from other types of liver disease. In most other types of hepatitis, the inflammatory infiltrate is composed of mononuclear cells predominately localized around the portal tracts.

2. In the past, alcoholic hepatitis was believed to be the prerequisite for alcoholic cirrhosis; however, it is now known that acetaldehyde may initiate fibrogenesis in the absence of demonstrable necroinflammation. Nevertheless, the severity of the clinical syndrome that occurs in some patients with alcoholic steatonecrosis and the potential of this lesion to progress to cirrhosis have made it a logical target in therapeutic trials.

CIRRHOSIS

1. Most patients with alcoholic fatty liver never progress to cirrhosis despite protracted and excessive consumption of alcohol. In other patients, deposition of fibrosis ensues. In some of these persons, features of all three histologic "stages" coexist.

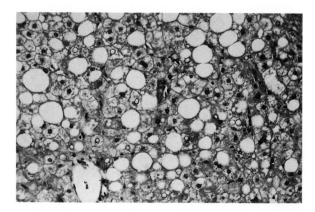

Fig. 8.1 Histopathology of fatty liver (steatosis) in alcoholic liver disease (hematoxylin and eosin [H&E]).

2. Alcoholic liver damage is typically associated with the deposition of collagen around the terminal hepatic vein (i.e., perivenular fibrosis) and along the sinusoids. This results in a "chicken wire" pattern of scarring that is rarely seen in other types of cirrhosis.
3. Long-term consumption of alcohol also impairs the regenerative response that is normally triggered by liver cell death. This results in small nodules of regenerating parenchyma. For this reason, **micronodular cirrhosis** is seen in actively drinking patients (Fig. 8.3).
4. Abstinence from alcohol releases the liver from the antiproliferative actions of alcohol and is associated with the development of **macronodular cirrhosis.**

Indices of Liver Dysfunction for Alcoholic Hepatitis

Formulae for estimating the **short-term prognosis** of patients with alcoholic hepatitis:
1. **Composite Clinical Laboratory Index (CCLI):** Orrego et al., in 1978, developed a formula to predict mortality in hospitalized patients with alcoholic hepatitis (Table 8.3).
2. **Maddrey discriminant function (DF):** Maddrey et al., in 1978, simplified the assessment of outcome of ALD by developing the DF:

$$DF = 4.6 \times \text{(the difference between the patient's and control prothrombin time)} + \text{serum bilirubin level}$$

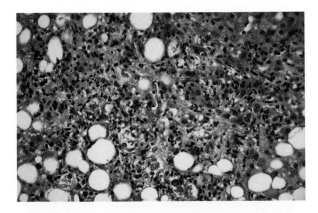

Fig. 8.2 Histopathology of alcoholic hepatitis. This histologic section shows macrovesicular steatosis, Mallory-Denk bodies, neutrophilic inflammation, and fibrosis (H&E).

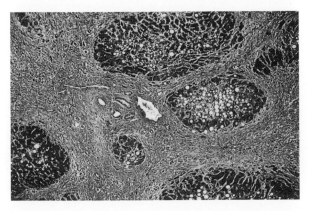

Fig. 8.3 Histopathology of alcoholic cirrhosis (H&E).

TABLE 8.3 ■ Composite Clinical Laboratory Index for Alcoholic Hepatitis

Parameter	Score
Hepatomegaly	1
Splenomegaly	1
Ascites	
1+	1
2+	2
3+	3
Encephalopathy	
Grade 1	1
Grade 2	2
Grade 3	3
Clinical bleeding	1
Spider telangiectasias	1
Palmar erythema	1
Collateral circulation	1
Peripheral edema	1
Anorexia	1
Weakness	1
AST >200 U/L	1
ALT (U/L)	
>100	1
>200	2
Alkaline phosphatase >80 IU/L	1
Albumin <2.59 g/dL	1
Prothrombin time (s prolonged)	
<3	1
3–5	2
>5	3
Bilirubin (mg/dL)	
1.2–2	1
2–5	2
>5	3

Initial CCLI ≥13 correlates with severe liver disease and/or cirrhosis.
The following normalization rate (NR) is used to assess effectiveness of therapy and/or follow disease progression:
NR = (Change in CCLI/days to reach lowest score) × 100
Example: Day   1   4   12   20   28
*   Score: 12   10   8   6   6*
NR = (12 − 6)/20 × 100 = 30
(The higher the NR, the faster the recovery.)

ALT, Alanine aminotransferase; *AST,* aspartate aminotransferase; *CCLI,* composite clinical laboratory index.

- **Patients with a DF >32 have a 50% mortality rate during their current hospitalization.** DF offers the advantage of few variables and easy computation (and therefore easy recall), but it is relatively imprecise.

3. **Model for End-stage Liver Disease (MELD) score:** The composite score uses a mathematical formula incorporating the patient's bilirubin, international normalized ratio, and creatinine. A MELD score >18 portends a poor prognosis in alcoholic hepatitis (see also Chapter 33).

4. **Early change in bilirubin level and Lille score:** A decrease in total bilirubin level at 7 days after initiation of glucocorticoids reflects improving liver function and predicts increased 6-month survival (82.8% versus 5.8%). If total bilirubin does not decrease at 7 days, the eventual response to glucocorticoids is low, and glucocorticoids can likely be discontinued. The Lille score is a composite score combining pretreatment parameters with response of bilirubin after 7 days of glucocorticoids. A score >0.45 indicates a lack of response and poor 6-month survival.

Treatment

GENERAL MEASURES

1. **Discontinuation of alcohol use and resumption of a nutritious diet remain the cornerstones of therapy for alcoholic patients even after progression to cirrhosis.**
2. Vigorous efforts to enroll patients in a detoxification program are essential.
3. Hospitalization benefits patients with significant extrahepatic complications of alcoholism, notably electrolyte abnormalities, cardiac dysfunction, pancreatitis, hemorrhagic gastropathy, major alcohol withdrawal syndromes, and infection.
4. The risk of hepatocellular carcinoma (HCC) is increased if alcoholic cirrhosis has developed (see Chapter 29). Surveillance with serial ultrasonography allows detection of HCC at a potentially curative stage. Chronic infection with hepatitis B or C increases the risk of HCC. Effective antiviral therapy may diminish the risk of HCC in alcoholic cirrhosis with concomitant viral hepatitis.

SPECIFIC THERAPY FOR ALCOHOLIC HEPATITIS

1. **Glucocorticoids:** Glucocorticoids have been the mainstay of pharmacologic treatment of severe alcoholic hepatitis. Two prospectively randomized, placebo-controlled trials demonstrated that patients with clinically severe alcoholic hepatitis benefit from treatment with glucocorticoids. Furthermore, a Cochrane systematic review confirmed that mortality was favorably impacted with the use of glucocorticoids in patients with a DF >32 or with hepatic encephalopathy:
   - **A 4-week (28-day) course of prednisolone 40 mg daily reduced the 1-month mortality rate by more than half in patients with a Maddrey DF >32 or hepatic encephalopathy.**
   - These results were obtained in carefully selected patients who did not have clinically significant diabetes mellitus, pancreatitis, cancer, or viral hepatitis. The efficacy of glucocorticoids in patients with these comorbid conditions and alcoholic hepatitis has not been established.
   - The efficacy of glucocorticoids (along with pentoxifylline [PTX]) in treating alcoholic hepatitis was reevaluated in a multicenter, double-blind, randomized trial (STeroids Or Pentoxifylline for Alcoholic Hepatitis [STOPAH]). The two-by-two factorial study design revealed a reduction in 28-day mortality that did not reach significance with glucocorticoid therapy. Additionally, no improvement in outcomes at 90 days or 1 year was noted with glucocorticoid therapy. These results cast doubt on the overall benefit of glucocorticoids in severe alcoholic hepatitis in light of risks associated with therapy.

2. **PTX:** This nonselective phosphodiesterase inhibitor was approved (at a dose of 400 mg orally three times daily) by the U.S. Food and Drug Administration for use as a rheologic agent. A benefit in the treatment of acute alcoholic hepatitis was initially suggested in 1991. A subsequent randomized double-blind placebo-controlled trial also suggested efficacy. In this study, 101 patients with a DF >32 were enrolled (49 in the PTX arm and 52 in the control arm):
   - **PTX significantly reduced 4-week mortality from 46.1% to 24.5%; it also reduced the frequency of hepatorenal syndrome from 34.6% to 8.2%.**
   - The mechanisms through which PTX exerted its effects were attributed, at least in part, to modification of cytokine (e.g., TNF) synthesis or effect.
   - On the other hand, **the STOPAH trial did not confirm that PTX improved survival in patients with alcoholic hepatitis.**

3. **Diet:** Alcohol ingestion interferes with intestinal absorption and storage of nutrients and reduces a person's appetite for nonalcoholic sources of calories, potentially leading to deficiencies of protein, vitamins, and minerals. **Malnutrition correlates with mortality in patients with ALD.**
   - Trials of supplemental amino acid therapy have yielded conflicting results.
   - Parenteral amino acids have been reported to help nutritional status, reduce serum bilirubin levels, and improve aminopyrine breath test results (a measure of liver function) but not short- or long-term survival.
   - Intensive enteral nutrition administered to patients with severe alcoholic hepatitis treated with glucocorticoids was evaluated in a randomized trial. The results of this study confirmed that low daily energy consumption increased mortality; however, intensive enteral nutrition proved to be difficult to implement and had no impact on survival.

4. **Other supplements:** Patients with severe alcoholic hepatitis who are actively drinking may be severely depleted of magnesium, potassium, and phosphate; these deficiencies contribute to multiorgan system dysfunction. Prompt electrolyte repletion is indicated.

5. **Thiamine:** This must be administered to prevent Wernicke encephalopathy.

6. **Strategies targeting the microbiome:** The use of antibiotics, probiotics, prebiotics, synbiotics, genetically modified bacteria, and fecal microbiota transplantation has been suggested to modulate the intestinal dysbiosis that contributes to the pathogenesis of alcoholic hepatitis. While promising, these therapeutic approaches remain largely unproven.

7. **Other treatments:** A variety of therapies have been employed in attempts to neutralize the proinflammatory cytokine TNF alpha (anti-TNF alpha antibodies), reduce oxidative stress (propylthiouracil and cyanidanol), improve hepatic regeneration (anabolic steroids), or prevent fibrosis (*D*-penicillamine and colchicine). None reproducibly improves short-term survival, and at least one (treatment with anti-TNF antibodies) increased mortality. None of these agents can be recommended. N-acetylcysteine in combination with prednisolone improved 1-month but not 6-month survival in one trial and remains of uncertain benefit in alcoholic hepatitis.

8. Liver transplantation improved survival in patients with severe alcoholic hepatitis unresponsive to medical therapy; however, concern about alcohol relapse following transplantation has limited access to liver transplantation for patients with alcoholic hepatitis and a short period of alcohol abstinence.

SPECIFIC THERAPY FOR ALCOHOLIC CIRRHOSIS

1. **Drug therapy:** Few long-term treatment trials of patients with ALD have been conducted and were generally confounded by noncompliance and high dropout rates.
   - A Cochrane systematic review concluded that, contrary to earlier reports, colchicine had deleterious effects on outcome in patients with fibrosis or cirrhosis of varying etiologies including alcoholic.

- Although a Canadian prospective, randomized controlled trial suggested that propylthiouracil improved long-term survival; a subsequent Cochrane systematic review of 6 randomized clinical trials could not confirm a significant impact on all-cause mortality, liver-related mortality, liver complications, or liver histology in ALD.

2. **Antioxidant therapy:** Several antioxidants have been evaluated for therapy of ALD, with or without cirrhosis, with varying, incompletely satisfying effects. Substantial benefit has yet to be proven with the following agents:
   - *S*-Adenosylmethionine (SAM-e)
   - Vitamin E
   - Silymarin (milk thistle–derived antioxidant)
   - Polyenylphosphatidylcholine (PPC)

3. **Liver transplantation** (see Chapter 33):
   - Liver transplantation clearly improves survival in patients with decompensated alcoholic cirrhosis.
   - **Patients with decompensated alcoholic cirrhosis should be considered for liver transplantation if abstinence from alcohol for at least 6 months has not resulted in spontaneous improvement and the patient has a commitment to long-term sobriety.**
   - Patients who abstain from alcohol for longer than 6 months and are determined to be at low risk for recidivism and noncompliance are good candidates for liver transplantation.
   - A signed contract stipulating abstinence may be helpful in maintaining commitment.
   - Although a variety of measures have been employed to reduce recidivism rates, alcohol use following transplantation is common, although it typically does not result in graft loss.
   - Patients who relapse after liver transplantation may, however, develop an accelerated form of ALD.

FURTHER READING

Akriviadis E, Bolta R, Briggs W, et al. Pentoxifylline improves short-term survival in severe acute alcoholic hepatitis: a double-blind, placebo-controlled trial. *Gastroenterology*. 2000;119:1637–1648.

Carithers RL, Herlong HF, Diehl AM, et al. Methylprednisolone therapy in patients with severe alcoholic hepatitis: a randomized multicenter trial. *Ann Intern Med*. 1989;110:685–690.

Fede G, Germani G, Gluud C, et al. Propylthiouracil for alcoholic liver disease. *Cochrane Database Syst Rev*. 2011:CD002800.

Hartmann P, Seebauer CT, Schnabl B. Alcoholic liver disease: the gut microbiome and liver cross talk. *Alcohol Clin Exp Res*. 2015;39:763–775.

Leclercq S, Matamoros S, Cani PD, et al. Intestinal permeability, gut-bacterial dysbiosis, and behavioral markers of alcohol-dependence severity. *Proc Natl Acad Sci U S A*. 2014;111:E4485–E4493.

Levy RE, Catana AM, Durbin-Johnson B, et al. Ethnic differences in presentation and severity of alcoholic liver disease. *Alcohol Clin Exp Res*. 2015;39:566–574.

Louvet A, Naveau S, Abdelnour M, et al. The Lille model: a new tool for therapeutic strategy in patients with severe alcoholic hepatitis with steroids. *Hepatology*. 2007;45:1348–1354.

Mathurin P, Moreno C, Samuel D, et al. Early liver transplantation for severe alcoholic hepatitis. *N Engl J Med*. 2011;365:1790–1800.

Mathurin P, O'Grady J, Carithers RL, et al. Corticosteroids improve short-term survival in patients with severe alcoholic hepatitis: meta-analysis of individual patient data. *Gut*. 2011;60:255–260.

Moreno C, Deltenre P, Senterre C, et al. Intensive enteral nutrition is ineffective for patients with severe alcoholic hepatitis treated with corticosteroids. *Gastroenterology*. 2016;150:903–910.

O'Shea RS, Dasarathy S, McCullough AJ, et al. AASLD practice guidelines: alcoholic liver disease. *Hepatology*. 2010;51:307–328.

Pereira SP, Howard LM, Muiesan P, et al. Quality of life after liver transplantation for alcoholic liver disease. *Liver Transpl*. 2000;6:762–768.

Rambaldi A, Saconato HH, Christensen E, et al. Systematic review: glucocorticosteroids for alcoholic hepatitis. A Cochrane Hepato-Biliary Group systematic review with meta-analyses and trial sequential analyses of randomized clinical trials. *Aliment Pharmacol Ther*. 2008;27:1167–1178.

Szabo G. Gut-liver axis in alcoholic liver disease. *Gastroenterology*. 2015;148:30–36.

Thursz MR, Richardson P, Allison M, et al. Prednisolone or pentoxifylline for alcoholic hepatitis. *N Engl J Med*. 2015;372:1619–1628.

CHAPTER 9

Fatty Liver and Nonalcoholic Steatohepatitis

Brent A. Neuschwander-Tetri, MD

KEY POINTS

1 Hepatic steatosis, the accumulation of triglyceride droplets in hepatocytes, is found in one third to one half of all adults in the United States and is an important cause of elevated serum aminotransferase levels (typically <250 U/L).

2 Steatosis without significant inflammation or fibrosis on biopsy is a benign hepatic condition, although it is associated with insulin resistance and indicates an increased risk for development of cardiovascular disease and type 2 diabetes mellitus.

3 Steatosis associated with substantial necroinflammatory changes identified on a liver biopsy specimen, called nonalcoholic steatohepatitis (NASH) when alcohol consumption is minimal or none, can cause progressive hepatic fibrosis, cirrhosis, and hepatocellular carcinoma.

4 Nonalcoholic fatty liver disease (NAFLD) is the umbrella term that includes both steatosis without inflammation and NASH.

5 A liver biopsy is warranted to diagnose NASH or other causes of occult liver disease when elevated aminotransferase levels are unexplained, especially in a patient with obesity or type 2 diabetes mellitus, because of the risk of advanced fibrosis and cirrhosis.

6 Hepatic steatosis is reliably identified by imaging techniques when the degree of fatty infiltration is substantial. Ultrasonography reveals increased liver echogenicity, whereas noncontrast computed tomography (CT) imaging reveals decreased liver density compared with the spleen. Magnetic resonance imaging (MRI) is the most sensitive test for detecting liver fat.

7 Focal steatosis is a variant typically detected incidentally during imaging of the abdomen. The appearance is usually characteristic, although biopsy confirmation is occasionally required to exclude malignancy when the imaging appearance is atypical.

8 Lipotoxic liver injury caused by metabolites of free fatty acids likely causes NASH; steatosis may be an adaptive mechanism with temporary storage of fatty acids as triglyceride to prevent lipotoxic injury.

Overview

TERMINOLOGY

1. *Nonalcoholic fatty liver disease* **(NAFLD) is the term used to describe excessive liver triglyceride accumulation when alcohol consumption is minimal (fewer than two to four drinks daily).**

2. No uniformly accepted term exists for NAFLD that is not NASH; terms such as *fatty liver, benign steatosis, simple steatosis,* and *nonalcoholic fatty liver* (NAFL) are commonly used.

3. NASH is diagnosed when a liver biopsy specimen shows steatosis and characteristic necroinflammatory changes in a patient who has fewer than two to four drinks per day; the presence

of fibrosis is not required, but characteristic perisinusoidal fibrosis supports a diagnosis of steatohepatitis.

4. NASH is *not* a diagnosis of exclusion; it can often be found in the presence of other liver diseases such as chronic hepatitis C.

Pathogenesis

- NASH is thought to be a disease of lipotoxic injury to hepatocytes caused by nontriglyceride metabolites of free fatty acids.
- Triglyceride in the lipid droplets may actually be a protective response to store fatty acids in an inert form.
- The specific metabolites of free fatty acids that cause lipotoxic injury have not been fully identified. Possibilities include ceramides, diacylglycerols, lysophosphatidylcholine species, omega-oxidized fatty acids, and phosphatidic acid species.

The causes of hepatic lipotoxicity are attributable to one or more of the following abnormalities in the trafficking of fatty acids in the body:

INCREASED PERIPHERAL MOBILIZATION OF FATTY ACIDS

- Adipose tissue releases free fatty acids in response to cyclic adenosine monophosphate (cAMP)–mediated signaling from glucagon, epinephrine, and adrenocorticotropic hormone; released fatty acids are transported to the liver bound to albumin in the circulation.
- Insulin is a major inhibitory signal that normally prevents adipose tissue lipolysis after meals; adipocyte insulin resistance allows inappropriate postprandial lipolysis in adipose tissue with release of free fatty acids into the circulation.
- Prolonged starvation is associated with appropriate release of fat from peripheral stores that can overwhelm the liver's ability to handle it, thereby leading to steatosis and NASH.

INCREASED HEPATIC SYNTHESIS OF FATTY ACIDS

- The liver disposes of excess carbohydrates, especially fructose, by converting carbohydrate to fatty acids through de novo lipogenesis.
- Excess carbohydrates from dietary sources (e.g., sugar-sweetened beverages) or provided parenterally (e.g., total parenteral nutrition) predispose to hepatic lipotoxicity.

IMPAIRED HEPATIC CATABOLISM OF FATTY ACIDS

- Impaired mitochondrial beta-oxidation of fatty acids is a major factor in alcoholic steatosis and has also been shown to contribute to the development of NASH.
- Factors that cause microvesicular steatosis may do so through impaired mitochondrial function (e.g., valproic acid, alcohol, acute fatty liver of pregnancy).
- Other oxidative pathways (cytochrome P-450 omega-oxidation, peroxisomal beta-oxidation) facilitate disposal of fatty acids.

IMPAIRED SYNTHESIS OF TRIGLYCERIDE AND SECRETION AS VERY-LOW-DENSITY LIPOPROTEINS (VLDL) FROM THE LIVER

- Fatty acids delivered to the liver but not metabolized are reesterified to form triglycerides.
- Fatty acid esterification to triglyceride ensures that the level of fatty acids within hepatocytes remains low, thus averting cellular injury from fatty acid metabolites.

- Monounsaturated fatty acids (MUFAs) are needed to make triglyceride; impaired MUFA synthesis in the liver may predispose to lipotoxicity.
- Once triglyceride is formed, various components are needed to form and secrete intact VLDL.
- Any deficiency or metabolic aberration that interferes with any one of these steps can cause accumulation of hepatic triglyceride and hepatic steatosis.
- Autophagy may be an important pathway for handling accumulated triglyceride to release free fatty acids by lysosomal lipases in hepatocytes.

Clinical Features

SYMPTOMS

1. Patients with benign steatosis or NASH are usually asymptomatic, whereas patients with alcoholic hepatitis are nearly always symptomatic.
2. Right upper quadrant pain or fullness of varying severity occurs in approximately a third of patients with NAFLD; liver capsule distention probably underlies the pain.
3. Patients occasionally present with right upper quadrant pain as a chief complaint; hepatic steatosis may be diagnosed as the cause only after imaging studies exclude other potential intrahepatic or biliary causes. Recognizing that the pain is due to NAFLD can reduce the chances of an unnecessary cholecystectomy.

PHYSICAL FINDINGS

1. Hepatomegaly is common but can be difficult to detect on physical examination of the obese patient.
2. Signs of chronic liver disease such as spider telangiectasias, muscle wasting, jaundice, and ascites suggest the presence of cirrhosis.
3. Acanthosis nigricans, identified as increased pigmentation around the neck and on the elbows, knuckles, or other joints, is associated with insulin resistance and may be seen, especially in children with NAFLD.

Risk Factors

1. **Insulin resistance** (Tables 9.1 and 9.2)
   - Most patients with NAFLD have underlying insulin resistance (Fig. 9.1).
   - NAFLD may be the first indication that a child or adult has insulin resistance.
   - Most risk factors for NAFLD are associated with insulin resistance.
   - Severe insulin resistance is a risk factor for NASH.
2. **Obesity**
   - An increased ratio of abdominal diameter to hip diameter predicts NAFLD.
   - NASH is found in 8% to 20% of obese persons with NAFLD.
   - NAFLD occurs in 90% to 95% of severely obese children and adults.

TABLE 9.1 ■ **Body Habitus and Frequency of Hepatic Steatosis**

Body Habitus	Hepatic Steatosis (%)
Normal	21
>10% over ideal body weight	75
Morbidly obese	90–95

TABLE 9.2 ■ **Causes of Nonalcoholic Steatohepatitis**

Nutritional Abnormalities

Obesity
Excessive calorie consumption
Excessive simple carbohydrate consumption (sucrose, fructose, glucose)
Total parenteral nutrition
Choline deficiency
Rapid weight loss
Kwashiorkor

Drugs

Tamoxifen
Chloroquine
Glucocorticoids

Metabolic Diseases

Insulin resistance
Abetalipoproteinemia
Hypobetalipoproteinemia
Wilson disease
Weber-Christian disease

Surgical Alteration of Gastrointestinal Anatomy

Jejunoileal bypass
Jejunocolic bypass
Extensive small bowel loss

Occupational Exposure

Hydrocarbons

3. **Type 2 diabetes mellitus**
   - NAFLD is unusual in type 1 diabetes mellitus unless glycemic control is poor or the patient is also obese and insulin resistant.
   - Type 2 diabetes mellitus is a risk factor for NASH in patients with NAFLD.
   - Type 2 diabetes mellitus is a risk factor for advanced fibrosis.
4. **Lipid abnormalities**
   - Fasting hypertriglyceridemia partially reflects increased trafficking of fat through the liver and increased hepatic secretion of VLDL and thus is commonly found in NAFLD but does not directly cause NAFLD.
   - The role of hypercholesterolemia in the causation of NAFLD is uncertain; the goal of treating hypercholesterolemia is to reduce cardiovascular risk.
5. **Gender**
   - Female gender is *not* a risk factor for NAFLD or NASH.
   - Estrogens may be protective; prepubertal girls and postmenopausal women may be at increased risk for NASH.
   - Steatosis is equally prevalent among male and female persons on CT and at autopsy.
6. **Medications**
   - Tamoxifen use is associated with NASH; the decision to stop tamoxifen should be individualized depending on the severity of liver disease and the risk of recurrent breast cancer.
   - Glucocorticoids have been implicated as contributing to NAFLD, but supporting data are weak.

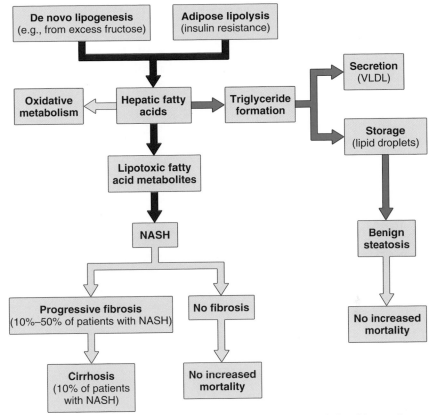

Fig. 9.1 Diagram showing the steps involved in substrate-overload lipotoxic liver Injury as the cause of nonalcoholic steatohepatitis (NASH) and the outcomes associated with lipotoxic liver injury. Accumulation of triglyceride as fat droplets, once thought to be a necessary step, is now considered to be a parallel but not pathogenic process and may actually be protective by drawing fatty acids away from the formation of lipotoxic intermediates. Dietary carbohydrates and inappropriate peripheral lipolysis are the major factors predisposing to an increased burden of fatty acids handled by the liver. Adipose insulin resistance is the major cause of inappropriate adipocyte lipolysis. Fatty acids are also disposed of through oxidative pathways (mitochondria, peroxisomes, cytochrome P-450); this generates reactive oxygen species (ROS), but the role of ROS in causing hepatocellular injury in NASH remains uncertain. Pathways predisposing to NASH are shown in red, and pathways preventing NASH are shown in green. *VDLD,* Very-low-density lipoprotein.

7. **Lifestyle**
   - Sedentary behavior is associated with insulin resistance and NAFLD.
   - Excessive consumption of high-fructose corn syrup, as in soft drinks, is associated with insulin resistance and NAFLD.
   - Animal data suggest that dietary *trans* fats may contribute to NASH.

Diagnosis

HISTORY

1. A patient suspected of having NASH should be interviewed regarding the following:
   - Alcohol consumption
   - Exercise habits and barriers to regular exercise

- Sugar-sweetened beverage consumption
- Frequency of consumption of fast food
- History of gestational diabetes mellitus
- Family history of type 2 diabetes mellitus
2. The nature and frequency of right upper quadrant abdominal pain should be ascertained.

LABORATORY FEATURES

1. No blood tests point unequivocally to steatosis or NASH.
2. Elevated aminotransferase (aspartate aminotransferase [AST], alanine aminotransferase [ALT]) levels are commonly the only biochemical indicators of steatosis and NASH.
3. Aminotransferase levels can be normal in both steatosis and NASH, as has been demonstrated in liver biopsy specimens of obese persons undergoing bariatric surgery.
4. The upper reference range for ALT and AST reported by clinical laboratories is often too high; healthy normal values for women are <19 U/L and for men <30 U/L.
5. The AST/ALT ratio can be helpful in distinguishing alcoholic hepatitis from NAFLD or NASH (Table 9.3): **An AST/ALT ratio >2 suggests alcoholic hepatitis, whereas patients with NASH typically have ALT levels that exceed AST levels in the absence of cirrhosis; AST is typically greater than ALT in NASH with cirrhosis.**
6. Serum aminotransferase levels and other liver biochemical tests are not helpful in identifying the presence of liver fibrosis or cirrhosis; aminotransferase levels often normalize as NASH progresses to cirrhosis.
7. Serum alkaline phosphatase may be elevated up to twice the upper limit of normal.
8. Viral, autoimmune, and metabolic causes of liver disease must be evaluated as potential contributors to elevated aminotransferase levels.

IMAGING

Imaging studies cannot distinguish benign steatosis from NASH, although NASH is usually diffuse and steatosis can be either focal or diffuse. Focal or diffuse steatosis is often an incidental imaging finding.
1. Ultrasonography
   - The liver is echogenic or "bright."
   - Ultrasonography detects steatosis only when fat accumulation is substantial.
   - Cirrhosis can also cause an echogenic appearance of the liver, but the texture is typically coarser.
2. CT
   - A liver with steatosis is low in density compared with the spleen on noncontrast images.
3. MRI
   - **MRI is the most sensitive noninvasive approach to detecting liver fat.**
   - Phase shifting can be useful for identifying focal fat based on its loss of intensity on T1-weighted images.

TABLE 9.3 ■ **Steatohepatitis and Serum Aminotransferase Patterns**

Alcoholic hepatitis	AST > ALT, typically >2 to 1 ratio
Nonalcoholic steatohepatitis	ALT > AST, sometimes >2 to 1 ratio

ALT, Alanine aminotransferase; *AST,* aspartate aminotransferase.

4. Focal fat
   - Focal fat is found in up to one third of patients with CT evidence of hepatic steatosis.
   - It can be peripheral (especially in the diabetic patient receiving insulin by peritoneal dialysis), central, or periportal.
   - It is typically aspherical or geometric in shape.
   - It does not exert a mass effect on adjacent structures.
   - Fine-needle biopsy occasionally is needed to establish the diagnosis.
5. Focal sparing
   - Focal sparing is defined as regions of normal liver in an otherwise steatotic liver on imaging.
   - It appears relatively hypoechoic by ultrasonography (compared with surrounding bright liver).
   - It appears relatively hyperdense by CT.
   - The shape is typically geometric.
   - The location is commonly in the caudate lobe or adjacent to the gallbladder.
   - It can be caused by an aberrant gastric vein draining directly into the liver that spares an area of the liver from receiving insulin-rich portal blood.
6. Problems identifying other lesions in a steatotic liver
   - Hemangiomas, which are usually characteristically hyperechoic by ultrasonography, can appear relatively hypoechoic in a steatotic liver.
   - Identifying dilatation of intrahepatic bile ducts can be difficult because of loss of contrast between the usually hyperechoic bile duct wall and the liver parenchyma.

LIVER BIOPSY (see also Chapter 1)

1. Liver biopsy is often needed to evaluate unexplained elevation of aminotransferase levels. Unless a therapeutic trial of discontinuance of specific medications, aggressive lifestyle modification, or avoidance of occupational exposures is planned, liver biopsy should not be delayed for arbitrary waiting periods.
2. Liver biopsy is usually not indicated when imaging suggests steatosis and aminotransferase levels are normal.
3. Histologic findings in NASH include:
   - *Steatosis*: Fat droplets (triglyceride) within hepatocytes can be large, displacing cellular contents to the periphery, small, or a mix of both types.
   - *Inflammation*: Mixed neutrophilic and mononuclear cell infiltrates are present within the lobule; portal chronic inflammation can occur, especially in children and after treatment, but is uncommon; ballooning enlargement of hepatocytes with rarefication of cytoplasmic contents is a marker of hepatocyte injury.
   - *Mallory-Denk bodies*: These eosinophilic cytoplasmic aggregates of keratins are typically smaller than those seen in alcoholic hepatitis and are usually found in ballooned hepatocytes.
   - *Glycogen nuclei*: These clear intranuclear vacuoles fill the nucleus.
   - *Fibrosis*: Similar to that seen in alcoholic liver disease, with perivenular deposition around the central vein and a "chicken wire" pattern of sinusoidal fibrosis; it signifies a risk for progression to end-stage liver disease. Fibrosis is staged as 1 (perisinusoidal *or* periportal only), 2 (perisinusoidal *and* periportal), 3 (bridging), or 4 (cirrhosis).

Prognosis (see Fig. 9.1)

STEATOSIS

Steatosis alone is a generally benign condition, although it may be associated with clinically significant right upper quadrant abdominal pain. Occasionally steatosis is associated with fibrosis.

NASH

- **The risk of developing fibrosis and cirrhosis is 10% to 50% in patients with NASH.**
- The risk of developing cirrhosis when fibrosis is absent on initial biopsy is low.
- Hepatocellular carcinoma is increasingly recognized in patients with advanced NASH with fibrosis or cirrhosis.

Treatment

WEIGHT LOSS AND EXERCISE

1. **For the overweight or obese person with hepatic steatosis or NASH, gradual and sustained weight loss can result in resolution of steatosis and normalization of aminotransferase levels.**
2. Weight loss achieved with protein malnutrition does not improve hepatic steatosis.
3. Weight loss achieved with bariatric surgery improves NASH, but patients must adhere to postoperative dietary guidance to achieve weight loss and avoid nutritional deficiencies.
4. Improved glycemic control in type 2 diabetes mellitus without weight loss is not helpful.
5. Regular exercise improves insulin sensitivity and improves NAFLD.

MEDICATIONS

No medications have been approved for the treatment of NASH; however, the following drugs have been examined in clinical trials:

- Pioglitazone appears to be beneficial for some patients, probably by improving adipocyte insulin sensitivity and preventing inappropriate lipolysis; side effects include weight gain, exacerbation of heart failure, and possibly osteoporosis.
- Vitamin E may be helpful in some patients.
- Many drugs are currently under evaluation for the treatment of NASH.
- **Statin use is not contraindicated in patients with NASH.**

FURTHER READING

Angulo P, Kleiner DE, Dam-Larsen S, et al. Liver fibrosis, but no other histologic features, is associated with long-term outcomes of patients with nonalcoholic fatty liver disease. *Gastroenterology*. 2015;149:389–397.

Bays H, Cohen DE, Chalasani N, et al. An assessment by the Statin Liver Safety Task Force: 2014 update. *J Clin Lipidol*. 2014;8:S47–S57.

Centis E, Marzocchi R, Di Domizio S, et al. The effect of lifestyle changes in non-alcoholic fatty liver disease. *Dig Dis Sci*. 2010;28:267–273.

Chalasani N, Younossi Z, Lavine JE, et al. The diagnosis and management of non-alcoholic fatty liver disease: practice guideline by the American Association for the Study of Liver Diseases, American College of Gastroenterology, and the American Gastroenterological Association. *Hepatology*. 2012;55:2005–2023.

Johnson NA, Keating SE, George J. Exercise and the liver: implications for therapy in fatty liver disorders. *Semin Liver Dis*. 2012;32:65–79.

Lassailly G, Caiazzo R, Buob D, et al. Bariatric surgery reduces features of nonalcoholic steatohepatitis in morbidly obese patients. *Gastroenterology*. 2015;149:379–388.

Marchesini G, Mazzella N, Forlani G. Weight loss for a healthy liver. *Gastroenterology*. 2015;149:274–278.

McKenney JM, Davidson MH, Jacobson TA, et al. Final conclusions and recommendations of the National Lipid Association Statin Safety Assessment Task Force. *Am J Cardiol*. 2006;97(8A):89C–94C.

Neuschwander-Tetri BA, Unalp A, Creer MH, et al. Influence of local reference populations on upper limits of normal for serum alanine aminotransferase levels. *Arch Intern Med*. 2008;168:663–666.

Neuschwander-Tetri BA. Hepatic lipotoxicity and the pathogenesis of nonalcoholic steatohepatitis: the central role of nontriglyceride fatty acid metabolites. *Hepatology*. 2010;52:774–788.

Neuschwander-Tetri BA. Carbohydrate intake and nonalcoholic fatty liver disease. *Curr Opin Clin Nutr Metab Care*. 2013;16:446–452.

Ratziu V. Pharmacological agents for NASH. *Nat Rev Gastroenterol Hepatol*. 2013;10:676–685.

Rinella ME. Nonalcoholic fatty liver disease: a systematic review. *JAMA*. 2015;313:2263–2273.

Sullivan S. Implications of diet on nonalcoholic fatty liver disease. *Curr Opin Gastroenterol*. 2010;26:160–164.

CHAPTER 10

Drug-Induced and Toxic Liver Disease

James H. Lewis, MD

KEY POINTS

1 The 10 most frequent causes of acute drug-induced liver injury (DILI) in the prospective Drug-Induced Liver Injury Network (DILIN) are amoxicillin-clavulanic acid (amox-clav), isoniazid (INH), nitrofurantoin, sulfamethoxazole-trimethoprim (SMX-TMP), minocycline, cefazolin, azithromycin, ciprofloxacin, levofloxacin, and diclofenac. These 10 drugs represent more than one third of the 190 agents reported to DILIN.

2 Although a rare event, acute DILI remains the most frequent overall cause of acute liver failure (ALF); the leading agent responsible is acetaminophen, followed by isoniazid and other antituberculosis (anti-TB) drugs, nonsulfa antibiotics, and sulfonamides.

3 Herbal and dietary supplements (HDS) leading to hepatotoxicity have become more frequent causes of hepatotoxicity in the United States and other developed nations. The incidence of HDS liver injury recorded in DILIN has nearly tripled since 2005 to 16%, so that HDS is the third most common class of implicated agents. Anabolic steroid-containing supplements used for body building are an important cause of prolonged jaundice in young men.

4 The clinical course and outcome of DILI ranges from mild self-limited elevations in serum alanine aminotransferase (ALT) levels to drug-induced ALF. Hy's law of drug-induced jaundice predicts a case-fatality rate or need for liver transplantation (LT) of 10% or higher and has been validated in several large national registries, including the ongoing U.S. DILIN study.

5 Since DILI can mimic all known causes of acute and chronic liver disease (CLD), establishing causality may be difficult. Knowledge of the biochemical injury pattern and clinical "signature" of a suspected drug is essential, because histopathologic findings are often nonspecific and rarely, if ever, considered pathognomonic.

6 Guidelines for the diagnosis and management of DILI have been published, although specific antidotes and therapies remain limited. N-acetylcysteine (NAC) is the mainstay of treatment for acetaminophen overdose; however, the value of NAC for nonacetaminophen drug-induced ALF may be limited to adults with early-stage coma.

7 The LiverTox.nih.gov website from the National Library of Medicine is an interactive, online, virtual textbook containing the latest information on several hundred agents that cause liver injury.

Overview

1. More than 670 drugs are currently listed in the LiverTox database (with >1000 compounds responsible if HDS and industrial chemicals are included).

2. **Nine of the top 10 causes of acute nonacetaminophen DILI in the U.S. DILIN are antimicrobial agents;** the three leading agents are amox-clav, INH, and nitrofurantoin. Collectively, these 10 drugs represent more than one third of all DILI cases. The most frequent 25 agents (including HDS) that cause DILI account for about 50% of the 190 individual causes.

3. Although liver injury caused by industrial chemicals is much less of an issue today than in the past, due in part to improved occupational safety procedures, liver injury due to certain household agents continues to be reported. For example, iron toxicity from inadvertent ingestion remains an issue with young children. Exposures to other heavy metals (e.g., phosphorus, copper) are largely a problem in the developing world.

4. Among botanical hepatotoxins, mushroom poisoning is one of the most common and requires prompt treatment if ALF is to be avoided.

5. HDS that cause liver injury are being recognized increasingly and are now the third leading class of drugs that cause DILI in the United States.

6. The low overall incidence of DILI is out of proportion to its potential severity and clinical significance. The risk of death or need for LT from drug-induced ALF is about 10%, and hepatotoxicity in clinical trials represents one of the most frequent reasons that new drugs are withdrawn during drug development.

7. Most agents that cause liver injury do so in an unpredictable, dose-independent manner (so-called metabolic idiosyncrasy). Host factors that convey an increased risk for DILI have included female gender, older age, obesity, underlying chronic hepatitis B or C or human immunodeficiency virus (HIV) infection, and chronic alcoholism. More recent studies suggest that the pharmacologic properties of the drug (i.e., higher daily dose, high degree of hepatic metabolism, high degree of lipophilicity), the patient's innate immune system, and the presence of certain genetic markers (human leukocyte antigen [HLA] and cytochrome P-450 [CYP] polymorphisms) are likely more important factors.

8. Clinical presentations of DILI range from asymptomatic elevations in serum levels of ALT to ALF. Some drugs are associated with characteristic clinical syndromes that can point the differential diagnosis in the direction of DILI and away from other causes of acute liver injury and CLD.

9. Diagnosing DILI can be extremely challenging because drug injury mimics all other forms of acute, chronic, benign, malignant, vascular, and granulomatous liver diseases, and there is no specific biomarker or pathognomonic histologic feature. **The diagnosis, therefore, remains one of exclusion of other causes.** Knowledge of the biochemical and clinicopathologic "signature" of known cases is essential when a drug suspected of causing liver injury is encountered. The extent of the evaluation is directly proportional to the ability to eliminate other more and less common etiologies.

10. Several causality assessment methods are available to help diagnose DILI. Roussel-Uclaf Causality Assessment Method (RUCAM) scoring is specifically designed to diagnose DILI but requires clinical expertise to calculate and interpret. **Until a specific biomarker is found that can accurately diagnose DILI, the opinion of a clinician skilled in the management of DILI will remain the most important diagnostic method.**

11. **Identification of suspected acute DILI requires prompt discontinuation of the putative culprit.** Typically, biochemical and clinical abnormalities should start to resolve soon after

its discontinuation. In cases in which hypersensitivity or autoimmune features fail to improve, treatment with glucocorticoids may be necessary. NAC is generally reserved for an acute acetaminophen overdose when the patient presents within 16 hours of ingestion. NAC can be given for nonacetaminophen drug-induced ALF but appears to be of benefit only in adults with early-stage hepatic coma (see Chapter 2).

Epidemiology

1. **Although severe DILI is a relatively rare event, drugs are the most common cause of ALF in the United States and other Westernized countries, with acetaminophen implicated in 40% to 50% of the estimated 2000 cases that occur annually in the United States.**
   - Other drugs (including HDS) are responsible for 11% to 12%, a percentage equal to that of ALF from acute viral hepatitis and greater than that seen with all other individually identified causes.
   - Drug-induced ALF accounts for approximately 15% of liver transplants performed for ALF. Acetaminophen accounts for most of these drug-induced cases, with all other idiosyncratic causes of drug-induced ALF accounting for a relatively small fraction.
2. Estimates of nonacetaminophen-related DILI range from 10 to 20 cases per 100,000 per year in Western nations. Among hospitalized patients, DILI is a relatively rare cause of jaundice.
3. Among hospitalized patients in Ireland with a serum ALT value >1000 U/L, ischemic liver injury was found to be the most common etiology (61%), and DILI was the next most common cause (16%), followed by acute viral hepatitis (12%), an undetermined cause (5%), and acute choledocholithiasis (4.4%). Acetaminophen toxicity accounted for almost one half of the DILI cases, with others caused by antituberculosis agents and other antibiotics.
4. The most common causes of DILI in the DILIN are listed in Table 10.1. The 10 most frequent causes represent about 35% of the 190 individual agents in the registry. The top 25 agents account for nearly one half of all cases.
5. The most common causes of ALF and drug-induced ALF from the U.S. ALF Study Group are listed in Table 10.2 (see also Chapter 2).
   - The definition of drug-induced ALF includes all of the following:
     - Encephalopathy: Any degree of mental alteration (e.g., day/night confusion, disorientation, sleepiness)
     - Coagulopathy (international normalized ratio [INR] >1.5)
     - Absence of preexisting cirrhosis
     - Injury of <26 weeks in duration
   - Nonacetaminophen drug-induced ALF has a poor prognosis, with a mortality rate of up to 75% without LT.
6. Hepatotoxicity due to HDS is increasingly recognized and reported. The DILIN reports HDS as a cause in 16% of cases, second only to antimicrobial agents as the most common reason for all-cause DILI. Similarly, HDS are a significant cause of drug-induced ALF. The more widespread use of HDS has also been associated with an increase in safety alerts issued by the U.S. Food and Drug Administration (FDA), as well as foreign regulatory bodies, for several products—most recently, the weight loss and muscle building compounds Hydroxycut and OxyELITE Pro. Among patients with HDS liver injury reported in the DILIN between 2003 and 2013, bodybuilding HDS accounted for 35% of the total. Many of these were anabolic steroids, nitric oxide boosters, and slimming aids. In addition, most patients were taking more than one compound, making causality difficult to ascertain in some cases. More than 200 products have been implicated (Table 10.3).

TABLE 10.1 ■ Drugs That Most Frequently Caused DILI in the U.S. DILI Network, 2004–2015

Rank	Drug	No. of Cases (%)
1	Herbal and dietary supplements	145 (16.1)
2	Amoxicillin-clavulanic acid	91 (10.1)
3	Isoniazid	48 (5.3)
4	Nitrofurantoin	42 (4.7)
5	Trimethoprim-sulfamethoxazole	31 (3.4)
6	Minocycline	28 (3.1)
7	Cefazolin	20 (2.2)
8	Azithromycin	18 (2.0)
9	Ciprofloxacin	16 (1.8)
10	Levofloxacin	13 (1.4)
11	Diclofenac	12 (1.3)
12	Phenytoin	12 (1.3)
13	Methyldopa	11 (1.2)
14	Azathioprine	10 (1.1)
15	Hydralazine	9 (1.0)
16	Lamotrigine	9 (1.0)
17	Mercaptopurine	9 (1.0)
18	Atorvastatin	8 (0.9)
19	Moxifloxacin	8 (0.9)
20	Allopurinol	7 (0.8)
21	Duloxetine	7 (0.8)
22	Rosuvastatin	7 (0.8)
23	Telithromycin	7 (0.8)
24	Terbinafine	7 (0.8)
25	Valproic acid	7 (0.8)

DILI, Drug-induced liver injury.
Adapted from Chalasani NP, Bonkovsky HL, Fontana RJ, et al. Drug-induced liver injury in the USA: a report of 899 instances assessed prospectively. *Gastroenterology.* 2015;148:1340–1352.

TABLE 10.2 ■ Specific Causes of Acute Liver Failure and Idiosyncratic DILI in the U.S. Acute Liver Failure Study Group Database

Cause of ALF (n = 2000)	No. of Cases (%)	Cause of Idiosyncratic DILI (n = 133)	No. of Cases (%)
AAP	916 (45.8)	Anti-TB drugs	25 (18.8)
Idiosyncratic DILI	220 (11)	Nonsulfa antibiotics	19 (14.3)
Hepatitis B	142 (7.1)	Sulfonamides	12 (9.0)
Hepatitis A	36 (1.8)	Antifungals	6 (4.5)
Autoimmune	137 (6.8)	HDS	14 (10.5)
Ischemic	112 (5.6)	Antiepileptics	11 (8.3)
Wilson disease	25 (1.25)	Psychotropics	4 (3.0)
Budd-Chiari syndrome	15 (0.075)	Antimetabolics	11 (8.3)
Pregnancy	18 (0.09)	NSAIDs	7 (5.3)
Other	134 (6.7)	Statins	6 (4.5)
Indeterminate	245 (12.25)	Biologics	4 (3.0)
		Others	8 (6.0)

AAP, Acetaminophen; *ALF,* acute liver failure; *DILI,* drug-induced liver injury; *HDS,* herbal, dietary, and weight loss supplements; *NSAIDs,* nonsteroidal antiinflammatory drugs; *TB,* tuberculosis.

TABLE 10.3 ■ **Potentially Hepatotoxic Herbal and Dietary Supplements**

Remedy	Popular Use	Source	Hepatotoxic Component	Type of Liver Injury Reported
Barakol	Anxiolytic	*Cassia siamea*	Uncertain	Reversible hepatitis or cholestasis
Black cohosh	Menopausal symptoms	*Cimicifuga racemosa*	Uncertain (mitochondrial damage?)	Acute hepatitis, ALF (unconfirmed)
"Bush tea"	Fever	*Senecio, Heliotropium, Crotalaria* spp.	Pyrrolizidine alkaloids	SOS causing a Budd-Chiari–like illness
Cascara	Laxative	*Cascara sagrada*	Anthracene glycoside	Cholestatic hepatitis
Chaso/onshido	Weight loss	—	*N*-nitro-fenfluramine	Acute hepatitis, ALF
Chaparral leaf (greasewood, creosote bush)	"Liver tonic," burn salve, weight loss	*Larrea tridentata*	Nordihydroguaiaretic acid	Acute cholestatic and chronic hepatitis, ALF
Comfrey	Herbal tea	*Symphytum officinale*	Pyrrolizidine alkaloid transformed into hepatotoxic adducts	Acute SOS, cirrhosis
Germander	Weight loss, fever	*Teucrium chamaedrys, Teucrium capitatum, Teucrium polium*	Diterpenoids, epoxides	Acute and chronic hepatitis, autoimmune injury(?), ALF
Greater celandine	Gallstones, IBS	*Chelidonium majus*	Uncertain	Cholestatic hepatitis, fibrosis
Herbalife products	Nutritional supplement	Multiple ingredients	Various	Severe hepatitis, ALF
Hydroxycut (initial formulation)	Weight loss	*Camellia sinensis*	Green tea extract	Acute hepatitis, ALF
Impila	Multiple uses	*Callilepis laureola*	Potassium atractylate	Hepatic necrosis
Jin bu huan	Sleep aid, analgesic	*Lycopodium serratum*	Levo-tetrahydropalmatine(?)	Acute or chronic hepatitis or cholestasis, steatosis
Kava kava	Anxiolytic	*Piper methysticum*	Kava lactones, pyrone	Acute hepatitis, cholestasis, ALF(?)
Kombucha	Weight loss	Lichen alkaloid	Usnic acid	Acute hepatitis
Lipokinetix	Weight loss	Lichen alkaloid	Usnic acid	Acute hepatitis, jaundice, ALF
Ma huang	Weight loss	*Ephedra* spp.	Ephedrine	Severe hepatitis, ALF
Mistletoe	Asthma, infertility	*Viscus album*	Uncertain	Hepatitis (in combination with skullcap)
OxyELITE Pro	Performance enhancement	Multiple ingredients	Uncertain (aegeline?, dimethylamylamine?)	Severe acute hepatitis, ALF
Pennyroyal (squawmint oil)	Abortifacient, insect repellent	*Hedeoma pulegioides, Mentha pulegium*	Pulegone, menthofurans, monoterpenes	Severe hepatocellular necrosis with seizures, circulatory collapse, and multiorgan failure

TABLE 10.3 ■ **Potentially Hepatotoxic Herbal and Dietary Supplements—cont'd**

Remedy	Popular Use	Source	Hepatotoxic Component	Type of Liver Injury Reported
Sassafras	Herbal tea	*Sassafras albidum*	Safrole	HCC (in animals)
Saw palmetto	Prostatism	*Serenoa repens*	Steroid-induced injury(?)	Chronic cholestasis
Senna	Laxative	*Cassia angustifolia*	Sennoside alkaloids; anthrone	Acute hepatitis
Shou-wu-pian	Traditional medicine	*Polygonum multiflorum*	Uncertain	Acute hepatitis or cholestasis
Skullcap	Anxiolytic, sedative	*Scutellaria*	Diterpenoids	Hepatitis (often in conjunction with other agents)
Syo-saiko-to	Multiple uses	*Scutellaria* root	Diterpenoids	Hepatocellular necrosis, cholestasis, steatosis, granulomas
Valerian	Sedative, sleep aid	*Valeriana officinalis*	Uncertain	Elevated serum ALT, AST (often in conjunction with other agents)

ALF, Acute liver failure; *ALT,* alanine aminotransferase; *AST,* aspartate aminotransferase; *HCC,* hepatocellular carcinoma; *IBS,* irritable bowel syndrome; *SOS,* sinusoidal obstruction syndrome.

Biochemical, Clinical, and Pathologic Features

1. DILI may present as asymptomatic elevations of serum ALT and aspartate aminotransferase (AST) levels. The usual threshold for a clinically significant elevation is >3 times the upper limit of normal (ULN).
   - Depending on the specific laboratory, the ULN for serum ALT and AST can vary considerably.
   - The true normal values for serum ALT in healthy subjects without liver disease are <30 U/L for men and <19 U/L for women (see Chapter 1).
2. If an ALT elevation does not worsen, and the patient remains free of any associated hepatitis-related symptoms despite continuing the drug, the term "drug tolerance" is applied, implying hepatic adaption to subclinical injury.
   - A list of drugs and the percentage of patients in whom tolerance occurs is shown in Table 10.4.
   - It is important to note that in some cases, ALT levels may continue to rise and overt hepatic injury can occur. As a result, careful biochemical and clinical monitoring is needed.
3. Recognition of **biochemical injury patterns (hepatocellular, cholestatic, mixed)** and how the absolute values (fold-elevation above normal) and the specific ratios of ALT, AST, alkaline phosphatase (AP), and bilirubin correlate with the various forms of DILI remain essential to the diagnosis of DILI. Alcoholic liver disease (ALD), in particular, has a unique biochemical profile that can often help distinguish it from DILI.

TABLE 10.4 ■ **Drugs Associated with Hepatic "Tolerance"**

Examples	Frequency of Drug Tolerance (%)
Tacrine	>25
Amiodarone, chlorpromazine, phenytoin, valproate	20–25
Androgens, disulfiram, erythromycin estolate, isoniazid, leflunomide, ketoconazole	10–20
NSAIDs (e.g., diclofenac)	5–10
Statins, sulfonamides, sulfonylureas, tricyclic antidepressants	<5

NSAIDs, Nonsteroidal antiinflammatory drugs.

- ■ R value to determine the biochemical injury pattern:
  - – This classification system uses the ratio of elevation above the ULN of ALT to AP to classify liver injury as hepatocellular, cholestatic, or a mixed pattern.
  - – First proposed as part of an International Consensus Meeting Criteria in 1990
  - – The serum bilirubin level is not a component of the pattern definition; if jaundice is present, the pattern is referred to as hepatocellular jaundice or cholestatic jaundice.

R value = ALT/ULN ÷ AP/ULN:

  - – Hepatocellular injury (R ≥5 and ALT >2× ULN)
  - – Cholestatic injury (R ≤2 and AP >2× ULN)
  - – Mixed injury (5 > R > 2 and ALT, AP both >2× ULN)
- ■ R values can help determine whether a specific drug is the cause of liver injury (Table 10.5).
  - – Example: ALT 500 U/L (ULN = 40 U/L); AP 230 U/L (ULN 115 U/L)

R value = ([500/40] = 12.5) ÷ ([230/115] = 2)
equals 6.25, signifying a hepatocellular pattern of injury

4. The absolute values (as times elevations above ULN) of ALT and AST and the ratio of ALT to AST can be helpful in differentiating idiosyncratic DILI from other causes of liver injury. Mean peak ALT values for acute idiosyncratic DILI are generally much lower than those seen with acute viral hepatitis, ischemic hepatitis, and acute poisoning from toxic mushrooms, acetaminophen, or chemicals. Certain non-DILI etiologies are associated with an AST > ALT (Table 10.6).

5. A serum gamma-glutamyltranspeptidase (GGTP) elevation can reflect inflammation or enzyme induction from multiple causes (GGTP is not considered a true liver injury–associated biochemical measure).
   - ■ GGTP rises in parallel with AP in cholestatic injury.
   - ■ Mild-to-moderate elevations of GGTP are seen in idiosyncratic DILI, nonalcoholic fatty liver disease (NAFLD), and other CLD.
   - ■ GGTP is elevated out of proportion to AST and ALT in ALD (because of enzyme induction).
   - ■ Isolated causes of a GGTP elevation are seen with anticonvulsants (e.g., phenytoin, barbiturates), alcohol ingestion, fatty liver, and heart failure.

6. Clinical syndromes associated with idiosyncratic DILI:
   - ■ Many instances of mild DILI are asymptomatic with self-limited ALT and AST elevations.
   - ■ Clinical features of severe DILI are often nonspecific and include nausea in 60%, abdominal pain in 40%, jaundice in 70%, and pruritus in 50% of cases.
   - ■ Clinical syndromes associated with DILI are shown in Table 10.7.

TABLE 10.5 ■ Causes of Drug-Induced Liver Injury According to Predominant Injury Patterns and R Value[a]

Drug Class	Hepatocellular (R ≥5)	Acute Cholestatic (R ≤2)	Chronic Cholestatic/VBDS (R ≤2)	Granulomatous (R ≤2 or mixed)	AIH (May be Hepatocellular, Cholestatic, or Mixed)
			Examples		
Anesthetics	Halothane				
Antibiotics	Sulfonamides Ketoconazole Dapsone	Erythromycin estolate Amoxicillin-clavulanic acid Flucloxacillin	Clindamycin Amoxicillin-clavulanic acid Thiabendazole SMX-TMP	—	Nitrofurantoin Minocycline
Anti-TB drugs	INH PYZ Rifampin	—	—	—	—
Anticonvulsants	Phenytoin VPA Carbamazepine	—	—	Phenytoin	—
Antiinflammatories/analgesics	Diclofenac AAP	Sulindac	—	Allopurinol Gold salts	Diclofenac
Psychotropics	TCAs	CPZ Haloperidol	CPZ Haloperidol Imipramine	Carbamazepine	—
Miscellaneous causes	Disulfiram Labetalol PTU Nicotinic acid	Anabolic and contraceptive steroids Captopril TPN	Tolbutamide Ethinyl estradiol Terbinafine	Hydralazine Quinidine Mineral oil	Fenofibrate Infliximab Ipilimumab Methyldopa Procainamide Statins

[a]R = ALT/ULN ÷ AP/ULN, where ALT is serum alanine aminotransferase level, AP is serum alkaline phosphatase level, and ULN is upper limit of normal.

AAP, Acetaminophen; AIH, autoimmune hepatitis; CPZ, carbamazepine; INH, isoniazid; PTU, propylthiouracil; PYZ, pyrazinamide; SMX-TMP, sulfamethoxazole-trimethoprim; TCAs, tricyclic antidepressants; TB, tuberculosis; TPN, total parenteral nutrition; VPA, valproic acid; VBDS, vanishing bile duct syndrome.

TABLE 10.6 ■ Peak ALT/AST Values and Ratios in Various Forms of Acute Liver Injury

Cause of Liver Injury	Peak Values	AST to ALT Ratio in Serum	Comment
Acute hepatocellular idiopathic DILI	<2000 U/L; median peak 500–800 U/L	ALT > AST	Jaundice implies impaired hepatic function
Alcoholic liver disease; alcoholic hepatitis (AH)	AST <300 U/L, ALT <100 U/L)	AST > ALT 2–3 to 1	RUQ pain, leukocytosis, and jaundice in AH
Acute hepatitis A or B	<6000 U/L	ALT > AST	Usually resolves over weeks
Acute hepatitis C	<2000 U/L	ALT > AST	Risk of chronicity with anicteric cases

Continued

TABLE 10.6 ■ Peak ALT/AST Values and Ratios in Various Forms of Acute Liver Injury—cont'd

Cause of Liver Injury	Peak Values	AST to ALT Ratio in Serum	Comment
Ischemic hepatitis (acute hypoxic hepatitis)	Can exceed 10,000 U/L	AST > ALT LDH > ALT	Rapid recovery within 10 days
Amanita and other toxic mushroom poisoning	Same range as ischemic hepatitis	ALT ≥ AST	Often results in ALF
Carbon tetrachloride and other chemical toxins	Same range as ischemic hepatitis	ALT ≥ AST	Often results in ALF

ALF, Acute liver failure; *ALT,* alanine aminotransferase; *AST,* aspartate aminotransferase; *LDH,* lactate dehydrogenase; *RUQ,* right upper quadrant.

TABLE 10.7 ■ Clinical Syndromes Associated with Acute Drug-Induced Liver Injury (DILI)

Clinical Syndrome	Manifestations	Drug Cause(s)
Acute viral hepatitis-like	Absence of hypersensitivity symptoms; presents with malaise, fatigue, anorexia, nausea, vomiting, RUQ pain	INH
Acute hypersensitivity	Fever, rash, and/or eosinophilia, usually with short latency and prompt rechallenge response	Allopurinol, amoxicillin-clavulanic acid, carbamazepine, halothane, phenytoin, SMX-TMP
Sulfone reaction	Fever, exfoliative dermatitis, lymphadenopathy, atypical lymphocytosis, eosinophilia, hemolytic anemia, methemoglobinemia	Dapsone
Pseudomononucleosis	Hypersensitivity syndrome with atypical lymphocytosis, lymphadenopathy, and splenomegaly	Phenytoin, dapsone, sulfonamides
DILI associated with severe skin injury	Stevens Johnson syndrome, toxic epidermal necrolysis	Phenytoin, carbamazepine, dapsone, nevirapine, allopurinol, SMX-TMP
AIH	Fatigue, anorexia, lethargy, arthralgias, positive autoantibodies (antinuclear and smooth muscle/anti-actin antibodies)	Nitrofurantoin, minocycline, methyldopa
Immune-mediated colitis with autoimmune hepatitis	Similar to AIH	Ipilimumab
Acute cholecystitis-like	Biliary pain	Erythromycin estolate, ceftriaxone
Reye syndrome–like	Hepatocellular injury, acidosis, hyperammonemia, encephalopathy, abdominal pain, nausea, vomiting, paradoxical worsening of seizure activity, microvesicular steatosis on biopsy	Valproic acid
Budd-Chiari–like	Acute onset ascites and jaundice due to SOS	Myeloablative treatment for bone marrow, stem cell transplant

TABLE 10.7 ■ **Clinical Syndromes Associated with Acute Drug-Induced Liver Injury (DILI)—cont'd**

Clinical Syndrome	Manifestations	Drug Cause(s)
Liver injury with atypical seizures	May present with worsening and more frequent seizures (including status epilepticus), and severe abdominal pain	Valproic acid
Noncirrhotic portal hypertension	Variceal bleeding and/or ascites due to nodular regenerative hyperplasia	Azathioprine, 6-mercaptopurine

AIH, Autoimmune hepatitis; *INH,* isoniazid; *RUQ,* right upper quadrant; *SOS,* sinusoidal obstruction syndrome; *SMX-TMP,* sulfamethoxazole-trimethoprim.

7. Clinicopathologic presentations of the most common causes of idiosyncratic DILI are shown in Table 10.8.
8. Clinical presentations of common chemical hepatotoxins are shown in Table 10.9.

Host Risk Factors for Developing Drug-Induced Liver Injury

1. Risk of DILI in patients with CLD and cirrhosis
   - 10% of U.S. DILIN series had CLD (mostly chronic hepatitis C, NAFLD, or unexplained baseline liver biochemical test abnormalities).
   - No differences were seen in the classes or agents implicated in DILI; the one exception was azithromycin (which was nearly four times as likely to cause DILI in patients with than without CLD).
   - The severity was greater in patients with CLD, and mortality was significantly increased (16% versus 5.2%), than in patients without CLD.
   - Patients with CLD and DILI had a higher frequency of diabetes mellitus (38% versus 23%) as a possible risk factor for DILI than those without CLD.
   - Drugs that should be avoided in patients with cirrhosis are shown in Box 10.1.
2. Effect of older age on DILI
   - 16.6% of U.S. DILIN patients are >65 years of age.
   - Older patients have more cholestatic DILI (36% versus 21%) than younger patients; however, they have no greater need for LT, nor are they more likely to have a fatal outcome than younger patients.
   - The risk of overt INH injury is especially age dependent (frequency of <0.5% in those age <20 years; 0.5% age 20 to 35; 1% to 2% age 35 to 50; 3% age >50 in the United States).
3. Other risk factors
   - Gender: Women are more prone to develop acute and chronic DILI, as well as drug-induced ALF, possibly because of higher rates of exposure to DILI-causing drugs (e.g., sulindac, diclofenac, nitrofurantoin, azathioprine, leflunomide), but for unclear reasons with other agents (e.g., halothane, INH). Men are at higher risk of DILI caused by amox-clav than women.
   - HLA polymorphisms: Several drugs have been shown to have a possible genetic basis for causing DILI (Table 10.10).

TABLE 10.8 ■ Clinicopathologic Features of Agents That Commonly Cause Drug-Induced Liver Injury

Drug	Time to Onset	Clinical Features	Histologic Features	Biochemical Injury Pattern	Comments
Amoxicillin-clavulanic acid	Mean 17 days (may be delayed for up to 6–7 weeks after treatment)	Hypersensitivity (fever, rash, eosinophilia) in two thirds; interstitial nephritis and sialadenitis may be seen	Acute and chronic cholestasis; may evolve into the VBDS	Acute hepatocellular injury in patients <55 years of age; cholestatic or mixed injury in those >55 years of age	Older men > women; risk higher after prior exposure
Isoniazid	2–4 months	Acute viral hepatitis-like (nausea, abdominal pain, jaundice, fatigue, malaise); may progress to ALF; usually resolves within 4 weeks	Diffuse degeneration and necrosis, and fatal cases have shown massive necrosis (often with eosinophilia)	Hepatocellular; serum ALT can exceed 1000 U/L; jaundice in some cases; 10%–20% have asymptomatic ALT elevation	Age-dependent risk; higher risk with elevated baseline ALT and concomitant use of rifampin
Nitrofurantoin	1–2 weeks (may be delayed after short course of treatment)	Acute hepatitis with hypersensitivity features; combined toxicity leading to pneumonitis and hepatitis may occur	—	Acute hepatocellular injury > cholestatic	Acute injury is quite rare
	Months to years	Insidious onset of fatigue, weakness, jaundice	Resembles chronic autoimmune hepatitis; less often granulomatous hepatitis	Acute/chronic hepatocellular injury; hyperglobulinemia, two thirds have positive ANA or SMA	Chronic injury common (1 in 1500), females > males
SMX-TMP	Few days to weeks	Acute hypersensitivity reaction with eosinophilia, atypical lymphocytosis	Acute cholestasis can evolve into chronic cholestasis with VBDS	Acute cholestasis > mixed injury; less often a mild reaction with granulomas	Higher incidence of hypersensitivity reactions in HIV-positive persons compared with the general population (up to 70% vs. 3%)
Minocycline	Mean of 15 days after administration	Rapid onset serum sickness–like illness associated with fever, myalgia, arthralgia, and rash	Typical features of autoimmune hepatitis	Acute hepatocellular injury	Women <40 years of age are most susceptible with a latency period about half as long as that seen in males
	3–4 weeks	Hypersensitivity syndrome with exfoliative dermatitis and eosinophilia			
	>1 year	Chronic drug-induced lupus-like syndrome with jaundice, malaise, polyarthralgia, fever, and the presence of autoantibodies (usually ANA)		Acute-on-chronic autoimmune hepatitis-like injury, positive ANA and or SMA	

TABLE 10.8 ■ **Clinicopathologic Features of Agents That Commonly Cause Drug-Induced Liver Injury—cont'd**

Drug	Time to Onset	Clinical Features	Histologic Features	Biochemical Injury Pattern	Comments
Cefazolin	Mean 20 days; can occur after a single dose; shorter latency on reexposure (3–6 days)	Most present with features of immunoallergy (jaundice, pruritus, nausea, fever, rash); generally mild-moderate severity and self-limited	Cholestatic hepatitis; chronic cholestasis less common; eosinophils in inflammatory infiltrate	Most cases cholestatic or mixed; mean peak serum ALT 409 U/L, alkaline phosphatase 409 U/L, bilirubin 9.8 mg/dL	Injury less severe than that due to other cephalosporins
Azithromycin	14 days (after mean treatment duration of 4 days [range 2–7 days])	Most present with jaundice (mean peak bilirubin 9.2 mg/dL); hypersensitivity skin injury in 10%; occasional death and need for liver transplantation in patients with underlying liver disease	Intrahepatic cholestasis; ductopenia and SOS in those with prolonged cholestasis	Hepatocellular in >50% (mean peak ALT 2127 U/L); cholestatic in ⅓ (mean peak alkaline phosphatase 481 U/L); mixed in 10%	Highest risk in patients with chronic liver disease
Fluoroquinolones (ciprofloxacin, levofloxacin)	Days to weeks	Typically presents with immunologic features suggestive of a hypersensitivity reaction	Focal necrosis, eosinophils	Hepatocellular, cholestatic, and mixed injury all reported	Acute and chronic liver failure reported with trovafloxacin
Diclofenac	1–3 months	Majority of patients present with fatigue, anorexia, and nausea, half of whom also have jaundice	Zone 3 hepatic necrosis or mixed injury; cases of intrahepatic cholestasis represent about 8% of the total	Mostly hepatocellular; instances resembling autoimmune hepatitis with ANA have been reported	The average age of affected patients is 60, and women with osteoarthritis appear to be most susceptible
Disulfiram	2–12 weeks (much shorter in cases of reexposure)	Can present with asymptomatic elevations in serum ALT in up to 25% of patients; more severe injury resembles acute viral hepatitis (malaise, anorexia, RUQ pain, jaundice) and can progress to ALF with a high mortality rate. Some patients present with fever, rash, and eosinophilia suggesting immunoallergy	Ranges from focal to severe necrosis; chronic inflammation with eosinophils in cases with rash and fever; no steatosis, polymorphonuclear leukocytes, or Mallory-Denk bodies (in contrast to alcoholic hepatitis)	Hepatocellular injury predominates; serum ALT >3× ULN in 4%–5%; peak values can be >1000 U/L (in contrast to alcoholic hepatitis); recovery generally occurs within 1–2 months after discontinuation	Risk of severe acute hepatitis estimated to be 1 in 10,000–30,000 patient-years of treatment

Continued

TABLE 10.8 ■ Clinicopathologic Features of Agents That Commonly Cause Drug-Induced Liver Injury—cont'd

Drug	Time to Onset	Clinical Features	Histologic Features	Biochemical Injury Pattern	Comments
Biologic agents (infliximab, ipilimumab)	3–9 weeks for ipilimumab	Can be associated with colitis and other immune-related symptoms	Findings consistent with autoimmune hepatitis	Immune-related hepatitis, may be severe (serum AST or ALT levels >8× ULN, or bilirubin levels >5× ULN)	Immune-related hepatitis
Phenytoin	Few days to 2 months	Acute generalized hypersensitivity and jaundice in approximately 30%; less dramatic hepatic injury also seen, as reflected by elevated aminotransferases, in about 20% of patients; may resemble "pseudolymphoma or mononucleosis-like syndrome" with lymphadenopathy and atypical lymphocytosis; almost all patients develop a generalized rash that may become exfoliative (as part of the anticonvulsant hypersensitivity syndrome)	Diffuse degeneration, multifocal or massive necrosis, and multiple apoptotic bodies; clusters of eosinophils or lymphocytes, and at times focal aggregates of hyperplastic Kupffer cells. Granulomatous inflammation has been described; the hepatic lesion, with lymphocyte "beading" in sinusoids, granulomatoid changes, and frequent hepatocyte mitoses, may resemble that of infectious mononucleosis	Mixed-hepatocellular damage, predominantly cytotoxic, although cholestasis may be prominent. Serum ALT levels up to 100× ULN, with lesser elevations of alkaline phosphatase	Alkaline phosphatase levels are elevated in almost all patients taking the drug
Dapsone	2–7 weeks	Erythematous maculopapular skin eruption, fever, hepatomegaly, pruritus, lymphadenopathy, edema, jaundice, methemoglobinemia, and hemolytic anemia	Inflammation with sinusoidal beading and nonzonal necrosis	Jaundice appears to be mixed-hepatocellular	2%–4% frequency in patients with leprosy and those treated for other indications; can be fatal
Valproic acid	1–3 months	Associated with lethargy, nausea, vomiting, abdominal pain, and increased seizure activity, including status epilepticus in 40%–60%; somnolence, hyperammonemia, coma, and coagulopathy can develop in fatal cases	Microvesicular steatosis, centrizonal necrosis, or both	Transient serum ALT elevations in 10%–15%; hyperammonemia may be seen	Children, and particularly infants <2 years, are more susceptible than adults

TABLE 10.8 ■ Clinicopathologic Features of Agents That Commonly Cause Drug-Induced Liver Injury—cont'd

Drug	Time to Onset	Clinical Features	Histologic Features	Biochemical Injury Pattern	Comments
Statins (e.g., atorvastatin)	1–4 months	Most patients have only asymptomatic elevations in serum ALT that usually do not progress and even normalize despite continued therapy; myalgias suggest myopathy	—	About 1% have a serum ALT >3× ULN; severe injury is rare; few cases of autoimmune hepatitis-like injury	Routine ALT monitoring is not needed
Total parenteral nutrition	Weeks to months to years	Ranges from asymptomatic elevations in serum alkaline phosphatase, ALT, and bilirubin to biliary pain from sludge or gallstones; may progress to biliary-type micronodular cirrhosis requiring liver transplantation	Intrahepatic cholestasis, ballooning and scattered apoptotic bodies, presence of lipofuscin pigment in hypertrophied Kupffer cells, variable periportal ductular proliferation, and fibrosis; steatosis is less common in infants than in adults	Often cholestatic or mixed injury	Risk factors in infants include prematurity, low birth weight, and sepsis
Azathioprine	1–3 months	Mild, asymptomatic, reversible serum ALT elevations; may resolve using lower doses	—	ALT usually <3–5× ULN	Obtain baseline TPMT levels; liver injury may occur with bone marrow suppression. Incidence of about 1 in 1000.
	2–12 months	Acute cholestatic jaundice and fatigue; hypersensitivity features rare	Bland cholestasis, scant inflammation; may progress to VBDS	Elevated alkaline phosphatase and bilirubin	Can progress if drug continued; some patients can develop lymphoma involving the liver
	Long-term use (years)	Noncirrhotic portal hypertension (e.g., variceal bleeding, ascites)	Nodular regenerative hyperplasia; sinusoidal dilatation	Mild elevations of serum ALT and alkaline phosphatase	Can progress if drug discontinued; some patients can develop lymphoma involving the liver

Continued

TABLE 10.8 ■ **Clinicopathologic Features of Agents That Commonly Cause Drug-Induced Liver Injury—cont'd**

Drug	Time to Onset	Clinical Features	Histologic Features	Biochemical Injury Pattern	Comments
Leflunomide	1–6 months	Can present as asymptomatic, self-limited ALT elevations; rarely presents as acute severe hepatitis with diarrhea, fever, and rash	May resemble acute viral hepatitis	Reversible serum ALT elevations, usually <3× ULN; severe injury can be hepatocellular or cholestatic; usually resolves but fatal cases reported	Severe organ toxicity treated with a bile acid washout regimen (see text)
Carbamaze-pine	Median 5 weeks	Can present as the anticonvulsant hypersensitivity syndrome similar to that seen with phenytoin. Fatal reactions in 10%–15% of cases in pretransplant era; SJS and TEN are reported	Cholestatic and hepatocellular injury as well as hepatic granulomas have all been reported; some of the cholestatic cases have shown prominent cholangitis; cholestatic injury may fail to subside for many months or even lead to chronic cholestasis with disappearance of intrahepatic bile ducts (VBDS)	Hepatocellular in about 25% of cases, cholestatic in about 30%, and mixed in the rest. Granulomatous hepatitis is present in up to 75% of biopsy specimens	Neonatal cholestasis from fetal exposure during pregnancy and breastfeeding has been reported

ALF, Acute liver failure; *ALT,* alanine aminotransferase; *ANA,* antinuclear antibodies; *HIV,* human immunodeficiency virus; *SJS,* Stevens Johnson syndrome; *SMA,* smooth muscle antibodies; *SOS,* sinusoidal obstruction syndrome; *TEN,* toxic epidermal necrolysis; *TPMT,* thiopurine methyltransferase; *ULN,* upper limit of normal; *VBDS,* vanishing bile duct syndrome.

TABLE 10.9 ■ **Clinicopathologic Features of Environmental Chemical Hepatotoxins**

Chemical	Clinical Features	Pathophysiology and Histopathology	Treatment	Prognosis	Comments
Iron	Severe injury is seen only with serum iron concentrations >700 μg/dL measured within the first 12 hours	Iron, per se, is not hepatotoxic, but ferric and ferrous ions acting through free radicals and lipid peroxidation can cause membrane disruption and necrosis; periportal necrosis may be seen in the most severe cases	Induce vomiting; administer activated charcoal after acute ingestion; iron chelators	Ingestion of <20 mg/kg of elemental iron is unlikely to produce serious toxicity, whereas doses >200 mg/kg can be fatal	Most cases occur in young children who mistake iron supplements for candy

TABLE 10.9 ■ **Clinicopathologic Features of Environmental Chemical Hepatotoxins—cont'd**

Chemical	Clinical Features	Pathophysiology and Histopathology	Treatment	Prognosis	Comments
Phosphorus	Poisoning by white phosphorus is rare because its use in fireworks and matches has been outlawed in the United States; current cases are usually due to the ingestion of rat or cockroach poison or firecrackers containing yellow phosphorus	The liver may show only steatosis, initially periportal and then diffusely; necrosis may be present	Supportive care	High mortality rate	Symptoms of severe gastrointestinal and neurotoxicity develop shortly after ingestion, with death occurring within 24 hours
Copper salts	Lead to a syndrome resembling iron toxicity; gastrointestinal erosions, renal tubular necrosis, and rhabdomyolysis often accompany hepatic injury that occurs by the second or third day	Perivenular necrosis and cholestasis in deeply jaundiced patients, but only focal necrosis or no changes in mildly jaundiced patients; noncirrhotic portal hypertension has been described	Supportive care, copper chelators (meso-2,3-dimercaptosuccinic acid [DMSA]) and D-penicillamine	Mortality rates in the past were around 15% after ingestion of toxic amounts (1–10 mg) with suicidal intent, especially on the Indian subcontinent	Serum copper as well as ceruloplasmin levels are markedly elevated in acute copper intoxication

BOX 10.1 ■ **Drugs Contraindicated or Restricted for Use in Patients with Cirrhosis Because of an Increased Risk of Drug-Induced Injury**

Agomelatine
Antituberculosis drugs
Azithromycin
Ketoconazole
Methotrexate (especially with leflunomide)
Pyrazinamide
Telithromycin
Tolvaptan
Trovafloxacin
Valproic acid

TABLE 10.10 ■ **Human Leukocyte Antigen Alleles That Predict Drug-Induced Liver Injury**

Drug	Risk Allele	Odds Ratio
Class I Alleles		
Amoxicillin-clavulanic acid	A*02:01	2.2
	B*18:01	2.8
Flucloxacillin	B*57:01	80.6
Ticlopidine	A*33:03	13
Class II Alleles		
Antituberculosis agents	DQB1*02:01	1.9
(isoniazid, rifampin, pyrazinamide)	DQA1*01:02	0.2[a]
Amoxicillin-clavulanic acid	DRB1*15:01 DQB1*06:02	2.3–10
	DRB1*07	0.18[a]
Flucloxacillin	DRB1*07:01–DQB1*03:03	7
	DRB1*15	a
Lapatinib	DRB1*07:01–DQA1*02:01	2.6–9
Lumiracoxib	DRB1*15:01–DQB1*06:02–	5
	DRB5*01:01–DQA1*01:02	
Nevirapine	DRB1*01:02	4.72
Ximelagatran	DRB1*07–DQA1*02	4.4

[a]Risk decreased.

Clues to Drug-Induced Liver Injury

1. Latency periods
   - Short onset (days to few weeks) with immunoallergic DILI (one third of drugs) and more prolonged (1 to 9 months) with metabolic idiosyncrasy
   - Most DILI associated with ultrashort latency periods (<7 days) involves an antibiotic or occurs after a deliberate (or unintentional) rechallenge with an agent known to cause DILI through a hypersensitivity (immunoallergic) mechanism.
   - A few drugs have a delayed onset (up to 6 weeks) after the drug has been stopped (e.g., amox-clav, cefazolin).
   - It is quite rare for acute DILI to occur after a drug is taken >12 months with no sign of liver dysfunction during that time.
   - Prolonged latency (>1 year) is seen with drugs that cause a form of chronic autoimmune-like hepatitis (e.g., nitrofurantoin, minocycline, methyldopa, statins), often associated with positive antinuclear or anti-actin antibodies.
2. Causality assessment of DILI (Box 10.2)
3. The RUCAM was proposed in the early 1990s as an objective means of diagnosing acute DILI. Although imperfect, RUCAM offers a validated method to assist in diagnosis but does not take into account histologic information and often requires the assistance of a clinician skilled in the field of DILI to interpret a number of its elements. Scoring of hepatocellular injury is shown in Table 10.11.
4. Liver biopsy findings in suspected DILI can be supportive of the diagnosis but may be more helpful in excluding competing etiologies. The histologic features of most cases of DILI are

---

BOX 10.2 ■ American College of Gastroenterology Guidelines for Diagnosing Drug-Induced Livery Injury (DILI)

Elements in Diagnostic Evaluation of DILI

Known duration of exposure (to determine latency)

Concomitant medications and diseases

Response to dechallenge (and rechallenge if performed)

Presence or absence of symptoms, rash, eosinophilia

Sufficient exclusionary testing (viral serology, imaging, etc.) to reflect the injury pattern and acuteness of liver biochemical tests (e.g., acute viral serology for hepatitis A, B, and C and AIH when presenting with acute hepatocellular injury; routine testing for hepatitis E virus is not recommended given limitations of current commercial assays; Epstein-Barr virus, cytomegalovirus, and other viral serology if lymphadenopathy, atypical lymphocytosis present)

Sufficient follow-up to determine the clinical outcome: Did the event resolve or become chronic?

Role of Liver Biopsy

Not required if acute injury resolves

Helpful in confirming a clinical suspicion of DILI, but rarely pathognomonic

Useful for differentiating drug-induced AIH from idiopathic AIH

Useful for excluding underlying chronic viral hepatitis, NAFLD, alcoholic liver disease, or other CLD

Used to exclude DILI when reexposure or ongoing use of an agent is expected

Rechallenge

Generally best avoided (especially if a hypersensitivity reaction occurred with initial exposure), unless there is no alternative treatment; desensitization can be attempted with antituberculosis drugs.

Use of Causality Assessment Methods

RUCAM is best considered an adjunct to expert opinion (it should not be the sole diagnostic method).

In patients with underlying chronic viral hepatitis, DILI requires a high index of suspicion, including knowledge of a stable clinical course prior to introduction of the new medication and monitoring of levels of viremia to rule out flares of an underlying viral disease.

Assigning causality to HDS products can be especially difficult and requires knowledge of all ingredients and their purity.

AIH, Autoimmune hepatitis; *CLD,* chronic liver disease; *HDS,* herbal and dietary supplements; *NAFLD,* nonalcoholic fatty liver disease; *RUCAM,* Roussel-Uclaf Causality Assessment Method.

---

nonspecific and rarely pathognomonic (Table 10.12). The photomicrographs in Fig. 10.1 illustrate a number of specific histopathologic forms of DILI.

5. The 3 broad phases of illness following the acute ingestion of various intrinsic hepatotoxins that cause ALF are shown in Table 10.13. A relatively asymptomatic second phase can be confused with clinical recovery, but close observation of such patients is crucial because liver (and other organ) damage often commences during that timeframe.

Prevention

1. Prevention of DILI caused by acetaminophen
   ■ Limiting access of acetaminophen through a reduction in pack size (to a total dose of 12 g or less) has been successful in reducing deaths from overdoses in the United Kingdom and in European Union countries.

TABLE 10.11 ■ Components of Roussel-Uclaf Causality Assessment Method Scoring

Criterion	Points Awarded
Time to onset of serum ALT level >2× ULN after drug start	+2 5–90 days +1 ≤15 days after stopping
≥50% decrease in serum ALT after stopping drug	+3 <8 days +2 <30 days
Negative hepatitis screen and ultrasonography	+2
Hepatotoxicity in product label or published reports	+2
No concomitant medication use	0
Use of concomitant medications that could be alternative causes of DILI	−1 to −3
Positive rechallenge (if performed)	+3
Alcohol use	+1
Age >55 years	+1
DILI RUCAM scoring: Highly probable >8 Probable 6–8 Possible 3–5 Unlikely 1–2 Excluded ≤0	

ALT, Alanine aminotransferase; *DILI,* drug-induced liver injury; *RUCAM;* Roussel-Uclaf Causality Assessment Method; *ULN,* upper limit of normal.

- Acetaminophen doses >2 to 3 g should be avoided in regular alcohol users and abusers to prevent a toxic interaction.
- Doses of 1 to 2 g are considered safe in patients with CLD, including cirrhosis (in whom nonsteroidal antiinflammatory drugs [NSAIDs] may be detrimental because of their effect on platelet function, renal function, and bleeding risk).

2. Potentially hepatotoxic agents that should be avoided in patients with underlying CLD are listed in Box 10.1.

3. Pharmacogenetic testing
   - A number of drugs (e.g., amoxicillin, amox-clav, flucloxacillin, INH) are associated with genetic risk factors (HLA and CYP polymorphisms) that predispose the host to an increased risk of DILI (see Table 10.10).
   - These pharmacogenetic associations may allow for the pre-prescription testing of individuals to prevent hepatotoxicity; to date, however, the cost of screening and the relatively low frequency of injury among affected persons limit the usefulness of such genome-wide association studies in predicting DILI. The one exception is **abacavir,** for which **HLA-B*5701 testing** is mandatory to prevent a severe hypersensitivity reaction in the 3% to 4% of persons who are positive for the at-risk alleles.

4. Serum ALT and other liver biochemical test level monitoring
   - Liver biochemical test level monitoring is frequently recommended by drug manufacturers on the advice of the FDA (Box 10.3). For most of the relevant agents, the latency periods for toxicity are 2 months or longer, and injury is not associated with hallmarks of hypersensitivity (fever, rash, eosinophilia).

TABLE 10.12 ■ **Histologic Findings That Suggest Possible Drug-Induced Liver Injury**

Finding	Examples
Steatosis	
Microvesicular	Didanosine, IV tetracycline, salicylates, valproic acid
Macrovesicular and phospholipidosis	Amiodarone, ethanol, glucocorticoids, lopitamide, methotrexate, tamoxifen
Necroinflammation	
Autoimmune hepatitis-like	Methyldopa, minocycline, nitrofurantoin, statins
Acute viral hepatitis-like	Diclofenac, isoniazid, sulfonamides
Mononucleosis-like	Dapsone, phenytoin, para-aminosalicylate
Cholestasis	
Intrahepatic (bland) cholestasis	C-17 alkylated anabolic, contraceptive steroids, TPN, warfarin
Acute cholestatic hepatitis	Amoxicillin-clavulanic acid, captopril, ciprofloxacin, CPZ, cyclosporine, D-penicillamine, erythromycin estolate, flucloxacillin, nevirapine, SMX-TMP, sulindac, telithromycin, terbinafine, TCAs
PBC-like ductopenia	Chlorpromazine, haloperidol, imipramine, thiabendazole
PSC-like biliary sclerosis	Floxuridine administered by hepatic artery infusion
VBDS	Amitriptyline, amoxicillin, carbamazepine, CPZ, flucloxacillin, thiabendazole
Vascular Injury	
Peliosis	Anabolic steroids, vinyl chloride
Sinusoidal dilatation	Contraceptive steroids
Sinusoidal obstruction syndrome	Busulfan, cyclophosphamide, pyrrolizidine alkaloids
Nodular regenerative hyperplasia	Arsenicals, azathioprine, copper sulfate, oxaliplatin, 6-mercaptopurine, 6-thioguanine, vinyl chloride
Hepatoportal sclerosis	Antineoplastic agents, arsenicals
Granulomas	
Fibrin-ring type	Allopurinol
Multinucleated giant cell type	Phenylbutazone
With associated cholangitis	Allopurinol, chlorpromazine, methyldopa
With associated vasculitis	Glibenclamide, phenytoin, sulfonamides
Lipogranuloma	Mineral oil
Neoplastic	
Hepatic adenoma	Contraceptive steroids
Angiosarcoma	Androgenic steroids, thorium dioxide, vinyl chloride
Hepatocellular carcinoma	Androgens, arsenicals, estrogens, methyltestosterone
Miscellaneous	
Mallory-Denk bodies	Amiodarone
Ground-glass change	Phenytoin
Hypertrophic stellate cells	Hypervitaminosis A

CPZ, Chlorpromazine; *IV,* intravenous; *PBC,* primary biliary cholangitis; *PSC,* primary sclerosing cholangitis; *SMX-TMP,* sulfamethoxazole-trimethoprim; *TCAs,* tricyclic antidepressants; *TPN,* total parenteral nutrition; *VBDS,* vanishing bile duct syndrome.

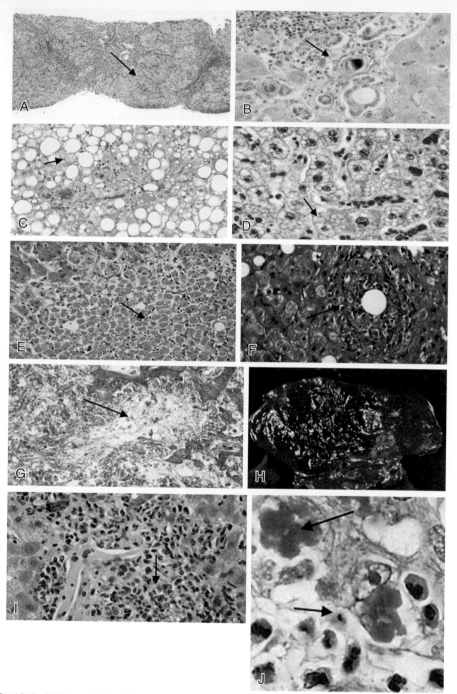

Fig 10.1 Pathology of drug-induced liver injury caused by various agents. A, Bridging fibrosis *(arrow)* and regeneration from pemoline. B, Bile plug *(arrow)* from ceftriaxone. C, Macrovesicular steatosis *(arrow)* from methotrexate. D, Microvesicular steatosis *(arrow)* from tetracycline. E, Confluent coagulative necrosis from acetaminophen; hepatocytes are shrunken, rounded, and eosinophilic and have lost their nuclei *(arrow)*. F, Fibrin ring ("donut hole") granuloma *(arrow)* from allopurinol. G, Sinusoidal obstruction syndrome from azathioprine and preconditioning radiation therapy; the central vein wall is thickened and the lumen totally occluded *(arrow)*. H, Ruptured adenoma from oral contraceptives. I, Autoimmune hepatitis from minocycline; portal inflammation with interface hepatitis and plasma cells *(arrow)*. J, Mallory-Denk bodies *(arrows)* from amiodarone. (From Lewis JH, Kleiner DE. Hepatic injury due to drugs, herbal compounds, chemicals, and toxins. In Burt A, Portmann B, Ferrell L, eds., *MacSween's Pathology of the Liver*, ed 6, Edinburgh/New York, 2012, Churchill Livingstone/Elsevier, 645–760.)

TABLE 10.13 ■ **Phases of Acute Liver Injury Following Acute Toxic Poisonings**

Phase	Toxin			
	Acetaminophen	**Amanita phalloides**	**Carbon tetrachloride**	**Phosphorus**
Phase I (1–24 hours)				
Onset of liver toxicity	Immediate	Delayed 6–20 hours after ingestion	Immediate	Immediate
Anorexia, nausea, vomiting, diarrhea	+	++++	+	++++
Shock	–	±	–	+
Neurologic symptoms	–	±	–	+ (convulsions)
Phase II (24–72 hours)				
Asymptomatic latent period	++	+	+	±
Phase III (>72 hours)				
Onset of jaundice	+	+	+	+
Hepatic failure	+	+	+	+
Renal failure	+	+	+	+
Maximum serum AST and ALT (×ULN)	1000	500	500	<10–100
Zonal necrosis	3	3	3	1
Steatosis	–	+	+	++++
Case-fatality rate (%)	5–15[a]	20–25	20–25	25–50

ALT, Alanine aminotransferase; *AST,* aspartate aminotransferase; *ULN,* upper limit of normal.

[a]Acetaminophen fatality depends on how soon *N*-acetylcysteine is administered.

- In contrast, drugs that cause DILI through immunoallergic mechanisms and have short latency periods (e.g., sulfa-containing compounds) tend to declare the toxicity clinically, and enzyme monitoring is of little additional clinical benefit.
5. Caveats
   - In many instances, monitoring is not performed as directed and is considered a burden by both patients and prescribers.
   - For many agents, it has been difficult to demonstrate that biochemical monitoring is an effective method to prevent serious DILI.
   - When performed, monitoring should continue through the anticipated latency period for toxicity of the drug in question to cover the period of time where patients are most susceptible to developing DILI.
   - Serum ALT monitoring is usually performed on no longer than a monthly basis; longer intervals are prone to miss early signals of liver injury.
   - The FDA states that for statin use, patients with normal baseline liver biochemical test levels do not require serum ALT monitoring.
   - Use of bosentan requires frequent serum ALT testing as part of a risk evaluation and management strategy program.
   - Monitoring for clinical symptoms of acute DILI (as is often recommended for INH) can lead to more severe injury if the drug is not promptly discontinued when clear-cut stopping rules are met (e.g., development of nausea, abdominal pain, fatigue, malaise, or jaundice).

BOX 10.3 ■ Drugs for Which Liver Enzyme Monitoring Is Recommended

Allopurinol	Mercaptopurine
Amiodarone	Methotrexate
Bosentan	Methyldopa
Carbamazepine	Mirtazapine
Clonazepam	Nicotinic acid
Cyclosporine	Nitrofurantoin
Diclofenac	Pemoline
Disulfiram	Pioglitazone
Fenofibrate	Pyrazinamide
Fluconazole	Ritonavir
Flutamide	Rosiglitazone
Gemfibrozil	Statins[a]
Isoniazid	Tamoxifen
Ketaconazole	Tretinoin
Labetalol	Valproic acid

[a]Not considered necessary if baseline liver biochemical test levels are normal.

Treatment (Box 10.4)

ACETAMINOPHEN POISONING

1. 60,000 cases, resulting in about 500 deaths, are reported annually in United States.
2. Accounts for 40% to 50% of all-cause ALF cases (adults and children)
3. 50% of the cases are attributed to inadvertent or unintentional overdose.
4. Many instances of less severe liver injury from acetaminophen likely go unrecognized; up to 44% of healthy subjects who ingest 4 g of acetaminophen daily for 14 days can develop asymptomatic elevations in ALT that may exceed 10 times ULN but resolve quickly when the drug is stopped.
5. The modified **Rumack-Matthew nomogram** for determining a toxic drug level is used in patients with a single ingestion *who present within the first 24 hours* (http://ars-informatica.ca/toxicity_nomogram.php?calc=acetamin).
6. The severity and risk of death should be determined based on the King College criteria, a Model for End-stage Liver Disease (MELD) score >30, or encephalopathy stage III or IV to gauge the patient's prognosis and need for referral to an LT center (see Chapters 2 and 11).
7. Newer biomarkers (e.g., microRNAs, keratin-18, CSF-1) are under evaluation to assist in predicting which patients are at risk of developing severe hepatotoxicity and require specific treatment.

Treatment

1. Induction of vomiting or nasogastric lavage followed by administration of activated charcoal should be considered for a patient presenting within 1 to 2 hours of an acute single overdose.
2. Treatment with NAC is initiated if the serum acetaminophen concentration is at or above 150 mg/L at 4 hours following ingestion on the Rumack-Matthew nomogram (or above the threshold level subsequently). NAC given within 8 hours reduces the mortality rate to <10% (and to 40% if given after 16 hours). No significant difference between oral and intravenous administration of NAC is seen in peak serum ALT levels >1000 U/L (12.6% versus 13.2%).
   - Oral NAC is administered in a dose of 140 mg/kg followed by 70 mg/kg every 4 hours × 17 doses, or until the INR is <1.5.

BOX 10.4 ■ Basic Principles for Diagnosing and Managing Drug-Induced Liver Injury

1. Determine the biochemical injury pattern (R values for hepatocellular, cholestatic, and mixed injury [see Table 10.5]).
2. Fractionate bilirubin (direct and indirect) to help differentiate DILI from Gilbert syndrome and hemolysis.
3. If cholestatic injury is present, determine whether an isolated alkaline phosphatase elevation is of hepatic, bone, intestinal, or placental origin.
4. Determine the pharmacologic properties of the suspect drug: Dose, degree of lipophilicity, degree of hepatic metabolism.
5. Determine if the injury fits the known clinicopathologic signature of other instances of DILI with the suspect drug (i.e., compatible latency, injury pattern, response to dechallenge, rechallenge, histology) as contained in the LiverTox database (www.livertox.nih.gov) or other resources.
6. Identify any associated signs of immunoallergy (fever, rash, eosinophilia, suggesting hypersensitivity); if present, look for associated DRESS reactions or severe skin injury (e.g., SJS, TEN).
7. Exclude other etiologies that may cause the same type of injury, such as the following:
   - Acute viral hepatitis: Serum AST or ALT >500 U/L—obtain serology for hepatitis A, B, C, E, cytomegalovirus, Epstein-Barr virus, herpes simplex virus.
   - Ischemic hepatitis: Serum AST > LDH > ALT >1000 to 10,000 IU—look for hypotension, shock, sepsis, with rapid resolution of liver enzyme elevations within 7 to 10 days.
   - Acute intrahepatic cholestasis: AP > 2× ULN; look for other causes of postoperative jaundice or hemolysis.
   - Obstructive jaundice: Obtain imaging (ultrasonography, MRCP or ERCP, EUS) to rule out gallstones or pancreatic or hepatobiliary malignancy.
   - Acute-on-chronic injury (e.g., underlying fatty liver disease or chronic viral hepatitis with previously stable baseline elevations in the serum ALT)
8. Monitor the patient for signs of impending ALF (e.g., INR >1.5, development of hepatic encephalopathy).
9. Refer the patient to a liver transplant center for evaluation and a higher level of care if ALF is suspected.
10. Consider what the risk of rechallenge is (generally not recommended after a severe hypersensitivity reaction); rechallenge may be considered as part of a desensitization approach for antituberculosis drugs.
11. Determine whether a specific antidote is available (e.g., NAC for acetaminophen overdose).
12. Assess whether nonspecific treatment measures are needed (e.g., glucocorticoids for immune-related hepatitis, ursodeoxycholic acid for cholestatic liver injury, liver assist devices).

ALF, Acute liver failure; *ALT,* alanine aminotransferase; *AP,* alkaline phosphatase; *AST,* aspartate aminotransferase; *DILI,* drug-induced liver injury; *DRESS,* drug rash with eosinophilia and systemic symptoms; *ERCP,* endoscopic retrograde cholangiopancreatography; *EUS,* endoscopic ultrasonography; *INR,* international normalized ratio; *LDH,* lactate dehydrogenase; *MRCP,* magnetic resonance cholangiopancreatography; *NAC,* N-acetylcysteine; *SJS,* Stevens Johnson syndrome; *TEN,* toxic epidermal necrolysis; *ULN,* upper limit of normal.

- Intravenous NAC is administered in a dose of 100 mg/kg in 250 mL 5% dextrose (D5W) over 1 hour, followed by 50 mg/kg in 500 mL D5W over 4 hours, followed by 100 mg/kg in 1000 mL D5W over 16 hours (may be extended to a total of 2 days), or until the INR is <1.5.
  – Common side effects of NAC are the following:
    - Anaphylaxis
    - Nausea and vomiting
    - Flushing
    - Skin rash

– Less common side effects of NAC are the following:
  ■ Stomatitis
  ■ Respiratory symptoms (cough, wheezing, stridor, bronchospasm)
  ■ Tachycardia, hypotension
  ■ Urticaria
  ■ Edema
  ■ Acidosis, hypokalemic
  ■ Syncope
  ■ Seizure
  ■ Sedation
  ■ Thrombocytopenia
■ The minimal duration of NAC treatment is 20 to 24 hours.
■ Intravenous NAC is preferred to oral NAC in pregnant women to maximize drug levels in the fetus and in patients with the short-bowel syndrome.
3. Urgent referral to a liver transplant center should be made for all cases with impending or suspected ALF.
4. Transplant-free survival is 70% compared with <25% for ALF from idiosyncratic DILI and <50% for non-DILI ALF.
5. One-year survival post-LT is 70% to 75%.

MUSHROOM POISONING

1. More than 90% of cases of fatal mushroom poisonings are due to *Amanita phylloides* ("death cap") or *Amanita verna* ("destroying angel").
2. A fatal dose can involve the ingestion of a single 50-g mushroom.
3. Alpha amatoxin is thermostable, can resist drying for years, and is not inactivated by cooking. It is rapidly absorbed via the gastrointestinal tract and is carried within the enterohepatic circulation to reach the hepatocytes, where it inhibits production of mRNA and protein synthesis and leads to necrosis.
4. A second toxin, phalloidin, is responsible for the gastrointestinal distress that precedes the hepatic and central nervous system injury.
5. The latent period for toxicity is often longer (6 to 20 hours) than that seen with the injury from CCl_4 and phosphorus.
6. Intense abdominal pain, vomiting, and diarrhea develop, with hepatocellular jaundice and renal failure occurring over the next 24 to 48 hours, followed by convulsions and coma by 72 hours.
7. The mean AST level is >5000 U/L and mean ALT >7000 U/L; the mean peak serum bilirubin level is >10 mg/dL at day 4 to 5.
8. Initial conservative management includes immediate nasogastric lavage (if the patient is seen within the first 1 to 2 hours after ingestion); otherwise, activated charcoal should be administered in multiple doses (regardless of the time after ingestion) to interrupt enterohepatic circulation of the amatoxin.
9. A number of therapies have been given to reduce the hepatic uptake or toxicity of alpha amatoxin, including the following:
  ■ Silymarin (milk thistle), given in a dose of 1 g orally four times daily, or as its purified alkaloid, silibinin, given intravenously in a dose of 5 mg/kg over 1 hour, followed by 20 mg/kg/day as a constant infusion
  ■ Intravenous benzyl penicillin
  ■ Cimetidine to inhibit toxin metabolite formation by CYP enzymes
  ■ NAC

10. LT has significantly lowered the 30% to 50% mortality observed in the pre-LT era.
11. Renal failure, convulsions, and muscarinic and other organ toxicities may signify ingestion of other mushroom toxins for which additional supportive and specific treatment measures may be indicated.

ROLE OF NAC IN NONACETAMINOPHEN ALF

■ Data from the U.S. ALF Study Group demonstrate that only adult patients with early-grade encephalopathy (grades I and II) show improved outcomes with NAC when compared with patients with grades III and IV encephalopathy.
■ Children have not been shown convincingly to benefit from NAC for nonacetaminophen ALF.

ROLE OF GLUCOCORTICOIDS

■ Glucocorticoids may be beneficial in cases of slow-to-resolve drug-induced autoimmune hepatitis (AIH) due to nitrofurantoin, minocycline, methyldopa, tyrosine kinase inhibitors, and others.
■ Cases of drug-induced AIH can be differentiated from those of idiopathic AIH by demonstrating resolution of the injury after the offending drug is stopped or after a short course of immunosuppression; idiopathic AIH would be expected to persist despite discontinuation of the drug and often relapses after short-term immunosuppressive therapy is ended.
■ Symptoms of and serum ALT elevations in severe ipilimumab-induced hepatitis may improve following a high-dose, pulsed glucocorticoid regimen (1 g of prednisolone intravenously daily for 3 to 5 days), followed by a slow glucocorticoid taper starting with methylprednisolone 1 to 2 mg/kg/day over at least 1 month.

LEFLUNOMIDE TOXICITY

■ Bile acid "washout" with cholestyramine for leflunomide toxicity takes advantage of the long terminal half-life and enterohepatic circulation of leflunomide.
■ Plasma concentrations of the active metabolite of leflunomide (teriflunomide) may be detectable in plasma for up to 2 years following discontinuation of the drug.
■ If urgent removal of leflunomide is needed because of severe hepatotoxicity, cholestyramine (8 g orally three times a day) should be given for 24 hours (with or without activated charcoal [50 g every 6 hours for 24 hours] either orally or via nasogastric tube); this method reduces leflunomide levels by 40% in the first 24 hours; treatment with cholestyramine should continue until drug levels are undetectable (<0.02 mg/L or 0.02 µg/mL).
■ For nonurgent removal, cholestyramine 8 g orally three times a day should be administered for 11 days (the 11 days do not need to be consecutive unless there is a need to lower the plasma levels rapidly).

ANTI-TB DRUG HEPATOTOXICITY

■ A method of desensitization and rechallenge has been proposed. After stopping INH, rifampin, and pyrazinamide for acute DILI, a modified anti-TB drug regimen of ethambutol, streptomycin, and a fluoroquinolone is administered.

- Patients are followed at weekly intervals until clinical and biochemical parameters of acute DILI have resolved and serum AST and ALT levels are <2 times ULN with a total bilirubin level <1 times ULN.
- Staged reintroduction is initiated starting with rifampin for 3 to 7 days before the next medication (INH) is added. Pyrazinamide can then be given (unless the patient had severe liver dysfunction, in which case pyrazinamide should be avoided).
- The medications should be reintroduced at doses lower than those used for initial therapy and gradually titrated up to the therapeutic range.
- During reintroduction, liver enzymes should be monitored closely (every few days) before a dose increase or introduction of the next drug.
- After reintroduction is complete, regular monitoring of liver biochemical test levels is performed weekly for the first month, every 2 weeks during the second and third months, and thereafter as clinically indicated.
- Although most patients can be expected to tolerate reintroduction of these agents, recurrence of DILI is anticipated in approximately 10% of cases.

LIVER ASSIST DEVICES (see Chapter 2)

- Liver assist devices are available outside the United States and are investigational in the United States.
- The molecular adsorbent recirculating systems (MARS) using albumin dialysis or plasma exchange devices offer a bridge to LT.

REFERRAL TO A LIVER TRANSPLANT CENTER

- Recommended for any patient in whom ALF is evident or considered imminent

FURTHER READING

Bjornsson ES. Epidemiology and risk factors for idiosyncratic drug-induced liver injury. *Semin Liver Dis.* 2014;34:115–122.

Chalasani NP, Bonkovsky HL, Fontana RJ, et al. Drug-induced liver injury in the USA: a report of 899 instances assessed prospectively. *Gastroenterology.* 2015;148:1340–1352.

Chalasani NP, Hayashi PH, Bonkovsky HL, et al. ACG clinical guideline: the diagnosis and management of idiosyncratic drug-induced liver injury. *Am J Gastroenterol.* 2014;109:950–986.

Chen M, Suzuki A, Borlak J, et al. Drug-induced liver injury: interactions between drug properties and host factors. *J Hepatol.* 2015;63:503–514.

Galvin Z, McDonough A, Ryan J, et al. Blood alanine aminotransferase levels >1000 IU/L: causes and outcomes. *Clin Med.* 2015;15:244–247.

Kleiner DE, Chalasani NP, Lee WM, et al. Hepatic histological findings in suspected drug-induced liver injury: systematic evaluation of and clinical associations. *Hepatology.* 2014;59:661–670.

Lee WM. Drug-induced acute liver failure. *Clin Liver Dis.* 2013;17:575–586.

Lewis JH. The art and science of diagnosing and managing drug-induced liver injury in 2015 and beyond. *Clin Gastroenterol Hepatol.* 2015;13:2173–2189.

Lewis JH. Causality assessment: which is best—expert opinion or RUCAM?. *AASLD Clinical Liver Disease.* 2014;4:S4–S8. Accessed at http://onlinelibrary.wiley.com/DOI:10.1002/cld.365.

Lewis JH, Stine JG. Review article: prescribing medications in patients with cirrhosis—a practical guide. *Aliment Pharmacol Ther.* 2013;37:1132–1156.

LiverTox. www.livertox.nih.gov.

Navarro VJ, Barnhart H, Bonkovsky HL, et al. Liver injury from herbals and dietary supplements in the U.S. Drug-induced Liver Injury Network. *Hepatology.* 2014;60:1399–1408.

Reuben A, Koch DG, Lee WM, et al. Drug-induced acute liver failure: results of the U.S. multicenter, prospective study. *Hepatology*. 2010;52:2065–2076.

Rumack BH. Acetaminophen hepatotoxicity: the first 35 years. *J Toxicol Clin Toxicol*. 2002;40:3–20.

Seeff LB, Bonkovsky HL, Navarro VJ, et al. Herbal products and the liver: a review of adverse effects and mechanisms. *Gastroenterology*. 2015;148:517–532.

Stine JG, Lewis JH. Current and future directions in the treatment and prevention of drug-induced liver injury: a systematic review. *Expert Rev Gastroenterol Hepatol*. 2016;10:517–536.

Urban TJ, Daly AK, Aithal GP. Genetic basis of drug-induced liver injury: present and future. *Semin Liver Dis*. 2014;34:123–133.

CHAPTER 11

Cirrhosis and Portal Hypertension

Emily D. Bethea, MD ■ Sanjiv Chopra, MBBS, MACP

KEY POINTS

1 The major causes of cirrhosis include chronic hepatitis B, chronic hepatitis C, alcoholic liver disease, nonalcoholic steatohepatitis (NASH), and hemochromatosis.

2 Etiologic classification of cirrhosis is more clinically relevant than morphologic classification (micronodular, macronodular, mixed), because morphologic appearance is relatively nonspecific with regard to etiology, and important management and treatment decisions are best addressed once the cause of cirrhosis has been determined.

3 Important and potentially life-threatening complications of cirrhosis include ascites, spontaneous bacterial peritonitis, variceal hemorrhage, hepatic encephalopathy, hepatorenal syndrome, hepatopulmonary syndrome, and hepatocellular carcinoma (HCC).

4 The Child-Pugh classification is useful in assessing prognosis and estimating the potential risk of variceal bleeding and operative mortality.

5 The Model for End-stage Liver Disease (MELD) combines international normalized ratio (INR), serum creatinine level, serum bilirubin level, and serum sodium levels to create a score that is used to predict prognosis and prioritize timing of liver transplantation.

Cirrhosis

DEFINITION

1. The word *cirrhosis* is derived from the Greek word *kirrhos*, meaning "orange or tawny," and *osis*, meaning "condition."
2. **The World Health Organization (WHO) definition of cirrhosis is a diffuse process characterized by fibrosis and the conversion of normal liver architecture into structurally abnormal nodules that lack normal lobular organization.**
3. Structural changes in the liver and resulting impairment of hepatic function may manifest as the development of
   - Jaundice
   - Portal hypertension
   - Varices
   - Ascites
   - Spontaneous bacterial peritonitis
   - Hepatorenal syndrome
   - Hepatic encephalopathy
   - Progressive hepatic failure
4. The WHO definition distinguishes cirrhosis from other types of liver disease that have either nodule formation or fibrosis, but not both. These other hepatic disorders may be characterized

by prehepatic or posthepatic portal hypertension, which occurs in the absence of cirrhosis. **Nodular regenerative hyperplasia,** for example, is characterized by diffuse nodularity without fibrosis, whereas chronic **schistosomiasis** is characterized by Symmers pipestem fibrosis with no nodularity.

CLASSIFICATION

1. **Morphologic classification** was historically used to describe cirrhosis as the following:
   - Micronodular cirrhosis, with uniform nodules <3 mm in diameter: Causes include alcohol, hemochromatosis, biliary obstruction, hepatic venous outflow obstruction, jejunoileal bypass, and Indian childhood cirrhosis.
   - Macronodular cirrhosis, with nodular variation ≥3 mm in diameter: Causes include chronic hepatitis C, chronic hepatitis B, alpha-1 antitrypsin deficiency, and primary biliary cholangitis.
   - Mixed cirrhosis, a combination of micronodular and macronodular cirrhosis: Micronodular cirrhosis frequently evolves into macronodular cirrhosis.

   Given limitations in morphologic grouping, including considerable overlap between categories, change in morphology with disease progression, need for invasive testing, and generally low specificity, this classification system has limited clinical utility.
2. **Etiologic classification** of cirrhosis is the most clinically useful and preferred approach for categorization.
   - This method of classification aims to ascertain the etiology of liver disease by combining clinical, biochemical, genetic, histologic, and epidemiologic data.
   - **The two most common causes of cirrhosis in developed countries are excessive alcohol use and viral hepatitis.** As the incidence of obesity and diabetes mellitus continues to rise, a parallel increase in NASH has been observed; by the year 2030, NASH is projected to be one of the leading causes of cirrhosis. Table 11.1 lists the etiologic classification and tests used to determine the cause.
   - Most cases of cryptogenic cirrhosis are felt to be "burned out" NASH.

PATHOLOGY

Liver biopsy is indicated in selected patients with chronic liver disease when the clinical, biochemical, and imaging data are not definitive for cirrhosis or its etiology.
1. Gross examination: The liver surface is irregular, with multiple yellowish nodules; depending on the severity of the cirrhosis, the liver may be enlarged because of multiple regenerating nodules or, in the final stages, small and shrunken.
2. Pathologic criteria for the diagnosis of cirrhosis
   - Nodularity (regenerative nodules)
   - Fibrosis (deposition of connective tissue creates pseudolobules)
   - Fragmentation of the sample
   - Abnormal hepatic architecture
   - Hepatocellular abnormalities
   - Pleomorphism
   - Dysplasia
   - Regenerative hyperplasia
3. Information obtained from histologic examination
   - Establishment of the presence of cirrhosis
   - Assessment of grade of histologic activity
   - Determination of the cause of cirrhosis in some cases

TABLE 11.1 ■ Etiology and Diagnostic Evaluation of the Common Causes of Cirrhosis

Etiology	Diagnostic Evaluation
Infection	
Hepatitis B	HBsAg, anti-HBs, anti-HBc, HBV DNA
Hepatitis C	Anti-HCV, HCV RNA
Hepatitis D	Anti-HDV
Toxins	
Alcohol	History, AST/ALT ratio, IgA level, liver biopsy
Cholestasis	
Primary biliary cholangitis	AMA, IgM level, liver biopsy
Secondary biliary cirrhosis	MRCP, ERCP, liver biopsy
Primary sclerosing cholangitis	MRCP, ERCP, liver biopsy
Autoimmune	
Autoimmune hepatitis	ANA, IgG level, smooth muscle antibodies, liver-kidney microsomal antibodies, liver biopsy
Vascular	
Cardiac cirrhosis	Echocardiogram, liver biopsy
Budd-Chiari syndrome	CT, US, MRI/MRA
Sinusoidal obstruction syndrome	History of offending drug use, liver biopsy
Metabolic	
Hemochromatosis	Iron studies, *HFE* gene mutation, liver biopsy
Wilson disease	Serum and urinary copper, ceruloplasmin, slit-lamp eye examination, liver biopsy
Alpha-1 antitrypsin deficiency	Alpha-1 antitrypsin level, protease inhibitor type, liver biopsy
NASH	History, risk factors (obesity, diabetes mellitus, hyperlipidemia), liver biopsy
Cryptogenic	Exclude NASH, celiac disease, drugs

AMA, Antimitochodrial antibodies; *anti-HBc,* antibody to hepatitis B core antigen; *anti-HBs,* antibody to hepatitis B surface antigen; *anti-HCV,* antibody to hepatitis C virus; *anti-HDV,* antibody to hepatitis D virus; *AST,* aspartate aminotransferase; *ALT,* alanine aminotransferase; *CT,* computed tomography; *ERCP,* endoscopic retrograde cholangiopan-creatography; *HBsAg,* hepatitis B surface antigen; *IgA,* immunoglobulin A; *IgM,* immunoglobulin M; *MRCP,* magnetic resonance cholangiopancreatography; *MRA,* magnetic resonance angiography; *MRI,* magnetic resonance imaging; *NASH,* nonalcoholic steatohepatitis; *US,* ultrasonography.

4. Histologic methods for determining the specific cause of cirrhosis
   - Immunohistochemistry (e.g., hepatitis B virus)
   - Polymerase chain reaction (PCR) techniques (e.g., hepatitis C virus)
   - Quantitative copper measurement (Wilson disease)
   - Periodic acid-Schiff (PAS)–positive, diastase-resistant globules (alpha-1 antitrypsin deficiency)
   - Quantitative iron measurement (hemochromatosis)

CLINICAL FEATURES

The manifestations of cirrhosis are protean. Patients with cirrhosis may come to clinical attention in numerous ways:

1. Stigmata of chronic liver disease on physical examination (e.g., palmar erythema, spider telangiectasias)

2. Abnormal serum chemistry test results and hematologic indices (e.g., serum aminotransferases, bilirubin, alkaline phosphatase, albumin, prothrombin time, platelet count)
3. Imaging abnormalities (e.g., small, shrunken, nodular liver or evidence of portal hypertension on cross-sectional imaging)
4. Complications of decompensated liver disease (e.g., ascites, variceal hemorrhage, encephalopathy)
5. Cirrhotic appearance of the liver at the time of laparotomy or laparoscopy
6. Autopsy

A patient with cirrhosis may present with none, some, or all of the following findings:

1. **General**
   - Fatigue
   - Anorexia
   - Malaise
   - Sleep-wake reversal
   - Weight loss
   - Muscle wasting
2. **Gastrointestinal**
   a. Parotid gland enlargement
   b. Diarrhea
   c. Cholelithiasis
   d. Gastrointestinal bleeding
      - Esophageal, gastric, duodenal, rectal, and/or stomal varices
      - Portal hypertensive gastropathy, enteropathy, and/or colopathy
3. **Hematologic**
   a. Anemia
      - Folate deficiency
      - Spur cell anemia (hemolytic anemia in the setting of severe alcoholic liver disease)
      - Splenomegaly with resulting pancytopenia
   b. Thrombocytopenia
   c. Leukopenia
   d. Impaired coagulation
   e. Disseminated intravascular coagulation
   f. Hemosiderosis
   g. Portal vein thrombosis
4. **Pulmonary**
   a. Decreased oxygen saturation
   b. Altered ventilation-perfusion relationships
   c. Portopulmonary hypertension
   d. Hyperventilation
   e. Reduced pulmonary diffusion capacity
   f. Hepatic hydrothorax
      - Accumulation of fluid within the pleural space in association with cirrhosis and in the absence of primary pulmonary or cardiac disease
      - Usually right sided (70%)
      - Typically associated with clinically apparent ascites, but can be found in patients without obvious ascites
   g. Hepatopulmonary syndrome
      - Triad of liver disease, an increased alveolar-arterial gradient while breathing room air, and evidence of intrapulmonary vascular dilatations
      - Wide range of reported prevalence rates in cirrhotic patients from approximately 5% to 50%

- Characterized by dyspnea, platypnea, orthodeoxia, digital clubbing, and severe hypoxemia (PO_2 <80 mm Hg, often <60 mm Hg)
- Intrapulmonary shunting demonstrated by contrast-enhanced ("bubble") echocardiography or technetium-99m macroaggregated albumin scanning; pulmonary arteriography rarely required
- Associated with significantly increased risk of mortality without liver transplantation; risk increases with severity of hypoxemia (see Chapter 33)
- MELD score exception points may be given to patients with significant hypoxemia (PO_2 <60 mm Hg).
- Complete resolution is typical after liver transplantation; the time course of improvement is variable and often delayed up to 1 year.

5. **Cardiac:** Hyperdynamic circulation, diastolic dysfunction
6. **Renal**
   - Secondary hyperaldosteronism leading to sodium and water retention
   - Renal tubular acidosis (more frequent in alcoholic cirrhosis, Wilson disease, and primary biliary cholangitis)
   - Hepatorenal syndrome
7. **Endocrinologic**
   a. Hypogonadism
      - Male patients: Loss of libido, testicular atrophy, impotence, decreased amounts of testosterone
      - Female patients: Infertility, dysmenorrhea, loss of secondary sexual characteristics
   b. Feminization (acquisition of estrogen-induced characteristics)
      - Spider telangiectasias
      - Palmar erythema
      - Gynecomastia
      - Changes in body hair patterns
   c. Diabetes mellitus
8. **Neurologic**
   a. Hepatic encephalopathy
      - Variants include spastic paraplegia and acquired non-Wilsonian hepatocerebral degeneration.
   b. Peripheral neuropathy
   c. Asterixis
9. **Musculoskeletal**
   - Reduction in lean muscle mass
   - Hypertrophic osteoarthropathy: Synovitis, clubbing, and periostitis
   - Hepatic osteodystrophy
   - Muscle cramping
   - Umbilical herniation
10. **Dermatologic**
    a. Spider telangiectasias
    b. Palmar erythema
    c. Nail changes
       - Azure lunules (Wilson disease)
       - Muercke nails: Paired horizontal white bands separated by normal color
       - Terry nails: White appearance of the proximal 2/3 of the nail plate
    d. Jaundice
    e. Pruritus
    f. Dupuytren contractures

    g. Clubbing

    h. Paper money skin

    i. Caput medusae

    j. Easy bruising

11. Infectious

    Infectious complications cause significant morbidity and mortality in patients with cirrhosis.

    a. Spontaneous bacterial peritonitis

    b. Urinary tract infection

    c. Respiratory tract infection

    d. Bacteremia

    e. Cellulitis

Certain infectious agents are more virulent and more common in patients with liver disease. These include *Vibrio vulnificus, Campylobacter jejuni, Yersinia enterocolitica, Plesiomonas shigelloides, Enterococcus faecalis, Capnocytophaga canimorsus,* and *Listeria monocytogenes,* in addition to organisms transmitted from other species. In patients with hemochromatosis, *L. monocytogenes, Y. enterocolitica,* and *V. vulnificus* may have enhanced virulence in the presence of excess iron.

COMPLICATIONS

- Ascites (see Chapter 13)
- Spontaneous bacterial peritonitis (see Chapter 13)
- Variceal hemorrhage (see Chapter 12)
- Hepatic encephalopathy (see Chapter 15)
- HCC (see Chapter 29)
- Hepatorenal syndrome (see Chapter 14)
- Portal vein thrombosis (see Chapter 21)

DIAGNOSIS

1. Physical examination

    a. Stigmata of chronic liver disease and/or cirrhosis

        - Spider telangiectasias
        - Palmar erythema
        - Dupuytren contractures
        - Gynecomastia
        - Testicular atrophy

    b. Features of portal hypertension

        - Ascites
        - Splenomegaly
        - Caput medusae
        - Evidence of hyperdynamic circulation (e.g., resting tachycardia)
        - Cruveilhier-Baumgarten murmur: Venous hum best auscultated in the epigastrium

    c. Features of hepatic encephalopathy

        - Confusion
        - Asterixis
        - Fetor hepaticus

    d. Others

        - Jaundice
        - Parotid gland enlargement
        - Scant chest and axillary hair

2. **Laboratory evaluation** (see also Chapter 1)
   a. Tests of hepatocellular injury
      - Aminotransferases (aspartate aminotransferase [AST] and alanine aminotransferase [ALT]): Most forms of chronic hepatitis other than alcohol have an AST/ALT ratio <1; however, as chronic hepatitis progresses to cirrhosis, the ratio of AST/ALT may reverse.
   b. Tests of cholestasis
      - Alkaline phosphatase
      - Serum bilirubin (conjugated and unconjugated): Also elevated in hepatocellular injury
      - Gamma-glutamyltranspeptidase (GGTP)
      - 5'-nucleotidase
   c. Tests of synthetic function
      - Serum albumin
      - Prothrombin time: Assesses status of coagulation factors (II, V, VII, X)
   d. Tests that aid in diagnosis
      - Viral hepatitis serology (see Chapters 3 to 6)
      - PCR techniques for detecting viral RNA or DNA
      - Serum iron, total iron binding capacity (TIBC), ferritin, genetic testing for the HFE gene mutation (hemochromatosis, see Chapter 18)
      - Ceruloplasmin, serum and urinary copper (Wilson disease, see Chapter 19)
      - Alpha-1 antitrypsin (A1AT) level and protease inhibitor type (A1AT deficiency, see Chapter 20)
      - Tissue transglutaminase (tTG) IgA (celiac disease)
      - Serum immunoglobulins (autoimmune hepatitis [see Chapter 7], alcoholic cirrhosis [see Chapter 8], primary biliary cholangitis [see Chapter 16])
      - Autoantibodies: Antinuclear antibodies (ANA), antimitochondrial antibodies (AMA), antiliver kidney microsomal antibodies (LKM), smooth muscle antibodies (SMA; autoimmune hepatitis, primary biliary cholangitis)
   e. Tumor marker and potential screening test in HCC: Serum alpha fetoprotein (see Chapter 29)
3. **Imaging studies** (see also Chapter 1)
   a. Abdominal ultrasonography
      - Noninvasive, relatively inexpensive
      - Can easily detect ascites, biliary dilatation
      - Preferred screening test for primary HCC
      - Duplex Doppler ultrasonography can further assess hepatic and portal vein patency.
   b. Computed tomography (CT)
      - Noninvasive, more expensive than ultrasonography
      - Often requires administration of potentially nephrotoxic contrast
      - Findings in cirrhosis are nonspecific.
      - May be helpful in the diagnosis of hemochromatosis; increased density of the liver is suggestive.
   c. Magnetic resonance imaging (MRI)
      - Noninvasive, high-expense imaging modality
      - Excellent for evaluation of hepatic masses; can help differentiate focal fat from a possible hepatic malignancy
      - Can easily assess hepatic vasculature without the need for nephrotoxic contrast agents; more reliable than Doppler ultrasonography

- May suggest iron overload states (black hypointense liver)
- Magnetic resonance cholangiography (MRC) is a noninvasive method to image the biliary tract.
  d. Radionuclide studies
  - Colloid liver spleen scan using technetium-99m sulfur colloid may aid in the detection of cirrhosis; uptake of colloid is increased in the bone marrow and spleen, with decreased uptake in the liver.
  - Seldom performed; has been supplanted by CT and MRI
  e. Esophagogastroduodenoscopy (EGD) to screen for gastroesophageal varices
4. **Noninvasive markers of hepatic fibrosis**
  a. AST-to-platelet ratio index and others (see Chapter 1)
  b. Ultrasound elastography
5. **Liver biopsy** (see also Chapter 1)
  a. The gold standard for the diagnosis of cirrhosis
  b. Usually performed percutaneously; occasionally obtained through a transjugular approach or at laparoscopy
  c. Relatively low-risk procedure
  d. Complications: Bleeding, infection, pneumothorax, pain

TREATMENT

1. Specific treatments are available in certain instances:
   - Avoidance of alcohol for alcohol-induced cirrhosis
   - Antiviral therapy for chronic hepatitis C
   - Antiviral agents for chronic hepatitis B
   - Weight loss and risk factor modification (management of diabetes mellitus and hyperlipidemia) in nonalcoholic fatty liver disease
   - Phlebotomy for hemochromatosis
   - Glucocorticoids for induction therapy and azathioprine for maintenance treatment of autoimmune hepatitis
   - D-Penicillamine or trientine for Wilson disease
   - Ursodeoxycholic acid and/or obeticholic acid for primary biliary cholangitis
2. In most cases, management focuses on the treatment of complications that arise in the setting of cirrhosis (e.g., variceal hemorrhage, hepatic encephalopathy, ascites, spontaneous bacterial peritonitis).
3. Surveillance for HCC with serial ultrasonographic examinations and serum alpha fetoprotein measurements at frequent intervals (e.g., every 6 months is recommended in patients with cirrhosis and in those with chronic hepatitis B).
4. Vaccination of cirrhotic patients against hepatitis A and B is recommended if patients lack serologic evidence of immunity.
5. All cirrhotic patients should be advised to avoid alcohol and other hepatotoxins.
6. **In end-stage cirrhosis, liver transplantation can be a lifesaving procedure if the patient is an appropriate candidate (see Chapter 33).**

PROGNOSIS

1. Prognosis depends on the development of cirrhotic-related complications.
2. A classification scheme proposed to assess survival, **Child classification** has undergone various modifications; the system currently used is the **Child-Turcotte-Pugh (CTP) scoring system** or **Child-Pugh classification** (Table 11.2).

TABLE 11.2 ■ **Modified Child-Turcotte-Pugh Scoring System for Cirrhosis**

	Numerical Score		
	1	**2**	**3**
Parameter			
Ascites	None	Slight	Moderate/severe
Encephalopathy	None	Slight/moderate	Moderate/severe
Bilirubin (mg/dL)	<2.0	2–3	>3.0
Albumin (mg/L)	>3.5	2.8–3.5	<2.8
Prothrombin time (seconds increased)	1–3	4–6	>6.0
Total Numerical Score	**Child-Pugh Class**		
5–6	A		
7–9	B		
10–15	C		

3. Patients with compensated cirrhosis may have a relatively good life expectancy in the absence of decompensation; estimated 10-year survival in compensated patients is 47%, but when decompensation occurs, estimated 5-year survival is only 16%.
4. In patients with cirrhosis and varices who have not yet had an index variceal hemorrhage, the risk of bleeding from varices can be predicted based on a scoring system that incorporates the Child-Pugh class, variceal size, and certain endoscopic stigmata such as red wale markings and cherry-red spots on varices (see Chapter 12).
5. In cirrhotic patients, the risk of general anesthesia and operative mortality also correlates with the Child-Pugh class (see Chapter 32).
6. The **MELD score** is a prognostic assessment based on serum bilirubin level, serum creatinine level, international normalized ratio (INR), and serum sodium level; it is used to predict prognosis and determine the optimal timing for liver transplantation (see Chapter 33).

EVALUATION

See Fig. 11.1.

Portal Hypertension

Definition: An increase in portal venous pressure
- Normal portal pressure results in a hepatic venous pressure gradient (HVPG) ≤5 mm Hg.
- Portal hypertension results in a HVPG ≥10 mm Hg.
- Normal portal blood flow is 1 to 1.5 L/minute.
- Increased resistance to portal blood flow leads to the formation of portosystemic collateral vessels that divert portal blood flow to the systemic circulation, thus effectively bypassing the liver.

CLASSIFICATION (Box 11.1)

1. Portal hypertension has causes other than cirrhosis.
2. The major classification scheme employed is based on the location of the block to portal flow: **Prehepatic, intrahepatic, and posthepatic**; intrahepatic causes are further separated into **presinusoidal, sinusoidal, and postsinusoidal** (Fig. 11.2).

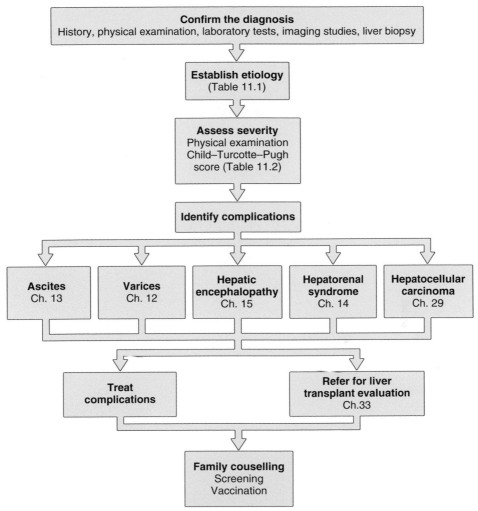

Fig. 11.1 Evaluation of the patient with cirrhosis.

CLINICAL CONSEQUENCES

1. Varices: Gastroesophageal, anorectal, retroperitoneal, stomal, other
2. Portal hypertensive gastropathy, enteropathy, colopathy
3. Caput medusae
4. Ascites and hepatic hydrothorax
5. Congestive splenomegaly
6. Hepatic encephalopathy

MEASUREMENT OF PORTAL PRESSURE

1. In most cases, the diagnosis of portal hypertension can be based on physical findings; however, in some instances direct measurement of the portal pressure is required.
2. Patency of the portal vein should be assessed before measurement of portal pressure; this may be accomplished by duplex Doppler ultrasonography or magnetic resonance angiography.

3. Direct measurement of portal pressure is invasive, expensive, complicated, and accurate.
   - Operative portal vein measurement: Requires laparotomy and is affected by many variables including anesthesia
   - Percutaneous transhepatic measurement
   - Transjugular measurement

BOX 11.1 ■ Causes of Portal Hypertension

Prehepatic

Portal vein thrombosis
Cavernous transformation of the portal vein
Splenic vein thrombosis
Splanchnic arteriovenous fistula
Idiopathic tropical splenomegaly

Intrahepatic (some overlap exists)

Presinusoidal: Affects portal venules
   Schistosomiasis (most common cause of portal hypertension worldwide)
   Congenital hepatic fibrosis
   Sarcoidosis
   Chronic viral hepatitis
   Primary biliary cholangitis (early)
   Myeloproliferative diseases
   Nodular regenerative hyperplasia
   Hepatoportal sclerosis (idiopathic portal hypertension)
   Malignant disease
   Wilson disease
   Hemochromatosis
   Polycystic liver disease
   Amyloidosis
   Toxic agents: Copper, arsenic, vinyl chloride, 6-mercaptopurine
Sinusoidal: Affects sinusoids
   All causes of cirrhosis (see Table 11.1)
   Acute alcoholic hepatitis
   Severe viral hepatitis
   Acute fatty liver of pregnancy
   Vitamin A intoxication
   Systemic mastocytosis
   Peliosis hepatis
   Cytotoxic drugs
Postsinusoidal: Affects central veins
   Sinusoidal obstruction syndrome
   Alcoholic central hyaline sclerosis

Posthepatic

Hepatic vein thrombosis
   Budd-Chiari syndrome
   Vascular invasion by tumor
Inferior vena caval obstruction
   Inferior vena cava web
   Vascular invasion by tumor
Cardiac disease
   Constrictive pericarditis
   Severe tricuspid regurgitation

4. Indirect measurement of portal pressure is the preferred method and is less invasive, safer, and less complicated than direct measurement.

  a. Hepatic vein catheterization

  ■ Involves cannulation of the hepatic vein with measurement of the free hepatic vein pressure (FHVP) and balloon occlusion of the hepatic vein with measurement of the wedged hepatic vein pressure (WHVP). WHVP is a measure of sinusoidal pressure, not a direct measure of portal pressure.

  ■ **HVPG is calculated by subtracting the FHVP from the WHVP; this value represents the difference between the portal pressure and that in the inferior vena cava. Portal hypertension is diagnosed when the HVPG is ≥10 mm Hg.**

  ■ Hepatic blood flow can also be measured.

  ■ In cases of presinusoidal and prehepatic portal hypertension, the measured HVPG may be artificially normal. In these instances direct portal pressures are sometimes obtained for diagnosis, because the WHVP and FHVP do not capture the higher upstream pressures that confirm the presence of portal hypertension.

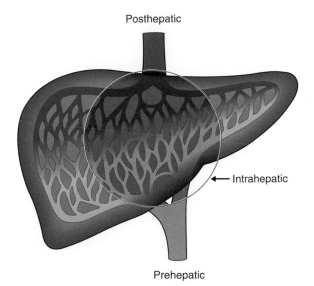

Posthepatic

Intrahepatic

Prehepatic

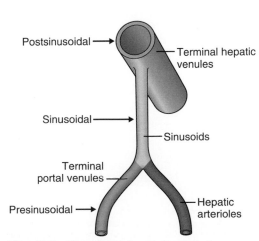

Postsinusoidal

Terminal hepatic venules

Sinusoidal

Sinusoids

Terminal portal venules

Presinusoidal

Hepatic arterioles

Fig. 11.2 Sites of block in portal hypertension.

b. Intrasplenic measurement
   ■ Involves percutaneous puncture of the spleen
   ■ Not routinely performed

TREATMENT OF COMPLICATIONS

See Chapters 12 to 15 and 33.

EVALUATION

See Fig. 11.3.

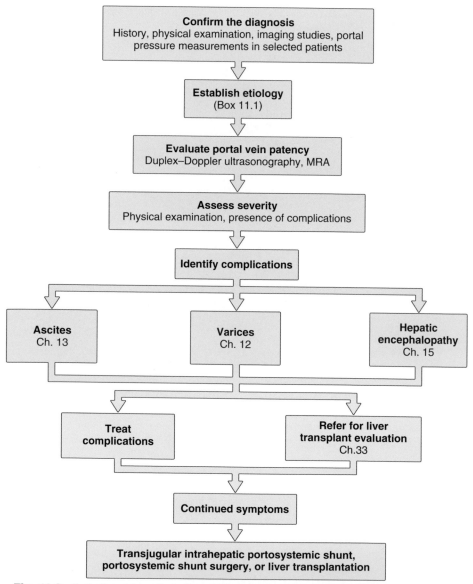

Fig. 11.3   Evaluation of the patient with portal hypertension. *MRA,* Magnetic resonance angiography.

FURTHER READING

Anthony PP, Ishak KG, Nayak NC, et al. The morphology of cirrhosis: recommendations on definition, nomenclature, and classification by a working group sponsored by the World Health Organization. *J Clin Pathol*. 1978;31:395–414.

Bosch J, Navasa M, Garcia-Pagan J, et al. Portal hypertension. *Med Clin North Am*. 1989;73:931–952.

Brann O. Infectious complications of cirrhosis. *Curr Gastroenterol Rep*. 2001;3:285–292.

Bunchorntavakul C, Chamroonkul N, Chavalitdhamrong D. Bacterial infections in cirrhosis: a critical review and practical guidance. *World J Hepatol*. 2016;8:307–321.

Chou R, Wasson N. Blood tests to diagnose fibrosis or cirrhosis in patients with chronic hepatitis C virus infection: a systematic review. *Ann Intern Med*. 2013;158:807–820.

Christensen E, Schicting P, Fauerholdt L, et al. Prognostic value of Child-Turcotte criteria in medically treated cirrhosis. *Hepatology*. 1984;4:430–435.

D'Amico G, Pagliaro L, Bosch J. The treatment of portal hypertension: a meta-analytic review. *Hepatology*. 1995;22:332–351.

Degos F, Perez P, Roche B, et al. Diagnostic accuracy of FibroScan and comparison to liver fibrosis biomarkers in chronic viral hepatitis: a multicenter prospective study (the FIBROSTIC study). *J Hepatol*. 2010;53:1013–1021.

Gines P, Quintero E, Arroyo V, et al. Compensated cirrhosis: natural history and prognostic factors. *Hepatology*. 1987;7:122–128.

Goldberg E, Chopra S. Cirrhosis in adults: etiologies, clinical manifestations, and diagnosis. *UpToDate*. 2017. Available at http://www.uptodate.com/contents/cirrhosis-in-adults-etiologies-clinical-manifestations-and-diagnosis. Accessed May 19, 2017.

Kamath P, Wiesner R, Malinchoc M, et al. A model to predict survival in patients with end-stage liver disease. *Hepatology*. 2001;33:464–470.

Lin Z, Xin Y, Dong Q, et al. Performance of the aspartate aminotransferase-to-platelet ratio index for the staging of fibrosis: an updated meta-analysis. *Hepatology*. 2011;53:726–736.

Londono MC, Cardenas A, Guevera M, et al. MELD score and serum sodium in the prediction of survival in patients with cirrhosis awaiting liver transplantation. *Gut*. 2007;56:1283–1290.

Wiesner R, Edwards E, Freeman R. Model for end-stage liver disease and allocation of liver donors. *Gastroenterology*. 2003;124:91–96.

Zarski JP, Sturm N, Guechot J, et al. Comparison of nine blood tests and transient elastography for liver fibrosis in chronic hepatitis C: the ANRS HCEP-23 study. *J Hepatol*. 2012;56:55–62.

CHAPTER 12

Portal Hypertension and Gastrointestinal Bleeding

Norman D. Grace, MD ■ Elena M. Stoffel, MD ■ James Puleo, MD

KEY POINTS

1   Patients with cirrhosis with clinically significant portal hypertension (hepatic venous pressure gradient [HVPG] >10 mm Hg) develop esophageal varices at a rate of 8% per year. This threshold is also required for development of other complications of portal hypertension, such as ascites.

2   Patients with cirrhosis in whom esophageal varices develop have a risk of a variceal hemorrhage of 5% to 15% per year, with patients having large varices at greater risk, and a 15% to 20% mortality rate associated with each bleeding episode. Mortality depends on the clinical status of the patient and the severity of the bleeding episode.

3   Treatment with a nonselective beta-adrenergic blocker (beta blocker) is effective in reducing portal pressure and is a first-line therapy for the primary prevention of variceal hemorrhage in patients with cirrhosis and portal hypertension. Endoscopic variceal ligation is an excellent alternative, especially for patients with varices who have contraindications to or cannot tolerate beta blockers.

4   Endoscopic therapy (variceal band ligation) and pharmacologic therapy (somatostatin, octreotide, vapreotide, lanreotide, terlipressin) are effective in controlling acute bleeding episodes. The combination of endoscopic and pharmacologic therapy offers an advantage over the use of either therapy alone.

5   The combination of endoscopic and pharmacologic treatment is the preferred option for prevention of recurrent variceal bleeding.

6   For patients in whom medical therapy fails to prevent recurrent variceal hemorrhage, options include transjugular intrahepatic portosystemic shunt (TIPS), surgical portosystemic shunt, and liver transplantation. Selection of the appropriate rescue procedure is dictated by the clinical status of the patient, the availability of expertise for performance of the procedure, and, in the case of liver transplantation, appropriateness of the candidate and availability of a donor organ.

Overview

PATHOPHYSIOLOGY

1. Portal hypertension is defined as an increase in the portal venous pressure gradient (PVPG) and is a function of portal venous blood flow and hepatic and portocollateral resistance.
2. In patients with cirrhosis, portal hypertension is initiated by an increase in hepatic and portocollateral resistance. This resistance is modulated by an increase in levels of intrahepatic endothelin, a potent vasoconstrictor, and a decrease in levels of intrahepatic nitric oxide, a vasodilator.

3. Hepatic resistance may be modified by changes in perivenular and presinusoidal myofibroblasts as well as the smooth muscle component of portocollateral vessels.
4. Portal hypertension is exacerbated by the development of systemic vasodilatation, which leads to plasma volume expansion, an increase in cardiac output, and a hyperdynamic circulation. Systemic vasodilatation is a result of an increase in systemic levels of nitric oxide and, to a lesser extent, increased circulatory levels of glucagon, prostaglandins, tumor necrosis factor (TNF) alpha, and other cytokines and alterations in the autonomic nervous system. Angiogenic factors modulate the development of collateral vessels secondary to increased portal vein pressure.
5. **Any increase in portal blood flow or hepatic or portocollateral resistance will increase portal pressure. Conversely, any decrease in portal blood flow or hepatic resistance will decrease portal pressure. This forms the basis for the pharmacologic treatment of portal hypertension.**

PHARMACOTHERAPY

1. Two classes of drugs—vasoconstrictors and vasodilators—are used for treatment of portal hypertension.
2. **Vasoconstrictors** (vasopressin, somatostatin, nonselective beta blockers) produce a decrease in splanchnic blood flow that leads to a reduction in portal venous blood flow and portal pressure. Carvedilol is a nonselective beta blocker with intrinsic anti-alpha-1 adrenergic activity. Clinical studies demonstrate a greater reduction in portal pressure with carvedilol when compared with propranolol or nadolol when used as monotherapy.
3. **Vasodilators** (nitroglycerin, long-acting nitrates, angiotensin inhibitors [losartan, irbesartan]) alter resistance by inducing changes in the intrahepatic perivenular and perisinusoidal myofibroblasts as well as the smooth muscle component of portocollateral vessels.
4. Combined use of vasoconstrictors and vasodilators offers the potential benefit of additive reductions in portal pressure, but their use may be limited by the side effects of treatment (i.e., systemic hypotension).

EPIDEMIOLOGY OF ESOPHAGOGASTRIC VARICEAL HEMORRHAGE

1. Patients with cirrhosis can be classified as compensated or decompensated. **Decompensation is defined as the appearance of ascites, variceal hemorrhage, hepatic encephalopathy, or jaundice.** Five stages have been proposed to account for the increased mortality associated with progressive decompensation. For patients with compensated cirrhosis, the 5-year mortality rate is 1.5% compared with 88% for patients with multiple complications of cirrhosis (stage 5) (Fig. 12.1). Therefore, a goal of therapy is to inhibit progression from compensated to decompensated cirrhosis.
2. Approximately 50% of patients with alcoholic cirrhosis will develop esophageal varices within 2 years of diagnosis, and 70% to 80% will do so within 10 years. In patients with cirrhosis due to chronic hepatitis C, the risk of varices is somewhat less; 30% will develop esophageal varices within 6 years of the initial diagnosis of cirrhosis.
3. Of patients with cirrhosis and large esophageal varices, 25% to 35% will experience an episode of variceal bleeding; most bleeding episodes occur within the first year after identification of varices.
4. In patients with cirrhosis who survive the initial episode of esophagogastric variceal hemorrhage (EVH) with medical management, the risk of recurrent EVH is 65% to 70%; most episodes of recurrent bleeding occur within 6 months of the index hemorrhage.
5. **EVH accounts for approximately 1/3 of deaths in patients with cirrhosis and portal hypertension**; the mortality rate for each episode of EVH is 15% to 20%, depending on the clinical status of the patient.

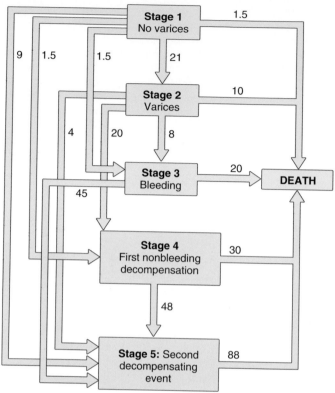

Fig. 12.1 Schematic representation of 5-year transitioning rate across stages and to death for a series of patients. Arrows represent transitions, and the numbers close to each arrow are the relevant transition rates (%). A fairly steady increase in death rate was found across stages. (From D'Amico G, Pasta L, Morabito A, et al. Competing risks and prognostic stages of cirrhosis: A 25-year inception cohort study of 494 patients. *Aliment Pharmacol Ther.* 2014;39:1180–1193.)

6. Treatment to prevent recurrent EVH should be initiated immediately following control of the acute EVH.

RISK FACTORS FOR FIRST VARICEAL HEMORRHAGE

■ Large esophageal varices
■ The presence of endoscopic red color signs (red weals, cherry-red spots, hematocystic spots); these are essentially small varices on the surface of large varices.
■ Hepatic decompensation as evaluated by the Child-Turcotte-Pugh score or the Model for End-stage Liver Disease (MELD) score; ascites is a particular risk factor (see Chapters 11 and 33).
■ Active alcohol consumption in patients with alcoholic liver disease

PREDICTIVE VALUE OF PORTAL HEMODYNAMIC MEASUREMENTS

1. Measurement of the HVPG is an easy and reproducible method for estimating portal pressure. HVPG is the difference between the wedged or occluded hepatic venous pressure and the free hepatic venous pressure. HVPG has a high correlation with portal pressure in patients with cirrhosis when hepatic resistance is sinusoidal or postsinusoidal, as in patients

with alcoholic cirrhosis. HVPG tends to underestimate portal pressure when the defect is presinusoidal, as in primary biliary cholangitis.

2. **An HVPG of 10 mm Hg or greater is necessary for esophageal varices to form and bleed.**
3. According to Laplace's law, variceal wall tension (T) is a function of the transmural pressure (TP) times the radius (r) of the varix divided by the variceal wall thickness (w):

$$T = (TP_1 - TP_2) \times r/w$$

   This calculation combines measurements of variceal size and pressure and has the highest predictive value for determining the risk of EVH.
4. The risk of recurrent EVH correlates with the level of HVPG: **The higher the HVPG, the greater the risk of recurrent EVH.**
5. HVPG also predicts survival: **The higher the HVPG, the lower the survival.** HVPG also predicts the development of hepatic decompensation and the development of hepatocellular carcinoma.
6. Serial measurements of HVPG are predictive of the risk of recurrent EVH. **Patients who achieve a decrease in HVPG to a level <12 mm Hg either spontaneously or in response to pharmacologic therapy are not at risk for recurrent EVH and other complications of portal hypertension. Patients in whom HVPG decreases by 20% or more over the first few months after the index hemorrhage, usually in response to pharmacologic therapy, have a marked decrease in the risk of recurrent EVH, whereas patients who have less than a 20% decrease in HVPG while receiving pharmacologic therapy maintain a high risk of recurrent EVH.**

Prevention of Initial Variceal Hemorrhage

PHARMACOLOGIC

1. **For patients with large esophageal varices and no prior history of EVH, therapy with a nonselective beta-adrenergic blocker has been shown to decrease the risk of initial variceal bleeding by approximately 40% and is the treatment of choice for the primary prevention of variceal hemorrhage.**
2. A nonselective beta blocker (propranolol, nadolol, timolol, carvedilol) should be offered to compliant patients who have no contraindications to the use of a beta blocker, such as severe chronic obstructive lung disease or heart failure.
3. For patients unable to tolerate beta-blocker therapy, no other drugs administered as monotherapy have benefit.
4. In routine practice, the dose of the nonselective beta-blocker should be achieved by a stepwise increase in dosage, adjusted to patient tolerance. If portal hemodynamic studies are readily available, serial measurements of HVPG in response to beta-blocker therapy may be of value in determining the therapeutic dose and potential clinical benefit of beta blockers.
5. **Therapy with a nonselective beta blocker should be continued indefinitely.** A follow-up study of persons with nonbleeding esophageal varices who discontinued propranolol after 2 to 3 years revealed that their risk of variceal hemorrhage increased to that of untreated persons, with increased mortality compared with an untreated population.

ENDOSCOPIC

1. **Endoscopic variceal band ligation (EVL)** to achieve variceal obliteration may prevent an initial episode of variceal hemorrhage with success rates comparable with those achieved with propranolol or nadolol.

2. Studies to date show no advantage to a combination of endoscopic and pharmacologic treatment with EVL and nonselective beta blockers for prevention of an initial variceal hemorrhage.

SURGICAL

1. Neither a TIPS nor prophylactic portosystemic shunt surgery is indicated for the prevention of initial variceal hemorrhage.
2. Decisions about candidacy for liver transplantation should be dictated by the overall clinical status of the patient. The presence of varices per se is not an indication for liver transplantation.

Treatment of Acute Variceal Hemorrhage

INITIAL

1. Resuscitation of the patient is critical in the management of the patient with cirrhosis and suspected EVH and should include the following measures:
   - Establish adequate venous access for blood and fluid replacement.
   - Insert a nasogastric or Ewald tube to assess the severity of bleeding and to lavage gastric contents before endoscopy.
   - Treatment of clotting factor deficiencies is controversial without clear evidence of efficacy. Fresh frozen plasma or recombinant factor VIIa has been used.
   - Administer blood transfusions to establish hemodynamic stability. Caution should be taken not to overtransfuse the patient. In general, patients should be kept slightly undertransfused, usually with a hematocrit value of approximately 24%, to avoid increasing portal pressure and exacerbating variceal bleeding unless comorbid conditions (i.e., cardiovascular events) require a higher hematocrit level.
   - Establish airway protection in patients with massive bleeding or evidence of hepatic encephalopathy.
   - Initiate antibiotic treatment to reduce the risk of infection (see Chapter 13). For patients with severe decompensation, ceftriaxone (1 g every 24 hours) is the antibiotic of choice. Before treatment, blood cultures, diagnostic paracentesis if ascites is present, and other studies as indicated should be performed.
   - Initiate pharmacologic therapy with vasoactive drugs (e.g., octreotide, terlipressin) as soon as possible and before endoscopy.
   - In the absence of contraindications (e.g., QT prolongation on electrocardiogram), infusion of erythromycin 250 mg intravenously 30 to 120 minutes before endoscopy promotes gastric emptying and may provide improved visualization of the bleeding site.
2. **Endoscopy is the only reliable means of establishing the source of bleeding and should be performed as soon as the patient is adequately resuscitated and no longer than 12 hours after admission.** The diagnosis of EVH is determined either by direct visualization of bleeding or, more often, by the detection of endoscopic stigmata in patients with varices and no other visible source of bleeding.

ENDOSCOPIC

1. **EVL is the endoscopic treatment of choice in the treatment of acute bleeding from esophageal varices.** EVL has been shown to have success rates of 80% to 90% in initial control of variceal hemorrhage and has few local complications, primarily mucosal ulceration.

2. The use of pharmacologic therapy in conjunction with endoscopic therapy improves the efficacy of endoscopic treatment in controlling acute bleeding.

PHARMACOLOGIC

1. The use of vasoactive drugs for the treatment of acute bleeding related to portal hypertension offers the following advantages:
   - Treatment can be started in the emergency department when variceal bleeding is suspected.
   - Unlike endoscopic therapy, in which the effects of treatment are local, vasoactive agents lower portal pressure.
   - The use of vasoactive agents before endoscopy may offer the endoscopist a clearer view of the varices because bleeding is less active.
   - Vasoactive agents can be useful for the treatment of sources of portal hypertensive bleeding other than esophageal varices, such as gastric varices more than 2 cm below the gastroesophageal junction or portal hypertensive gastropathy.
   - Vasoactive drugs should be continued for up to 5 days after initiation of treatment.
2. Pharmacologic agents include somatostatin, octreotide, vapreotide, lanreotide, and terlipressin (Table 12.1). Although in common use throughout the world, none of these agents is approved by the U.S. Food and Drug Administration for this indication.
   - **Somatostatin,** given intravenously by bolus followed by continuous infusion, has been effective in controlling variceal bleeding in 60% to 80% of patients and has no serious side effects associated with its use.
   - Because somatostatin is not generally available in the United States, **octreotide,** its synthetic analogue with a longer half-life, is widely used instead in this country. A meta-analysis concluded that octreotide was superior to vasopressin or terlipressin in controlling acute variceal bleeding. Vapreotide and lanreotide are somatostatin analogues not currently available in the United States.
   - **Terlipressin,** a synthetic analogue of vasopressin, has a longer half-life than vasopressin and therefore can be given by intravenous bolus infusion. Randomized controlled trials have shown that this drug is more effective than vasopressin, with far fewer side effects. It is used widely in Europe, and approval by the Food and Drug Administration is expected.

   The combination of endoscopic and pharmacologic therapy (octreotide) offers clinical advantages over the use of either therapy alone, with less rebleeding in the acute period (first 5 days) and lower transfusion requirements; however, combination therapy has not been shown to improve survival.

TABLE 12.1 ■ **Pharmacologic Treatment of Acute Variceal Bleeding**

Drug	Route	Dose
Terlipressin	IV	Initially 1–2 mg every 4 hours until control of bleeding; then 1 mg every 4 hours maintenance
Somatostatin	IV	Initial bolus of 250 µg followed by continuous infusion of 250–500 µg/hr
Octreotide	IV	Initial bolus of 50 µg followed by continuous infusion of 50 µg/hr
Treatment should be continued for 5 days		

IV, Intravenous.

TIPS

In high-risk patients (Child-Pugh class C or Child-Pugh class B with active bleeding at endoscopy), the placement of TIPS using a coated stent within 24 hours of admission may result in less morbidity and improved survival compared with standard medical therapy.

BALLOON TAMPONADE

1. Endoscopic therapy has replaced balloon tamponade as initial therapy for variceal bleeding; however, balloon tamponade may still be of value as a temporizing treatment for failures of pharmacologic and endoscopic therapy, before more definitive treatment for the control of acute variceal bleeding is undertaken.
2. Success with balloon tamponade can often be achieved with inflation of the gastric balloon alone, thereby avoiding the additional complications associated with inflation of the esophageal balloon.
3. Complication rates with the use of balloon tamponade relate to the experience of the team using the balloon. Specific precautions are required to minimize the risk of aspiration and asphyxiation. The balloon should not be kept inflated for more than 24 hours because of the risk of esophageal necrosis.
4. The use of endoscopically placed self-expandable esophageal stents offers a safer alternative to balloon tamponade and may be used for a longer period of time.

TREATMENT FOR FAILURES OF MEDICAL THERAPY

1. **A National Institutes of Health consensus conference supported the use of TIPS for the rescue of the 10% to 20% of patients in whom medical therapy fails to control acute variceal hemorrhage.**
2. In experienced hands, TIPS can be successful in 90% to 95% of patients, with relatively low immediate mortality compared with the use of a surgical portosystemic shunt.
3. Rebleeding and hepatic encephalopathy are long-term complications of TIPS but are less of a risk since the advent of coated stents.

Prevention of Recurrent Variceal Hemorrhage

Because of the high recurrence rate of variceal bleeding after control of initial bleeding, it is not surprising that medical therapy for the control of acute variceal bleeding has not been associated with improved survival. Treatment to prevent recurrent variceal bleeding has a greater potential to influence long-term survival.

1. The risk of recurrent variceal bleeding is highest in the first few weeks, and the risk of rebleeding remains significantly elevated during the first 6 months after the index hemorrhage.
2. **It is crucial that therapy to prevent recurrent bleeding be initiated as soon as the acute bleeding episode is adequately controlled.**

ENDOSCOPIC

1. **EVL is the endoscopic therapy of choice for the prevention of recurrent variceal bleeding.** When compared with sclerotherapy, EVL is associated with lower rates of recurrent bleeding, mortality, and complications and requires fewer sessions for variceal obliteration.
2. The combination of EVL and sclerotherapy offers no advantage over EVL alone.

TABLE 12.2 ■ Pharmacologic Treatment for Prevention of Variceal Bleeding

Drug	Initial Dose	Therapeutic Dose Range
Propranolol	40 mg twice/day	40–320 mg/day
Nadolol	40 mg/day	40–160 mg/day
Timolol	10 mg/day	5–40 mg/day
Carvedilol	6.25 mg/day	6.25–12.5 mg/day
Isosorbide 5-mononitrate	20 mg twice/day	20 mg 3–4 times/day

3. Patients who have had a variceal bleeding episode should undergo EVL at regular intervals (every 1 to 2 weeks) until the varices are obliterated, followed by regular surveillance (6- to 12-month intervals), with repeat endoscopic treatment if varices recur. The combination of endoscopic and pharmacologic therapy may decrease the risk of recurrent varices.

PHARMACOLOGIC (Table 12.2)

1. **Nonselective beta-adrenergic blockers (propranolol, nadolol, carvedilol) have been shown to reduce the risk of recurrent variceal bleeding and to reduce mortality associated with bleeding.**
2. Beta-blocker therapy is indicated for patients
   - With good hepatic function (Child-Pugh classes A and B)
   - Deemed to be compliant with taking medication
   - With no contraindications to use of beta blockers (e.g., heart failure, severe chronic lung disease)
3. The therapeutic dose of the beta blocker is adjusted to the highest tolerated dose.
4. In centers where hepatic hemodynamic measurements are readily available, serial measurements of the HVPG (baseline and at 1 to 3 months) are predictive of the efficacy of treatment. Recurrent variceal bleeding is significantly reduced when HVPG decreases to <12 mm Hg or at least a 20% decrease in HVPG from baseline is noted.
5. If therapy with a beta blocker does not achieve one of these end points, the addition of a second drug (e.g., a long-acting nitrate) may be considered in an attempt to reduce HVPG further. Carvedilol, a nonselective beta blocker with intrinsic anti–alpha-1-adrenergic activity, has been shown to decrease portal pressure to a greater extent than nonselective beta blockers (e.g., propranolol) and is reasonably well tolerated. Clinical studies have shown mixed results as to whether this drug is superior to traditional nonselective beta-blockers.

COMBINED ENDOSCOPIC AND PHARMACOLOGIC

Combination endoscopic and pharmacologic treatment is the preferred therapy for the prevention of recurrent variceal bleeding. A meta-analysis of randomized controlled trials has shown endoscopic therapy plus a nonselective beta blocker is more effective than either drug treatment or EVL alone for the prevention of rebleeding.

TREATMENT FOR FAILURES OF MEDICAL THERAPY

1. **TIPS** is effective at reducing portal pressure and is currently the preferred treatment for patients in whom initial medical therapy fails, especially for those patients who are poor operative risks.

2. For low-risk patients (Child-Pugh class A), portosystemic shunt surgery remains an alternative in selected centers with experience in portosystemic shunt surgery. In patients with nonalcoholic cirrhosis, a distal splenorenal shunt is preferable to a portacaval shunt because of the lower frequency of hepatic encephalopathy associated with the selective shunt.
3. Liver transplantation should always be considered for patients with end-stage liver disease. Selection of candidates is dictated by the patient's clinical status, the cause of cirrhosis, abstinence from alcohol in patients with alcoholic cirrhosis, and absence of severe nonhepatic comorbidities (see Chapter 33).
4. For patients who are candidates for liver transplantation, a TIPS procedure can be used as a bridge to transplantation.

Management of Nonesophageal Variceal Sources of Bleeding Related to Portal Hypertension

GASTRIC VARICES

1. Gastric varices that extend more than 5 cm below the gastroesophageal junction or are isolated to the fundus are at high risk of bleeding.
2. Endoscopic treatment for gastric varices is less effective than for esophageal varices. Use of **cyanoacrylate glue** has been effective in the management of bleeding gastric varices and is the treatment of choice. Complications of therapy include bacteremia and glue embolization. The efficacy of other therapies, such as clips, snares, and thrombin, is under investigation.
3. Pharmacologic therapy (e.g., octreotide) should be considered for initial treatment of acute bleeding and prevention of recurrent bleeding.
4. Patients in whom pharmacologic therapy fails should be considered for TIPS or, for appropriate candidates, liver transplantation.

PORTAL HYPERTENSIVE GASTROPATHY

1. Portal hypertensive gastropathy is a common complication of cirrhosis and portal hypertension, but clinically significant gastrointestinal bleeding from this source is relatively uncommon.
2. Endoscopically, portal hypertensive gastropathy ranges from a mild form characterized by a diffuse mosaic ("snakeskin") mucosal pattern to more severe forms characterized by brown spots, cherry-red spots, granular mucosa, and diffuse mucosal hemorrhages.
3. Prior treatment of esophageal varices with endoscopic therapy has been implicated in increasing the severity of portal hypertensive gastropathy.
4. Pharmacologic therapy is the only medical option for treating acute bleeding or preventing recurrent bleeding from portal hypertensive gastropathy. Endoscopic therapy has no role.
5. For failures with medical therapy, TIPS and liver transplantation are potential options.

FURTHER READING

Abraczinskas DR, Ookubo R, Grace ND, et al. Propranolol for the prevention of first esophageal variceal hemorrhage: a lifetime commitment? *Hepatology*. 2001;34:1096–1102.
Abraldes JG, Vellanueva C, Banares R, et al. Hepatic venous pressure gradient and prognosis in patients with acute variceal bleeding treated with pharmacologic and endoscopic therapy. *J Hepatol*. 2008;48:229–236.
Augustin S, Muntaner L, Altamirano JT, et al. Predicting early mortality after acute variceal hemorrhage based on classification and regression tree analysis. *Clin Gastroenterol Hepatol*. 2009;7:1347–1354.
Castera l, Chan HLY, Arrese M, et al. EASL-ALEH Clinical Practice Guidelines: non-invasive tests for evaluation of liver disease severity and prognosis. *J Hepatol*. 2015;63:237–264.

D'Amico G, Pasta L, Morabito A, et al. Competing risks and prognostic stages of cirrhosis: a 25-year inception cohort study of 494 patients. *Aliment Pharmacol Ther.* 2014;39:1180–1193.

deFranchis R. Expanding consensus in portal hypertension. Report of the Baveno VI consensus workshop: stratifying risk and individualizing care for portal hypertension. *J Hepatol.* 2015;63:743–752.

Garcia-Pagan JC, Caca K, Bureau C, et al. Early use of TIPS in patients with cirrhosis and variceal bleeding. *N Engl J Med.* 2010;362:2370–2379.

Garcia-Tsao G, Bosch J. Varices and variceal hemorrhage in cirrhosis: a new view of an old problem. *Clin Gastroenterol Hepatol.* 2015;13:2109–2117.

Garcia-Tsao G, Sanyal J, Grace ND, et al. Prevention and management of gastroesophageal varices and variceal hemorrhage in cirrhosis. *Hepatology.* 2007;46:922–938.

Gonzalez R, Zamora J, Gomez-Camarera J, et al. Combination endoscopic and drug therapy to prevent variceal rebleeding in cirrhosis. *Ann Intern Med.* 2008;149:109–122.

Groszmann RJ, Garcia-Tsao G, Bosch J, et al. Beta-blockers to prevent gastroesophageal varices cirrhosis. *N Engl J Med.* 2005;353:2254–2261.

Lo GH, Lai KH, Cheng JS, et al. Endoscopic variceal ligation plus nadolol and sucralfate compared with ligation alone for the prevention of variceal rebleeding: a prospective, randomized trial. *Hepatology.* 2000;32:461–465.

Lui HF, Stanley AJ, Forrest EH, et al. Primary prophylaxis of variceal hemorrhage: a randomized controlled trial comparing band ligation, propranolol, and isosorbide mononitrate. *Gastroenterology.* 2002;123:735–744.

Sanyal AJ, Fontana RJ, DiBisceglie AM, et al. The prevalence and risk factors associated with esophageal varices in subjects with hepatitis C and advanced fibrosis. *Gastrointest Endosc.* 2006;64:855–864.

Tan PC, Hou MC, Lin HC, et al. A randomized trial of endoscopic treatment of acute gastric variceal hemorrhage: N-butyl-2-cyanoacrylate injection versus band ligation. *Hepatology.* 2006;43:690–697.

CHAPTER 13

Ascites and Spontaneous Bacterial Peritonitis

Kavish R. Patidar, DO ■ Arun J. Sanyal, MD

KEY POINTS

1 Cirrhosis accounts for 85% of the cases of ascites in the United States; the development of ascites is associated with a 50% 2-year survival rate.

2 Abdominal paracentesis with ascitic fluid analysis is a safe and cost-effective strategy in the differential diagnosis of ascites. Routine ascitic fluid tests include cell count, inoculation of fluid into blood culture bottles, albumin, and total protein, with additional testing depending on the clinical setting.

3 Treatment of cirrhotic ascites involves dietary sodium restriction and diuretic therapy.

4 Refractory ascites develops in 10% of cirrhotic patients with ascites. Management includes intermittent large-volume paracentesis (LVP) and insertion of a transjugular intrahepatic portosystemic shunt (TIPS).

5 All patients who develop ascites caused by cirrhosis should be considered for liver transplantation.

6 Spontaneous bacterial peritonitis (SBP) is ascitic fluid infection that develops in the setting of cirrhotic ascites in the absence of a perforated viscus. The morbidity and mortality of SBP is high, and prompt diagnosis by paracentesis with appropriate ascitic fluid analysis and prompt treatment with a nonnephrotoxic antibiotic intravenous infusion of albumin are crucial.

Overview of Ascites

DEFINITION

Ascites is defined as the pathologic accumulation of fluid in the peritoneal cavity.

EPIDEMIOLOGY

1. **Cirrhosis accounts for 85% of the cases of ascites in the United States.** Infectious etiologies, most notably tuberculosis, predominate in the developing world.
2. Ascites is the most common complication of cirrhosis and marks the transition from compensated cirrhosis to decompensated cirrhosis.
3. Ascites is present in 20% to 60% of patients with cirrhosis at the time of diagnosis.
4. Ascites develops in approximately 50% of patients with cirrhosis within 10 years of diagnosis.
5. **Once ascites occurs, the survival of patients is significantly reduced to 50% at 2 years.**
6. Patients with ascites are susceptible to the development of ascites-related complications such as SBP, acute kidney injury, and hepatorenal syndrome.

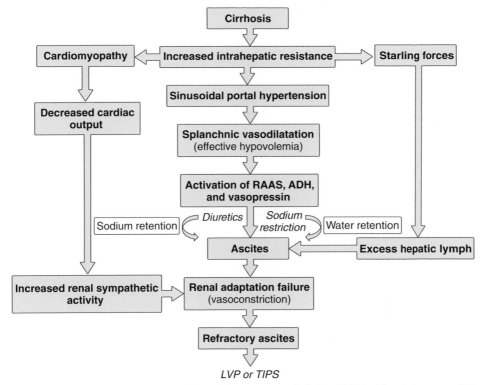

Fig. 13.1 Pathophysiology of ascites. Potential treatments are in italics. *ADH,* Antidiuretic hormone; *LVP,* large-volume paracentesis; *RAAS,* renin-angiotensin-aldosterone system; *TIPS,* transjugular intrahepatic portosystemic shunt.

PATHOPHYSIOLOGY OF CIRRHOTIC ASCITES

1. The major contributing factors leading to the development of ascites is portal hypertension resulting from increased intrahepatic resistance to blood flow and splanchnic vasodilation that lead to a decrease in effective arterial blood volume (Fig. 13.1).
2. Portal hypertension also increases translocation of gut bacteria and bacterial products, which stimulate cytokine synthesis, thereby leading to further arterial vasodilation.
3. In response to the decrease in effective arterial blood volume and to maintain arterial blood pressure, the sympathetic nervous system, renin-angiotensin-aldosterone system (RAAS), antidiuretic hormone, and, in later stages, arginine vasopressin are activated, thereby causing avid renal sodium and water retention.
4. Starling forces in the hepatic sinusoids (increased sinusoidal pressure and decreased oncotic pressure) drive excess sodium and water into hepatic lymph.
5. When the capacity of hepatic lymphatics is exceeded, the excess hepatic lymph spills into the peritoneal cavity to form ascites.

Diagnosis

HISTORY

1. The patient's history often reveals clues to the cause of the underlying liver disease (e.g., viral hepatitis, alcoholic liver disease, nonalcoholic fatty liver disease).

TABLE 13.1 ■ **Causes of Ascites**

Portal Hypertension
Presinusoidal, sinusoidal, and postsinusoidal

Neoplastic Diseases
Hepatocellular carcinoma, peritoneal carcinomatosis, lymphoma, ovarian cancer, mesothelioma

Inflammatory Disorders
Allergic, chemical, immunologic, infectious

Renal Disorders
Nephrotic syndrome, dialysis-associated ascites

Miscellaneous Causes
Ovarian hyperstimulation syndrome, thoracic duct obstruction

2. Other etiologies, including intraabdominal malignancy and cardiovascular, renal, and pancreatic disease, should be considered (Table 13.1).
3. Patients may complain of increased abdominal girth, which is often accompanied by lower extremity edema.

PHYSICAL EXAMINATION

1. The aim of the physical examination is to identify signs of portal hypertension in addition to the physical signs of cirrhosis (i.e., spider telangiectases, palmar erythema, abdominal wall collateral vessels, splenomegaly) (see Chapter 11).
2. Physical findings in patients with ascites
    ■ Full and bulging abdomen
    ■ Flank dullness on percussion
    ■ Shifting dullness, which usually suggests the presence of >1500 mL of ascites fluid.
    ■ Commonly, abdominal wall hernias such as umbilical and ventral wall hernias.
    ■ An obese abdomen can mimic ascites; abdominal ultrasonography is useful for confirming the presence of ascites (see later).

LABORATORY AND IMAGING FEATURES

1. Laboratory values to be obtained include the following:
    ■ Complete blood count, renal function panel (electrolytes, serum creatinine, blood urea nitrogen), coagulation panel (prothrombin time and international normalized ratio), and hepatic panel (serum aminotransferases, bilirubin, total protein, albumin, alkaline phosphatase)
2. Abdominal ultrasonography
    ■ **The most cost-effective and least invasive method to confirm the presence of ascites**
    ■ Can detect as little as 100 mL of ascites
    ■ Can determine the optimal site for diagnostic or therapeutic paracentesis
    ■ Helpful for the diagnosis of portal hypertension (e.g., spleen larger than 12 cm, portal vein >1.3 cm, enlarged periumbilical vein)
    ■ Can differentiate ascites from obesity and from ovarian and mesenteric masses
3. Computed tomography or magnetic resonance imaging
    ■ Not recommended for the initial evaluation of cirrhosis

■ Helpful for identifying an alternative diagnosis to cirrhosis if the initial workup is not conclusive (e.g., hepatic vein thrombosis)

ASSESSMENT OF THE SEVERITY OF ASCITES

1. The International Ascites Club classifies ascites according to severity (grade), presence or absence of complications (uncomplicated or complicated), and response to diuretic treatment (diuretic resistant or diuretic intractable).
   a. Grade
      ■ Mild: Detectable only on ultrasonography
      ■ Moderate: Moderate distention of abdomen
      ■ Large: Marked distension of abdomen ("tense")
   b. Complication
      ■ Uncomplicated: Ascites with no infection and hepatorenal syndrome
      ■ Complicated: Ascites with infection or hepatorenal syndrome
   c. Response to diuretic treatment
      ■ **Diuretic resistant:** No response to a sodium-restricted diet and high-dose diuretic treatment (see later)
      ■ **Diuretic intractable:** Side effects induced by diuretics preclude optimal dosing

Ascitic Fluid Analysis

DIAGNOSTIC PARACENTESIS

1. Diagnostic paracentesis (at least 30 mL of fluid) is required in all patients presenting with the new onset of ascites, on hospital admission, or experiencing clinical deterioration (fever, hepatic encephalopathy, renal failure).
2. With the use of the "Z-track" approach, the left lower quadrant of the abdomen (i.e., two fingerbreadths cephalad and two fingerbreadths medial to the anterior superior iliac spine) is the best location for paracentesis because the abdominal wall is thinner at this location and generally overlies a large pocket of ascites.
   ■ If this location is not feasible, an alternative site is the midline between the pubic symphysis and umbilicus.
3. Coagulopathy (i.e., prolonged prothrombin time) should not be an absolute contraindication in patients with cirrhosis, because the risk for bleeding is <1% after paracentesis. Thrombocytopenia is also not an absolute contraindication.
   ■ Other coagulopathic states, such as disseminated intravascular coagulation or hyperfibrinolysis, should preclude paracentesis.
4. Complications of paracentesis include abdominal wall hematoma, bowel perforation, and fluid leak at the site of paracentesis (which may occur if the Z-track approach is not used).

ASCITES FLUID TESTS AND INTERPRETATION

1. The most commonly ordered ascitic fluid tests are shown in Table 13.2.
2. **The serum-ascites albumin gradient (SAAG) is necessary to determine if a patient's ascites is due to portal hypertension**.
   ■ Calculation of SAAG is performed by measuring the serum albumin and ascitic fluid albumin concentrations simultaneously and then subtracting the ascitic fluid albumin from the serum albumin.

TABLE 13.2 ■ **Ascitic Fluid Tests**

Routine	Optional	Unusual	Not Helpful
Albumin	Gram stain	Tuberculosis culture/smear	Alpha fetoprotein
Total protein	Lactate dehydrogenase	Cytology	Cholesterol
Cell count with differential	Glucose	Triglycerides	pH and lactate
Culture	Amylase	Bilirubin	Fibronectin

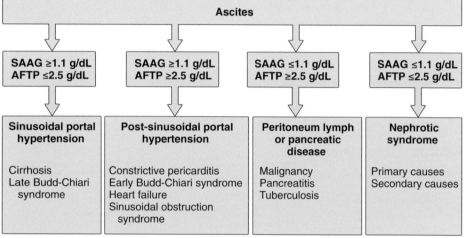

Fig. 13.2   Cause of ascites according to the serum-ascites albumin gradient and ascitic fluid total protein concentration. *AFTP,* Ascitic fluid total protein concentration; *SAAG,* serum-ascites albumin gradient.

■ **A SAAG of >1.1 g/dL is 97% accurate in detecting portal hypertension** (Fig. 13.2).
3. Ascitic fluid total protein measurements help further define the etiology of ascites and the risk for SBP (increased when the total protein concentration is <1 g/dL).
4. **Ascites containing ≥250 polymorphonuclear neutrophils (PMNs)/mm³ is presumed to be infected.**
   ■ The sensitivity of the ascitic fluid culture can be enhanced with immediate (bedside) inoculation 10 mL of fluid into aerobic and anaerobic bottles (sensitivity of 90%).
   ■ For bloody ascites (see definition later), the PMN count can be corrected by subtracting 1 PMN for every 250 red blood cells in ascites fluid.
   ■ Lactate dehydrogenase and glucose levels can help differentiate SBP from secondary peritonitis (see later discussion)
5. Additional features of ascites:
   ■ Bloody ascites: Red blood cell count >10,000/m³ in ascites fluid
      – Hepatocellular carcinoma is the cause of bloody ascites in about 30% of patients with cirrhosis.
   ■ Chylous ascites: Ascitic fluid that has the appearance of milk, with a triglyceride concentration >200 mg/dL
6. The yield of ascitic fluid is low for malignancy (approximately 7%). However, in peritoneal carcinomatosis, if an adequate amount of ascitic fluid (three samples) is sent promptly for analysis, the sensitivity is approximately 97%.

TABLE 13.3 ■ **Differential of Causes of Ascites Based on Ascites Fluid Clues**

Cause	Clues
Cirrhotic ascites	SAAG ≥1.1 g/dL ATFP <2.5 g/dL
Cardiac ascites	SAAG ≥1.1 g/dL AFTP ≥2.5 g/dL
Peritoneal carcinomatosis	SAAG ≤1.1 g/dL AFTP ≥2.5 g/dL Malignant cells on cytology
Tuberculous ascites	SAAG ≤1.1 g/dL AFTP ≥2.5 g/dL WBC >500/m³, lymphocyte predominance
Chylous ascites	SAAG ≤1.1 g/dL AFTP ≥2.5 g/dL Ascites TG > serum TG (>200 mg/dL)
Nephrotic syndrome	SAAG ≤1.1 g/dL AFTP <2.5 g/dL
Pancreatic ascites	SAAG ≤1.1 g/dL AFTP ≥2.5 g/dL Ascites amylase > serum amylase (>1000 U/L)

AFTP, Ascitic fluid total protein; *SAAG,* serum-ascites albumin gradient; *TG,* triglycerides; *WBC,* white blood cell count.

7. The yield of a smear and culture for mycobacterial infections is 0% and 50%, respectively
8. The differential diagnosis of the causes of ascites based on ascitic fluid analysis is shown in Table 13.3.

Treatment of Cirrhotic Ascites

GENERAL PRINCIPLES

1. **The goal of management is to induce a negative sodium balance** (Table 13.4).
2. The International Ascites Club recommends dietary sodium restriction to 88 mmol sodium per day.
   - Stringent sodium restriction mobilizes ascites in patients with cirrhosis.
   - The average North American Diet contains 100 to 150 mmol of sodium per day.
   - In the absence of diuretics, a cirrhotic patient without ascites will excrete <20 mmol of sodium per day.
   - The resulting positive sodium balance of 80 to 130 mmol/day equates to the formation of 4 to 7 L of ascites per week, hence the need for dietary sodium restriction.
3. **To achieve negative sodium balance, urinary sodium excretion should exceed 78 mmol per day.**
4. If satisfactory weight loss with a decrease in ascites does not occur, a 24-hour urine sodium collection to determine dietary adherence may be helpful.
   - A 24-hour urine collection is cumbersome, and a "spot" urine sodium-to-potassium concentration ratio may be done instead.
   - A urinary sodium-to-potassium ratio >1 indicates adequate sodium excretion, and the patient should lose weight.
   - There is significant diurnal variation to renal sodium excretion, which is maximal at night.

5. There is no need for routine fluid restriction, unless the serum sodium concentration drops below 125 to 130 mEq/L.

DIURETIC THERAPY

1. Sodium restriction alone can eliminate ascites in only 10% of patients, and therefore diuretic therapy is usually required. Diuretics are generally required in patients with grades 2 (moderate) and 3 (severe) ascites.
2. In general, only aldosterone antagonists/distal convoluted tubule-acting diuretics and loop diuretics are used.
3. Because the RAAS plays an important role in the formation of ascites, **spironolactone, an aldosterone antagonist/distal convoluted tubule-acting diuretic, is the diuretic of choice.**
   - Loop diuretics, such as furosemide, have shown less efficacy when used alone as compared with spironolactone alone.
   - When furosemide is used alone, sodium that is not absorbed in the ascending loop is taken up in the distal tubule as a result of the hyperaldosteronism that is present in cirrhosis.
4. **Spironolactone can be used alone or in combination with furosemide,** and if natriuresis is not achieved (i.e., weight loss of <1.5 kg/week), the dose can be increased in a stepwise fashion until maximum doses of 400 mg of spironolactone and 160 g of furosemide daily are reached.
   - For example, 100 mg of spironolactone and 40 mg of furosemide can be started and can be titrated up initially to 200 mg of spironolactone and 80 mg of furosemide.
   - Dose adjustments should only be made every 3 to 4 days because the effect of spironolactone takes several days to occur.
   - Serum electrolyte and creatinine levels should be monitored before starting and after adjusting the dose of diuretics.
5. The recommended rate of weight (and thus fluid) loss is ≤0.5 kg/day. Once ascites is controlled, it may be necessary to decrease the diuretic doses, especially in patients in whom the underlying liver disease improves (e.g., a patient with alcoholic cirrhosis who abstains from alcohol).
6. Monitoring for excessive diuresis and dehydration is important. **Diuretic therapy should be interrupted if renal impairment, hyponatremia (serum sodium <125 mEq/L), or hepatic encephalopathy develops.** Because of diminished muscle mass, serum creatinine levels may

---

TABLE 13.4 ■ **Management of Ascites**

General Principals

   Sodium restriction (88 mmol/day)
   Maintain adequate nutrition
   Immunizations: Influenza, pneumococcal, others

Treatment of Underlying Disease

   Direct-acting antiviral agents, alcohol abstinence, weight loss, etc.

Pharmacotherapy

   Aldosterone antagonists/distal convoluted tubule-acting diuretics (i.e., spironolactone)
   Loop diuretics (i.e., furosemide)

Liver Transplantation Evaluation

Transjugular Intrahepatic Portosystemic Shunt/Large-Volume Paracentesis

   Refractory ascites

inadequately reflect renal function, and even an apparently small rise in the creatinine level may indicate a substantial decrease in the glomerular filtration rate.

7. Use of spironolactone is associated with tender gynecomastia. If this occurs, patients can be switched to amiloride (initial dose of 5–10 mg daily, which can be increased ultimately to 60 mg daily), although amiloride tends to induce a less effective diuresis.

8. It is important to ensure that patients with cirrhotic ascites do not take nonsteroidal antiinflammatory drugs such as ibuprofen and aspirin because they blunt the natriuretic effect of diuretics and may cause nephrotoxicity.

REFRACTORY ASCITES
Epidemiology

1. Ascites may become refractory in 10% of cirrhotic patients with ascites, with a 50% 1-year mortality rate.

2. Refractory ascites is associated with dilutional hyponatremia, type 2 hepatorenal syndrome (see Chapter 14), SBP, and muscle wasting

Definition and Diagnostic Criteria

1. Refractory ascites is defined as failure to mobilize ascites despite high-dose diuretic therapy or the early recurrence of ascites after an LVP that cannot be prevented by medical therapy (Table 13.5).

2. Two categories
   - **Diuretic resistant:** Inability to mobilize ascites or prevent the early recurrence of ascites after an LVP due to lack of response to dietary sodium restriction and intensive diuretic therapy (typically at maximum doses)
   - **Diuretic intractable:** Inability to mobilize ascites or prevent the early recurrence of ascites after an LVP due to the development of diuretic-induced complications that preclude the use of an effective diuretic dose

Management

1. Management is with either periodic LVPs or consideration of a TIPS.

2. LVP
   - Removal of more than 5 L of fluid

TABLE 13.5 ■ **Definition and Diagnostic Criteria of Refractory Ascites**

Diuretic-resistant ascites: Inability to mobilize ascites or prevent the early recurrence of ascites after a large-volume paracentesis because of the lack of response to dietary sodium restriction and intensive diuretic therapy (maximum doses of spironolactone and furosemide).

Diuretic-intractable ascites: Inability to mobilize ascites or prevent the early recurrence of ascites after a large-volume paracentesis due to the development of diuretic-induced complications that preclude the use of an effective diuretic dose.

Diagnostic Criteria

- *Treatment duration*: Patients must be on intensive diuretic therapy for at least 1 week and on a salt-restricted diet of <88 mmol/day.
- *Lack of response*: Mean weight loss of <0.8 kg over 4 days and urinary sodium output less than the sodium intake (i.e., urine sodium-to-potassium ratio <1)
- *Early ascites recurrence*: Recurrence of grade 2 or 3 ascites within 1 month of initial mobilization
- *Diuretic-induced complications*: Hepatic encephalopathy, renal impairment, and diuretic-induced hyponatremia (<125 mEq/L)

- An intravenous infusion of albumin (6 to 8 g/L of ascites removed for paracentesis of more than 5 L) is recommended to prevent postparacentesis circulatory dysfunction.
  - **Postparacentesis circulatory dysfunction** is characterized by worsening vasodilatation, hyponatremia, sodium retention, and renal insufficiency.
- The need for an LVP more frequently than once every 2 weeks implies that the patient is nonadherent to salt and fluid restriction.

3. TIPS
  - A TIPS decompresses the portal vein through the creation of a low-resistance channel between the hepatic vein and the portal vein.
  - The goal of TIPS is to reduce the portosystemic pressure gradient to <12 mm Hg.
  - A TIPS help reduce ascites by increasing natriuresis through reductions in both proximal tubular sodium reabsorption and activity of the RAAS.
  - TIPS is effective in 90% of patients with refractory ascites, and improvement is noted in 1 to 3 months.
  - Outcomes after TIPS placement depend on the patient's Model for End-stage Liver Disease (MELD) score (see Chapter 33); the outcomes are better when the MELD score is ≤18 than when it is >18.
  - The ideal candidate is one with preserved hepatic synthetic function, no contraindications to TIPS placement, and no hepatic encephalopathy.
  - Most patients need continued diuretic use after TIPS.
  - Compared with repeated LVP, a TIPS is associated with the following:
    - Decreases in ascites in about 64% of patients versus 24% in those undergoing repeated LVP
    - Lack of a survival advantage for TIPS in most clinical trials, but one meta-analysis suggested an overall benefit (49% versus 32.5% 2-year survival)
    - Higher frequency of hepatic encephalopathy (40%)

4. Peritoneovenous shunting is as effective as LVP and does not improve survival. This procedure has been abandoned because of numerous complications and poor long-term patency.

5. An experimental automated low-flow ascites pump system to mechanically remove ascites from the peritoneal cavity into the bladder is being studied as a palliative approach.

6. Liver transplantation
  - Liver transplantation is the only lifesaving therapy for patients with refractory ascites, in whom the 1-year survival rate is 25% without treatment.
  - Better outcomes occur when patients undergo liver transplantation before the onset of the hepatorenal syndrome.

Spontaneous Bacterial Peritonitis and Other Ascitic Fluid Infections

OVERVIEW

1. **Patients with cirrhosis and ascites have a 10% annual risk of ascitic fluid infection.**
2. Variants of ascitic fluid infection may have different prognostic significance and require different management strategies (Table 13.6). SBP is the most common type of ascitic fluid infection.
3. A high index of suspicion is necessary to prompt early diagnosis of infection and initiation of antibiotics; paracentesis must be performed to diagnose ascitic fluid infection.
4. **Early initiation of appropriate broad-spectrum nonnephrotoxic antibiotics has significantly decreased the mortality rate (currently 5%) of ascitic fluid infection.**
5. The MELD score correlates with risk of SBP; in one study, for every 1-point increase in MELD score, the risk of SBP increased by 11%.
6. Use of proton pump inhibitors has been associated with an increased risk of SBP in patients with cirrhosis and ascites.

TABLE 13.6 ■ **Classification of Ascitic Fluid Infection**

Category	Ascites Fluid Analysis
Spontaneous bacterial peritonitis	PMNs ≥250/mm³, single organism
Culture-negative neutrocytic ascites	PMNs ≥250/mm³, negative culture
Monomicrobial nonneutrocytic bacterascites	PMNs <250/mm³, single organism
Polymicrobial bacterascites	PMNs <250/mm³, multiple organisms
Secondary bacterial peritonitis	PMNs ≥250/mm³, multiple organisms

PMN, Polymorphonuclear neutrophils.

PATHOGENESIS

1. Bacterial seeding of ascitic fluid is the common denominator of ascitic fluid infections; the two most likely routes are as follows:
   a. Translocation of bacteria through the intestinal wall
      - This accounts for >70% of ascitic fluid infections in patients with cirrhosis.
      - It is promoted by abnormal gut flora, mucosal edema, and altered gut permeability.
   b. Hematogenous seeding of ascites fluid
      - 50% of SBP episodes are accompanied by bacteremia with the same organism isolated from the ascitic fluid.
      - The causative organism can sometimes be cultured from urine or sputum.
2. Colonization of ascitic fluid ("bacterascites")
   - Bacterascites may have one of two different outcomes: Clearance by intraperitoneal phagocytic cells or progressive bacterial growth with peritonitis (i.e., SBP).
   - Bacterascites normally resolves as a result of opsonization of the bacteria and subsequent clearance by intraperitoneal phagocytic cells.
3. Bacterial flora of SBP
   a. *Escherichia coli* (43%), *Streptococcus* spp. (23%), and *Klebsiella pneumoniae* (11%) caused 80% of SBP cases in the past; in the current era of selective intestinal decontamination, gram-positive organisms cause more than 50% of bacterial infections.
   b. Anaerobes cause only 1% of cases of SBP.
4. **Risk factors for ascitic fluid infection**
   - A prior episode of SBP: This is the most important risk factor; two thirds of patients will develop a recurrence within the following year.
   - Gastrointestinal bleeding (specifically variceal hemorrhage)
   - Ascitic fluid total protein <1.0 g/dL

CLINICAL FEATURES AND DIAGNOSIS

1. Ascitic fluid infections develop primarily in patients with preexisting ascites in the setting of cirrhosis.
2. Approximately 87% of patients with SBP have symptoms or signs of infection, including fever (69%), abdominal pain (59%), and a change in mental status (54%).
3. **The occurrence of any symptoms and/or signs of infection in a patient with ascites should prompt diagnostic paracentesis.**

4. Lactoferrin is a product of activated PMNs that acts as a surrogate marker for PMNs and may provide a simple and rapid test for diagnosing SBP, if it becomes commercially available.
5. Dipsticks that measure leukocyte esterase can detect an elevated PMN count in 90 to 180 seconds at the bedside and permit immediate initiation of antibiotics; most of the studies performed to date have used a dipstick designed for urine, but an ascitic fluid–specific dipstick shows promise.

CLASSIFICATION (See Table 13.6)

1. **SBP** is characterized by a positive ascitic fluid culture (almost always a single organism) and a PMN count in the ascitic fluid of at least 250 cells/mm^3 in the absence of an intraabdominal surgical source of infection.
2. **Culture-negative neutrocytic ascites (CNNA)** is characterized by a negative ascitic fluid culture, an ascitic fluid neutrophil count of at least 250 cells/mm^3, and no apparent intraabdominal source of infection.
   - It most commonly reflects a suboptimal culture technique.
   - With an adequate culture technique, it most commonly represents resolution of transient bacterial colonization of the ascitic fluid because of the fluid's inherent antibacterial properties.
   - Bacterial growth may continue, leading to SBP and positive fluid culture.
   - Recent antibiotic exposure (even one dose) may suppress bacterial growth in the culture.
   - **CNNA and SBP have comparable mortality rates; therefore, similar management is warranted.**
   - Other than SBP, the following causes of neutrocytic ascites should be considered:
     - Peritoneal carcinomatosis
     - Pancreatitis
     - Tuberculous peritonitis
     - Peritonitis due to connective tissue disease
     - Hemorrhage into ascitic fluid
3. **Monomicrobial nonneutrocytic bacterascites (MNB)** is a variant of SBP with a positive ascitic fluid culture (single organism) associated with a normal ascitic fluid PMN count (<250 cells/mm^3).
   - Patients with MNB generally have less severe liver disease than do those with SBP.
   - The outcome of bacterascites is determined by the presence or absence of associated clinical symptoms or signs; asymptomatic bacterascites typically resolves spontaneously without antibiotic treatment; symptomatic bacterascites should be managed in the same manner as SBP.
   - When an ascitic fluid culture unexpectedly yields an organism, paracentesis should be repeated promptly to evaluate for the development of a neutrocytic response, which mandates antibiotic treatment.
4. **Polymicrobial bacterascites** indicates inadvertent perforation of the bowel by the paracentesis needle, with an ascitic fluid culture demonstrating multiple organisms in the setting of a normal neutrophil count (<250 cells/mm^3).
   - Inadvertent bowel perforation by paracentesis occurs rarely, typically in the setting of an extremely difficult paracentesis, and may be obvious when air or stool is aspirated during the tap.
   - Most inadvertent bowel perforations resolve spontaneously without development of secondary peritonitis; however, paracentesis should be repeated to evaluate the patient for a neutrocytic response and the need for antibiotics.

- Management of patients with a neutrocytic ascitic fluid response is with empiric broad-spectrum antibiotics to cover gram-negative enteric, gram-positive, and anaerobic organisms.
5. **Secondary bacterial peritonitis** is differentiated from SBP by the presence of a known or suspected surgically treatable intraabdominal source of infection (e.g., perforated viscus or intraabdominal abscess). The ascitic fluid PMN count is at least 250 cells/mm^3, and the culture grows multiple gut organisms.
   - Other ascitic fluid findings ("Ruynon criteria") indicate secondary bacterial peritonitis are the following (requires two of the three features):
     1. Total protein >1.0 g/dL
     2. Glucose <50 mg/dL
     3. Lactate dehydrogenase greater than the upper limit of normal for serum
   - Secondary peritonitis should also be suspected if repeat paracentesis performed after 48 hours of appropriate antibiotic treatment reveals an ascitic fluid PMN count higher than the baseline value.
   - Management includes empiric broad-spectrum antibiotics to cover gram-negative enteric, gram-positive, and anaerobic bacteria; evaluation to localize the perforation is indicated.
   - Prompt surgical intervention is mandatory; medical therapy alone is insufficient.

TREATMENT

1. **Empiric treatment is indicated before culture results become available when the ascitic fluid PMN count is ≥250 cells/mm^3.**
   - The flora responsible for ascitic fluid infections continues to evolve, presumably as a result of antibiotic pressures.
   - Anaerobic organisms rarely lead to ascitic fluid infections except in secondary peritonitis.
   - Aminoglycosides carry an unacceptable risk of nephrotoxicity and are contraindicated in cirrhotic patients with ascites.
   - Fungi do not cause SBP except in patients with acquired immunodeficiency syndrome; fungi are usually cultured from ascitic fluid only in cases of secondary peritonitis.
2. Third-generation cephalosporins are the recommended treatment.
   - **Cefotaxime, a nonnephrotoxic broad-spectrum third-generation cephalosporin, provides coverage for more than 94% of the flora responsible for SBP and is the antibiotic of choice for empiric treatment.**
   - The recommended dose is 2 g intravenously every 8 hours over 5 days.
   - Ascitic fluid cultures rapidly become sterile after even one dose of cefotaxime.
   - The antibiotic spectrum may be narrowed once culture results become available and the sensitivities of the causative organism are known.
   - Alternative antibiotic regimens include amoxicillin-clavulanic acid (in Europe) and fluoroquinolones.
   - Lack of a response at 48 hours suggests infection with a resistant pathogen. The addition of an alternative antibiotic or switching to a broad-spectrum antibiotic is indicated.
3. A follow-up paracentesis is indicated for either of the following:
   - Secondary (surgical) bacterial peritonitis is suspected.
   - The typical clinical response to cefotaxime (i.e., fall in serum white cell count, defervescence) does not occur.
4. Secondary bacterial peritonitis or SBP caused by an organism resistant to cefotaxime can lead to persistently positive ascitic fluid cultures and ascitic fluid PMN counts higher than pretreatment values.
5. Survival rates in patients with SBP have improved, reflecting early recognition and treatment.

6. **Intravenous volume expanders in patients with SBP have shown benefit.**
   - SBP is associated with marked increases of cytokines, including tumor necrosis factor alpha and interleukin-6, and production of nitric oxide, a potent vasodilator.
   - These changes are associated with clinical deteriorations in blood pressure, renal function, coagulation, and hepatic function.
   - Intravenous volume expanders (specifically albumin) increase central volume and maintain renal perfusion.
   - One study reported that administration of **intravenous albumin 1.5 g/kg at the time SBP is diagnosed and 1.0 g/kg on day 3 of antibiotic treatment** decreased the risk of renal insufficiency and SBP-related mortality; it is reasonable to administer albumin in this setting while awaiting additional studies.

Prophylaxis of Ascitic Fluid Infection

INDICATIONS

1. Patients at high risk for development of SBP include those with (1) a prior episode of SBP, (2) gastrointestinal hemorrhage, and (3) ascitic fluid total protein concentration <1.0 g/dL during hospitalization.
2. Selective intestinal decontamination to prevent SBP has been recommended in these situations (Table 13.7).

ANTIBIOTIC REGIMENS

1. Norfloxacin, a poorly absorbed fluoroquinolone, has been used to achieve selective intestinal decontamination in cirrhotic patients; norfloxacin has several characteristics that make it suitable for prophylaxis.
   - Poor absorption when taken orally
   - Effectiveness against enteric gram-negative organisms
   - Sparing of gram-positive and anaerobic organisms to maintain their protective role in the normal gut flora
     a. Norfloxacin reduces the frequency of SBP, delays progression to hepatorenal syndrome, and improves overall survival.

TABLE 13.7 ■ **Indications for Prophylaxis of Ascites Fluid Infection**

Indication	Duration of Prophylaxis
Recovery from an episode of SBP	Indefinitely, or until ascites disappears
Gastrointestinal bleeding in a patient with cirrhosis	7 days
Ascitic fluid total protein <1.0 g/dL	During hospitalization (controversial)
Ascitic fluid protein <1.5 g/dL plus one of the following parameters: Child-Turcotte-Pugh score >9 and bilirubin >3 mg/dL Creatinine >1.2 mg/dL Blood urea nitrogen >25 mg/dL Serum sodium <130 mEq/L	Continue until decompensated liver disease improves or liver transplant performed

SBP, Spontaneous bacterial peritonitis.

b. In patients who have survived an episode of SBP:
- The recurrence rate can be as high as 68% at 1 year without antibiotic prophylaxis.
- Norfloxacin, 400 mg orally daily, has been shown to decrease the probability of recurrent SBP to 20% at 1 year.
- Norfloxacin prophylaxis is cost effective in reducing recurrent SBP.
- However, norfloxacin treatment does not alter the overall mortality in these patients.

c. Norfloxacin has not been available in the United States since 2014.

2. In patients with cirrhosis and gastrointestinal hemorrhage:
- The incidence of SBP can be as high as 45% to 66% at 1 year without antibiotic prophylaxis.
- Antibiotic prophylaxis started immediately and continued for 7 days decreases the incidence of SBP to 10% to 20%.
- Antibiotic prophylaxis may improve survival in these patients.
- Intravenous ceftriaxone has been shown to be more effective than oral norfloxacin for SBP prophylaxis in patients with advanced cirrhosis and gastrointestinal hemorrhage.

3. In hospitalized patients with ascitic fluid total protein <1.0 g/dL:
- The overall probability of new-onset SBP is 20% in 1 year.
- Prophylaxis with norfloxacin 400 mg orally daily decreases in-hospital incidence of SBP from 22% to 0% without an effect on in-hospital mortality.

4. **Trimethoprim-sulfamethoxazole,** one double-strength tablet orally daily, has also been reported to be effective in preventing SBP and has supplanted norfloxacin in the United States.

FUTURE CONSIDERATIONS

1. Routine long-term use of prophylactic norfloxacin leads to the rapid development of fluoroquinolone-resistant organisms in the fecal flora.

2. Long-term norfloxacin prophylaxis is associated with:
- Fluoroquinolone-resistant gram-negative bacilli in 50% of SBP cultures
- A high frequency of urinary tract infection by fluoroquinolone-resistant gram-negative bacilli

3. Future study should focus on effective prophylaxis with minimal risk for development of bacterial resistance.
- Antibiotic cycling
- Use of nonabsorbable antibiotics such as rifaximin
- Use of nonantibiotic treatments such as prebiotics and probiotics, prokinetics, nonselective beta receptor antagonists, and bile acids

FUTHER READING

Bajaj JS, Zadvornova Y, Heuman DM, et al. Association of proton pump inhibitor therapy with spontaneous bacterial peritonitis in cirrhotic patients with ascites. *Am J Gastroenterol.* 2009;104:1130–1134.

Bellot P, Welker MW, Soriano G, et al. Automated low flow pump system for the treatment of refractory ascites: a multi-center safety and efficacy study. *J Hepatol.* 2013;58:922–927.

Fernandez J, Arbol LR, Gomez C, et al. Norfloxacin vs ceftriaxone in the prophylaxis of infections in patients with advanced cirrhosis and hemorrhage. *Gastroenterology.* 2006;131:1049–1056.

Fernandez J, Navasa M, Planas R, et al. Primary prophylaxis of spontaneous bacterial peritonitis delays hepatorenal syndrome and improves survival in cirrhosis. *Gastroenterology.* 2007;133:818–824.

Gines P, Cardenas A, Arroyo V, et al. Management of cirrhosis and ascites. *N Engl J Med.* 2004;350:1646–1654.

Moore KP, Wong F, Gines P, et al. The management of ascites in cirrhosis: report on the consensus conference of the International Ascites Club. *Hepatology.* 2003;38:258–266.

Obstein KL, Campbell MS, Reddy KR, et al. Association between model for end-stage liver disease and spontaneous bacterial peritonitis. *Am J Gastroenterol.* 2007;102:2732–2736.

Rössle M, Ochs A, Gülberg V, et al. A comparison of paracentesis and transjugular intrahepatic portosystemic shunting in patients with ascites. *N Engl J Med.* 2000;342:1701–1707.

Runyon BA. Ascites and spontaneous bacterial peritonitis. In: Feldman M, Friedman LS, Sleisenger MH, eds. *Sleisenger and Fordtran's Gastrointestinal and Liver Disease: Pathophysiology, Diagnosis, Management.* 10th ed. Philadelphia: Saunders Elsevier; 2016:1553–1576.

Runyon BA. Management of adult patients with ascites due to cirrhosis: an update. AASLD Practice Guideline. *Hepatology.* 2009;49:2087–2107.

Sanyal AJ, Genning C, Reddy KR, et al. The North American study for the treatment of refractory ascites. *Gastroenterology.* 2003;124:634–641.

Sort P, Navasa M, Arroyo V, et al. Effect of intravenous albumin on renal impairment and mortality in patients with cirrhosis and spontaneous bacterial peritonitis. *N Engl J Med.* 1999;341:403–409.

Wiest R, Krag A, Gerbes A. Spontaneous bacterial peritonitis: recent guidelines and beyond. *Gut.* 2012;62:297–310.

CHAPTER 14

Hepatorenal Syndrome

Andres Cardenas, MD, MMSc, PhD, AGAF, FAASLD ■ Pere Ginès, MD

KEY POINTS

1 The term *hepatorenal syndrome* (HRS) refers to kidney failure in patients with decompensated cirrhosis.

2 HRS is characterized by a rapid decline of kidney function and is associated with a poor prognosis and high resource utilization.

3 In 1996, the International Ascites Club proposed the first diagnostic criteria to define HRS, and with time these criteria have evolved to incorporate an updated definition of acute kidney injury (AKI) in cirrhosis.

4 In 2015, these criteria were revised.

Definition

1. In the past, renal failure in cirrhosis was defined by a level of serum creatinine >1.5 mg/dL in persons with advanced liver disease and portal hypertension. A drawback of this definition was that creatinine may overestimate glomerular filtration rate (GFR) in persons with cirrhosis due to decreased creatinine production resulting from reduced muscle mass. Therefore, a serum creatinine level ≤1.5 mg/dL does not necessarily exclude renal dysfunction in patients with cirrhosis.

2. Instead of relying on a specific creatinine level, more recent definitions of renal failure (AKI) in patients with cirrhosis are based on a change in serum levels of creatinine. **An increase in serum creatinine >50% from baseline or a rise in serum creatinine ≥0.3 mg/dL (≥27 μmol/L) in less than 48 hours reflects significant renal dysfunction and has the advantage of detecting kidney dysfunction at an early stage (Table 14.1).**

3. Minor increases in serum creatinine detected by the AKI criteria are independently associated with mortality in hospitalized patients with cirrhosis.

4. HRS is characterized by the following:
   ■ Marked decreases in GFR (usually <30 mL/hour) and renal blood flow in the absence of other identifiable causes of renal failure
   ■ Marked circulatory abnormalities
   ■ Activation of endogenous vasoactive systems
   ■ Absence of histologic changes in the kidneys

5. The diagnosis of HRS relies on the exclusion of other conditions that may cause renal failure in cirrhosis (see Table 14.1).

Pathogenesis

The pathogenesis of HRS is not completely understood (Fig. 14.1). However, it is clear that **marked vasoconstriction of the renal circulation is a major pathophysiologic factor.**

TABLE 14.1 ■ **Definitions of Terms**

Term		Definition
Acute kidney injury (AKI)	Stage 1	Increase in serum creatinine ≥0.3 mg/dL within 48 hours or ≥50% from baseline
	Stage 2	Increase in serum creatinine 2- to 3-fold from baseline
	Stage 3	Increase in serum creatinine >3-fold from baseline or a serum creatinine >4 mg/dL
Hepatorenal syndrome	Cirrhosis and ascites are present. AKI (as above) No improvement in the serum creatinine level after 2 consecutive days of diuretic withdrawal and plasma volume expansion with albumin (1 g/kg/day) Absence of shock, no recent use of nephrotoxins (e.g., nonsteroidal antiinflammatory drugs, iodinated contrast) Exclusion of structural renal disease: No hematuria (≤50 RBC per high-power field) No proteinuria (≤500 mg/24 hours) No obstructive nephropathy	

1. Important functional renal disturbances in patients with cirrhosis are sodium and solute-free water retention, which are reflected in the development of ascites and hypervolemic hyponatremia. In advanced cirrhosis, intense renal vasoconstriction leads to the development of HRS.
2. The following mechanisms are implicated.
   ■ Severe disturbances in systemic hemodynamics
   ■ Increased activity of endogenous vasoconstrictor systems
   ■ Decreased activity of vasodilatory factors
3. Systemic circulatory disturbances
   ■ Hemodynamic alterations result from severe splanchnic arterial vasodilatation.
   ■ This vasodilatation is due mainly to an increased production or activity of vasodilatory factors, such as nitric oxide (NO), inflammatory cytokines, carbon monoxide, and endocannabinoids, in patients with portal hypertension.
   ■ The hemodynamic profile is characterized by low arterial pressure, low systemic vascular resistance, and high cardiac output.
   ■ Due to increased activity of vasoconstrictor systems, marked renal vasoconstriction develops.
   ■ Vasoconstriction occurs not only in the renal circulation, but also in the brachial, femoral, and cerebral circulation, probably as a compensatory mechanism to counteract splanchnic vasodilatation.
   ■ In patients with decompensated cirrhosis, a hyperdynamic circulation is usual; although cardiac output is initially high, in advanced stages, when HRS supervenes, cardiac output drops.

VASOCONSTRICTOR FACTORS

1. Renin-angiotensin-aldosterone system (RAAS) and sympathetic nervous system (SNS)
   ■ The activity of the RAAS and SNS is typically increased in cirrhotic patients with ascites, especially in patients with HRS.
   ■ Plasma renin activity and plasma norepinephrine levels are significantly elevated in patients with HRS.

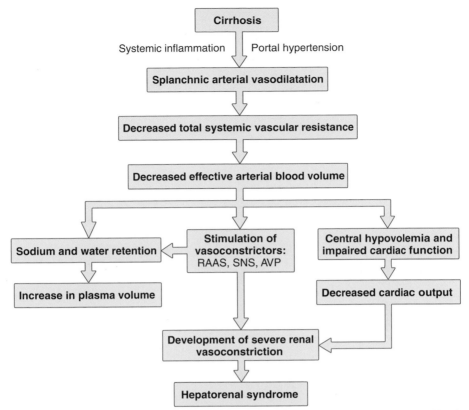

Fig. 14.1 Proposed pathogenic mechanism of hepatorenal syndrome (HRS). Splanchnic vasodilatation arising from portal hypertension, an increased plasma volume, and a decreased cardiac output seem to play equally important roles in the decrease in renal perfusion that leads to HRS. The impairment in effective arterial blood volume responsible for the activation of vasoconstrictor systems that act on the renal circulation is a consequence of both a low systemic vascular resistance that causes an abnormal distribution of blood volume and a low cardiac output relative to the markedly dilated arterial bed secondary to cirrhotic cardiomyopathy. *AVP,* Arginine vasopressin; *RAAS,* renin-angiotensin-aldosterone system; *SNS,* sympathetic nervous system.

- The activity of both systems, RAAS and SNS, correlates inversely with renal blood flow.
- Pharmacologic blockade of the effectors of these systems induces a reduction in systemic vascular resistance and arterial hypotension, findings that suggest that their increased activation is crucial to maintain systemic hemodynamics.

2. Arginine vasopressin (AVP)
   - AVP is also activated in patients with HRS; it has a vasoconstrictor effect that contributes to the maintenance of arterial pressure in advanced cirrhosis.
   - This hormone also contributes to solute-free water retention and hypervolemic hyponatremia.

3. Endothelin (ET)
   - Levels of this endothelial-derived peptide, a powerful vasoconstrictor, is also increased in cirrhosis.
   - The most important effect of ET is renal vasoconstriction, which can decrease renal blood flow and GFR.

■ In patients with cirrhosis, ET levels are highest in those with HRS.
■ The role of ET in the pathogenesis of HRS remains to be clarified.

VASODILATORY FACTORS

1. Renal prostaglandins (PGs)
   ■ PGs have important vasodilatory effects in patients with advanced liver disease; they help counteract the vasoconstrictor effects of RAAS, SNS, and AVP.
   ■ PGs help maintain renal perfusion in cirrhotic patients.
   ■ The use of nonsteroidal antiinflammatory drugs (NSAIDs), which inhibit PG synthesis, is a common cause of kidney failure in cirrhotic patients.
   ■ Patients with advanced cirrhosis and HRS have reduced production of renal PGs.
2. Nitric oxide (NO)
   ■ NO is locally synthesized within the kidney.
   ■ Under normal conditions, NO plays a role in the regulation of the glomerular microcirculation, sodium excretion, and renin release.
   ■ Inhibition of NO does not induce renal vasoconstriction because of a compensatory increase in renal PGs.
   ■ Inhibition of both NO and PGs induces renal vasoconstriction in patients with cirrhosis and ascites.
   ■ NO interacts with PGs to maintain renal perfusion in cirrhotic patients with ascites.
3. Natriuretic peptides
   ■ Natriuretic peptides are vasodilators involved in the maintenance of renal perfusion.
   ■ Atrial natriuretic peptide (ANP) is the major natriuretic hormone.
   ■ Levels of ANP are elevated in decompensated cirrhosis, and patients with HRS have the highest levels.
   ■ Increased ANP levels may act as a homeostatic mechanism to counteract the effect of vasoconstrictor systems.
4. Systemic inflammation
   ■ Systemic inflammation is implicated in the pathogenesis of HRS.
   ■ Bacterial translocation (i.e., the passage of bacteria from the intestinal lumen to the mesenteric lymph nodes) contributes to impaired circulatory function in cirrhotic patients in whom HRS develops.
   ■ Bacterial translocation induces an inflammatory response, with increased production of proinflammatory cytokines (particularly interleukin-6 and tumor necrosis factor-α) and vasoactive factors (i.e., NO), thereby leading to further splanchnic vasodilatation.
   ■ Cirrhotic patients with increased levels of lipopolysaccharide (LPS)–binding protein or circulating levels of bacterial DNA (a surrogate marker of bacterial translocation) have increased levels of circulating cytokines, reduced systemic vascular resistance, and high cardiac output.

SUMMARY

1. Fig. 14.1 summarizes the most widely accepted theory of the pathogenesis of HRS.
2. Portal hypertension, the initial event, induces arterial vasodilatation by mechanisms not completely understood.
3. Arterial vasodilatation occurs mainly in the splanchnic circulation.
4. Vasodilatation induces decreased effective arterial blood volume and increased activity of vasoconstrictor systems.
5. Activation of the vasoconstrictor system compensates for circulatory dysfunction.
6. HRS is the extreme manifestation of circulatory dysfunction and may be the result of:

- Marked activation of vasoconstrictor systems
- Decreased activity of vasodilatory factors
- Increased production of intrarenal vasoconstrictors

Other Causes of Acute Kidney Injury in Cirrhosis

Besides HRS, cirrhotic patients may develop renal dysfunction for other reasons, including bacterial infections, hypovolemia, administration of nephrotoxic drugs, or intrinsic kidney diseases, including glomerulonephritis associated with hepatitis B or C viral infection or alcoholic cirrhosis.

ACUTE TUBULAR NECROSIS

1. Acute tubular necrosis (ATN) is characterized by abrupt impairment of renal function.
2. Cirrhotic patients frequently experience complications that predispose to the development of ATN, such as gastrointestinal bleeding, hypovolemic shock, or bacterial sepsis.
3. Although no specific markers for ATN have been described, the presence of the following criteria may be useful, albeit often inconclusive or nonspecific.
   - High urine sodium concentration
   - Urine/serum osmolality ratio <1
   - Abnormal urine sediment, with epithelial cells and casts
4. There is considerable interest in diagnostic urinary biomarkers such as neutrophil gelatinase-associated lipocalin (NGAL), a protease expressed in the distal convoluted tubule. Elevated NGAL levels are consistent with ATN, and levels >300 to 400 μg/g have high sensitivity and specificity for the diagnosis.

GLOMERULAR DISEASE

1. Intrinsic renal diseases in cirrhotic patients may be related to the cause of liver disease, notably chronic hepatitis B or C and alcoholic liver disease. Kidney disease in this setting typically reflects deposition of circulating immune complexes in the glomeruli.
2. Despite the high frequency of glomerular abnormalities on histologic examination in patients with cirrhosis, symptoms or signs of glomerular dysfunction seldom develop.
3. The most common forms of glomerulonephritis in hepatitis C are membranoproliferative glomerulonephritis, membranous glomerulonephritis, and focal segmental glomerular sclerosis. Membranous nephropathy is encountered in patients with hepatitis B, and immunoglobulin (Ig)A nephropathy occurs in patients with alcoholic cirrhosis.
4. Intrinsic renal disease is considered if there is either proteinuria >500 mg/24 hours, an abnormal urine sediment with >50 red blood cells per high-power field, or abnormal renal ultrasonographic findings in the absence of other causes of renal failure.

DRUG-INDUCED KIDNEY INJURY

1. Aminoglycosides and NSAIDs are the most common drugs implicated in renal failure in cirrhotic patients.
2. Drug-induced renal failure has a clinical profile similar to that of ATN.
3. The use of nonselective beta receptor antagonists in patients with established AKI and cirrhosis is controversial, but it is recommended that these drugs should be temporarily withheld in patients with HRS.

PRERENAL AZOTEMIA

1. Intravascular volume depletion can lead to prerenal azotemia.
2. Causes of intravascular volume depletion include vomiting, diarrhea, and overvigorous diuresis.
3. Improvement in renal function after albumin expansion (intravenous infusion of albumin, 1 g/kg/d, for 2 days) allows differentiation of prerenal azotemia from HRS.
4. Absence of a response to albumin expansion is a major diagnostic criterion of HRS (see Table 14.1).

Clinical Features and Classification of Hepatorenal Syndrome

HRS is classified as type 1 or type 2 according to both the intensity and the pace of progression of renal failure. These types exhibit different prognoses and survival rates.

TYPE 1

1. Type 1 HRS is characterized by severe and rapidly progressive renal failure, defined as doubling of the serum creatinine level, with a peak >2.5 mg/dL reached in less than 2 weeks.
2. Patients usually have severe liver disease (with jaundice, encephalopathy, and coagulopathy).
3. Type 1 HRS may occur following a precipitating factor, such as a severe bacterial infection, gastrointestinal hemorrhage, or therapeutic paracentesis without plasma expansion.
4. Type 1 HRS is the complication with the poorest prognosis in patients with cirrhosis.
5. **The median survival time is only 2 weeks.**

TYPE 2

1. Type 2 HRS is associated with steady impairment of renal function and serum creatinine levels usually ranging from 1.5 to 2.5 mg/dL.
2. Patients with type 2 HRS have a median survival time of 6 months if they do not undergo liver transplantation.
3. Patients with type 2 HRS may progress to type 1 HRS, either due to progression of the liver and kidney disease or an additional insult such as bacterial sepsis.
4. The main clinical consequence is refractory ascites.

Treatment

1. **Liver transplantation is definitive treatment for HRS.** The main objective in the management of HRS is to mitigate renal failure until liver transplantation can be performed.
2. Adequate management depends on the timely detection of renal failure and of its underlying cause.
   - If bacterial infection is suspected, antibiotics, such as third-generation cephalosporins, should be given pending the results of appropriate cultures.
   - Patients with renal failure and hypovolemia usually respond to albumin (1 g/kg body weight up to a maximum of 100 g/day for up to 2 days).
   - In patients with suspected drug-induced renal disease, NSAIDs and diuretics should be withheld.

TABLE 14.2 ■ **Pharmacologic Treatment of Hepatorenal Syndrome**

Vasoconstrictors	
Terlipressin	1 mg/4–6 hours intravenously; the dose is increased up to a maximum of 2 mg/4–6 hours after 3 days if there is no response to therapy as defined by a reduction of the serum creatinine >25% of pretreatment values. Response to therapy is considered when there is a marked reduction in the high serum creatinine levels, at least below 1.5 mg/dL (133 μmol/L). Treatment is usually given for 5–15 days.
Midodrine and octreotide	Midodrine 7.5 mg orally 3 times daily, increased to 12.5 mg 3 times daily if needed. Octreotide 100 μg subcutaneously 3 times daily, increased to 200 μg 3 times daily if needed.
Norepinephrine	0.5–3 mg/hour as a continuous intravenous infusion aimed at increasing the mean arterial pressure by 10 mm Hg. Treatment is maintained until the serum creatinine level decreases below 1.5 mg/dL.
Albumin	Concomitant administration of albumin together with a vasoconstrictor drug: 1 g/kg body weight at day 1 followed by 20–50 g/day.

3. **The mainstay of therapy for patients with HRS, other than liver transplantation, consists of the administration of splanchnic vasoconstrictors (terlipressin, octreotide plus midodrine, or norepinephrine) and intravenous albumin** (Table 14.2).
   - By causing selective vasoconstriction of the extremely dilated splanchnic arterial bed, these drugs improve arterial underfilling and reduce the activity of the endogenous vasoconstrictor systems.
   - Intravenous albumin is given at an initial dose of 1 g/kg of 20% to 25% albumin, followed by daily doses of 20 to 50 g.
   - A response to therapy is defined as a reduction in serum creatinine levels <1.5 mg/dL, usually associated with increased urine output and improvement in hyponatremia.
2. Other modalities such as transjugular intrahepatic portosystemic shunts (TIPS), renal replacement therapy (RRT), and albumin dialysis may be useful in some patients.
3. Patients with type 2 HRS usually have a sufficiently prolonged survival to allow liver transplantation.

TYPE 1 HEPATORENAL SYNDROME (Fig. 14.2)

1. **Terlipressin** (not yet licensed in the United States)
   - Type 1 HRS is reversible following treatment with terlipressin, a specific splanchnic vasoconstrictor analogue of vasopressin, and intravenous albumin.
   - Numerous studies, including meta-analyses and several randomized, controlled trials, have demonstrated the efficacy of terlipressin in the treatment of HRS.
   - Approximately 50% to 70% of patients with HRS respond to treatment with terlipressin and albumin.
   - Terlipressin can be given by bolus (1 mg/4 to 6 hours intravenously, and the dose is increased to a maximum of 2 mg/4 to 6 hours after 3 days) or by continuous infusion without a bolus at 3 mg/24 hours titrated to 12 mg/24 hours if the serum creatinine fails to decrease by >25% of the initial value.
   - Concurrent systemic vasoconstriction may potentially cause ischemic side effects in approximately 10% of patients.
   - Responders have an increased survival compared with nonresponders.
   - Recurrence of HRS after withdrawal of therapy occurs in <10% of patients, and retreatment with terlipressin is effective in most cases.

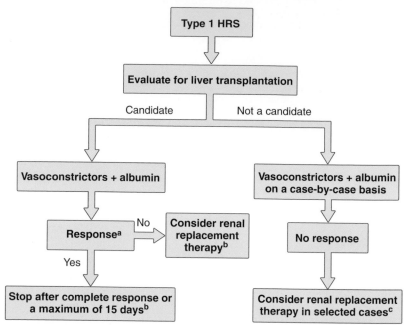

Fig. 14.2 Management strategy for patients with type 1 hepatorenal syndrome (HRS). [a]Response to therapy with vasoconstrictors plus albumin is considered when the serum creatinine level is reduced to <1.5 mg/dL. [b]If HRS recurs, patients should be retreated. [c]Renal replacement therapy should be reserved for patients with severe volume overload, intractable acidosis, or severe hyperkalemia.

- Factors associated with poor response include a total serum bilirubin ≥10 mg/dL, failure to increase mean arterial pressure >5 mm Hg, and lack of an absolute serum creatinine reduction >0.5 mg/dL by the third day of therapy.

2. **Midodrine and octreotide**
    - The combination of oral midodrine and subcutaneous octreotide with intravenous albumin may improve renal function in patients with HRS.
    - A controlled study that compared intravenous terlipressin and albumin with octreotide and midodrine plus albumin in patients with type 1 HRS showed that renal function was significantly more likely to improve in patients who received terlipressin and albumin (70.4%) than in those treated with midodrine and octreotide plus albumin (28.6%).
    - For centers without access to terlipressin, the standard therapy for HRS should include oral midodrine in doses up to 12.5 mg three times per day and octreotide titrated from 100 to 200 µg subcutaneously three times daily.
    - In a study of 87 patients with type 1 HRS, 21 of whom received no intervention and 66 of whom received midodrine and octreotide, sustained reductions in the serum creatinine level were observed in 40% of patients who received therapy compared with 5% of those who did not receive therapy.
    - Octreotide administered alone is ineffective.

3. **Norepinephrine**
    - Norepinephrine in combination with albumin is effective for treating patients with HRS.
    - Two randomized trials comparing terlipressin with norepinephrine showed no significant differences in safety or efficacy between the two agents. Nearly 40% of patients treated with terlipressin and 43% treated with norepinephrine responded to therapy.

- The adverse event profile was similar with both drugs.
- A limitation of norepinephrine is that it must be given in an intensive care unit (ICU); therefore, the cost, including ICU care, is similar or higher than that for terlipressin.

4. **TIPS**
   - By reducing portal pressure, TIPS reduces sympathetic and RAAS activity.
   - TIPS results in improved renal function—including HRS, demonstrated by an increase in urinary sodium excretion—and urinary volume and a decrease in serum creatinine levels.
   - TIPS leads to improvement in both type 1 and type 2 HRS, a decrease in recurrence rates of HRS, and resolution of ascites.
   - The applicability of TIPS in patients with HRS is low, because TIPS is considered contraindicated in patients with features of severe liver failure and a high Model for End-stage Liver Disease (MELD) score, which are common findings in patients with type 1 HRS (see Chapter 33).

5. **Renal replacement therapy**
   - RRT may be indicated in patients with HRS who do not respond to medical therapy as a bridge to liver transplantation.
   - In those in whom liver transplantation is not an option, either initiation or continuation of RRT is controversial because of the lack of long-term benefit.
   - The data are limited, and many patients develop side effects, including severe arterial hypotension, bleeding, and infections, that may contribute to death during RRT. Additionally, standard indications for RRT (severe fluid overload, acidosis, or hyperkalemia) are uncommon in patients with type 1 HRS, at least in the early stages.

6. **Extracorporeal albumin dialysis,** a system that uses an albumin-containing dialysate that is recirculated and perfused through a charcoal and anion-exchanger column, has been shown to improve renal function in patients with type 1 HRS. However, one study showed that molecular adsorbent recirculating system (MARS) treatment does not improve the GFR.

TYPE 2 HEPATORENAL SYNDROME

- Management of type 2 HRS is focused mainly on the treatment of refractory ascites that is usually found in these patients (see Chapter 13).
- Uncontrolled trials support the efficacy of therapy in improving kidney function, but recurrence after treatment withdrawal is common.
- In one study, 60% of patients with type 2 HRS treated with terlipressin and albumin responded to therapy, but half of them relapsed after withdrawal of treatment.
- Among those who underwent liver transplantation, there were no significant differences in serum creatinine levels among those with reversal of type 2 HRS and those without reversal of type 2 HRS before transplantation.
- In addition, there were no significant differences in frequency of AKI, need for RRT, frequency of chronic kidney disease 1 year after transplantation, length of hospitalization, and survival.
- Therefore, therapy of patients with type 2 HRS with terlipressin and albumin does not appear to improve either pretransplantation or posttransplantation outcomes.

Prevention

HRS may be prevented in the following three situations.

1. **Therapeutic paracentesis:** The administration of plasma volume expanders, specifically albumin, after total paracentesis (>5 L) in patients with cirrhosis and ascites decreases the frequency of renal failure and hyponatremia.

2. **Spontaneous bacterial peritonitis (SBP):** The administration of albumin (1.5 g/kg intravenously and 1 g/kg intravenously 48 hours later) together with intravenous cefotaxime 1 g twice daily for 5 to 7 days in patients with cirrhosis and SBP markedly reduces the frequency of impairment in circulatory function and the occurrence of type 1 HRS (see Chapter 13). The frequency of HRS in patients with SBP who receive albumin and antibiotic therapy is 10% compared with 33% in those who do not receive albumin. More importantly, survival is improved in those who receive albumin (10%) than in those who do not receive albumin (30%).

3. **Primary prophylaxis of SBP:** Long-term oral norfloxacin (or several other antibiotics) reduces the risk of SBP in patients with an ascitic total protein concentration <1.5 mg/dL and serum bilirubin >4 mg/dL, associated with a Child-Pugh score >9 (see Chapter 11), or a serum creatinine level >1.2 mg/dL. Both the 1-year probabilities of SBP (7% versus 61%) and of type 1 HRS (28% versus 41%) are reduced, and the 3-month and 1-year probabilities of survival (94% versus 62% and 60% versus 48%, respectively) are increased significantly.

FURTHER READING

Angeli P, Gines P, Wong F, et al. Diagnosis and management of acute kidney injury in patients with cirrhosis: revised consensus recommendations of the International Club of Ascites. *J Hepatol.* 2015;62:968–974.

Boyer TD, Sanyal AJ, Wong F, et al. Terlipressin plus albumin is more effective than albumin alone in improving renal function in patients with cirrhosis and hepatorenal syndrome type 1. *Gastroenterology.* 2016;150:1579–1589.

Cavallin M, Kamath PS, Merli M, et al. Terlipressin plus albumin versus midodrine and octreotide plus albumin in the treatment of hepatorenal syndrome: a randomized trial. *Hepatology.* 2015;62:567–574.

Cavallin M, Piano S, Romano A, et al. Terlipressin given by continuous intravenous infusion versus intravenous boluses in the treatment of hepatorenal syndrome: a randomized controlled study. *Hepatology.* 2016;63:983–992.

EASL clinical practice guidelines on the management of ascites. spontaneous bacterial peritonitis, and hepatorenal syndrome in cirrhosis. *J Hepatol.* 2010;53:397–417.

Francoz C, Nadim MK, Durand F. Kidney biomarkers in cirrhosis. *J Hepatol.* 2016;65:809–824.

Ginès P. Management of hepatorenal syndrome in the era of acute-on-chronic liver failure: terlipressin and beyond. *Gastroenterology.* 2016;150:1525–1527.

Ginès P, Schrier RW. Renal failure in cirrhosis. *N Engl J Med.* 2009;361:1279–1290.

Gluud LL, Christensen K, Christensen E, et al. Terlipressin for hepatorenal syndrome. *Cochrane Database Syst Rev.* 2012;9. CD005162.

Gonwa TA, Wadei HM. The challenges of providing renal replacement therapy in decompensated liver cirrhosis. *Blood Purif.* 2012;33:144–148.

Martin-Llahi M, Pepin MN, Guevara M, et al. Terlipressin and albumin vs albumin in patients with cirrhosis and hepatorenal syndrome: a randomized study. *Gastroenterology.* 2008;134:1352–1359.

Salerno F, Gerbes A, Gines P, et al. Diagnosis, prevention and treatment of hepatorenal syndrome in cirrhosis. *Gut.* 2007;56:1310–1318.

Solà E, Cárdenas A, Ginès P. Results of pretransplant treatment of hepatorenal syndrome with terlipressin. *Curr Opin Organ Transplant.* 2013;18:265–270.

Tapper EB, Bonder A, Cardenas A. Preventing and treating acute kidney injury among hospitalized patients with cirrhosis and ascites: a narrative review. *Am J Med.* 2016;129:461–467.

Wong F, O'Leary JG, Reddy KR, et al. New consensus definition of acute kidney injury accurately predicts 30-day mortality in patients with cirrhosis and infection. *Gastroenterology.* 2013;145:1280–1288.

CHAPTER 15

Hepatic Encephalopathy

Sanath Allampati, MD ■ Kevin D. Mullen, MD, FRCPI, FAASLD

KEY POINTS

1 Hepatic encephalopathy (HE) occurs only in the setting of significant liver disease. Any neuropsychiatric symptom or sign in a patient with severe liver dysfunction should be considered HE until proven otherwise.

2 HE may be covert or overt.

3 HE associated with acute liver failure is uncommon; its clinical course and treatment are distinct from those of encephalopathy complicating chronic liver disease.

4 Although several hypotheses exist to explain the pathogenesis of HE, ammonia is clearly implicated.

5 The diagnosis of HE is mainly on clinical grounds and is not based on blood ammonia levels.

6 Patients with suspected overt HE are managed by a four-pronged strategy: General care of the unconscious patient, exclusion of other causes of encephalopathy, correction of precipitating factors, and initiation of empiric therapy.

Definition and Classification

1. **Overt HE:** A wide spectrum of neurologic and neuropsychiatric abnormalities in patients with advanced chronic liver dysfunction
2. **Covert HE:** A disorder in which patients with cirrhosis have normal mental and neurologic status on routine clinical examination but exhibit reversible and quantifiable neuropsychologic and/or neuropsychiatric abnormalities
Table 15.1 shows the working party classification of HE.

Pathophysiology

1. Failure of hepatic detoxification of neuroactive compounds arising from the gut; cross-circulation experiments in an animal model favor this theory.
2. **Specific hypotheses for the pathogenesis of HE**
   a. **Ammonia**
      ■ Predominantly derived from nitrogenous products in the diet, bacterial metabolism of urea, and deamination of glutamine by the enzyme glutaminase. Ammonia enters the portal circulation from the gut and is converted to urea in the liver.
      ■ In the presence of significant portosystemic shunting, with or without hepatocellular dysfunction, ammonia concentration rises in blood and crosses the blood-brain barrier.

TABLE 15.1 ■ 1998 Hepatic Encephalopathy Working Party Proposed Classification of Hepatic Encephalopathy

Type	Description	Subcategory	Subdivision
A	Encephalopathy associated with acute liver failure	—	—
B	Encephalopathy with portosystemic bypass and no intrinsic hepatocellular disease	—	—
C	Encephalopathy associated with cirrhosis or portal hypertension/portosystemic shunts	Episodic	Precipitated Spontaneous Recurrent
		Persistent	Mild Severe Treatment dependent
		Covert	—

- Exposure to increased brain ammonia results in structural alterations in astrocytes that cause swelling and low-grade brain edema. Over a long period of exposure to high ammonia levels, brain cells develop structural changes, including Alzheimer type II astrocytes.

b. **Inflammation**
   - Inflammatory mediators and cytokines play an important role along with hyperammonemia in the pathogenesis of HE.
   - Possible mechanisms include cytokine-mediated changes in blood-brain barrier permeability, microglial activation and the subsequent production of neurosteroids, and altered activity of peripheral benzodiazepine binding sites, now called translocator protein receptor.

c. **Increased benzodiazepine-like compounds in the brain**

d. **Accumulation of manganese in the basal ganglia:** This is implicated in altered dopaminergic neurotransmission and extrapyramidal symptoms.

e. **Alterations in central nervous system (CNS) tryptophan metabolites** (e.g., serotonin): These changes may underlie altered sleep-wake cycles seen in early stages of encephalopathy.

Clinical Features

The clinical presentation of HE is categorized as follows:

1. **Type A,** which is associated with acute liver failure (see Chapter 2)
2. **Type B,** which is associated with portosystemic shunting
3. **Type C,** which is associated with cirrhosis and chronic liver disease. **Type C is the most common type of HE** and can be subdivided into single or recurrent episodes of HE (2 episodes of HE within 1 year).
4. **Persistent HE,** which is defined as mental status changes lasting >2 weeks
   - Low-grade HE (minimal HE + grade I HE): Mental status changes without disorientation for which the term *covert HE* has been adopted.
   - High-grade HE (stages II to IV): Mental status changes with disorientation.
5. Acquired hepatocerebral degeneration
6. Spastic paraparesis

The last 2 presentations are rare and are exceptions to the rule that HE is usually reversible; they generally occur in the background of fluctuating HE and major long-standing portosystemic shunts.

Diagnosis

1. **A diagnosis of HE needs to be considered in a patient with neurologic dysfunction and known or suspected liver dysfunction.** Clinical or laboratory evidence of hepatocellular dysfunction and/or portal hypertension are usually obvious. However, in a minority of patients, evidence of significant liver disease may be subtle, as in the following scenarios.
   a. Well-compensated cirrhosis (e.g., chronic hepatitis C, remote alcohol abuse)
   b. Noncirrhotic portal hypertension
      ■ Splanchnic vein thrombosis
      ■ Schistosomiasis
      ■ Noncirrhotic portal fibrosis
      ■ Idiopathic portal hypertension
   c. Congenital hepatic fibrosis
   d. Congenital intrahepatic and extrahepatic portosystemic shunts
2. **Clues to occult liver disease and/or portosystemic shunting**
   a. History of injection drug use
   b. Family history of cirrhosis (e.g., hemochromatosis)
   c. Residence in areas endemic for schistosomiasis
   d. History of umbilical sepsis (splanchnic vein thrombosis)
   e. History of pancreatitis (splenic vein thrombosis)
   f. History of hepatitis (hepatitis B or C, alcoholic hepatitis)
   g. History of use of hepatotoxic drugs (e.g., methotrexate, nitrofurantoin)
3. **Physical signs suggesting underlying significant liver disease** (see also Chapter 11)
   a. Upper extremities
      ■ Clubbing, leukonychia
      ■ Dupuytren contracture, palmar erythema
      ■ Spider telangiectasias, tattoos, injection marks, asterixis
      ■ Scratch marks, pigmentation, ecchymoses
      ■ Loss of muscle mass
   b. Eyes and face
      ■ Conjunctival icterus, cyanosis, parotid enlargement
      ■ Kayser-Fleischer rings
   c. Chest
      ■ Spider telangiectasias, loss of axillary hair, gynecomastia
   d. Abdomen
      ■ Splenomegaly (usually <5 cm below the left costal margin)
      ■ Hepatomegaly
      ■ Caput medusae
      ■ Ascites
   e. Testicular atrophy
   f. Loss of escutcheon
   g. Loss of hair on the shins
   h. Pedal edema
4. **Laboratory test abnormalities**
   a. Hepatic synthetic dysfunction: Increased prothrombin time, low serum albumin
   b. Elevated ammonia levels (not routinely recommended; see discussion later in chapter)
   c. Hypergammaglobulinemia
   d. Pancytopenia, leukopenia, thrombocytopenia
   e. Elevated cerebrospinal fluid glutamine levels (rarely needed)
   f. Decreased plasma branched-chain/aromatic amino acid ratio

The history, physical signs, and laboratory tests can individually or in combination indicate the presence of underlying liver disease even when results of standard tests of hepatic function, such as serum albumin and prothrombin times, are normal. **Patients with well-preserved synthetic function of the liver do not frequently develop overt HE; a major precipitating factor is needed to induce an episode.**

COVERT HEPATIC ENCEPHALOPATHY

1. Covert HE is defined as **abnormal performance on psychometric testing** when standard neurologic examination is completely normal.
2. It is present in 30% to 50% of patients with cirrhosis.
3. **Covert HE has a significant negative impact on quality of life and is associated with poor driving skills, impaired navigational skills, and increased traffic violations and accidents.**
4. It can increase the risk of progression to overt HE.
5. The International Society for Hepatic Encephalopathy recommends the **Psychometric Hepatic Encephalopathy Score (PHES)** as the gold standard for diagnosis of covert HE; impairment of >2 SD in two or more of the following tests is necessary for the diagnosis of covert HE.
   - Number Connection Test A (NCT A): Measures concentration, mental tracking, and visuomotor speed
   - Number Connection Test B (NCT B): Measures concentration, mental tracking, and visuomotor speed
   - Digit Symbol Test (DST): Assesses psychomotor and visuomotor speed
   - Line Tracing Test (LTT): Measures both speed and accuracy and has visuomotor and visuospatial components
   - Serial Dotting Test (SDT): Assesses psychomotor speed

   The PHES has failed to gain popularity because of the lack of availability of testing material and normative data for comparison in the United States.
6. Drawbacks of paper and pencil tests
   - Difficulty in interpretation and scoring
   - Overreliance on fine motor skills
   - Poor test of memory
7. The following computerized tests are being evaluated for the diagnosis of covert HE.
   - Inhibitory control test (ICT)
   - Cognitive Drug Research Factor Score
   - Critical Flicker/Fusion Frequency (CFF) Test (see discussion later in chapter)
   - Stroop smartphone app test (EncephalApp)

Overt Hepatic Encephalopathy

1. The diagnosis of overt HE should be suspected when alterations in consciousness occur in a patient with known or suspected significant liver dysfunction.
2. **The West Haven Criteria for Classification of Hepatic Encephalopathy** is a diagnostic tool.
3. Recommended tests that allow better distinction among the different grades of HE are shown in Table 15.2.
4. Associated motor disorders
   - Slow, monotonous speech pattern
   - Loss of fine motor skills
   - Extrapyramidal-type movement disorders
   - Hyperreflexia, extensor plantar response (Babinski sign), clonus
   - Asterixis

TABLE 15.2 ■ West Haven Criteria for the Classification of Hepatic Encephalopathy

Grade	Description	Recommended Tests
0	No abnormality detected	—
Minimal (covert)	Normal mental status and neurologic examination Abnormal psychometric tests	>2 SD on 2 or more tests in PHES ICT: >5 lures CFF: Cutoff frequency 39 Hz
I	Trivial lack of awareness Euphoria or anxiety Shortened attention span Impairment of addition or subtraction	Naming ≤7 animals in 120 s Orientation in time and space

II	Lethargy or apathy
	Disorientation for time
	Obvious personality change
	Inappropriate behavior
		Disorientation in time (≥3 items incorrect):
		  Day of the week
		  Day of the month
		  The month
		  The year
		Orientation to place

III	Somnolence to semistupor
	Responsiveness to stimuli
	Confusion
	Gross disorientation
	Bizarre behavior
		Disorientation to place (≥2 items incorrect):
		  State/country
		  Region/county
		  City
		  Place
		  Floor/ward
		Disorientation to time (as above)
		Reduction of Glasgow coma score (8–14)

IV	Coma, inability to test mental state	Unresponsiveness to pain stimuli (Glasgow coma score <8)

CFF, Critical Flicker/Fusion Frequency; *HE*, hepatic encephalopathy; *ICT*, inhibitory control test; *PHES*, Psychometric Hepatic Encephalopathy Score; *SD*, standard deviation.

- Hyperventilation
- Seizures
- Confusion, coma
- Decerebrate/decorticate posturing

5. **The diagnosis of overt HE remains a diagnosis of exclusion.** Other possible etiologies of disordered mentation need to be considered.

Laboratory Tests

1. **Blood ammonia: Routine measurement is not recommended because it does not change the approach to the diagnosis or treatment of patients with suspected HE.**
   a. Venous ammonia has the same correlation with the severity of HE as does arterial ammonia.
   b. Measures that should be used while collecting blood for ammonia assay
      - Blood must be collected from a stasis-free vein; fist clenching or application of a tourniquet can falsely elevate ammonia levels by release of ammonia from skeletal muscle.
      - Care must be taken to avoid turbulence or hemolysis.
      - Blood must be collected in a green-top glass Vacutainer that contains lithium or sodium heparin; heparin inhibits the release of ammonia from red blood cells.
      - Blood must be stored in an ice bath and immediately transported for assay within 20 minutes of collection.

- An enzymatic assay is used most commonly by laboratories to test ammonia over a broad range from as low as 12 μmol/L to as high as 1 mmol/L.

c. The five most common sources of laboratory error are the following:
  - Improper collection technique
  - Delay in transportation
  - Hemolysis or use of heparin lock during venipuncture
  - Smoking by the patient
  - Pollution of the laboratory atmosphere or laboratory glassware with ammonium-containing detergents

2. **Electroencephalography (EEG)**
   a. EEG is rarely used clinically to make a diagnosis of HE but may be useful to exclude causes of disordered mentation, such as a postictal state.
   b. The main EEG criterion for HE is slowing of mean frequency.
   c. The reported sensitivity varies from 43% to 100%.
   d. Advances in automated EEG measurements require further validation.
   - Artificial neural network expert system software (ANNESS)
   - Spatiotemporal decomposition, designated short epoch, dominant activity, cluster analysis (SEDACA)

3. **CFF Test**
   - The CFF is based on the hypothesis that retinal gliopathy (hepatic retinopathy) could serve as a marker of cerebral gliopathy in HE.
   - It correlates well with paper and pencil psychometric tests used to diagnose covert HE.
   - It enables discrimination of stage 0 HE from covert HE and overt HE at a cutoff frequency of 39 Hz, with a sensitivity of 55% and a specificity of 100%.
   - It allows quantification of HE and is not affected appreciably by training.
   - It is useful for monitoring fluctuations in the severity of HE in response to precipitating factors or therapeutic interventions.

4. **Magnetic resonance imaging (MRI)**
   a. MRI may show evidence of cortical atrophy, which is most pronounced in patients with alcoholic liver disease.
   b. Hyperintensity of basal ganglia is seen on T1-weighted images.
   - Signal abnormalities may reflect manganese deposition in basal ganglia.
   - These abnormalities resolve following liver transplantation.
   c. Proton MR spectroscopy detects a consistent increase in the glutamine/glutamate signal along with depletion of *myo*-inositol in the brain that normalizes after liver transplantation.
   d. Newer techniques to assess brain edema in HE
   - Magnetization transfer ratio (MTR)
   - Fast fluid attenuated inversion recovery (FLAIR) T2-weighted image
   - Diffusion weighted imaging (DWI)
     - The MTR and T2/FLAIR techniques provide an indirect measure of total cerebral water content.
     - These techniques are helpful in demonstrating that varying degrees of astrocyte swelling occur in chronic liver disease and may be partially responsible for HE; this swelling correlates somewhat with the severity of neuropsychiatric impairment.
     - Excessive cerebral water content is reduced with lactulose treatment or liver transplantation (see discussion later in the chapter).
     - T2/FLAIR imaging has shown a higher signal intensity in the white matter in and around the corticospinal tract that reverses following liver transplantation.
     - DWI can differentiate between intracellular and extracellular edema; some studies have shown an increase in interstitial edema in the brain.

Treatment

1. **Response to treatment confirms the diagnosis of HE post hoc.**
2. **Four-pronged strategy for acute treatment**
   - General supportive care of the unconscious patient
   - Exclusion of other causes of encephalopathy and treatment of any that are discovered
   - Identification and treatment of correctable precipitating factors
   - Initiation of empiric treatment for HE
3. **Exclusion of other causes of encephalopathy**
   a. Patients with significant liver dysfunction are susceptible to many causes of encephalopathy other than HE.
      - Sepsis
      - Hypoxia
      - Hypercapnia
      - Acidosis
      - Uremia
      - Sensitivity to CNS drugs
      - Gross electrolyte abnormalities
      - Postictal confusion
      - Delirium tremens
      - Wernicke-Korsakoff syndrome
      - Intracerebral hemorrhage
      - CNS sepsis
      - Pancreatic encephalopathy
      - Drug intoxication
      - Cerebral edema/intracranial hypertension (usually seen in acute liver failure)
      - Hypoglycemia (usually seen in acute liver failure)
   b. Many patients have other causes of encephalopathy as well as HE, a situation contributing to difficulty in diagnosing HE.
4. **Identification of precipitating factors**
   a. Most patients with significant liver disease (except for type A HE) have a precipitating factor that is responsible for inducing the onset of an episode of HE. Some precipitating factors can be easily envisaged to enhance the production and/or absorption of gut-derived compounds (e.g., ammonia). Correcting these conditions is a key aspect of the treatment of HE.
   b. Other precipitating factors are less obvious but may act by reducing hepatic function. Sepsis and CNS-active drugs can independently cause encephalopathy or precipitate HE. Precipitating factors include the following:
      - Sepsis
      - Gastrointestinal hemorrhage
      - Constipation
      - Dietary protein overload
      - Dehydration
      - CNS-active drugs
      - Hypokalemia/alkalosis
      - Poor compliance with lactulose therapy
      - Postanesthesia
      - Postportal decompression procedure
      - Intestinal obstruction or ileus
      - Uremia

- Superimposed hepatic injury
- Development of hepatocellular carcinoma

5. **Empiric therapy**
   a. Gut cleansing with enemas and gastric aspiration or lavage
   b. Low-protein or zero-protein diet
   c. Lactulose 15 mL orally or by nasogastric tube every 2 hours until loose bowel movements are initiated and then 30 mL orally two to three times daily titrated to produce two to three bowel movements per day. Lower doses may suffice if the patient is not comatose; higher doses are not more efficacious, and overtreatment can cause dehydration and electrolyte abnormalities that can aggravate HE.
   d. Empiric therapy may be effective by correcting precipitating factors; however, because the response to correcting precipitating factors cannot be predicted, **all patients should receive full empiric therapy.**

6. **Response to treatment**
   a. **In virtually all cases of overt HE in chronic liver disease, encephalopathy should be reversible.** Failure to reverse HE after 72 hours of treatment and cathartic agents may indicate the following:
      - Another cause of encephalopathy has been missed or treated inadequately.
      - A precipitating factor has been missed or treated inadequately or remains uncorrected.
      - Effective empiric therapy has not been instituted.
      - Excessive lactulose therapy has induced dehydration.
   b. **The most common reason for ineffective therapy is lack of delivery of lactulose into the small intestine or right colon.** Only intestinal obstruction or ileus should prevent adequate delivery. Reluctance to use nasogastric tube delivery of lactulose in the comatose patient because of fear of precipitating variceal bleeding is unwarranted.

7. **Second-line therapy, if needed**
   a. Rifaximin: 550 mg orally twice daily
   b. Metronidazole: 250 mg orally four times daily (recommend only short term)
   c. Neomycin: 500 mg orally four times daily (use higher doses with caution)
   d. Vancomycin: 250 mg orally four times daily
   e. Sodium benzoate (not approved for use in the United States)
   f. Flumazenil (may be effective but has a very short duration of action)
   g. Other agents such as branched-chain amino acids, ornithine aspartate, and cathartic agents like polyethylene glycol have been shown to be beneficial in the treatment of overt HE but have not been approved by the U.S. Food and Drug Administration.

8. **Type A HE** (see Chapter 2)
   a. Type A accounts for a small fraction of HE cases per year.
   b. Treatment follows the same principles as in chronic liver disease, except for the following:
      - Precipitating factors are often not obvious, and, even if these factors are present, correction is usually not effective.
      - The overall response to empiric therapy is poor.
      - If deep coma occurs, the prognosis is poor without liver transplantation.
      - Cerebral edema and intracranial hypertension are common and often lethal.
      - Other concurrent causes of encephalopathy are common (e.g., hypoglycemia, acidosis, sepsis).
      - Approximately 20% of patients have an agitated delirium or seizure phase.
      - Cathartic agents are ineffective.

9. **Long-term treatment**
   a. Lactulose
   b. Rifaximin

    c. Vegetable-based protein diet

    d. Diet enriched with branched-chain amino acids

    e. Bromocriptine

    f. Zinc repletion

    g. Sodium benzoate

    h. Ornithine aspartate

10. If an approach fails, compliance should be confirmed and another agent added. A long-term low-protein diet is not ideal because protein restriction to avoid HE does not allow adequate maintenance of nitrogen balance.

11. Options for intractable or recurrent HE

    a. Liver transplantation

- Treatment for intractable HE
- Treatment for recurrent HE or HE responsive only to a low-protein diet
- Once a patient has had a bout of overt HE, he or she should be referred for liver transplantation evaluation.

    b. Modification of an existing portosystemic shunt

- Surgical portosystemic shunts or transjugular intrahepatic portosystemic shunts (TIPS) may be amenable to closure or a reduction in shunt diameter, possibly in combination with other measures to prevent recurrent variceal bleeding.
- Acquired spontaneous portosystemic shunts are often amenable to occlusion (by embolization) or a reduction in flow (e.g., splenic artery embolization). The results of such interventions can be striking and may delay the need for liver transplantation for years.
- Congenital portosystemic shunts are amenable to closure in some cases.

    c. Other options

- Colonic exclusion: Virtually abandoned
- Arterialization or portal venous stump: Abandoned
- Radiologic portal vein thrombolysis plus TIPS
- TIPS in Budd-Chiari syndrome

FURTHER READING

Allampati S, Duarte-Rojo A, Thacker LR, et al. Diagnosis of minimal hepatic encephalopathy using Stroop EncephalApp: a multicenter US-based norm-based study. *Am J Gastroenterol.* 2016;111:78–86.

Atluri DK, Asgeri M, Mullen KD. Reversibility of hepatic encephalopathy after liver transplantation. *Metab Brain Dis.* 2010;25:111–113.

Bajaj JS. The modern management of hepatic encephalopathy. *Aliment Pharmacol Ther.* 2010;31:537–547.

Bajaj JS, Hafeezullah M, Franco J, et al. Inhibitory control test for the diagnosis of minimal hepatic encephalopathy. *Gastroenterology.* 2008;135:1591–1600.

Bajaj JS, Saeian K, Schubert CM, et al. Minimal hepatic encephalopathy is associated with motor vehicle crashes: the reality beyond the driving test. *Hepatology.* 2009;50:1175–1183.

Bajaj JS, Schubert CM, Heuman DM, et al. Persistence of cognitive impairment after resolution of overt hepatic encephalopathy. *Gastroenterology.* 2010;138:2332–2340.

Bajaj JS, Wade JB, Sanyal AJ. Spectrum of neurocognitive impairment in cirrhosis: implications for the assessment of hepatic encephalopathy. *Hepatology.* 2009;50:2014–2021.

Bass NM, Mullen KD, Sanyal A, et al. Rifaximin treatment in hepatic encephalopathy. *N Engl J Med.* 2010;362:1071–1081.

Ferenci P, Lockwood A, Mullen KD, et al. Hepatic encephalopathy: definition, nomenclature, diagnosis and quantification: final report on the Working Party at the 11th World Congress of Gastroenterology, Vienna, 1998. *Hepatology.* 2002;35:716–721.

Haussinger D, Schliess F. Pathogenetic mechanisms of hepatic encephalopathy. *Gut.* 2008;57:1156–1165.

Mardini H, Saxby BK. Record CO. Computerized psychometric testing in minimal hepatic encephalopathy and modulation by nitrogen challenge and liver transplant. *Gastroenterology.* 2008;135:1582–1590.

Mullen KD, Amodio P, Morgan MY. Therapeutic studies in hepatic encephalopathy. *Metab Brain Dis.* 2007;22:407–423.

Prasad S, Dhiman RK, Duseja A, et al. Lactulose improves cognitive functions and health–related quality of life in patients with cirrhosis who have minimal hepatic encephalopathy. *Hepatology.* 2007;45:549–559.

Rahimi RS, Singal AG, Cuthbert JA, et al. Lactulose vs polyethylene glycol 3350—electrolyte solution for treatment of overt hepatic encephalopathy: the HELP randomized clinical trial. *JAMA Intern Med.* 2014;174:1727–1733.

Rovira A, Alonso J, Córdoba J. MR findings in hepatic encephalopathy. *Am J Neuroradiol.* 2008;29:1612–1621.

CHAPTER 16

Primary Biliary Cholangitis

Gwilym J. Webb, BM BCh, MA, MRCP ■ Gideon M. Hirschfield, MB BChir, PhD, FRCP

KEY POINTS

1 Primary biliary cholangitis (PBC, formerly known as primary biliary cirrhosis) is a chronic cholestatic liver disease that typically affects middle-aged women. Its pathogenesis includes a combination of environmental and genetic factors.

2 Genetic studies suggest that the human leukocyte antigen (HLA) and type 1 helper T-cell (Th1)/interleukin-12 signaling axis are particularly relevant biologically in the origin of this autoimmune small-duct lymphocytic cholangitis.

3 Most patients are asymptomatic at the time of diagnosis; symptom severity does not always correlate with disease severity, and symptom burden can markedly impair quality of life.

4 The combination of persistently cholestatic liver biochemical test levels, normal biliary imaging, and the presence of antimitochondrial antibodies (AMA) or specific antinuclear antibodies is usually sufficient to diagnose PBC. Liver biopsy is not recommended by consensus guidelines unless doubt exists about the diagnosis or antibodies are absent.

5 Treatment guidelines recommend that ursodeoxycholic acid (UDCA) be offered to all patients with PBC. The absence of a biochemical response to treatment is associated with a poorer outcome. Alternative therapies have been difficult to identify. Randomized data failed to provide support for the use of methotrexate or colchicine. The efficacy of fenofibrate and bezafibrate remains anecdotal, with concern over safety.

6 The farnesoid X–receptor agonist obeticholic acid (OCA) has biochemical efficacy in UDCA nonresponders and has successfully completed phase 2 and 3 randomized-controlled trials, with long-term evaluation of efficacy in advanced liver disease patients underway. OCA is now licensed in the United States and recommended as therapy for patients who do not have a biochemical response to UDCA or who are intolerant of UDCA.

7 Liver transplantation (LT) is an effective treatment for PBC in patients meeting standard transplant indications; intractable pruritus is occasionally an indication for LT in the absence of liver failure; fatigue is not.

Nomenclature

Consensus statements driven by patient feedback have supported a change in name from primary biliary *cirrhosis* to primary biliary *cholangitis*. Ultimately, a high proportion of patients do progress to cirrhosis and require surveillance for hepatocellular carcinoma (HCC).

Epidemiology

1. **PBC is a female-predominant (90% to 95%) disease recognized in all ethnicities.** It appears less frequent among African Americans but is reported to be more frequent in some populations such as Canadian First Nations.
2. An estimated 1 in 1000 women older than 40 years of age have PBC. A meta-analysis has suggested an incidence of 0.33 to 5.8 per 100,000 persons/year and a prevalence of 1.91 to 40.2 per 100,000 persons, with an increasing prevalence over time.
3. The age of onset ranges from 30 to 70 years, and the diagnosis of PBC is increasingly made when screening or investigation for other conditions reveals abnormal serum liver biochemical test levels. Although AMA reactivity in children is recognized, a diagnosis of PBC before menarche has not been reported. Younger age at onset (<50) is typically associated with more aggressive UDCA-nonresponsive disease.
4. The rate of LT for PBC has been reduced by widespread use of UDCA, but some patients, typically younger at onset, continue to progress to decompensation.

Genetics

1. Genetic factors play a role in PBC, although the disorder is not solely the consequence of a single genetic mutation.
2. Approximately 1 in 20 patients has a family member affected with PBC. Patients and their family members are more likely to have other autoimmune diseases, particularly celiac disease and scleroderma.
3. Lack of complete concordance for PBC in identical twins suggests that environmental factors are also important; plausible factors proposed include xenobiotic exposure and molecular mimicry from infection. Smoking is an important risk factor for disease severity and progression.
4. An association with variations in the class II HLA locus is established but not understood mechanistically.
5. Genome-wide association testing and replication studies have identified variations in genes important in the Th1/interleukin-12 pathway (*IL12A, IL12RB2, IRF5, NFKB1, TYK2, STAT4*) as particularly relevant to the pathogenesis of PBC. Variations in other genes involved in T-cell activation, B- and T-cell development, B-cell positioning, and antigen presentation are also reported.
6. Many of the genetic associations of PBC—including HLA antigens—are shared with other autoimmune conditions (e.g., multiple sclerosis, ulcerative colitis, rheumatoid arthritis, type 1 diabetes mellitus, celiac disease).
7. Suggestions that changes in X chromosome function and number affect disease susceptibility have not been supported by genome-wide studies; however, differences in disease severity between men and women are reported.

Immunology

Genetic studies of PBC support the concept that immunologic aberrations underlie this archetypal autoimmune disease. Immunologic changes identified in patients with PBC include the following:
1. **AMA**
   a. Detected in 95% of patients with PBC
   b. Do not affect the course or response to treatment of PBC
   c. Can be seen in other liver diseases, including acute liver failure, drug injury, and autoimmune hepatitis

   d. Persist after LT
   e. A family of antibodies that react with different antigens within the mitochondria
      ■ AMA PDH-E2
         – The major autoantibody found in PBC
         – Directed principally against the dihydrolipoamide acyltransferase component (E2) of the ketoacid dehydrogenase complexes on the inner mitochondrial membrane
         – Pyruvate dehydrogenase is the best known of these enzyme complexes.
      ■ Anti-M4, anti-M8, and anti-M9
         – Other AMA are described in PBC but not considered relevant to clinical care.
         – Their existence was not confirmed in a study that used highly purified cloned human mitochondrial proteins as antigens.
   f. Significance
      ■ The relationship between AMA and immunologic bile duct injury remains unclear.
      ■ AMA typically precede clinically apparent disease.
      ■ Biochemical changes to the pyruvate dehydrogenase complex during biliary epithelial cell apoptosis appear important in explaining the relevance of AMA in PBC.
      ■ Pyruvate dehydrogenase and the other mitochondrial antigens are aberrantly expressed on the luminal surface of biliary epithelial cells from patients with PBC but not from control subjects or patients with primary sclerosing cholangitis.
      ■ Pyruvate dehydrogenase E2 is expressed in bile duct epithelial cells before T-lymphocyte cytotoxicity occurs.
      ■ Mitochondrial antigens are not tissue specific.
      ■ No correlation exists between the presence or titer of AMA and the severity of the course of PBC; antibody titers can fall with treatment.
      ■ High titers of AMA can be induced in experimental animals by immunization with pure human pyruvate dehydrogenase, but these animals do not develop liver disease; induction of autoimmune cholangitis with AMA following a chemical (2-octynoic acid) xenobiotic immunization or *Escherichia coli* infection in autoimmunity-prone mice has been reported.
      ■ Genetic manipulation of mice (e.g., NOD.c3c4 congenic or multiple different defects affecting the T-regulatory pathway including FOXP3 deficiency; IL2 receptor alpha dysfunction; expression of dominant negative transforming growth factor [TGF] β receptor on CD4+ T cells; anion exchanger 2 knockouts) leads to AMA production and autoimmune biliary disease with some features reminiscent of PBC.
2. Other circulating autoantibodies
   a. Antinuclear antibodies (ANA)
      ■ The pattern of immunofluorescence is highly specific for PBC, thus making the presence of multiple nuclear dot ANA (sp100) or the membrane rim ANA pattern (gp210) potentially diagnostic in AMA-negative patients.
   b. Anticentromere antibodies
      ■ Studies suggest that gp210-positive patients tend to have a more aggressive disease course with liver failure, whereas anticentromere antibody-positive patients tend to have a portal hypertensive phenotype.
3. Serum immunoglobulins
   a. Increased concentrations of serum immunoglobulin M (IgM), which is immunoreactive and highly cryoprecipitable
   b. Possible false-positive results with assays to detect immune complexes
4. Association with other autoimmune diseases
   a. Scleroderma
   b. Sjögren syndrome

    c. Celiac disease

    d. Thyroiditis or hypothyroidism

    e. Rheumatoid arthritis or systemic lupus erythematosus

5. **Abnormalities of cellular immunity**

    a. Reduced T-regulatory cell function and number have been reported.

    b. Decreased numbers of circulating T lymphocytes but increased numbers of T follicular helper cells

    c. Increased Th17 cells in the liver

    d. Sequestration of T lymphocytes within hepatic portal triads

Pathogenesis

1. **Chronic nonsuppurative granulomatous cholangitis** is a more accurate description of the disease than PBC, with at least two related processes leading to hepatic damage (Fig. 16.1).

2. The first process is **chronic, often granulomatous, destruction of small bile ducts**, presumably mediated by activated lymphocytes. The initial destructive bile duct lesion in PBC is caused by cytotoxic T lymphocytes. Interface hepatitis can be present (5% to 10%), but whether this is just a facet of PBC or coexistent autoimmune hepatitis remains controversial. It is, however, clear that younger, UDCA-nonresponsive patients can have a more hepatic presentation of disease, although not typically glucocorticoid responsive.

3. Bile duct cells in patients with PBC express increased amounts of class I HLA-A, HLA-B, and HLA-C and class II HLA-DR antigens.

4. The bile duct lesion resembles disorders mediated by cytotoxic T lymphocytes, such as graft-versus-host disease and hepatic allograft rejection.

5. The second process includes **chemical damage to hepatocytes** in areas of the liver where bile drainage is impeded by destruction of the small bile ducts.

    ▪ Retention of bile acids, bilirubin, copper, and other substances that are normally secreted or excreted into bile occurs; absorption of lipids and lipid-soluble substances is also impaired.

    ▪ The increased concentration of some of these substances, such as bile acids, may further damage liver cells.

    ▪ Consequences of bile duct destruction include portal inflammation and scarring, which progress to cirrhosis and eventual liver failure.

Pathology

GROSS FINDINGS

1. The liver is initially enlarged but smooth.

2. With disease progression, the liver enlarges further, becoming nodular and grossly cirrhotic with bile staining. Eventually its size may diminish in size in end-stage disease.

3. An increased frequency of gallstones is noted (approximately 40% of patients).

4. An increased frequency of nodular regenerative hyperplasia (NRH) is observed in the early stage of PBC. Although varices and portal hypertension typically reflect cirrhosis, presinusoidal portal hypertension can develop due to NRH in patients with PBC who are not yet cirrhotic.

5. Enlarged lymph nodes resulting from benign reactive hyperplasia may be seen in the porta hepatis and around the aorta and inferior vena cava; this finding should be distinguished from lymphoma.

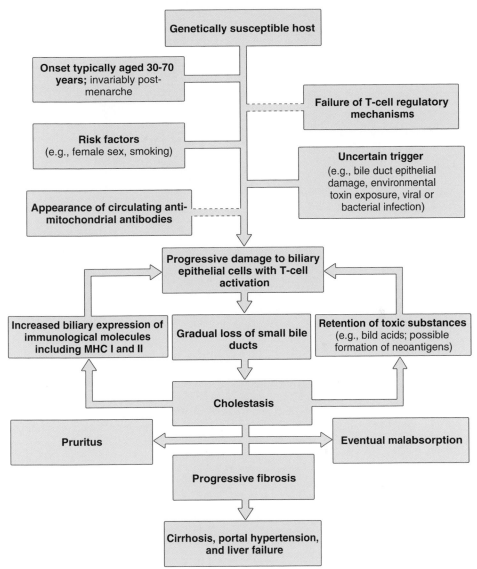

Fig. 16.1 Sequence of events in the possible pathogenesis of primary biliary cholangitis (PBC). The cause of PBC remains unknown, although genetic and immunologic factors appear to play a role. *MHC*, Major histocompatibility complex.

HISTOLOGIC FINDINGS

1. Four histologic stages of PBC are recognized.
2. Histologic staging has been superseded as a prognostic tool by the biochemical response to treatment, thereby reducing the need for liver biopsy, which is therefore not recommended in clinical practice. Increasingly, noninvasive markers of fibrosis, particularly ultrasound elastography, are being used.

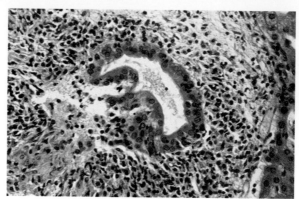

Fig. 16.2 Histopathology of stage I florid bile duct lesion of primary biliary cholangitis. The epithelial cell lining of a small duct is infiltrated with lymphocytes (hematoxylin and eosin [H&E]).

3. Considerations in interpreting liver biopsy staging
   a. Disease involvement may not be uniform and may be affected by sampling variation.
   b. Several stages may be seen on a single biopsy specimen; by convention, staging is based on the most advanced lesion seen on the biopsy specimen.
   c. Because PBC is increasingly diagnosed at an early stage, it is less likely now than in the past that characteristic pathologic findings will be present on needle biopsy specimens.
4. Standard histologic stages
   a. **Stage I**
      ■ Injured bile ducts are usually surrounded by a dense infiltrate of mononuclear cells, most of which are lymphocytes (Fig. 16.2).
      ■ These florid, asymmetric destructive lesions of interlobular bile ducts are irregularly scattered throughout the portal tracts and are often seen only on large surgical biopsy specimens of the liver in which adequate representation of small bile ducts occurs.
      ■ Inflammation is confined to the portal tracts.
   b. **Stage II**
      ■ The lesion is more widespread but less specific.
      ■ Reduced numbers of normal bile ducts within portal tracts and increased numbers of atypical, poorly formed bile ducts with irregularly shaped lumens may be evident (Fig. 16.3).
      ■ Diffuse portal fibrosis and mononuclear cell infiltrates are seen within portal tracts.
      ■ Inflammation may spill into the surrounding periportal areas.
      ■ **A diminished number of bile ducts in an otherwise unremarkable needle biopsy specimen of the liver should alert one to the possibility of PBC.**
   c. **Stage III**
      ■ This is similar to stage II, except fibrous septa extend beyond portal tracts and form portal-to-portal bridges (Fig. 16.4).
   d. **Stage IV**
      ■ This represents the end stage of the lesion, with frank cirrhosis and regenerative nodules (Fig. 16.5).
      ■ Findings may be indistinguishable from other types of cirrhosis; however, a paucity of normal bile ducts in areas of scarring suggests the possibility of PBC.
5. Newer pathologic scoring systems assess the amount of fibrosis (portal/periportal fibrosis/few septa/numerous septa/cirrhosis); grades of lymphocytic interface hepatitis and ductopenia

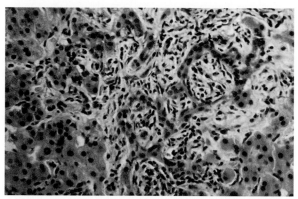

Fig. 16.3   Histopathology of stage II primary biliary cholangitis. Atypical bile duct hyperplasia is seen. Tortuous bile ducts are visible, with an inflammatory cell infiltrate consisting of primarily lymphocytes and few neutrophils (H&E).

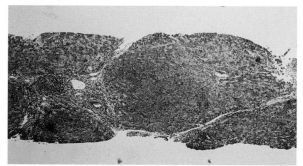

Fig. 16.4   Histopathology of stage III primary biliary cholangitis. A portal-to-portal fibrous septum is shown on this low-power view (Masson trichrome).

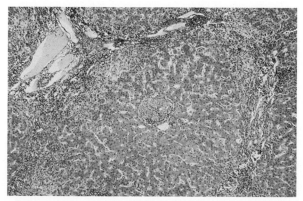

Fig. 16.5   Histopathology of stage IV primary biliary cholangitis. A noncaseating granuloma is visible in the center of a nodule. Portal tracts are linked by bands of connective tissue and inflammatory cells (Masson trichrome).

(bile duct ratio—i.e., the ratio of the number of portal tracts with ducts to the total number of portal tracts); or stage of PBC (fibrosis, bile duct loss, and the deposition of copper-binding protein) and grade of necroinflammatory activity (cholangitis and hepatitis).

Clinical Features

SYMPTOMS

Approximately two thirds of patients are asymptomatic at the time of initial diagnosis. Symptoms and signs of PBC partly reflect cholestasis.

1. **Fatigue**
   - Most common symptom, but variably reported depending on the method of ascertainment
   - Not specific for PBC; seen in other hepatic and nonhepatic disease
   - Other explanations, such as depression, anemia, sleep apnea, hypothyroidism, iron deficiency, and hypoadrenalism, should be considered.
2. **Pruritus**
   - Pathogenesis unknown; itching is not solely from retention of the naturally occurring primary and secondary bile acids but likely caused by another substance normally secreted into bile.
   - Increased opioidergic tone related to chronic cholestasis has been suggested as a potential etiologic factor.
   - Serum autotaxin activity and lysophosphatidic levels have been correlated with the intensity of pruritus and may be potential therapeutic targets.
   - Characteristically worse at bedtime
   - May initially develop during the third trimester of pregnancy and persist after delivery
   - Paradoxically, pruritus often improves as disease progresses.
   - UDCA is not a treatment for pruritus and may exacerbate pruritus. Farnesoid X–receptor agonists such as obeticholic acid may also exacerbate pruritus; dose titration and concomitant symptomatic treatment of pruritus have proved effective in ameliorating pruritus in patients taking obeticholic acid.
3. **Osteoporosis**
   - Osteopenic bone disease occurs in at least 25% of patients with PBC; the pathogenesis is still unclear but seems to reflect low bone turnover as well as the severity of liver disease.
   - Osteomalacia is uncommon.
   - Clinical symptoms of osteoporosis are unusual, but when present they relate to spontaneous or low-impact fractures.
4. **Malabsorption**
   - A now uncommon clinical manifestation; previously it was recognized in patients with long-standing cholestasis.
   - Impaired secretion of bile results in diminished concentration of bile acids within the intestinal lumen; bile acid concentration may fall to less than the critical micellar concentration and be inadequate for complete digestion and absorption of neutral triglycerides in the diet.
   - Patients may experience nocturnal diarrhea, foul-smelling bulky stools, or weight loss despite a good appetite and increased caloric intake.
   - Malabsorption of the fat-soluble vitamins A, D, E, and K and calcium may be present; night blindness is a particularly important symptom of vitamin A deficiency.
   - Pancreatic insufficiency may also contribute to malabsorption; this is most likely in patients with concomitant sicca syndrome.
5. **Sicca complex**
   - This combination of dry eyes, dry mouth, and vaginal dryness is a frequent complaint in patients with PBC.
   - Some patients have primary Sjögren syndrome, although most with sicca complex do not.

6. **Right-sided abdominal pain**
   - Nonspecific pain is described by up to one third of patients without an obvious clinical or radiologic explanation.
7. **Arthralgia and bone pain**
   - Frequently reported; may also indicate concomitant inflammatory arthritis

PHYSICAL EXAMINATION

1. Findings vary depending on the stage of the disease; examination is typically unremarkable in asymptomatic patients.
2. **Hepatomegaly and splenomegaly** are detected with progressive disease; a few patients may have splenomegaly early as a result of portal hypertension related to NRH.
3. **Skin abnormalities**
   - Hyperpigmentation, if seen, may resemble tanning and is caused by melanin, not bilirubin, in early-stage PBC.
   - Excoriations may be diffuse from scratching caused by intractable pruritus.
   - Jaundice usually manifests later in the course of the disease.
   - Xanthelasma and xanthomata reflect hypercholesterolemia; xanthelasma are more common than xanthomata (Figs. 16.6 and 16.7). Less than 5% of patients will eventually develop xanthomata, which are found on the palms of the hands and soles of the feet, over extensor surfaces of the elbows and knees, in tendons of the ankles and wrists, and on the buttocks.
4. **Eye abnormalities:** Kayser-Fleischer rings are rarely detected and result from copper retention from prolonged cholestasis.
5. **End-stage PBC:** Spider telangiectasias, temporal and proximal limb muscle wasting, ascites, and edema usually occur with cirrhosis and portal hypertension.

Diagnosis

LABORATORY TESTS

1. Liver biochemical tests
   - A **cholestatic pattern** is usual (alkaline phosphatase [ALP] to aspartate aminotransferase [AST] or alanine aminotransferase [ALT] ratio usually more than 3 and serum AST or ALT level less than five times the upper limit of normal [ULN])

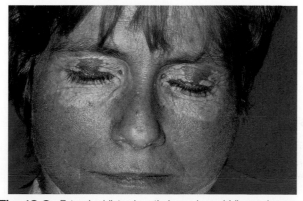

Fig. 16.6 Extensive bilateral xanthelasma in a middle-aged woman.

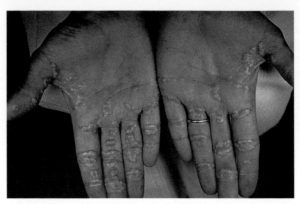

Fig. 16.7   Bilateral plantar xanthomata in the palms of a patient with PBC.

- Biochemical tests alone are never diagnostic of PBC.
- Elevation of serum ALP and gamma-glutamyltranspeptidase levels are the earliest abnormalities; the degree of elevation may relate to the severity of duct injury and likelihood of treatment response.
- Serum aminotransferase activity is often elevated during the course of the disease; persistent elevation on treatment is associated with poorer long-term outcomes (see discussion later in chapter).
- **Serum bilirubin** is usually normal early in the course but becomes elevated if the disease progresses; it remains the **best predictor of outcome** (even within the normal range), and with ALP values, is a validated biomarker of outcome and a commonly applied surrogate of treatment efficacy.

2. **AMA are present in 95% of patients.** In those in whom AMA are absent, many have specific ANA, including gp100 and sp210.
3. Other associated findings
   - Serum albumin concentration and prothrombin time are normal in the early stages and abnormal in the late stage.
   - Serum IgM levels are elevated polyclonally.
   - Serum cholesterol levels are elevated in at least 50% of patients, due to cholestasis, without an increase in cardiovascular events in this female-predominant condition; treatment of hyperlipidemia, if concomitant risk factors exist, is safe. High-density lipoprotein levels are elevated.
   - Hepatic and urinary copper levels are elevated.
   - Hypothyroidism with increased thyroid-stimulating hormone levels is frequent.
   - Evidence of other concomitant autoimmune conditions (e.g., tissue transglutaminase antibodies in celiac disease) may be found.

LIVER BIOPSY

1. Liver biopsy is no longer routinely performed but can aid in confirming the diagnosis of PBC and providing an estimate of disease severity at presentation.
2. In patients without AMA (and when specific ANA testing is not available) or in those with potential alternative explanations for liver biochemical test findings, liver biopsy

should be considered. Such cases include so-called "overlap" or "cross-over" syndromes in which liver histology is essential to review in the context of the overall clinical features (see Chapter 7).

IMAGING TESTS

Imaging tests are useful for ruling out bile duct obstruction and screening for gallstones if abdominal pain is present.
1. Ultrasonography: Noninvasive and usually adequate to exclude biliary obstruction
2. Cholangiography: Indicated only in AMA-negative patients in whom primary sclerosing cholangitis is a possible diagnosis; magnetic resonance cholangiography is the preferred technique.

PRINCIPLES OF DIAGNOSIS

1. The diagnosis of PBC is based on history, physical findings, laboratory tests, and histology, if available.
2. **The combination of cholestatic liver biochemical test levels and presence of AMA have a high positive predictive value for a histologic diagnosis of PBC.**
3. The diagnosis of PBC is now generally based on laboratory findings. Rising rates of obesity, however, may necessitate additional investigation: 0.5% of the healthy population is AMA positive, and up to 30% of healthy persons may have fatty liver, which biochemically can be reflected by a rise in ALP.

DIFFERENTIAL DIAGNOSIS

1. Gallstones
2. Mechanical, extrahepatic bile duct obstruction, such as tumors, cysts, and postsurgical strictures
3. Primary sclerosing cholangitis
4. Nonalcoholic or alcoholic fatty liver
5. Cholestatic viral hepatitis
6. Granulomatous hepatitis
7. Autoimmune hepatitis
8. Vanishing bile duct syndrome
9. Benign recurrent intrahepatic cholestasis
10. Drug-induced cholestasis
11. IgG4 disease

Natural History and Prognosis

1. Median survival of symptomatic patients has ranged from 7.5 to 10 years and is 7 years for histologic stages III and IV PBC.
2. Median survival of asymptomatic patients in historic, nonstratified cohorts has ranged from 10 to 16 years.
3. Most asymptomatic patients will develop symptoms, usually within 2 to 4 years of diagnosis.
4. The presence or titer of AMA does not influence survival.
5. If patients achieve a biochemical response to treatment with UDCA (see Risk Stratification later in chapter), then 10-year survival is excellent at >90%.
6. Younger age at presentation and male sex are associated with decreased rates of response to UDCA.

TABLE 16.1 ■ **Drug Treatment of Pruritus**

Drug	Mechanism of Action	Dose	Side Effects
Cholestyramine	Bile acid resin	4–16 g orally/day	Unpalatability, constipation, interference with absorption of other medications
Colestipol	Bile acid resin	5 g orally 3 times/day	Constipation, interference with absorption of other medications
Rifampin	Competes with bile acids for hepatic uptake	300–600 mg orally/day	Idiosyncratic hepatotoxicity
Sertraline	SSRI	50–100 mg/day	Dry mouth
Naloxone	Opioid antagonist	0.2 µg/kg IV/min for 24 hours	Self-limited opioid withdrawal-like symptoms
Nalmefene	Opioid antagonist	60–120 mg orally/day	Self-limited opioid withdrawal-like symptoms
Naltrexone	Opioid antagonist	50 mg orally/day	Self-limited opioid withdrawal-like symptoms

IV, Intravenously; *SSRI,* selective serotonin reuptake inhibitor.

Treatment

SYMPTOMS OF CHRONIC CHOLESTASIS

1. **Pruritus** (Table 16.1)
   a. Antihistamines
      ■ These are occasionally helpful early in the course of PBC when itching is not severe; the sedative side effects of nonselective antihistamines may be useful.
   b. Cholestyramine
      ■ This nonabsorbed resin binds bile acids and relieves pruritus in many patients.
      ■ Therapy should be directed at symptomatic relief, with a usual dose of 4 g twice daily, generally taken mixed with water or juice before and after breakfast.
      ■ Depending on the severity of cholestasis, it may take up to 14 days before itching remits.
      ■ Other medications need to be taken 1 hour before or 2 to 4 hours after cholestyramine, to avoid impaired intestinal absorption.
   c. Colestipol hydrochloride (ammonium resin)
      ■ This may be considered in patients who find cholestyramine unpalatable; however, some patients find colestipol equally unpalatable. Colesevelam is also an option.
   d. Other antipruritogenic agents that may control itching in some patients (in order of suggested use)
      ■ Rifampin (150 to 300 mg twice daily)
      ■ Sertraline (50 to 100 mg once daily)
      ■ Naloxone (opioid antagonist): Based on data suggesting that itching may be mediated by opioidergic neurotransmission
      ■ Nalmefene (opioid antagonist)
      ■ Naltrexone (opioid antagonist)
      ■ Phototherapy with ultraviolet B light
      ■ Plasmapheresis (almost always helpful but inconvenient and expensive)
      ■ Molecular adsorbents recirculation system (MARS; effective where available)
      ■ LT
      ■ Trials of apical sodium codependent bile acid transporter inhibitors are ongoing.

2. **Malabsorption of fat-soluble vitamins**
   a. The frequency of malabsorption is roughly proportional to the severity and duration of cholestasis and is now rarely a clinical concern.
   b. Vitamin A, D, E, and K levels should be measured in jaundiced patients with PBC; supplementation should be prescribed to patients with low levels.
   c. Treatment: Vitamins should be administered orally as far apart from cholestyramine as possible.
      - Oral vitamin K: 5 mg/day
      - Vitamin A: 10,000 to 25,000 IU/day
      - 25-OH vitamin D: 20 µg three times weekly; check serum levels of 25-OH vitamin D after several weeks
      - Supplemental calcium
      - Vitamin E: 400 to 1000 IU/day
3. **Steatorrhea**
   a. Treated by a low-fat diet supplemented with medium-chain triglycerides (MCT) to maintain a reasonable caloric intake
   b. Most patients tolerate 60 mL of MCT oil per day.
   c. Some patients with PBC and the sicca syndrome may have concomitant pancreatic insufficiency, which can be treated with pancreatic enzyme replacement therapy.
   d. Patients may develop iron deficiency anemia, which reflects unrecognized gastrointestinal blood loss usually from gastric manifestations of portal hypertension (gastropathy or gastric antral vascular ectasia). Colonoscopy to exclude a lower gastrointestinal cause and exclusion of concomitant celiac disease are required.
4. **Osteoporosis**
   a. Osteoporosis is a manifestation of PBC but is also a frequent finding in otherwise healthy women of similar age.
   b. Bone mineral density and associated fracture risk should be assessed with dual x ray absorptiometry on diagnosis of PBC.
   c. A retrospective study has suggested beneficial effects of hormone replacement therapy in postmenopausal women with PBC.
   d. LT is effective in increasing bone mineral density, with improvement often delayed until 1 year after transplantation. Bone mineral density decreases initially for up to 6 months after transplantation because of immunosuppression with glucocorticoids and physical inactivity.

UNDERLYING DISEASE (Table 16.2)

1. **UDCA**
   - **UDCA is the initial agent used for PBC.** It reduces hepatic dysfunction and may retard disease progression. The greatest overall benefit is in patients with early disease, although a survival benefit is demonstrable only in those with advanced disease.
   - UDCA is safe and well tolerated; mild weight gain (averaging 3 kg), bloating, and thinning of the hair are side effects. If a patient has a biochemical response to treatment, it is typically maintained; however, if UDCA therapy is interrupted, hepatic dysfunction returns.
   - In four controlled trials, UDCA, 13 to 15 mg/kg body weight/day orally, reduced serum bilirubin, ALP, aminotransferase, and IgM concentrations.
   - Individual studies also indicate UDCA can favorably affect survival, slow histologic deterioration, and diminish progression of portal hypertension.
   - When data were pooled from three major studies, UDCA prolonged time to LT compared with placebo.
   - In a multicenter study conducted in the United States, efficacy was limited to a subgroup of patients with stage I and II disease whose initial serum bilirubin levels were <2 mg/dL.

TABLE 16.2 ■ **Drug Treatment of Primary Biliary Cholangitis**

Drug	Mechanism of Action	Dose	Benefits	Side Effects	Comments
Ursodeoxycholic acid	Choleretic	13–15 mg/kg/day orally	Improves liver biochemistries, slows histologic progression, and probably improves long-term survival	Diarrhea, weight gain, thinning of hair, increased pruritus	Most widely used agent
Obeticholic acid	Farnesoid-X-receptor agonist	5 mg per day, titrated to 10 mg per day at 3 months, if tolerated	Improves liver biochemistries	Dose-dependent pruritus	Approved by the FDA and EMA for patients who have an inadequate response to UDCA or who are intolerant of UDCA

EMA, European Medicines Agency; *FDA*, U.S. Food and Drug Administration; *UDCA*, ursodeoxycholic acid.

- Meta-analyses have provided conflicting results because of the challenge of combining studies of short duration with inadequate UDCA dosing with studies of longer duration with appropriate UDCA dosing.
- Multiple studies, however, clearly show that **patients with a biochemical response to UDCA have a normal life expectancy;** the definition of response to therapy varies but generally includes improvement in the serum ALP value.
- The decreased number of patients with PBC requiring LT reflects the widespread use of UDCA.

2. **Obeticholic acid**
   - Obeticholic acid (OCA) is a semisynthetic farnesoid-X-receptor agonist that is administered orally. It acts to reduce hepatocyte bile acid synthesis and also has an antifibrotic effect.
   - OCA reduces serum alkaline phosphatase activity when compared with placebo in controlled trials in which it is administered in combination with UDCA or as monotherapy. Reductions in serum alkaline phosphatase levels correlate with improved survival in PBC, but a direct survival benefit has not yet been demonstrated for OCA.
   - OCA is licensed in the United States for use in patients without a biochemical response to UDCA or who are intolerant of UDCA. The initial dose is 5 mg per day orally, with titration to 10 mg per day at 3 months, if tolerated.
   - Pruritus may be seen with OCA; management includes dose adjustment as well as standard therapy with cholestyramine or rifampin.

3. **Other agents**
   - Colchicine: Although early data were encouraging, a Cochrane review failed to confirm efficacy.
   - Methotrexate: Although early data were encouraging, a Cochrane review failed to confirm efficacy.

■ Others
  — Candidate agents have included budesonide, fenofibrates, and rituximab; however, data are not available to support routine off-label use of these drugs.
  — Other drugs that act on the farnesoid X receptor axis (in addition to OCA) may become available.
  — For patients without a biochemical response to therapy with UDCA, new drugs are needed.
4. Smoking appears to increase the rate of progression of PBC and should be discontinued.

SURVEILLANCE FOR COMPLICATIONS OF CIRRHOSIS

1. Varices can occur in patients with PBC in the absence of cirrhosis due to presinusoidal portal hypertension caused by NRH. If cirrhosis is suspected or if there is a reduction in platelet count, endoscopy to screen for varices is indicated. Patients with fatigue may find therapy with a beta receptor antagonist troublesome, thus necessitating prophylactic banding of varices.
2. HCC can occur in cirrhotic patients with PBC; guidelines recommend ultrasound surveillance every 6 months in patients with cirrhosis.

Risk Stratification

1. **Transplant-free survival may be predicted by a biochemical response to UDCA.** A range of response definitions for UDCA response derived from clinical cohorts exist including the Paris-1, Barcelona, and Toronto criteria.
   ■ With the Paris-1 criteria, if after 1 year of treatment the serum bilirubin level is <ULN, AST or ALT <2×ULN, and ALP <3×ULN, then the 10-year transplant-free survival rate is >90%.
   ■ In clinical trial settings, the Toronto criteria have been used (e.g., a target after intervention of ALP <1.67×ULN, with a 15% drop in ALP, and a serum bilirubin level within the normal range).
   ■ Similarly, the UK-PBC and GLOBE risk scores are composite risk scores based on baseline and post-UDCA-therapy variables from large clinical cohorts. Both accurately predict transplant-free survival at several time points. Both scores variably combine markers of disease risk (e.g., age, AST, ALP, bilirubin) and stage (e.g., albumin, platelets).
2. Varices
   ■ The optimal timing for determining when to screen by endoscopy is debated; in general, a reduced platelet count or increased spleen size are indicators.
   ■ The Newcastle Varices in PBC Risk Score uses several variables (albumin, ALP, platelets, splenomegaly on ultrasonography) to predict a composite risk of varices in patients with PBC.
3. HCC
   ■ Risk is increased in patients who do not achieve a biochemical response to UDCA.
   ■ The risk is increased with male gender, elevated serum aminotransferase levels, thrombocytopenia, and decompensated disease.
4. In general, male gender, younger presentation, and the presence of specific ANA are predictors of poorer outcomes. Less than 50% of women presenting under 40 years of age achieve a biochemical response.
5. Risk scores do not adjust for comorbidity, may underestimate the impact of established cirrhosis in a late presentation of PBC, and require a year of full-dose UDCA therapy to calculate.

Liver Transplantation

1. Patients with decompensated cirrhosis due to PBC are excellent candidates for LT; the Model for End-stage Liver Disease (MELD) score is generally an appropriate way to identify patients likely to benefit (see Chapter 33).
2. End-stage PBC is generally defined as cirrhosis complicated by at least one of the following:
   a. Gastroesophageal variceal hemorrhage
   b. Intractable ascites
   c. Hepatic encephalopathy
   d. Serum albumin <3.5 g/dL
   e. Serum bilirubin >4 mg/dL
3. 1-year survival after LT in patients with PBC is approximately 90%.
4. PBC may recur in the allograft, although recurrence is relatively infrequent and rarely compromises graft survival.
5. Use of cyclosporine-based immunosuppression, as compared with tacrolimus, may protect against recurrent disease.

FURTHER READING

Boonstra K, Beuers U, Ponsioen CY. Epidemiology of primary sclerosing cholangitis and primary biliary cirrhosis: a systematic review. *J Hepatol.* 2012;56:1181–1188.

Carbone M, Mells GF, Pells G, et al. Sex and age are determinants of the clinical phenotype of primary biliary cirrhosis and response to ursodeoxycholic acid. *Gastroenterology.* 2013;144:560–569.

Carbone M, Sharp SJ, Flack S, et al. The UK-PBC risk scores: derivation and validation of a scoring system for long-term prediction of end-stage liver disease in primary biliary cholangitis. *Hepatology.* 2016;63:930–950.

European Association for the Study of the Liver. EASL Clinical Practice Guidelines: the diagnosis and management of patients with primary biliary cholangitis. *J Hepatol.* 2017 Apr 18. Epub ahead of print.

Gong Y, Huang ZB, Christensen E, et al. Ursodeoxycholic acid for primary biliary cirrhosis. *Cochrane Database Syst Rev.* 2008. CD000551.

Hirschfield GM, Gershwin ME. The immunobiology and pathophysiology of primary biliary cirrhosis. *Annu Rev Pathol.* 2013;8:303–330.

Huet PM, Vincent C, Deslaurier J, et al. Portal hypertension and primary biliary cirrhosis: effect of long-term ursodeoxycholic acid treatment. *Gastroenterology.* 2008;135:1552–1560.

Lammers WJ, Hirschfield GM, Corpechot C, et al. Development and validation of a scoring system to predict outcomes of patients with primary biliary cirrhosis receiving ursodeoxycholic acid therapy. *Gastroenterology.* 2015;149:1804–1812.

Nevens F, Andreone P, Mazzella G, et al. A placebo-controlled trial of obeticholic acid in primary biliary cholangitis. *N Engl J Med.* 2016;7:631–643.

Patanwala I, McMeekin P, Walters R, et al. A validated clinical tool for the prediction of varices in PBC: the Newcastle Varices in PBC Score. *J Hepatol.* 2013;59:327–335.

Pollheimer MJ, Fickert P. Animal models in primary biliary cirrhosis and primary sclerosing cholangitis. *Clin Rev Allergy Immunol.* 2015;48:207–217.

Tang R, Chen H, Miao Q, et al. The cumulative effects of known susceptibility variants to predict primary biliary cirrhosis risk. *Genes Immun.* 2015;16:193–198.

Trivedi PJ, Corpechot C, Pares A, et al. Risk stratification in autoimmune cholestatic liver diseases: opportunities for clinicians and trialists. *Hepatology.* 2016;63:644–659.

Webb GJ, Siminovitch KA, Hirschfield GM. The immunogenetics of primary biliary cirrhosis: a comprehensive review. *J Autoimmun.* 2015;64:42–52.

Yang CY, Ma X, Tsuneyama K, et al. IL-12/Th1 and IL-23/Th17 biliary microenvironment in primary biliary cirrhosis: implications for therapy. *Hepatology.* 2014;59:1944–1953.

CHAPTER 17

Primary Sclerosing Cholangitis

Christopher L. Bowlus, MD

KEY POINTS

1 Primary sclerosing cholangitis (PSC) is a chronic cholestatic disease that frequently occurs in association with inflammatory bowel disease (IBD), usually ulcerative colitis.

2 The diagnosis of PSC is based on clinical, biochemical, and, most importantly, cholangiographic findings in the absence of secondary causes of sclerosing cholangitis.

3 The etiology of PSC remains unknown, but both genetic and environmental factors are involved and evidence points toward a defective inflammatory response to intestinal microbial antigens.

4 The progression of PSC is highly variable but typically leads to dominant biliary strictures, cirrhosis, and cholangiocarcinoma (CCA). The risk of colon cancer is increased in patients with PSC and ulcerative colitis.

5 Medical, endoscopic, and surgical therapies have not had a major impact on survival or the prevention of complications of PSC.

6 Liver transplantation is associated with a 5-year survival rate of 85%. Although recurrence of PSC after liver transplantation has been described and appears to be increasing in frequency, graft failure is uncommon.

Overview

1. **Primary sclerosing cholangitis (PSC) is a chronic cholestatic liver disease characterized by inflammation and fibrosis of the intrahepatic or extrahepatic biliary tract, or both.**

2. The evolution of PSC results in damage to the bile ducts and can ultimately lead to cholestasis, biliary cirrhosis, and hepatocellular failure.

3. Long-term follow-up of patients with PSC has revealed a high frequency of bile duct, gallbladder, and colon cancers, which may be related to chronic inflammation and bile acid exposure.

4. Although multiple medical, endoscopic, and surgical therapies have been evaluated for the treatment of PSC, no therapy apart from liver transplantation has demonstrated improvement in survival.

Terminology and Diagnostic Criteria

1. PSC is an idiopathic entity of biliary sclerosis that is distinguished from secondary sclerosing cholangitis by the absence of an obvious etiology (Box 17.1).
    - Diagnosis is based on a cholestatic biochemical profile, with cholangiography by magnetic resonance cholangiography (MRC), endoscopic retrograde cholangiography (ERC), or

> **BOX 17.1 ■ Secondary Causes of Sclerosing Cholangitis**
>
> Cholangiocarcinoma
> Diffuse intrahepatic malignancy (lymphoma)
> Histiocytosis X
> IgG4-related sclerosing cholangitis
> Infectious disorders (AIDS cholangiopathy, recurrent pyogenic cholangitis)
> Intraarterial chemotherapy
> Ischemia resulting from surgical complication, trauma, or vasculitis
> Sarcoidosis
>
> ───────
>
> *AIDS,* Acquired immunodeficiency syndrome; *IgG4,* immunoglobulin G4.

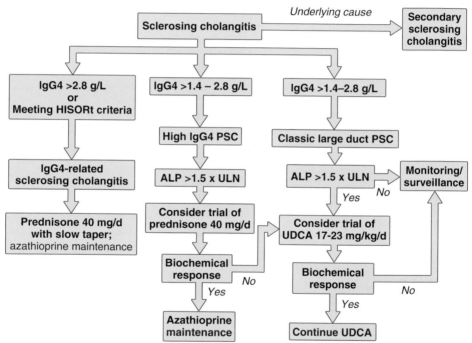

Fig. 17.1 Algorithm for the evaluation and management of patients with cholestatic liver biochemistry test results, nondiagnostic ultrasonography, and negative antimitochondrial antibodies (AMA). Magnetic resonance cholangiography (MRC) of good quality has a specificity greater than 95%. Although the sensitivity of MRC is high (approximately 85%), endoscopic retrograde cholangiography (ERC) should be pursued if the quality of MRC is poor or if the index of suspicion is high, as in patients with inflammatory bowel disease (IBD). *ALP,* Alkaline phosphatase; *HISORt,* histology, imaging, serology, other organ involvement, and response to therapy; *IgG4,* immunoglobulin G 4; *PSC,* primary sclerosing cholangitis; *UDCA,* ursodeoxycholic acid; *ULN,* upper limit of normal.

percutaneous transhepatic cholangiography demonstrating multifocal strictures and segmental dilatations in the absence of secondary causes of sclerosing cholangitis. **MRC is sufficient for diagnosis in most cases,** but ERC may be indicated in cases where MRC is inadequate and clinical suspicion for a diagnosis of PSC is high.

■ Liver biopsy is not indicated in cases with typical cholangiographic findings (Fig. 17.1).

2. **Small duct PSC** refers to histologic changes consistent with PSC but without abnormal bile ducts on cholangiogram.

3. PSC/autoimmune hepatitis (AIH) overlap has features of both PSC and AIH and typically affects children and young adults. In some cases, AIH precedes the development of PSC.

4. Immunoglobulin G4 (IgG4)–related sclerosing cholangitis is a disease related to autoimmune pancreatitis and is a separate entity from PSC; however, approximately 10% of patients with PSC have serum IgG4 levels >1.5 times the upper limit of normal (see also Chapter 24).

Epidemiology

1. The incidence and prevalence of PSC vary geographically and appear to correlate with the prevalence of IBD.
   - The reported incidence (0.9 to 1.3 per 100,000/year) and prevalence (8.5 to 14.2 per 100,000) of PSC are similar in Oslo, Norway, Wales, and Olmsted County, Minnesota.
   - The prevalence of PSC appears to be lower in southern Europe, Asia, and Alaska.
   - The incidence of PSC appears to be increasing, but this observation may reflect a secondary ascertainment bias resulting from the increased use of ERC and MRC.

2. The frequency of PSC in IBD cohorts is 2.4% to 7.5% and varies by geography.
   - The highest rates are in northern Europe and North America (75% to 98%), whereas rates are lower in southern Europe and Asia (21% to 44%).
   - The frequency of IBD in PSC is decreasing.

Etiology and Pathogenesis

The etiology of PSC is unknown, but genetic and acquired factors are likely involved. Although PSC has often been regarded as an autoimmune disorder, several characteristics, such as an absence of a female predilection, lack of a disease-specific autoantibody, and a poor response to glucocorticoids and other immunosuppressive therapies, are not supportive of this hypothesis. By contrast, PSC may be more likely to be an inflammatory disease similar to IBD, in which aberrant innate immune responses to bacterial pathogens are implicated.

1. Genetic factors
   a. A 100-fold increased risk of PSC in first-degree relatives suggests an important genetic component.
   b. Genome-wide association studies have demonstrated that the human leukocyte antigen (HLA) region has the greatest effect on PSC risk.
      - Approximately 40% of patients with PSC carry the HLA-B8 DR3 haplotype, compared with 20% of the unaffected population.
      - HLA-B8, but not HLA-DR3, is associated with PSC in African Americans listed for liver transplantation, suggesting that the causative variant is closer to the HLA B gene.
      - Several, but not all, genes that predispose to IBD also increase the risk of PSC.
      - Genes involved in signaling by bile acids have been associated with PSC risk and disease progression (*TGR5* and *SXR*, respectively).

2. Immunologic mechanisms
   a. Aberrant lymphocyte homing
      - Lymphocytes in livers from patients with PSC express the chemokine receptor CCR9 and $\alpha_4\beta_7$ integrin, which are markers of intestinal lymphocytes.
      - CXCL21 and MAdCAM-1 are ligands for CCR9 and $\alpha_4\beta_7$ integrin and are aberrantly expressed in livers from patients with PSC.
      - These cells have a memory phenotype, suggesting that they are generated in the gut during inflammation and then circulate to the liver, where they are recruited by chemokine

receptors and adhesion molecules expressed in the liver. This may help explain why PSC can develop after colectomy.

b. Activation of innate immune responses to bacterial pathogen-associated molecular patterns (PAMPs) likely circulating from an inflamed intestinal epithelium

- PAMPs activate macrophages, dendritic cells, and natural killer (NK) cells through pattern recognition receptors, including Toll-like receptors (TLRs) and CD14, leading to the secretion of cytokines, which, in turn, activate NK cells (interleukin-12 [IL-12]) and promote recruitment and activation of lymphocytes.
- IgG directed against biliary epithelial cells (BECs) has been detected in the sera of some patients with PSC and induces the expression of TLR4 and TLR9 on BEC secretion of granulocyte-macrophage colony-stimulating factor, IL-1β, and IL-8, which, in turn, may lead to the recruitment of neutrophils, macrophages, and T cells.
- BECs can also secrete inflammatory cytokines by activation of TLRs.

3. Toxic bile

- The absence of phospholipids in bile results not only in unopposed bile acid toxicity, but also in cholesterol supersaturated bile, which could facilitate oxidation of BECs.
- Whether this is a primary insult or a secondary factor leading to progression of disease is unclear.

Clinical Features

1. Demographic features

a. The median age at diagnosis of PSC is 35 to 40 years of age, but PSC can occur in children and older adults.

b. Of patients, two thirds are male.

- In patients with PSC, 60% to 80% have IBD, most commonly ulcerative colitis and less commonly Crohn colitis, with features including extensive colitis, rectal sparing, backwash ileitis, or a quiescent course of disease.
- Female patients are typically diagnosed at an older age and with less frequent IBD.

c. Although best characterized in Caucasians, PSC occurs with a similar frequency in African Americans but with less of a male predominance and a lower frequency of IBD.

2. Symptoms and signs of PSC at the time of presentation are highly variable, as outlined in Table 17.1.

3. Tables 17.2 and 17.3 show the frequencies of abnormal biochemical test results and autoantibodies, respectively, at the time of diagnosis.

4. Hepatic histologic features of PSC are nonspecific but typically include periductal fibrosis, inflammation, and bile duct proliferation alternating with ductal obliteration and ductopenia. Due to the patchy nature of PSC, liver biopsy specimens frequently lack diagnostic features.

5. Radiologic features most commonly seen in PSC include the following:

- Diffusely distributed multifocal annular strictures with intervening segments of normal or slightly ectatic ducts
- Short, bandlike strictures
- Diverticulum-like sacculations

Diseases Associated With Primary Sclerosing Cholangitis

1. Various other autoimmune disorders are associated with PSC (Table 17.4).

2. **IBD is the most common and most important of these associations.**

- The diagnosis of IBD usually precedes the diagnosis of PSC; however, PSC may occur before the diagnosis of IBD or years after proctocolectomy. Furthermore, IBD can present for the first time after liver transplantation for PSC.

TABLE 17.1 ■ **Symptoms and Signs of Primary Sclerosing Cholangitis at Diagnosis**

		Frequency (%)
Symptom	Fatigue	75
	Weight loss	40
	Abdominal pain	37
	Pruritus	30–70
	Jaundice	30–65
	Fever	17–35
	Variceal bleeding	4–15
	Ascites	4–5
	None	44
Sign	Hepatomegaly	34–62
	Jaundice	30–65
	Hyperpigmentation	25
	Splenomegaly	20–30
	Xanthomata	4

TABLE 17.2 ■ **Liver Biochemical Test Results in Primary Sclerosing Cholangitis at Diagnosis**

Test	Abnormal Result (%)
Serum alkaline phosphatase	91–99
Serum aminotransferases	95
Serum bilirubin	41–65
Hypergammaglobulinemia	30
Serum albumin	20
Prothrombin time	10

TABLE 17.3 ■ **Autoantibodies in Primary Sclerosing Cholangitis**

Antibody	Frequency (%)
Perinuclear antineutrophil cytoplasmic antibodies (pANCA)	50–80
Antinuclear antibodies (ANA)	35
Smooth muscle antibodies (SMA)	15
Antiendothelial cell antibodies	13–20
Anticardiolipin antibodies	7–77
Thyroperoxidase	7–16
Thyroglobulin	4–66
Rheumatoid factor	4

TABLE 17.4 ■ **Diseases Associated With Primary Sclerosing Cholangitis**

Disease	Frequency (%)
Inflammatory bowel disease	~80
Type 1 diabetes mellitus	10
Thyroid disorders	8
Psoriasis	4
Rheumatoid arthritis	3
Celiac disease	2
Systemic lupus erythematosus	2
Sarcoidosis	1
Autoimmune hemolytic anemia	<1[a]
Systemic sclerosis/retroperitoneal fibrosis	<1[a]
Immune thrombocytopenic purpura	<1[a]
Any autoimmune disease	24

[a]Limited to case reports.

- PSC associated with Crohn disease appears to have a more favorable course.
- Patients with PSC and ulcerative colitis who undergo proctocolectomy and who have an ileal pouch–anal anastomosis have an increased risk of pouchitis compared with patients who have ulcerative colitis alone.
- The risk of colorectal cancer is increased 5- to 10-fold in patients with PSC and ulcerative colitis compared with those with ulcerative colitis alone (Fig. 17.2). The risk of colon cancer is not increased above that in the general population in patients with PSC who do not have IBD. Surveillance colonoscopy is recommended once the diagnosis of PSC and IBD is established.

Natural History

1. **The natural history of PSC is variable with some patients progressing slowly while others appear not to progress at all.** Early studies had suggested a median survival from time of diagnosis of 12 to 16 years, but more recent studies in nontransplant centers suggest a median survival of greater than 20 years.
   - Without liver transplantation, 70% of deaths in PSC are related to liver failure, whereas 10% to 20% are due to related malignancies.
   - Several prognostic models have been developed to define independent variables associated with survival, but none is sufficiently accurate to be used clinically.
   - Ultrasound elastography and magnetic resonance elastography may more accurately predict clinical outcomes.
   - A more favorable prognosis is seen in patients with small duct PSC or normal serum alkaline phosphatase (Fig. 17.3).
2. Advanced PSC is associated with typical complications of portal hypertension including ascites, spontaneous bacterial peritonitis, and hepatic encephalopathy. As in other biliary types of liver injury, esophageal varices tend to appear early, even before cirrhosis.

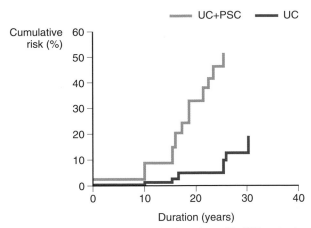

Fig. 17.2 Risk of colorectal cancer in patients with ulcerative colitis (UC) and primary sclerosing cholangitis (PSC), compared with UC alone. (From Jayaram H, Satsangi J, Chapman RW. Increased colorectal neoplasm in chronic ulcerative colitis complicated by primary sclerosing cholangitis: fact or fiction? *Gut.* 2001;48:430–434.)

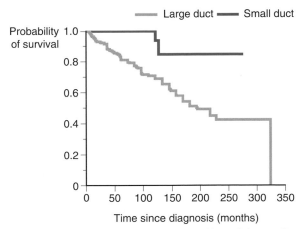

Fig. 17.3 Kaplan-Meier estimated survival curves for patients with small duct and large duct primary sclerosing cholangitis. (From Bjornsson E, Boberg KM, Cullen S, et al. Patients with small duct primary sclerosing cholangitis have a favourable long-term prognosis. *Gut.* 2002;51:731–735.)

3. CCA was originally reported to occur in up to 30% of patients. More recent studies reported a 10-year cumulative frequency of 7% to 9%, with the highest frequency within the first year of diagnosis.

4. Patients with PSC are also at increased risk of gallbladder carcinoma, and gallbladder polyps in PSC have a high rate of dysplasia and cancer.

5. Dominant strictures are defined as strictures with a diameter <1.5 mm in the bile duct or <1.0 mm in a hepatic duct within 2 cm of the bifurcation. They occur with a cumulative frequency of 36% to 57% of patients with PSC and predict diminished survival, largely due to an increase in CCA.

6. Nearly half of patients with PSC who are listed for liver transplantation will experience an episode of bacterial cholangitis.

Treatment

1. **Medical therapy has been disappointing, and no controlled clinical trial has shown a benefit in survival.**
   - Ursodeoxycholic acid (UDCA) has been the most extensively studied medication in large, long-term, randomized, placebo-controlled trials at doses of 13 to 15 mg/kg/day, 17 to 23 mg/kg/day, and 28 to 30 mg/kg/day. Although treatment with UDCA was associated with an increase in death and liver transplantation, a subgroup of patients in whom the serum alkaline phosphatase level normalizes may benefit from treatment (Fig. 17.4).
   - Glucocorticoids and other immunosuppressive medications have been studied but only in small trials and without evidence of a clear benefit. Benefit has been seen in pediatric patients with PSC/AIH overlap, in whom immunosuppression resulted in reversal of biliary strictures on ERC; adult patients with PSC/AIH overlap, in whom glucocorticoids may also be beneficial; and patients with IgG4-related cholangitis.
   - Reports of beneficial effects of antibiotics in PSC include a randomized trial of vancomycin in adults and a case series of open-label vancomycin in pediatric patients with PSC.
2. Although dilation of strictures has been demonstrated to lessen jaundice and to relieve bacterial cholangitis, a long-term benefit of these interventions in halting disease progression has not been demonstrated.
3. Biliary reconstructive surgical procedures have also been shown to relieve symptoms and have the advantage of excluding CCA; however, a long-term impact on prolonging disease progression has not been shown. Moreover, biliary reconstructive surgery has been associated with increased morbidity in patients who subsequently undergo liver transplantation and should be avoided if possible.
4. **Liver transplantation is currently the treatment of choice for patients with end-stage PSC.** Liver transplantation in patients with PSC is associated with patient survival rates of up to 90% at 1 year and 85% at 5 years (see Chapter 33).

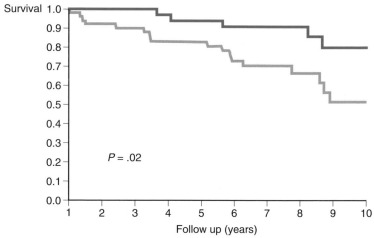

Fig. 17.4 Kaplan-Meier analysis of end point–free survival (cholangiocarcinoma, liver transplantation, or death) for patients in whom the serum alkaline phosphatase level normalized (blue line, $n = 35$) and those with a persistently elevated alkaline phosphatase (gold line, $n = 52$) demarcated by years ($P = .02$). (From Stanich PP, Bjornsson E, Gossard AA, et al. Alkaline phosphatase normalization is associated with better prognosis in primary sclerosing cholangitis. *Dig Liver Disease.* 2011;43:309–313.)

- Indications for liver transplantation are similar to those for other chronic liver diseases. Additional indications related to PSC include intractable pruritus, recurrent cholangitis, and early CCA.
- PSC recurs in up to 20% to 25% of patients after 5 to 10 years; however, the diagnosis of recurrent PSC is difficult because of lack of standard diagnostic criteria and potential confounding factors that can mimic PSC, including chronic rejection, cytomegalovirus infection, and hepatic artery thrombosis.

Complications and Their Treatment

1. The management of complications related to portal hypertension is similar to that for other forms of chronic liver disease.
2. Dominant strictures
   - The most common site is the perihilar region. A dominant stricture raises concern about CCA, although most dominant strictures are benign.
   - **Dominant strictures should be treated endoscopically or radiologically with balloon dilation and stenting.** In all cases, biliary histology and brush cytology should be obtained to attempt to exclude CCA. Long-term stenting is rarely necessary.
3. Bacterial cholangitis frequently occurs in patients who have had a previous biliary procedure and who have an obstructing dominant stricture.
   - Bacterial cholangitis should be treated with broad-spectrum intravenous antibiotics and, in the case of a dominant stricture, drainage.
   - For patients with frequent episodes of bacterial cholangitis unresponsive to dilation of a dominant stricture, prophylactic or on-demand therapy with ciprofloxacin, which achieves high biliary concentrations, is often effective in reducing the frequency of episodes.
4. CCA carries a poor prognosis and does not respond well to chemotherapy or radiation therapy. Most liver transplant programs consider CCA associated with PSC to be an absolute or relative contraindication to liver transplantation; however, protocols incorporating combined radiotherapy and chemotherapy offer acceptable survival in a subset of patients with CCA who undergo liver transplantation. Distinguishing a benign stricture from CCA remains difficult (see Chapters 35 and 36).
   - CA19-9 levels are often elevated in CCA but are also elevated in bacterial cholangitis. In addition, variants in the *FUT2* gene influence serum CA19-9 levels. At a cutoff of 130 U/mL, the sensitivity and specificity of CA19-9 for CCA are 79% and 98%, respectively.
   - Imaging studies rarely detect CCA but can be virtually diagnostic in patients with typical features of delayed venous enhancement.
   - Brush cytology has low sensitivity, ranging from 18% to 40%, but very high specificity. The presence of polysomy by fluorescence in situ hybridization may increase the sensitivity.
   - Positron emission tomography (PET) has no proven role in the diagnosis of CCA in PSC.
   - Evidence to recommend routine screening is insufficient, but annual ultrasonography or MR imaging and CA19-9 measurement are often performed.
5. The new onset of pruritus should prompt an evaluation for a dominant stricture or CCA. Identifying an effective agent in an individual patient often requires trials of several different medications.
   - Cholestyramine 4 to 16 g daily in divided doses (should be used as first-line therapy); separate from UDCA by at least 2 hours
   - Rifampin 150 to 300 mg twice daily
   - Oral opiate antagonists (e.g., naltrexone 50 mg daily)
   - Sertraline 75 to 100 mg daily
   - Antihistamines and phenobarbital are not recommended.

6. Gallbladder disease
   - Among patients with PSC, 25% will develop gallstones, usually black pigment stones. No association exists with disease stage or use of UDCA.
   - Patients with PSC are at increased risk of gallbladder carcinoma and should be screened annually with ultrasonography. Cholecystectomy should be considered in any patient with PSC who has a gallbladder polyp or mass.
7. Steatorrhea can be caused by a decrease in duodenal concentration of bile acids, and thus a reduction in micellar formation, or concurrent conditions such as chronic pancreatitis and celiac disease.
8. Fat-soluble vitamin deficiencies (A, D, E, and K) can be related to steatorrhea, but levels of fat-soluble vitamins A, D, and E should be measured even in the absence of steatorrhea and deficiencies treated with replacement therapy.
9. Peristomal varices are common in patients who have undergone a proctocolectomy for underlying IBD and who have an ileal stoma.
   - Bleeding from peristomal varices can be controlled by a transjugular intrahepatic portosystemic shunt.
10. Patients with PSC should be screened for hepatic osteodystrophy with bone density testing at diagnosis and every 2 to 3 years thereafter. Treatment is as follows:
    - Osteopenia: Calcium, 1.0 to 1.5 g; and vitamin D, 1000 IU daily
    - Osteoporosis: Calcium and vitamin D, with consideration given to administration of a bisphosphonate

Acknowledgment

Dr. Bowlus acknowledges the contribution of Dr. Russell H. Wiesner, who authored this chapter in the second edition of the *Handbook of Liver Disease*.

FURTHER READING

Bjornsson E, Olsson R, Bergquist A, et al. The natural history of small-duct primary sclerosing cholangitis. *Gastroenterology*. 2008;134:975–980.

Boonstra K, Weersma RK, van Erpecum KJ, et al. Population-based epidemiology, malignancy risk, and outcome of primary sclerosing cholangitis. *Hepatology*. 2013;58:2045–2055.

Chapman R, Fevery J, Kalloo A, et al. Diagnosis and management of primary sclerosing cholangitis. *Hepatology*. 2010;51:660–678.

Claessen MM, Vleggaar FP, Tytgat KM, et al. High lifetime risk of cancer in primary sclerosing cholangitis. *J Hepatol*. 2009;50:158–164.

Corpechot C, Gaouar F, El Naggar A, et al. Baseline values and changes in liver stiffness measured by transient elastography are associated with severity of fibrosis and outcomes in patients with primary sclerosing cholangitis. *Gastroenterology*. 2014;146:970–979.

European Association for the Study of the Liver. EASL Clinical Practice Guidelines: management of cholestatic liver diseases. *J Hepatol*. 2009;51:237–267.

Gotthardt DN, Rudolph G, Kloters-Plachky P, et al. Endoscopic dilation of dominant stenosis in primary sclerosing cholangitis: outcome after long-term treatment. *Gastrointest Endosc*. 2010;71:527–534.

Graziadei IW. Recurrence of primary sclerosing cholangitis after liver transplantation. *Liver Transpl*. 2002;8:575–581.

Lindor KD, Kowdley KV, Harrison ME. ACG Clinical Guideline: primary sclerosing cholangitis. *Am J Gastroenterol*. 2015;110:646–659.

Liu JZ, Hov JR, Folseraas T, et al. Dense genotyping of immune-related disease regions identifies nine new risk loci for primary sclerosing cholangitis. *Nat Genet*. 2013;45:670–675.

Loftus Jr EV, Harewood GC, Loftus CG, et al. PSC-IBD: a unique form of inflammatory bowel disease associated with primary sclerosing cholangitis. *Gut*. 2005;54:91–96.

Sarkar S, Bowlus CL. Primary sclerosing cholangitis: multiple phenotypes, multiple approaches. *Clin Liver Dis*. 2016;20:67–77.

CHAPTER 18

Hemochromatosis

Nicholas J. Procaccini, MD, JD, MS ■ Kris V. Kowdley, MD, FACP

KEY POINTS

1. Hereditary hemochromatosis (HH) is an inherited disorder characterized by iron-mediated tissue injury reflecting impaired regulation of intestinal iron absorption.

2. Classic HH is most commonly associated with autosomal recessive inheritance of mutations in the *HFE* gene that create unregulated intestinal iron absorption.

3. Mutations in other genes such as hemojuvelin, hepcidin, transferrin receptor 2, and ferroportin are rare causes of HH.

4. Although the *HFE* gene mutation is most prevalent in the Caucasian population (0.4% in northern Europeans), its clinical penetrance is low. Relatively few patients homozygous for the C282Y mutation in the *HFE* gene manifest the complete phenotype.

5. Consequences of iron overload are often unrecognized until features of advanced disease, including cirrhosis, diabetes mellitus, or cardiomyopathy, develop.

6. Patients in whom hemochromatosis is detected early and who are treated with iron depletion therapy (phlebotomy) have an excellent prognosis with normal life expectancy.

7. If suspected, HH should be evaluated with biochemical markers of iron overload (serum transferrin saturation and ferritin), *HFE* gene mutation analysis, and, in selected cases, liver biopsy (for confirmation of diagnosis and staging).

8. Once confirmed, HH should be treated with iron depletion therapy to maintain the serum ferritin level in the range of 50 to 100 μg/L.

Epidemiology and Genetics

1. In Caucasians, approximately 1 in 200 to 1 in 250 are homozygous, and 1 in 8 to 1 in 12 are heterozygous, for the C282Y mutation of the *HFE* gene, the most common genetic defect in HH.
2. The clinical penetrance of the C282Y mutation is low (Table 18.1).
3. HH associated with other mutations such as juvenile HH and mutations of the ferroportin transfer gene are rare (Table 18.2).

Classification

HFE HEMOCHROMATOSIS (TYPE 1)

1. The *HFE* gene is a major histocompatibility complex (MHC) class I–like gene and is located on the short arm of chromosome 6 telomeric to the A3 MHC class 1 histocompatibility locus.
   ■ **Homozygous mutation of C282Y accounts for approximately 85% to 90% of individuals with HH.**

TABLE 18.1 ■ Penetrance of the C282Y Mutation

Type of Penetrance	Definition	Frequency Among C282Y Homozygotes (%)	
		Women	Men
Biochemical	Elevated serum transferrin saturation and ferritin level	50	75
Clinical	Hepatocellular carcinoma, hepatic fibrosis or cirrhosis, meta-carpophalangeal arthritis, or elevated serum aminotransferase levels	Rare	28

TABLE 18.2 ■ Genes Mutated in Each Type of Hereditary Hemochromatosis

Type	Common Name	Gene (and Gene Product)
1	Classic hemochromatosis	*HFE* (HFE)
2A	Juvenile hemochromatosis	*HFE2* (hemojuvelin)
2B	Juvenile hemochromatosis	*HAMP* (hepcidin)
3	*Tfr2*-related hemochromatosis	*Tfr2* (transferrin receptor-2)
4	Ferroportin-related iron overload	*SLC40A1* (ferroportin)

- Homozygosity for H63D, another mutation of the *HFE* gene, is associated with less severe iron overload and rarely results in expression of the clinical phenotype of HH.
- C282Y/H63D compound heterozygosity accounts for 5% to 7% of clinically expressed HH.

2. The *HFE* gene is expressed primarily in the crypt cells of the duodenum, where it interacts with the transferrin receptor and beta-2 microglobulin.
3. Hepcidin is a protein thought to play a role in iron metabolism by binding to ferroportin and decreasing iron export from enterocytes and macrophages. In HH, hepcidin expression is decreased, resulting in increased iron absorption from enterocytes and increased release from macrophages.
4. There is variable penetrance and clinical expression for C282Y homozygotes. Less than 10% will develop end-organ disease.
5. An effect of modifying genes has also been postulated to contribute to the variable phenotypic disease expression.

NON-HFE HEMOCHROMATOSIS

1. HH associated with mutations in other genes is rare (see Table 18.2).
2. Unlike HFE HH, numerous different mutations are associated with each type of non-HFE HH.
3. **Type 2 HH** (juvenile hemochromatosis) is associated with more severe iron overload and tissue damage that develops earlier in life than HFE HH.
4. **Type 3 HH** has clinical manifestations that are similar to those of HFE HH.
5. **Type 4 HH** has distinct clinical and histologic manifestations.
   - The serum transferrin saturation may be normal with an elevated serum ferritin level.

- Iron is deposited predominantly in cells of the reticuloendothelial system in the liver.
- Patients may tolerate phlebotomy poorly.

6. All forms of HH are inherited as autosomal recessive traits, except for type 4 HH, which is inherited as an autosomal dominant trait.

Pathophysiology

IRON ABSORPTION

1. Dietary iron is absorbed primarily in the crypt enterocytes of the duodenum. **Only approximately 10% of dietary iron is absorbed in physiologically normal persons,** with absorption regulated in accordance with body iron stores.
2. In normal persons, iron absorption is downregulated when serum transferrin saturation is high and following high dietary iron intake.
3. In persons with HH, iron absorption is increased and is not downregulated as in normal persons, thereby resulting in a positive iron balance.
4. Small bowel mucosal ferritin and ferritin mRNA levels are inappropriately decreased in HH; this pattern is typically associated with iron deficiency and is corrected by iron repletion.
5. Iron absorption involves the uptake of iron from the intestinal lumen into the enterocytes with subsequent transfer from enterocytes to plasma. Both processes are increased in HH. In vivo kinetic studies indicate that increased transport of iron from the serosal side of the intestine into plasma drives the increased iron absorption.
6. **The effect of the *HFE* mutation is thought to be mediated by lack of sufficient expression of hepcidin in the liver in response to iron stores at the level of the hepatocyte; this leads in turn to a failure to inhibit iron absorption in the duodenum, thereby resulting in iron overload.**

PARENCHYMAL IRON DEPOSITION IN TYPES 1 TO 3 HEREDITARY HEMOCHROMATOSIS

1. **Iron is deposited in multiple organs including liver, heart, pancreas, joints, skin, gonads, and other endocrine organs.**
2. The major site of iron deposition in HH is the liver, consistent with the liver's role as the major storage organ for iron.
3. Iron is deposited primarily in hepatocytes as ferritin and subsequently also as hemosiderin, with a decreasing gradient of iron absorption from periportal (zone 1) to pericentral (zone 3) hepatocytes.
4. Late in the disease, iron may be deposited in Kupffer and bile duct cells.
5. Saturation of serum transferrin precedes hepatic iron accumulation and is responsible for an initial increase in iron delivery to the tissues.
6. Later, non–transferrin-bound iron may play a role in iron delivery and toxicity.
7. A defect of iron storage in reticuloendothelial cells is also possible.

EFFECT OF ALCOHOL INTAKE

1. Excessive alcohol intake is associated with higher serum iron levels, increased severity of clinical disease, and an increased risk of cirrhosis and hepatocellular carcinoma (HCC) in C282Y homozygotes.
2. Liver fibrosis and cirrhosis occur at an earlier age and at lower levels of hepatic iron in these persons.
3. Similarly, HH can accentuate development of alcoholic liver disease (ALD), potentially through excess free radical formation in the presence of iron overload.

EFFECT OF NONALCOHOLIC FATTY LIVER DISEASE

1. Similar to ALD, coexistent nonalcoholic fatty liver disease (NAFLD) is associated with increased serum iron levels and transferrin saturation.
2. This can accelerate the progression of fibrosis in HH.
3. Patients with nonalcoholic steatohepatitis (NASH) with higher iron indices have higher NASH activity scores and more rapid progression of fibrosis (see Chapter 9).

LIVER DAMAGE

1. Excess iron may mediate liver damage or promote liver fibrosis by several mechanisms.
   - Iron may catalyze the formation of free radicals, which may damage cell organelles.
   - Iron may damage DNA directly and thus lead to mutations and carcinogenesis.
   - Iron may stimulate development of hepatic fibrosis by increasing collagen synthesis.
2. Excessive alcohol intake may cause liver damage through accelerated tissue injury mediated by oxidative and nonoxidative mechanisms.
3. Liver disease in HH is characterized by progressive fibrosis, although histology characteristically does not show significant inflammation.
4. The presence of hepatitis (inflammatory changes) can suggest a coexistent viral infection, NASH, or ALD.
5. Cirrhosis and HCC develop with long-standing iron overload; however, HCC without cirrhosis is rare.
6. Higher liver iron concentrations increase the risk of fibrosis and ultimately cirrhosis.
7. The risk of fibrosis and cirrhosis increases as men reach age 40 and in women over 50, although potentially earlier if coexisting factors (e.g., viral hepatitis, NASH, excessive alcohol intake) are present.

Clinical Features

1. Before 1960, HH was typically recognized clinically late in its course with end-organ damage including "bronze diabetes mellitus," arthritis, liver disease, and heart failure.
2. With increased awareness of the disease, the diagnosis is now made most commonly in the asymptomatic phase through laboratory testing.
3. The diagnosis of asymptomatic HH is often made following discovery of abnormal serum iron markers in the following clinical situations:
   - Elevated serum aminotransferase levels
   - Elevated iron stores
   - Family or population screening
4. When the diagnosis is made after the onset of symptoms, the most common symptoms now at the time of diagnosis include:
   - Weakness, lethargy, or fatigue
   - Arthralgia or arthritis (women more commonly than men)
   - Nonspecific right upper quadrant pain
   - Loss of libido or potency (men)
5. Other manifestations include:
   - Increased skin pigmentation
   - Diabetes mellitus
   - Amenorrhea (women)
   - Liver disease
   - Heart failure

LIVER DISEASE

1. An increased hepatic iron concentration is present in patients with HFE HH and an elevated serum ferritin level.
2. Liver disease is the most common form of end-organ damage seen in HH.
3. **The severity of liver disease generally correlates with the severity of hepatic iron overload,** although coexisting liver diseases can increase liver injury.
4. The level of serum aminotransferase elevation is generally modest, and serum aminotransferase levels frequently normalize once excess iron stores are removed.
5. If iron depletion is achieved and maintained before the development of hepatic fibrosis or cirrhosis, further hepatic complications are prevented.
6. Once cirrhosis has developed, patients remain at increased risk of HCC even after iron depletion.
7. Increased prevalence rates of chronic hepatitis B and C, NASH, and excessive alcohol intake have been reported in patients with phenotypic HH.
8. Excessive alcohol use is associated with increased morbidity in patients with HH.

CARDIAC DISEASE

1. **HH (especially type 2) can be associated with cardiac dysfunction and arrhythmias.**
   - Cardiac dysfunction can manifest as a restrictive or dilated cardiomyopathy.
   - Atrial and ventricular dysrhythmias can occur.
2. Cardiac involvement occurs relatively late in the course of HFE HH, and iron depletion before the development of dilated cardiomyopathy improves cardiac function. Cardiac dysfunction has become less common with earlier diagnosis and treatment of HH.
3. Cardiomyopathy is a major cause of postoperative morbidity and mortality after liver transplantation for HH.

DIABETES MELLITUS

1. Diabetes mellitus probably results from iron deposition in the pancreas.
2. It may be associated with increased plasma insulin levels, a finding that suggests peripheral insulin resistance (type 2), particularly in association with liver disease.

JOINT DISEASE

1. **Joint disease is a major cause of morbidity.**
2. It characteristically involves the second and third metacarpophalangeal joints; other metacarpophalangeal joints and wrist joints are also frequently involved. Less commonly affected joints include shoulders, hips, knees, and ankles.
3. Pathologic features include joint space narrowing, chondrocalcinosis, subchondral cyst formation, and osteopenia.
4. Arthropathy does not improve with iron depletion.

INFECTIONS

1. Patients with HH have an increased risk of bacterial, viral, and fungal infections.
2. The mechanism for the increased risk of infections is unknown but is postulated to relate to iron-mediated impairment of innate and acquired immune responses.

3. Infections may be caused by the following uncommon bacteria:
   - *Vibrio vulnificus*
   - *Yersinia enterocolitica*
   - *Yersinia pseudotuberculosis*
   - *Listeria monocytogenes*

Natural History and Prognosis

1. Liver disease is slowly progressive but is usually mild (except with concomitant viral hepatitis or alcohol abuse) when the hepatic iron concentration is <200 μmol/g dry weight of liver.
2. Hepatic decompensation and HCC are the most common end-organ manifestations of HH and account for 60% of iron overload–related mortality.
3. Patients with HH and cirrhosis have a significantly increased (20- to 200-fold) risk of HCC and should undergo routine surveillance for HCC.
4. An increased risk of mixed HCC-cholangiocarcinoma has also been reported.
5. Concern exists about an increased risk of nonhepatobiliary cancers in HH, but the data are conflicting.
6. Some manifestations improve with iron depletion (malaise, fatigue, skin pigmentation, diabetes mellitus, abdominal pain, cardiac dysfunction, reduced energy, elevated serum aminotransferase levels, noncirrhotic hepatic fibrosis), whereas others do not (arthropathy, hypogonadism, cirrhosis).
7. Patients without cirrhosis or diabetes mellitus have a normal life expectancy if iron depletion is maintained.
8. Patients with cirrhosis or diabetes mellitus have a significantly decreased life expectancy, but the prognosis is improved after iron depletion therapy.
9. Patients with HH may need liver transplantation for end-stage liver disease or HCC.
10. Liver transplantation in patients with HH is associated with an increased risk of infections, especially fungal infections, cardiac events, and decreased survival.
11. HH has been reported to be associated with even worse posttransplant outcomes than other causes of iron overload; however, outcomes of liver transplantation appear to have improved.

Diagnosis

CLINICAL SUSPICION AND LABORATORY TESTS

1. HH should be considered in the following conditions (Fig. 18.1):
   - Degenerative arthropathy
   - Unexplained hepatomegaly or liver disease
   - Unexplained hypogonadism
   - Elevated serum transferrin saturation or ferritin levels
   - Elevated serum aminotransferase levels
2. **The serum transferrin saturation and ferritin level are the initial tests if HH is suspected.**
3. The serum transferrin saturation is more sensitive and specific than the serum ferritin level for HH.
   - Elevation of the transferrin saturation is the earliest manifestation of HH.
   - Serum ferritin is an acute phase reactant and can be elevated in inflammatory conditions and other chronic liver diseases (e.g., NASH, chronic hepatitis C, ALD).
4. Circadian and postprandial variations of the transferrin saturation can be a source of laboratory error; therefore patients should fast before testing.
5. A transferrin saturation of more than 45% warrants further evaluation for HH.
6. Isolated elevation of the serum ferritin with a normal transferrin saturation may indicate type 4 HH, particularly in non-Caucasian patients.

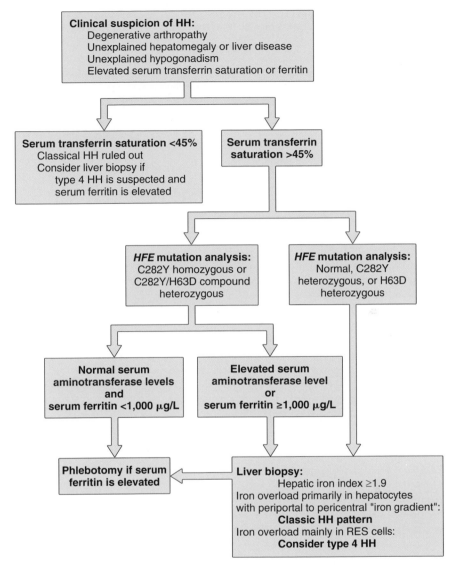

Fig. 18.1 Proposed algorithm for the diagnosis and treatment of hereditary hemochromatosis (HH). *RES,* Reticuloendothelial system.

GENOTYPING

1. *HFE* mutation analysis should be performed in all persons with a persistently elevated transferrin saturation, especially if the serum ferritin level is also elevated.
2. The presence of C282Y homozygosity or C282Y/H63D compound heterozygosity confirms the diagnosis of HFE HH in the appropriate clinical setting.
3. Genetic tests for non-HFE HH are not currently available for clinical use.

TABLE 18.3 ■ **Tests Used to Assess Hepatic Iron Overload in Liver Biopsy Specimens**

Test	Comment
Hepatic iron index (hepatic iron concentration in μmol/g dry weight divided by the patient's age in years) measured in fresh or preserved tissue	Hepatic iron index ≥1.9 is frequently observed in patients with phenotypic HH, but in many C282Y homozygotes the index is <1.9.
Staining for hepatic iron (Perls Prussian blue stain)	Staining for hepatic iron is important because sampling variability can yield a low hepatic iron index.

HH, Hereditary hemochromatosis.

LIVER BIOPSY

1. The current indications for liver biopsy are limited.
   - For diagnosis when HFE genotyping is negative in a patient with suspected non-HFE HH
   - For staging (presence or absence of cirrhosis) in a patient with confirmed HFE HH when the serum ferritin level exceeds 1000 μg/L or when the serum alanine or aspartate aminotransferase level is elevated
2. Liver biopsy for diagnosis involves two studies (Table 18.3): The hepatic iron index and staining for hepatic iron.
3. Liver biopsy for staging is important because of the following:
   - Histopathology remains the gold standard for establishing the presence of cirrhosis in the absence of overt evidence such as portal hypertension.
   - The presence of cirrhosis is associated with increased risks of mortality and HCC.
   - Knowledge of the presence or absence of cirrhosis may influence management (e.g., patients with cirrhosis require surveillance for HCC).

OTHER TESTS

1. Magnetic resonance imaging can estimate hepatic iron quantitatively in a noninvasive fashion.
2. Quantitative phlebotomy is useful for estimation of iron overload when liver biopsy is not required. Each phlebotomy usually removes 500 mL of blood (approximately 250 mg of iron); the need to remove 4 g or more of iron before the onset of iron-limited erythropoiesis with anemia indicates the presence of significant iron overload.

Differential Diagnosis

1. **Secondary iron overload** can occur in the following situations:
   - Increased red blood cell turnover (e.g., disorders of ineffective erythropoiesis)
   - Repeated blood transfusions
   - A combination of these factors
2. Major causes of secondary iron overload can be classified as follows:
   a. Iron-loading anemias with or without transfusion
      - Thalassemia major
      - Sideroblastic anemia
      - Chronic hemolytic anemias
   b. Dietary iron overload (rare)
   c. Iron overload associated with chronic liver disease including

- ALD
- Chronic hepatitis B and C
- NAFLD
  d. Miscellaneous causes
  - Porphyria cutanea tarda
  - African iron overload
  - Neonatal hemochromatosis
  - Aceruloplasminemia
  - Atransferrinemia

3. The following features are helpful in differentiating secondary iron overload associated with chronic anemias from HH:
   - Liver biopsy in secondary iron overload shows iron overload primarily in Kupffer and other reticuloendothelial cells, with a paucity of iron in hepatocytes. A periportal to pericentral "iron gradient" is also not observed in these conditions; however, a similar pattern may be observed in type 4 HH.
   - Secondary iron overload is typically milder (1+ to 2+).
   - Quantitative phlebotomy demonstrates the onset of iron-limited erythropoiesis with anemia before removal of 4 g or more of iron.

Treatment

1. **Iron depletion by serial phlebotomy remains the cornerstone of therapy for HH.** Suggested protocol for serial phlebotomy:
   - Phlebotomy is performed, with removal of 500 mL of blood (approximately 250 mg of iron) weekly or biweekly until the serum ferritin declines to 50 to 100 µg/L.
   - The hematocrit or hemoglobin value should be checked before each session, and the serum ferritin level should be assessed every 3 months (after every 10 to 12 phlebotomies).
   - If the hematocrit value is <32%, phlebotomy should be postponed, and the frequency should be decreased to once every 2 weeks.
   - Once the serum ferritin level is <50 µg/L, it should be tested every 3 to 4 months, with phlebotomy repeated as required to maintain the serum ferritin level at 50 to 100 µg/L.
   - The required frequency of maintenance phlebotomy depends on the rate of iron accumulation as is generally required once in 2 to 4 months.
2. Precautions during phlebotomy:
   - Anemia should be prevented by monitoring the hematocrit value before each phlebotomy and ensuring adequate dietary protein, vitamin B12, and folate intake.
   - High doses of ascorbic and citric acid, as well as a diet rich in iron, should be avoided. Moderate consumption of red meat is permissible.
   - Alcohol should be avoided while iron depletion therapy is in progress.
   - During maintenance phlebotomy, gastric acid suppression with a proton pump inhibitor may allow a reduction in the frequency of phlebotomies, presumably by decreasing iron absorption in the duodenum.
3. Because of increased susceptibility to *V. vulnificus* infection, patients should avoid eating uncooked seafood and exposing open wounds to warm coastal seawater. Susceptibility to *V. vulnificus* infection does not resolve with iron depletion therapy.
4. Iron chelators (deferoxamine, deferiprone, deferasirox) are less effective and more expensive than phlebotomy and associated with adverse effects. These drugs are used only in patients with anemia or those who cannot tolerate phlebotomy.

Screening

FAMILY SCREENING

1. All first-degree relatives of patients with confirmed HH should undergo screening for HH.
2. *HFE* mutation analysis or a fasting transferrin saturation and ferritin is suggested for screening.
3. Relatives of patients with HFE HH who are negative for an *HFE* mutation do not require further testing.
4. Relatives who are positive for an *HFE* mutation should be monitored with an annual serum ferritin level, and phlebotomy should be initiated when appropriate.

POPULATION SCREENING

1. Population screening for HH is not generally recommended.
2. Several economic models have not found population screening to be cost effective.
3. Phenotypic screening (transferrin saturation) could be considered in high-risk populations, but negative results in young adults should be interpreted with caution because the transferrin saturation may become elevated with aging.

FURTHER READING

Adams PC, Barton JC. Haemochromatosis. *Lancet*. 2007;370:1855–1860.

Allen KJ, Gurrin LC, Constantine CC, et al. Iron-overload-related disease in HFE hereditary hemochromatosis. *N Engl J Med*. 2008;358:221–230.

Bacon BR, Adams PC, Kowdley KV, et al. Diagnosis and management of hemochromatosis: 2011 practice guidelines by the American Association for the Study of Liver Diseases. *Hepatology*. 2011;54:328–343.

Fix OK, Kowdley KV. Hereditary hemochromatosis. *Minerva Med*. 2008;99:605–617.

Franchini M. Hereditary iron overload: update on pathophysiology, diagnosis, and treatment. *Am J Hematol*. 2006;81:202–209.

Kowdley KV, Brandhagen DJ, Gish RG, et al. Survival after liver transplantation in patients with hepatic iron overload: the national hemochromatosis transplant registry. *Gastroenterology*. 2005;129:494–503.

Olynyk JK, Trinder D, Ramm GA, et al. Hereditary hemochromatosis in the post-HFE era. *Hepatology*. 2008;48:991–1001.

Online Mendelian Inheritance in Man (OMIM). Johns Hopkins University, Baltimore. MIM No. 235200. 2010 Jan 7. Available at http://www.ncbi.nlm.nih.gov/omim/235200.

Pietrangelo A. Hemochromatosis: an endocrine liver disease. *Hepatology*. 2007;46:1291–1301.

Weiss G. Genetic mechanisms and modifying factors in hereditary hemochromatosis. *Nat Rev Gastroenterol Hepatol*. 2010;7:50–58.

CHAPTER 19

Wilson Disease and Related Disorders

Michael L. Schilsky, MD

KEY POINTS

1 Wilson disease (WD) is an autosomal recessive disorder of copper metabolism caused by disease-specific defects in the *ATP7B* gene that encodes a copper-transporting P-type adenosine triphosphatase (ATPase) expressed primarily in the trans-Golgi network of hepatocytes.

2 Loss of *ATP7B* function is responsible for defective biliary excretion of copper by liver cells that leads to pathologic accumulation of hepatic copper and secondary organ injury as well as defective copper incorporation into ceruloplasmin, which is a phenotypic marker in most patients with WD.

3 Most patients with symptomatic WD present clinically in the second or third decades of life with hepatic disease and in the third or fourth decades with neuropsychiatric features; however, patients have been diagnosed even into the eighth decade of life.

4 Liver disease due to WD ranges from asymptomatic to chronic hepatitis, cirrhosis, and even acute liver failure (ALF).

5 The diagnosis of WD requires a combination of clinical signs and biochemical testing or detection of two disease-specific mutations of *ATP7B* by molecular testing.

6 Family screening of first-degree relatives is mandatory, and genetic screening for the *ATP7B* mutation with use of the index patient's DNA as a reference should be performed if possible.

7 Initial treatment of symptomatic patients with WD should be with copper chelation therapy: D-penicillamine or trientine; maintenance therapy or treatment of asymptomatic patients may be with a chelating agent or zinc salts, which induce a blockade of copper absorption.

8 Liver transplantation (LT) is indicated for patients with WD and ALF or decompensated cirrhosis unresponsive to medical therapy.

Copper Metabolism (Figs. 19.1 and 19.2)

1. Approximately 1 to 2 mg of dietary copper is absorbed by the proximal small intestinal epithelial cells daily. The copper transporter CTR1 is responsible for copper uptake by intestinal epithelial cells, and the Menkes disease protein ATP7A participates in copper transfer from epithelial cells into the circulation.

2. Copper that is transferred into the portal circulation is bound to serum albumin and amino acids. The remaining intraepithelial copper is mostly bound to the endogenous chelating peptide metallothionein and is subsequently excreted as intestinal epithelial cells are sloughed. No significant enterohepatic circulation of copper occurs.

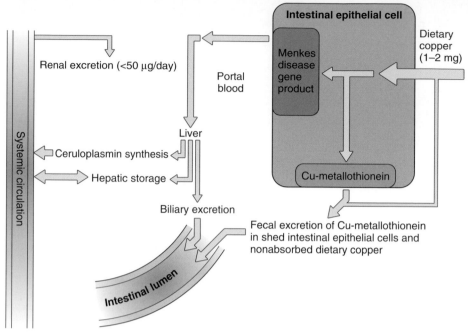

Fig. 19.1 Copper (Cu) absorption and excretion. Dietary copper (1 to 2 mg/day) is transported into the intestinal epithelial cell, with the Menkes gene product regulating transport into the portal circulation (25% to 60%). The remaining intraepithelial copper is bound to metallothionein and is subsequently excreted in stool as the intestinal epithelial cells are sloughed. A small amount of the absorbed copper is excreted in urine, but the majority is taken up by the hepatocyte, synthesized into ceruloplasmin, and stored in the liver or excreted in bile.

3. Only a small fraction of circulating copper (<50 µg/24 hours) is normally excreted by the kidney; most is taken up by hepatocytes, and excess is excreted into bile.
4. In the hepatocyte, copper is complexed with and detoxified by metallothionein or glutathione and is used as a cofactor for specific cellular enzymes, incorporated into ceruloplasmin that is excreted into the circulation, or excreted into bile.
5. The site of hepatocellular copper incorporation into ceruloplasmin is the trans-Golgi apparatus. ATP7B is presumed to be responsible for copper transport in this compartment and subsequent incorporation into ceruloplasmin.
6. The delivery of cytosolic copper to specific intracellular locations is mediated by small proteins termed *copper chaperones.*
7. Relocation of ATP7B from the trans-Golgi network to a vesicular compartment adjacent to the canalicular membrane in response to increased hepatocellular copper content facilitates canalicular and biliary copper excretion. A secondary route for biliary copper excretion of hepatocellular copper is via transport of copper-glutathione. In addition, some intracellular copper transports back across the hepatocyte basolateral plasma membrane into the circulation.

Genetics

1. WD is an autosomal recessive disease with an incidence of 1/20,000 to 30,000 in most populations. Gene frequency for WD is estimated to be 0.3% to 0.7%, thus accounting for a heterozygote carrier rate of slightly >1 in 150 to 200.

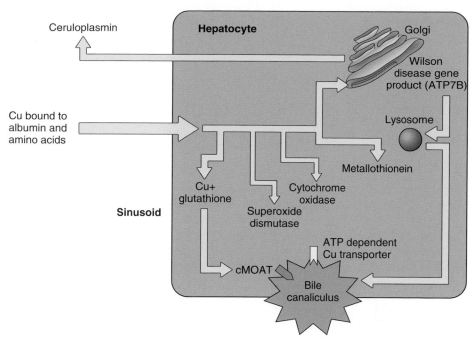

Fig. 19.2 Hepatocellular copper metabolism. Copper (Cu) is taken up by the hepatocytes, where it interacts with glutathione and metallothionein. A portion of the intracellular copper is incorporated into metalloenzymes (e.g., superoxide dismutase, cytochrome oxidase), and some is transported into the trans-Golgi network by the WD gene protein (ATP7B), where it is incorporated into ceruloplasmin. It is postulated that copper is also routed from the trans-Golgi apparatus to a vesicular compartment in lysosomes for subsequent excretion in bile. Copper bound to glutathione is also excreted into the bile canaliculus through the organic anion transporter (cMOAT [or MRP2]). It is uncertain if ATP7B is at or near the apical canalicular membrane, but this is the critical pathway affected in Wilson disease. *cMOAT*, Canalicular multispecific organic anion transporter 1; *MRP2*, multidrug resistance-associated protein 2.

2. In 1985, the WD gene was shown to be linked to the red cell enzyme, esterase D, an association that established the location on **chromosome 13.** In 1993, three different groups of investigators identified the **WD gene as encoding a copper-transporting ATPase designated *ATP7B.*** This gene spans an 80-kb region of the chromosome that encodes a 7.5-kb transcript expressed primarily in the liver, with some smaller amount of expression in kidney and placenta.

3. ATP7B is a 1466-amino acid protein that is a member of the cation-transporting P-type ATPase subfamily that is highly preserved in evolution. ATP7B is highly homologous to the Menkes gene *(ATP7A)* product and the copper-transporting ATPase (cop A) found in copper-resistant strains of *Enterococcus hirae.*

4. **Over 600 disease-causing mutations of the WD gene** have been identified to date. Most of the mutations are missense mutations. Comparatively few patients are homozygous for the same mutation; however, **most are compound heterozygotes** (i.e., bearers of different mutations on each allele).

5. Despite the clinical diversity of WD, allelic heterogeneity at the *ATPB7* locus does not appear to account for the marked phenotypic and clinical variability observed in patients.

6. Although one normal *ATP7B* allele is adequate to prevent clinical disease, heterozygotes with one mutation of the WD gene may demonstrate subclinical abnormalities in copper metabolism such as a mild elevation in liver copper above normal levels and, in 20%, a reduced level of circulating ceruloplasmin.

Pathogenesis

1. Maintenance of normal copper homeostasis depends on a balance between gastrointestinal absorption and biliary excretion. Intestinal copper absorption in patients with WD does not differ from that of nonaffected individuals.
2. **Biliary excretion of copper is reduced in WD** due to defective or absent ATP7B function, which may cause defective entry of cytosolic copper into the vesicular component of the excretory pathway to bile.
3. Reduced biliary copper excretion in WD leads to pathologic hepatocellular copper accumulation via free radical–induced oxidative injury to lipids, proteins, and nucleic acids; depletion of antioxidants; and polymerization of copper-metallothionein. Therefore, copper-induced injury leads to hepatocellular necrosis and apoptosis. Morphologic abnormalities from oxidant damage have been identified, particularly in mitochondria (i.e., enlargement, dilatation of cristae, and crystalline deposits).
4. Hepatic copper accumulation and hepatocellular injury lead to increased circulating non-ceruloplasmin-bound copper, which is responsible for extrahepatic copper accumulation. Copper toxicity plays a primary role in the pathogenesis of extrahepatic manifestations of WD. Affected organs, in particular the central nervous system, invariably exhibit elevated copper levels.
5. Pathologic copper deposition in the brain, mostly in the caudate nucleus and the putamen of the basal ganglia, results in the neurologic and psychiatric manifestations of the disease. Excessive deposition of copper in the Descemet membrane of the cornea gives rise to Kayser-Fleischer (KF) rings and rarely sunflower cataracts.
6. Deficiency of the plasma copper protein ceruloplasmin does not have a role in the pathogenesis of WD. The low serum ceruloplasmin level in patients with WD is the result of reduced incorporation of copper into the ceruloplasmin peptide without copper (aceruloplasmin), which has a shorter half-life than copper-bound ceruloplasmin (holoceruloplasmin).

Clinical Features

1. Patients may be asymptomatic, although most present with hepatic or neurologic manifestations. Less commonly, patients present with renal, skeletal, cardiac, ophthalmologic, endocrinologic, or dermatologic symptoms.
2. Clinical symptoms are rarely observed before age 3 to 5 years, and most untreated patients become symptomatic by the age of 40 years. Hepatic symptoms usually are present in the second or third decade of life, and neurologic in the third and fourth decades.
3. In a large series, the initial clinical manifestations were hepatic in 42%, neurologic in 34%, psychiatric in 10%, and hematologic in 12%. Fewer patients presented with WD after 50 years of age; the oldest reported siblings presented at 70 and 72 years of age.

HEPATIC

1. **Hepatic manifestations tend to occur at a younger age (mean, 10 to 12 years) than neurologic manifestations.** The rate of progression of liver disease is variable in WD patients. Patients with asymptomatic disease typically have abnormalities of liver biochemical tests that correlate histologically with hepatic steatosis and inflammation. Young patients may present with features that are indistinguishable from chronic viral or autoimmune hepatitis.
2. Ongoing inflammation leads to progression of fibrosis and eventual cirrhosis with progressive hepatic insufficiency and liver failure. Complications of portal hypertension become evident with advancing cirrhosis.

3. ALF develops in a minority of patients (see discussion later in chapter).
4. Hepatocellular carcinoma, once considered rare, has been reported in patients with WD.
5. Treated patients have a good prognosis even if they have developed cirrhosis. Treatment may even permit regression of fibrosis in some cases. Discontinuation of treatment leads to disease progression and development of ALF or progressive liver failure.

Acute Liver Failure

1. Patients tend to be young, in their second decade of life, and the clinical picture may be indistinguishable from that of viral-induced massive hepatic necrosis. This same clinical picture may also appear in patients who discontinue therapy for WD.
2. **Although serum aminotransferase levels are only mildly to moderately elevated, there is marked elevation of the serum bilirubin, a low serum alkaline phosphatase level, and evidence of Coombs-negative hemolytic anemia.** Serum ceruloplasmin levels are poorly predictive of WD in the acute setting; however, 24-hour urinary copper and circulating copper levels are markedly elevated.
3. Characteristic clinical features include coagulopathy, nonimmune hemolysis, splenomegaly, KF rings, and a fulminant course; patients rarely survive longer than days to weeks unless LT is performed. Only rare patients may be rescued with medical therapy alone.
4. Liver biopsy, if performed (generally via a transjugular route due to coagulopathy), demonstrates an elevated hepatic copper content and usually advanced fibrosis or cirrhosis with severe hepatocellular injury. Apoptosis and necrosis may be apparent.

NEUROLOGIC

1. Neurologic involvement tends to occur in the third to fourth decades of life. The diagnosis of WD is often delayed for 1 to 2 years in patients in whom neurologic features predominate.
2. **Common early neurologic symptoms are dysarthria, clumsiness, tremor, drooling, gait disturbance, masklike facies, and deterioration of handwriting.**
3. Rigidity with overt Parkinsonian features, flexion contractures, and spasticity are seen less often and in the later stages of the disease. Athetosis (involuntary writhing movements) or a more severe movement disorder may be present. Rarely, generalized seizures may occur.
4. Autonomic dysfunction may be present, most commonly in association with other advanced neurologic findings.
5. Cognitive ability usually remains normal but may be impaired in patients with severe neurologic impairment.
6. Neurologic symptoms may improve markedly with medical treatment or after LT, although residual deficits are common, especially in those with long-standing symptoms before the onset of therapy.
7. Magnetic resonance imaging (MRI) shows focal lesions in the putamen and globus pallidus, and in some cases additional lesions in the pons and brainstem.

PSYCHIATRIC

1. Of all patients with WD, one third may present with psychiatric symptoms. Patients may be mistakenly diagnosed with a progressive psychiatric illness, thereby delaying a diagnosis of WD and increasing the odds of concurrent neurologic or progressive hepatic disease.
2. Early symptoms in teenagers may be limited to subtle behavioral changes and deterioration of academic and work performance.

3. Patients may present later with personality changes, lability of mood, emotionalism, impulsive and antisocial behavior, depression, and increased sexual preoccupation. Frank psychosis may occur.
4. Psychiatric symptoms may resolve with medical therapy or after LT.

OPHTHALMOLOGIC
Kayser-Fleischer Rings
1. Electron-dense granules rich in copper and sulfur are deposited in the Descemet membrane of the cornea, creating the KF ring. The KF ring is golden brown or has a greenish discoloration in the limbus that is evident initially at the superior and inferior corneal poles on slit-lamp examination of the cornea. The ring eventually becomes circumferential, and the width of the ring increases in untreated patients. KF rings diminish in size and may disappear with treatment, typically over months to years.
2. The presence or absence of KF rings should be confirmed by an experienced ophthalmologist using slit-lamp examination.
3. **KF rings are present in most symptomatic patients with WD and nearly always in those with neurologic manifestations; they are often absent in asymptomatic cases and in 40% to 50% of patients with hepatic disease.**
4. The reappearance after regression or new appearance of KF rings suggests nonadherence to medical therapy.
5. KF rings are not pathognomonic of WD because they also are seen occasionally in patients with long-standing cholestasis from other causes.

Sunflower Cataracts
1. Typically observed in association with KF rings, but less frequently overall
2. Vision is unimpaired.
3. Resolve with treatment of WD

RENAL
1. Findings include proximal renal tubular acidosis or features of Fanconi syndrome in patients with a chronic disease presentation. Acute tubular injury may occur in ALF due to WD from the large release of copper and copper complexes from injured liver cells.
2. Distal renal tubular acidosis also may occur and may be responsible for the increased incidence of renal calculi in WD.
3. Hematuria, mostly microscopic, may be caused by nephrolithiasis or glomerular disease.
4. Proteinuria has been noted as a manifestation of WD, although nephrotic syndrome and Goodpasture syndrome are more likely to be a side effect of therapy with D-penicillamine or less commonly trientine (see discussion later in chapter).
5. Chelation therapy usually results in marked improvement in renal function.

SKELETAL
1. More than one half of patients with WD exhibit osteopenia caused by osteomalacia, osteoporosis, or both.
2. Symptomatic arthropathy occurs in 25% to 50% of patients; this degenerative joint disease resembles osteoarthritis and involves the spine and large joints.
3. Osteochondritis dissecans, chondromalacia patellae, and chondrocalcinosis have also been described.

OTHERS

1. An episode of acute intravascular hemolysis may be the presenting feature in up to 15% of patients; it is often transient and self-limited but can be associated with ALF due to WD.
2. The frequency of cardiac involvement was underestimated in the past; electrocardiographic abnormalities are present in one third of cases. Dysautonomia may cause dysrhythmia.
3. Azure lunulae (bluish discoloration of the lunules [bases] of fingernails) are an uncommon but characteristic finding.
4. Delayed puberty, gynecomastia, and amenorrhea have been noted. They occur most often in patients with advanced liver disease and may be due to hormonal imbalance from the liver disease and not to WD itself.

Diagnosis

WD should be considered in persons with:

- **Unexplained serum aminotransferase elevations, chronic hepatitis with steatosis, poorly responsive autoimmune hepatitis, cirrhosis, and ALF**
- **Neurologic features of unexplained origin** (abnormal behavior, incoordination, tremor, dyskinesia)
- A neurologic or psychiatric disorder with signs of concurrent hepatic disease
- KF rings detected on routine eye examination
- Unexplained, acquired Coombs-negative hemolytic anemia
- A sibling or parent with a diagnosis of WD

TESTS

1. **Ceruloplasmin**
   - Normal serum concentration is 20 to 40 mg/dL (consult the local laboratory for reference ranges, as minor variations are common).
   - 95% of all patients with chronic WD have levels lower than the normal range.
   - **Normal levels are found in at least 5% of patients with WD.**
   - Ceruloplasmin may be elevated to normal or near normal in WD patients with an acute phase response to hepatic injury and in patients with elevated serum estrogen levels secondary to pregnancy or exogenous administration.
   - A decreased level of ceruloplasmin is not pathognomonic of WD. The following non-Wilsonian causes also should be considered:
     - Up to 20% of asymptomatic heterozygotes
     - Children younger than 6 months of age (physiologically low levels)
     - Diminished synthetic function as a consequence of severe liver disease
     - Nephrotic syndrome, protein-losing enteropathy, and intestinal malabsorption
     - Hereditary aceruloplasminemia, which is unrelated to WD and may be associated with iron overload
2. **Nonceruloplasmin serum copper**
   - In unaffected patients copper in ceruloplasmin accounts for approximately 90% of the total serum copper. In untreated patients with WD, total serum copper is usually decreased due to reduced levels of circulating ceruloplasmin (except in patients with ALF due to WD, in whom massive amounts of copper are present in the circulation).
   - An estimate of the "free" (nonceruloplasmin) serum copper concentration can be calculated by subtracting the amount of ceruloplasmin copper (0.047 µmol copper/mg of

ceruloplasmin) from the total serum copper concentration. A rough approximation of this formula is: [total serum copper (μg/dL) – (3.15 × ceruloplasmin [mg/dL])].

- Patients with WD have an elevated proportion of copper bound to serum albumin, amino acids, or other peptides (nonceruloplasmin copper) compared with unaffected persons (in whom approximately 10% of total circulating copper is nonceruloplasmin copper). In untreated patients with WD, nonceruloplasmin-bound copper exceeds 25 μg/dL; in patients with liver failure caused by WD, levels are markedly elevated and may exceed 200 μg/dL.
- **The nonceruloplasmin serum copper concentration is useful for monitoring the adequacy of chelation therapy during maintenance treatment. The proportion of nonceruloplasmin copper is reduced in treated patients, and levels are typically 5 to 15 μg/dL.**
- Newer assays for "exchangeable copper" measure nonceruloplasmin copper directly from plasma samples and may in the future be useful for monitoring treatment.

3. **Urinary copper excretion**
   - Normal urinary copper excretion is <40 μg/24 hours.
   - **Most patients with symptomatic WD have a urinary copper excretion greater than 100 μg/24 hours, and patients with ALF often have levels that exceed 1000 μg/24 hours.**
   - Asymptomatic patients with WD may exhibit normal urinary copper excretion, and 16% to 23% of patients with WD who present with liver disease excrete <100 μg/24 hours. Therefore, the predictive value of this test in isolation is limited.
   - Elevated levels may be seen in other hepatic disorders, such as primary biliary cholangitis and chronic hepatitis, and in severe proteinuria from ceruloplasmin loss in urine.
   - The test is useful in confirming the diagnosis of WD and in monitoring compliance and response to chelation therapy.
   - The D-penicillamine stimulation test, administered in a dose of 0.5 g before and 12 hours later during a 24-hour urine collection, has been shown to increase urinary copper excretion, but it does not reliably distinguish patients with WD from heterozygotes and persons with other liver diseases and therefore has limited utility in adult populations. Lowering the threshold of basal urine copper excretion (without D-penicillamine) to 40 μg from 100 μg increases the sensitivity of the test for the diagnosis of WD.

4. **Liver biopsy**
   - Histologic changes on light microscopy are often nonspecific in WD. Early features may include glycogen inclusions in the nuclei of periportal hepatocytes (glycogenated nuclei) and moderate fatty infiltration that may be both microsteatotic and macrosteatotic. At this stage, ultrastructural alterations of mitochondria are observed.
   - In more advanced cases, fibrosis or cirrhosis is present.
   - In severe acute hepatitis and chronic hepatitis, submassive necrosis with Mallory hyaline, (Mallory-Denk bodies) and cirrhosis or advanced fibrosis is seen. Evidence of apoptosis as well as necrosis may be apparent in these specimens.
   - Histochemical staining of liver biopsy specimens for copper using rhodanine or rubeanic acid is of limited value unless results are positive, because during the initial stages of hepatocellular copper accumulation the metal is distributed diffusely in the cytosol and does not stain histochemically by these methods. Timm sulfide staining can detect cytosolic copper binding protein, but this test in not routinely performed.
   - **A hepatic copper concentration >250 μg/g dry liver (normal, 15 to 55 μg/g) accompanied by a low serum ceruloplasmin establishes the diagnosis of WD**, with two caveats:
     - The biopsy needle and the specimen container should be free of copper. A disposable needle made of steel is acceptable. In older reusable needles that may be made of brass, such as a Klatskin or Menghini needle, recommendations were to wash the needle in 0.1 M ethylenediaminetetraacetic acid (EDTA) and rinse with demineralized water before use. Using sterile plastic containers avoids the need for EDTA washing of glass specimen containers that may be contaminated with metal.

    – The finding of **a normal hepatic copper concentration excludes the diagnosis,** but an elevated level alone may also be found in other liver diseases.

       ■ Cholestatic disorders (e.g., primary biliary cholangitis, primary sclerosing cholangitis, intrahepatic cholestasis of childhood, biliary atresia)

       ■ Non-Wilsonian hepatic copper toxicosis (e.g., Indian childhood cirrhosis, endemic Tyrolean infantile cirrhosis, idiopathic copper toxicosis)

5. Incorporation of orally administered radiocopper into ceruloplasmin

    ■ Serum radioactivity (mainly as radiocopper-containing ceruloplasmin) is measured after oral administration of radiolabeled copper (^{64}Cu or ^{67}Cu) at 1, 2, 4, and 48 hours. Normally, one sees the prompt appearance of radiolabeled copper in serum, followed by its disappearance over time. This early peak is absent in patients with WD.

    ■ This test was used mainly for suspected WD patients with normal serum levels of ceruloplasmin; however, due to the difficulties in obtaining the radiocopper and the increased availability of molecular genetic testing, this test is now used infrequently.

6. **Genetic diagnosis**

    ■ In family studies, haplotype analysis is available for the diagnosis in siblings of identified patients, with a <1% to 2% error rate (errors can occur with double recombination).

    ■ Use of direct mutational analysis of *ATP7B* in the diagnosis of WD is markedly improved with advances in DNA sequencing technology and analysis. The test is now widely available at commercial laboratories; however, limitations to testing still exist.

    – The cost of the analysis is still relatively expensive.

    – WD is caused by many different disease-specific mutations, now numbering over 600. There are many other polymorphisms with unknown effects on protein function.

    – Family screening of siblings can be performed less expensively when the diagnosis of WD is already established in one family member by using the index patient's known mutations as a reference.

    ■ Biochemical evaluation may still be performed when the diagnosis of WD is established by either haplotype analysis or by mutation analysis to help characterize the patient phenotypically.

SCORING SYSTEMS

1. A scoring system (the **Leipzig criteria**) was developed by Ferenci and colleagues to assist clinicians in determining when WD should be considered and in helping to establish the diagnosis.

2. The system uses a weighted score of a combination of disease signs and symptoms, laboratory values, and finally mutational analysis (Table 19.1). A score of <3 suggests that another diagnosis should be considered; a score of 3 suggests that further diagnostic testing should continue; and a score of ≥4 establishes the diagnosis of WD.

3. This scoring system has been incorporated into guidelines published by the European Association for the Study of the Liver (EASL) in 2012.

4. An index for predictive mortality (Nazer score) has been developed (Table 19.2).

DIAGNOSTIC APPROACH

See Fig. 19.3.

Treatment

DIET

1. **A low-copper diet is recommended.** Foods with a high copper content (e.g., liver, chocolate, nuts, mushrooms, legumes, and shellfish) should be avoided.

TABLE 19.1 ■ **Leipzig Criteria for the Diagnosis of Wilson Disease**

Typical Clinical Symptoms and Signs		Other Tests	
Kayser-Fleischer rings:		Liver copper (in the absence of cholestasis):	
Present	2	>5× ULN (>4 µmol/g)	2
Absent	0	0.8–4 µmol/g	1
		Normal (<0.8 µmol/g)	−1
		Rhodanine-positive granules[a]	1
Neurologic symptoms[b]:		Urinary copper (in the absence of acute hepatitis):	
Severe	2	Normal	0
Mild	1	1–2× ULN	1
Absent	0	>2× ULN	2
		Normal, but >5× ULN after D-penicillamine	2
Serum ceruloplasmin:		Mutation analysis:	
Normal (>0.2 g/L)	0	Mutations detected on both chromosomes	4
0.1–0.2 g/L	1	Mutations detected on 1 chromosome	1
<0.1 g/L	2	No mutations detected	0
Nonimmune-mediated hemolytic anemia:			
Present	1		
Absent	0		

Total Score	Interpretation
≥4	Diagnosis established
3	Diagnosis possible, more tests needed
≤2	Diagnosis unlikely

[a]If no quantitative liver copper available, [b]or typical abnormalities on brain magnetic resonance imaging. *ULN,* Upper limit of normal.

From Ferenci P, Caca L, Loudianos G, et al. Diagnosis and phenotypic classification of Wilson disease. *Liver Int.* 2003;23:139–142.

TABLE 19.2 ■ **Modified Nazer Score for Predicting Mortality in Wilson Disease[a]**

Points	Bilirubin (µmol/L)	INR	AST (U/L)	WBC (10⁹/L)	Albumin (g/L)
0	0–100	0–1.29	0–100	0–6.7	>45
1	101–150	1.3–1.6	101–150	6.8–8.3	34–44
2	151–200	1.7–1.9	151–300	8.4–10.3	25–33
3	201–300	2.0–2.4	301–400	10.4–15.3	21–24
4	>300	>2.5	>400	>15.4	<20

[a]Patients with a total score ≥10 should be considered for liver transplantation.

AST, Aspartate aminotransferase; *INR,* international normalized ratio; *WBC,* white blood cell count.

Adapted from Dhawan A, Taylor RM, Cheeseman P, et al. Wilson's disease in children: 37-year experience and revised King's score for liver transplantation. *Liver Transpl.* 2005;11:441–448.

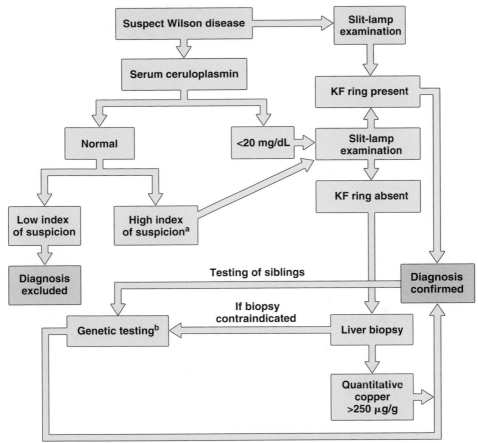

Fig. 19.3 Diagnostic algorithm for Wilson disease (WD). In the past, radioactive copper testing was used, with lack of incorporation of orally administered radiocopper into ceruloplasmin supporting the diagnosis of WD; this test is rarely used now. [a]Example: Presence of Kayser-Fleischer (KF) ring, high urinary copper excretion, and neuropsychiatric symptoms with liver involvement. [b]Genetic testing is performed for siblings in whom the diagnosis was already established in a family member by using the index patient's DNA as a reference. Other family members may be screened with clinical and biochemical studies.

2. A list of foods and their copper and other nutrient contents is available at the U.S. Department of Agriculture website: https://ndb.nal.usda.gov/ndb/search.

3. Use deionized or distilled water if the home drinking water copper content is >0.2 ppm.

DRUGS

1. **D-Penicillamine**
   - D-penicillamine is an amino acid derivative identified in the urine of patients taking penicillin.
   - Its mechanisms of action include copper chelation, detoxification, and possibly induction of cellular metallothionein synthesis, which enhances the proportion of nontoxic Cu-metallothionein.

- **Initial dose: Approximately 20 mg/kg in divided doses daily starting with a fraction of this dosage ramped up to the full 20 mg/kg over the course of 2 to 4 weeks, with a standard maintenance dose of 10 to 15 mg/kg daily; it is best absorbed if taken on an empty stomach.**
- Small doses of pyridoxine (25 mg/day) should be given daily, because of the weak antipyridoxine effect of D-penicillamine.
- Side effects develop in approximately 20% of patients within the first month of therapy, most commonly a hypersensitivity reaction, consisting of fever, malaise, rash, and occasionally lymphadenopathy. Most patients can be desensitized for these symptoms by gradual reintroduction of the drug. Bone marrow suppression or significant (>1 g/24 hours) or worsening proteinuria usually requires withdrawal of the drug.
- The drug may also cause significant worsening of neurologic features or precipitate autoimmune features such as myasthenia, polymyositis, or systemic lupus erythematosus. If these side effects occur, D-penicillamine should be discontinued and appropriate alternative therapy instituted. Dermatologic side effects include pemphigus, acanthosis nigricans, and elastosis perforans serpiginosa.

2. **Trientine**
- Trientine was introduced in 1969 as an alternative chelation agent to D-penicillamine.
- Its mechanisms of action include copper chelation and detoxification.
- **Daily dose (similar to that of penicillamine): Initial treatment dose approximately 20 mg/kg in divided doses daily starting with a fraction of this dosage ramped up to the full 20 mg/kg over the course of 2 to 4 weeks, with a standard maintenance dose of 10 to 15 mg/kg daily in divided dosages; best absorbed if taken on an empty stomach.**
- New pilot data suggest that this medication may possibly be given as a single daily dosage, thereby improving adherence and reducing inconvenience related to avoiding taking the medication with meals.
- Sideroblastic anemia is the only major side effect of this agent and occurs with overtreatment; other infrequently reported side effects include skin rash, gastrointestinal distress and colitis, and, rarely, rhabdomyolysis. Most of the side effects of D-penicillamine, with the exception of elastosis perforans serpiginosa, subside when the patient is converted to trientine.
- **Due to its improved safety profile compared with D-penicillamine, this drug has been recommended as first-line therapy for patients with WD who start with chelation therapy; however, it is expensive.**

3. **Zinc**
- Zinc salts administered orally in divided doses can be used for treatment of WD. Zinc works by inducing intestinal epithelial metallothionein synthesis, thereby reducing intestinal copper absorption. Intestinal cell copper is excreted when intestinal epithelial cells are shed, which occurs every 24 to 48 hours, thereby yielding a negative copper balance over time.
- Zinc is relatively safe; side effects include gastrointestinal upset and elevated amylase and lipase without clinical or imaging evidence of pancreatitis.
- **Dose: 150 mg daily of zinc acetate in adults, divided into three doses between meals; pediatric dose: 75 mg divided into three doses between meals**
- **The role of zinc in therapy is mainly in presymptomatic WD and as a maintenance therapy in patients.**
- May be used during pregnancy without dose reduction
- Zinc monotherapy is not recommended as initial therapy for symptomatic patients, but good outcomes have been shown in patients with predominately neurologic disease, even when zinc is used as initial therapy. Outcomes are less satisfactory when zinc is used as a single agent to maintaining patients with primarily hepatic disease.

4. **Ammonium tetrathiomolybdate (TM)**
   - The use of TM is still experimental in the United States. Treatment trials for patients using a stabilized form of the medication are ongoing (see https://clinicaltrials.gov/ct2/show/NCT02273596?term=wilson%27s+disease&rank=1).
   - Following absorption, TM forms nontoxic complexes with serum copper and albumin and prevents copper uptake by tissue.
   - Because its affinity for copper is higher than that of metallothionein, TM can remove copper bound to metallothionein, thereby potentially making it a more potent chelator than D-penicillamine and trientine.
   - Older clinical trials using a less stable form of TM suggest that it may be more effective in preventing neurologic deterioration than either penicillamine or trientine during initial therapy for patients with neurologic disease.
   - Potential side effects of TM appear to be dose related and reversible; these include bone marrow suppression and abnormal liver biochemical test levels.

PREFERRED REGIMENS

1. **Initial therapy**
   - A baseline 24-hour urinary copper determination, serum copper, ceruloplasmin, blood counts with platelets, international normalized ratio (INR), liver biochemical tests, and urinalysis should be obtained.
   - D-penicillamine or trientine should be initiated in divided doses at 25% to 50% of the initial target dosage of 20 mg/kg over 2 to 4 weeks with monitoring.
   - Patients intolerant of D-penicillamine may be treated with trientine or zinc.
   - **Evidence of improvement in liver synthetic function or neurologic and psychiatric symptoms often begins within 6 to 12 months of uninterrupted therapy.**
   - Patients with severe hepatic insufficiency unresponsive to pharmacotherapy, typically defined as 3 months of treatment, if possible, with a modified **Nazer score** (based on the serum bilirubin, serum aspartate aminotransferase, international normalized ratio, white blood cell count, and serum albumin; range 0 to 20) of 10 or greater, should be considered for LT (see Table 19.2 and discussion later in chapter).
2. **Maintenance therapy**
   - Once clinical symptoms and signs have stabilized, urinary excretion of copper is declining from baseline values, and the nonceruloplasmin copper is reduced to <15 µg/dL, the dose of chelating agents should be reduced to maintenance ranges.
   - A fall in the nonceruloplasmin copper to <5 µg/dL may indicate severe copper depletion, which may result in bone marrow suppression with anemia and thrombocytopenia and even lead to reduced ferroxidase activity with toxic hepatic iron accumulation; in this situation, the chelating agent or zinc should be temporarily stopped or reduced in dose.
   - Treatment of asymptomatic patients with WD, diagnosed by screening of family members, may be started as early as age 2 to 3 years.
   - **Lifelong therapy without interruption is essential in all patients with WD;** cessation of therapy may result in rapid and irreversible hepatic and neurologic deterioration.
3. Pregnancy
   - **Therapy should be continued throughout pregnancy.**
   - Teratogenicity has been reported in animal studies with pharmacologic doses of D-penicillamine and trientine; however, successful pregnancies have been reported on these medications. Zinc is also safe during pregnancy.
   - To reduce the risk of teratogenicity, in patients well maintained on chelation therapy, **the dose of D-penicillamine or trientine should be reduced by 50% during the time that conception is anticipated and throughout pregnancy.** The patient should be monitored

more frequently, approximately once every 3 months or during each trimester if pregnancy is achieved, until after delivery.

■ Maintenance therapy with zinc does not require dose adjustment during pregnancy.

4. Neurologic disease

■ **Approximately 20% of patients presenting with neurologic disease have worsening of neurologic symptoms during initial treatment with D-penicillamine or trientine;** this is most likely caused by the mobilization and redistribution of copper in the brain during initial treatment. A slow ramping up of the medication may reduce the frequency of this complication.

– Dose reduction or discontinuation of chelation treatment may be necessary if neurologic worsening occurs. Patients may be placed on zinc during this time.

– Alternatively, combination therapy with zinc and a lower dose of the chelating agent temporally spaced may prove to be an alternative treatment for these patients but has not been tested in clinical trials.

■ Clinical trials are evaluating the use of TM for patients with an initial presentation with neurologic disease. One trial has suggested a benefit of TM over trientine in preventing the initial worsening of neurologic disease during treatment initiation.

■ Case reports of the use of combination therapy with a chelating agent (D-penicillamine or trientine) separated temporally from zinc given in divided dosages indicate encouraging results in symptomatic patients and in those with severe liver disease. In some patients with an elevated Child-Turcotte-Pugh score (see Chapter 32), clinical and biochemical improvement eliminated the need for liver transplantation.

LIVER TRANSPLANTATION (see also Chapter 33)

1. **LT is curative for WD** because the defect of the disease resides within hepatocytes. A complete reversal of the metabolic defect in copper metabolism is seen, as is improvement in hepatic and neurologic manifestations in most patients.

2. The majority of adults transplanted for WD have chronic liver failure. ALF is a more common indication in the pediatric population. In an analysis of LT in the U.S. database for transplantation from the United Network for Organ Sharing (UNOS) from 1997 to 2008, 400 adults and 170 children underwent LT for WD. Patient and graft survival for adult and pediatric patients transplanted for WD were excellent. One- and 5-year survival rates, respectively, were 90% and 89% for children, compared with 88% and 86% for adults.

3. WD in patients with ALF can be identified with the use of simple biochemical testing and blood counts even before the results of testing for copper in blood, urine, and liver tissue are available. **Patients with ALF due to WD have a relatively low alkaline phosphatase value that declines as the liver failure progresses.** Because these patients have hemolysis and elevations in the bilirubin occur rapidly, **the ratio of alkaline phosphatase to serum bilirubin is typically <4, and the AST to ALT ratio is >2.** If patients have these two biochemical parameters and a low hemoglobin level due to hemolysis, the sensitivity and specificity for the diagnosis of WD as the etiology for the ALF is nearly 100%.

4. **Patients with ALF due to WD should be referred immediately for LT.** Measures to stabilize the patient are directed at lowering the marked elevated levels of copper in the circulation. This has been accomplished by several means, including exchange transfusion, plasmapheresis coupled with hemofiltration, albumin hemodialysis, and molecular adsorbent recirculating system (MARS) (see Chapter 2). Only rare WD patients with ALF survive without LT, and the previous measures serve to stabilize the patient while awaiting a new organ but are usually inadequate in providing enough support for liver regeneration to occur.

5. Studies of the natural history of patients with hepatic WD in the era before LT led to development of the Nazer score (see Table 19.2 and discussion earlier in chapter). The score was later modified to include other parameters of hepatic insufficiency and systemic inflammation. Patients with a score above 10 did not survive without LT, whereas those with a lower score improved with medical therapy. Although the prognostic score is not perfect in predicting the outcome of treatment for all patients, it is a helpful guide.

6. **In the absence of severe hepatic disease, LT for refractory neurologic manifestations should still be considered experimental;** however, several reports have noted improvement in these patients after LT. Patients with severe neurologic involvement do not always improve after LT, and poorer posttransplantation outcomes have been reported with respect to survival and complications from use of calcineurin inhibitors to prevent graft rejection.

FUTURE THERAPIES

1. Identification of the *ATP7B* gene and the mechanism of disease should make molecular-based therapies, including gene repair and gene therapy, possible.

2. A report of adeno-associated virus-mediated gene transfer of *ATP7B* with long-term expression of the protein in an animal model of WD is encouraging and should lead to future clinical trials.

3. Another potential therapy is hepatocyte cell transplantation, which has been applied in the animal model of WD, the Long Evans Cinnamon (LEC) rat, and a mouse model lacking *ATP7B*, in which complete metabolic correction was achieved. Limitations of this approach for human trials are the need to achieve adequate cell repopulation with transplanted normal cells and the need for immunosuppression to prevent rejection of the transplanted cells.

Other Copper-Related Disorders

INDIAN CHILDHOOD CIRRHOSIS

1. Environmental ingestion of excessive amounts of copper, resulting from the use of copper and brass vessels, is the likely cause of copper overload in this disorder, although a genetic predisposition appears to coexist in some patients.

2. Rapidly progressive cirrhosis manifests at 6 months to 5 years of age; the disorder is generally restricted to the Indian subcontinent.

3. Grossly increased hepatic, urinary, and serum copper concentrations are noted.

4. This entity was once a common cause of chronic liver disease in India, but it is rarely seen now because of health education and avoidance of the use of brass vessels.

IDIOPATHIC COPPER TOXICOSIS

1. This is a rare disorder, with sporadic cases occurring worldwide.

2. Severe, progressive cirrhosis occurs in the absence of neurologic disease, with clinical onset usually by 2 years of age.

3. Serum ceruloplasmin levels are normal; liver biopsy specimens reveal cirrhosis with Mallory-Denk bodies and a hepatic copper concentration >400 µg/g dry weight.

4. The disorder may be caused by an unidentified genetic defect or excessive environmental copper exposure (e.g., contaminated spring water in endemic Tyrolean infantile cirrhosis).

MENKES DISEASE

1. Menkes disease is an X-linked recessive neurodegenerative disorder that presents typically at <3 months of age and is fatal in most cases by 3 to 6 years of age.
2. It is caused by mutations in the *ATP7A* gene, which encodes a p-type ATPase, homologous to ATP7B, that causes impaired copper transport across the placenta, intestine, and blood-brain barrier and thereby leads to a severe copper deficiency state (with deficient activity of essential cuproenzymes).
3. Affected infants may develop hypotonia, seizures, and failure to thrive.
4. The reduced function of the copper-dependent enzyme lysyl oxidase leads to reduced collagen cross-linking and the "kinky hair" that is characteristic. Other features are hypopigmentation, osteoporosis, and arterial vascular tortuosity.
5. Newborn screening is not routinely available. Experimentally, a high ratio of dopamine to norepinephrine as well as of dihydroxyphenylacetic acid to dihydroxyphenylglycol can identify patients before the onset of severe symptoms. Eventually serum markers of a low copper and ceruloplasmin are indicative of relative copper deficiency. Molecular genetic testing for *ATP7A* mutations can be performed, but there is genetic diversity and not all mutations are well characterized.
6. Treatment with daily injections of copper histidine, if instituted early in the disease course, may partially improve outcomes. Trials of gene therapy in animal models are ongoing.

FURTHER READING

Ala A, Aliu E, Schilsky ML. Prospective pilot study of a single daily dosage of trientine for the treatment of Wilson disease. *Dig Dis Sci.* 2015;60:1433–1439.

Beinhardt S, Leiss W, Stättermayer AF, et al. Long-term outcomes of patients with Wilson disease in a large Austrian cohort. *Clin Gastroenterol Hepatol.* 2014;12:683–689.

Brewer GJ, Askari F, Lorincz MT, et al. Treatment of Wilson disease with ammonium tetrathiomolybdate: IV. Comparison of tetrathiomolybdate and trientine in a double-blind study of treatment of the neurologic presentation of Wilson disease. *Arch Neurol.* 2006;63:521–527.

Ferenci P, Czlonkowska A, Stremmel W, et al. EASL clinical practice guidelines: Wilson's disease. European Association for Study of Liver. *J Hepatol.* 2012;56:671–685.

Kaler SG. Translational research investigations on ATP7A: an important human copper ATPase. *Ann N Y Acad Sci.* 2014;1314:64–68.

Koppikar S, Dhawan A. Evaluation of the scoring system for the diagnosis of Wilson's disease in children. *Liver Int.* 2005;25:680–681.

Korman JD, Volenberg I, Balko J, et al. Screening for Wilson disease in acute liver failure by serum testing: a comparison of currently used tests. *Hepatology.* 2008;48:1167–1174.

Murillo O, Luqui DM, Gazquez C, et al. Long-term metabolic correction of Wilson's disease in a murine model by gene therapy. *J Hepatol.* 2016;64:419–426.

Roberts E, Schilsky ML. A practice guideline on Wilson disease. *Hepatology.* 2008;47:2089–2111.

Schilsky ML. Liver transplantation for Wilson disease. *Ann NY Acad Sci.* 2014;1315:45–49.

Zimbrean PC, Schilsky ML. The spectrum of psychiatric symptoms in Wilson's disease: treatment and prognostic considerations. *Am J Psychiatry.* 2015;172:1068–1072.

CHAPTER 20

Alpha-1 Antitrypsin Deficiency and Other Metabolic Liver Diseases

Christine E. Waasdorp Hurtado, MD, MSCS ■ Ronald J. Sokol, MD ■
Hugo R. Rosen, MD, FACP

KEY POINTS

1. **Alpha-1 antitrypsin deficiency** (α-1 ATD) is the most common metabolic liver disease in childhood. The diagnosis should be considered in all adults and children with chronic hepatitis or cirrhosis of unknown origin. α-1 ATD is associated with chronic liver disease in 10% of affected adults and in 10% to 15% of affected children.

2. **Hereditary tyrosinemia** is characterized by progressive liver failure, renal tubular dysfunction, and hypophosphatemic rickets. Patients are at high risk for hepatocellular carcinoma (HCC) if the disease is untreated. Treatment is available if the disease is identified early in life.

3. **Gaucher disease** is the most common lysosomal storage disease. The clinical presentation and severity of liver involvement are variable.

4. **Cystic fibrosis** is the most common potentially fatal autosomal recessive disease in the white population. The prevalence of cirrhosis with portal hypertension is 5% to 10%.

5. **Porphyrias** are a heterogeneous group of genetic and acquired disorders of heme biosynthesis. The diagnosis should be considered in patients with abdominal pain and other gastrointestinal, renal, and neurologic complaints without an identified cause.

Overview

1. Acute and chronic liver diseases are increasingly identified as inherited, at least in part.
2. In most cases, a diagnosis can be made with a complete history, physical examination, and appropriate laboratory studies; some diagnoses require genetic testing or a liver biopsy.
3. Genetic and metabolic liver diseases account for approximately 10% of liver transplants in children.
4. Liver transplantation (LT) should be considered in children with metabolic liver disease associated with failure to thrive, extrahepatic organ dysfunction (e.g., central nervous system, kidneys) caused by a toxic metabolic product, or progressive liver failure.
5. The presence of one genetic mutation for a specific liver disease can modify the severity of other diseases. The heterozygous state of α-1 ATD may increase the risk of progression in hepatitis B virus (HBV) and hepatitis C virus (HCV) infections, nonalcoholic fatty liver disease (NAFLD), cystic fibrosis (CF), and cryptogenic cirrhosis. Genetic polymorphisms are potential modifiers of hepatic cirrhosis.

269

TABLE 20.1 ■ **Findings in Patients with Alpha-1 Antitrypsin Deficiency (PiZZ or PiSZ Phenotype)**

	Infancy (1–4 mo) (%)	At 18 Yr of Age (%)
Elevated serum alanine aminotransferase levels	48	10
Elevated serum gamma-glutamyltranspeptidase levels	60	8
Clinical signs of liver disease	17	0

From Sveger T, Eriksson S. The liver in adolescents with alpha 1-antitrypsin deficiency. *Hepatology* 1995;22:514–517.

Alpha-1 Antitrypsin Deficiency

GENETICS

1. Alpha-1 antitrypsin (α-1 AT), a serine protease of the SERPIN superfamily, inhibits tissue proteases such as neutrophil elastase and proteinase 3.
2. α-1 AT is encoded by the *SERPINA1* gene on the long arm of chromosome 14 (14q31-32.2); α-1 ATD is an autosomal codominant disorder affecting up to 1 in 1800 live births.
3. PiMM (Pi = protease inhibitor), the normal variant, is the phenotype present in 95% of the population and is associated with normal serum levels of α-1 AT.
4. >100 allelic variants of α-1 AT are recognized. Not all variants are associated with clinical disease.
5. The Z α-1 AT protein is caused by a single nucleotide substitution (Glu to Lys). The variant is most common in persons of northern European descent.
6. **PiZZ and PiSZ phenotypes are associated with severe deficiency and liver disease,** whereas the PiMZ phenotype leads to an intermediate deficiency and rarely causes liver disease. Low circulating levels of α-1 AT cause emphysema, whereas liver disease is caused by retention of the abnormally folded protein in the endoplasmic reticulum.

CLINICAL FEATURES

1. α-1 ATD predisposes children and adults to liver disease.
2. Liver involvement is often first identified in the newborn period as a result of persistent cholestatic jaundice. Affected infants tend to be small for gestational age. From 10% to 15% of persons with the PiZZ phenotype present with liver disease in the first years of life (Table 20.1).
   ■ Of those presenting with neonatal liver disease, 10% to 30% develop moderate to severe liver disease with coagulopathy, poor growth, and ascites in childhood.
   ■ In a prospective study from Sweden of children identified by newborn screening, 85% of PiZZ children demonstrated improvement in both clinical and laboratory signs of liver disease over an 18-year period. Only 5% to 10% of all PiZZ children developed significant liver disease (Fig. 20.1).
3. Serum aminotransferase, alkaline phosphatase, and gamma-glutamyltranspeptidase (GGTP) levels may all be elevated.
4. Emphysema develops in 60% to 70% of adults with α-1 ATD older than 25 years of age, especially in those who smoke tobacco, with a peak in the fourth and fifth decades.
5. Vascular abnormalities, including spontaneous carotid artery dissection and neutrophilic panniculitis, are also associated with α-1 ATD.

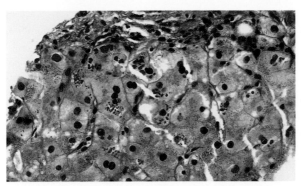

Fig. 20.1 Histopathology of liver involvement in alpha-1 antitrypsin deficiency. Periportal hepatocytes contain numerous eosinophilic diastase-resistant globules that are periodic acid–Schiff (PAS) positive.

PATHOGENESIS

1. Liver disease is associated with retention of abnormally folded Z protein in the endoplasmic reticulum of hepatocytes. Liver disease occurs in the PiZZ and PiSZ phenotypes but rarely in persons with PiMZ. Liver disease does not occur with the other variants (e.g., PiSS).
2. Far fewer patients exhibit liver and lung disease associated with α-1 ATD than estimated by population human genetic estimations, a finding that suggests involvement of unidentified genetic and environmental factors and modifier genes in the development of tissue damage.
3. The pathogenesis of α-1 ATD–associated liver disease is not completely understood. The following theories have been proposed:
   - Accumulation of mutant protein in the endoplasmic reticulum may result in hepatotoxicity. This theory is supported by a transgenic mouse model and a study demonstrating delayed protein degradation of mutant α-1 AT Z protein in persons with liver disease compared with those without liver disease.
   - Autophagy, a cellular mechanism for disposal of accumulated proteins, has been suggested to be defective in those with liver disease.
   - Other inherited traits for protein degradation and environmental factors (e.g., viral hepatitis) may increase accumulation of the defective protein and result in increased liver injury.
   - Liver disease is unlikely to be a consequence of a "proteolytic attack" mechanism, which is the likely mechanism responsible for lung injury.
4. The PiMZ state may predispose to more severe liver injury in various hepatic disorders (HBV and HCV infections, alcoholic liver disease, CF-associated liver disease, NAFLD).

DIAGNOSIS

1. The diagnosis of α-1 ATD is established by a serum α-1 AT level, phenotype (Pi typing), or genotype.
2. Serum levels of α-1 AT are generally decreased in affected patients; however, α-1 AT is an acute phase reactant and can be falsely elevated. Serum concentrations are rarely higher than 50 to 60 mg/dL in patients with the PiZZ phenotype. The PiMZ or PiSZ phenotype correlates with an α-1 AT level that is 50% of normal.
3. Liver histology showing diastase-resistant globules that are periodic acid–Schiff positive in the endoplasmic reticulum of periportal hepatocytes is classic for the disease, but these features should not be used for diagnosis because some patients with PiMZ also have these findings (see Fig. 20.1).

4. The diagnosis should be considered in all adults and children with chronic hepatitis or cirrhosis of unknown origin, children presenting with portal hypertension of unknown origin, and infants with neonatal cholestasis.

TREATMENT AND SCREENING

1. No specific therapies are available for α-1 ATD–associated liver disease at this time.
2. Infants with cholestasis may benefit from fat-soluble vitamin supplements (vitamins A, D, E, and K) and infant formula containing medium-chain triglyceride oil. In addition, treatment with ursodeoxycholic acid may increase bile flow and reduce liver injury associated with cholestasis, although no evidence indicates a direct long-term benefit in α-1 ATD.
3. **Avoidance of cigarette smoking,** including secondhand smoke, and of environmental pollution exposure is mandatory to delay the onset or slow the progression of lung disease. Replacement therapy with purified or recombinant α-1 AT by infusion has been successful in slowing the decline in forced expiratory volume in a nonrandomized trial, and this therapy is often used.
4. **LT** is the recommended treatment for α-1 ATD–associated end-stage liver disease and liver failure.
5. The recipient assumes the donor Pi phenotype and is no longer at risk for emphysema. Long-term survival is excellent. LT should be pursued before lung decompensation precludes LT.
6. Somatic gene therapy, in which a normal α-1 ATD gene is transferred to an organ capable of synthesizing the mature protein that could be secreted into the circulation, is potentially useful for the treatment of lung disease. Gene therapy for treatment of liver disease requires delivery of peptides to the endoplasmic reticulum to prevent polymerization of mutant protein or manipulation of the degradation system in those at risk for liver disease. The technology is currently limited by poor transfer of gene products and unknown safety risks.
7. Small molecule pharmacologic chaperone therapy, RNA interference of PiZZ gene translation, and manipulation of autophagy are being evaluated as possible future treatment strategies.
8. Screening is recommended for all relatives of patients with α-1 ATD to identify PiZZ or PiSZ family members and is mandatory for siblings of affected patients. Universal newborn screening has not been instituted.

Hereditary Tyrosinemia

GENETICS

1. This disease is caused by a deficiency of fumarylacetoacetate hydrolase (FAH), the terminal enzyme in phenylalanine and tyrosine degradation.
2. This autosomal recessive defect has an incidence of 1 in 100,000. The disorder is most prevalent in French Canadians in Quebec, Canada, where it has an incidence of 1 in 1800.
3. Many mutations of the FAH gene have been identified; no correlations exist between the genotype and the severity of disease. A founder mutation has been found in Quebec.

CLINICAL FEATURES

1. The disorder is characterized by **progressive cholestasis and liver failure, renal tubular dysfunction, and hypophosphatemic rickets.**

2. It may manifest as acute hepatic failure in infancy, neonatal cholestasis, rickets, or failure to thrive, or, later in childhood, as compensated or decompensated cirrhosis. The acute form usually manifests with poor growth, irritability, and vomiting. Death from liver failure by 1 to 2 years of age is not uncommon in untreated patients.
3. Patients have a characteristically prolonged prothrombin time despite mild elevations in aminotransferase and bilirubin levels and may have hypoglycemia with fasting. Serum alkaline phosphatase levels may be disproportionately elevated because of rickets caused by renal tubular involvement.
4. Neurologic crises develop and resemble acute intermittent porphyria, presumably from competitive inhibition of δ-aminolevulinic acid (ALA) dehydratase by succinylacetone.
5. Cardiomyopathy, particularly interventricular septal hypertrophy, is found in 30% of newly diagnosed patients. This complication resolves during treatment in most patients.
6. The incidence of **HCC** in untreated persons is high, even in the first 2 to 3 years of life.

PATHOGENESIS

1. Tyrosine metabolites, including tyrosine and succinylacetone, proximal to the FAH blockage accumulate.
2. Succinylacetone and succinylacetoacetate inhibit enzymes, including porphobilinogen synthase, and this process results in increased levels of ALA, which is responsible for acute neurologic crises.
3. The pathogenesis of liver injury caused by the accumulation of toxins is not understood.
4. Liver histology is characterized by macrovesicular steatosis, pseudoacinar formation of hepatocytes, hemosiderosis, and variable hepatocyte necrosis and apoptosis. Periportal fibrosis progresses to micronodular cirrhosis with regenerative nodules.

DIAGNOSIS

1. The diagnosis of hereditary tyrosinemia is established by the presence of elevated levels of succinylacetone in the urine or by genotyping.
2. Other features include elevated plasma levels of tyrosine, methionine, and alpha fetoprotein, which are nonspecific findings.
3. The diagnosis should be considered in patients with cirrhosis who have diminished hepatic synthetic function with mildly elevated aminotransferase levels.
4. Renal tubular dysfunction results in glycosuria, proteinuria, amino aciduria, and hyperphosphaturia.

TREATMENT AND SCREENING

1. **Nutritional restrictions** are important, although they do not prevent or reduce the progression of liver disease. **Phenylalanine, tyrosine, and methionine** are restricted, with close monitoring of serum amino acids to ensure that levels remain in the normal range. Nutritional restrictions may benefit the kidneys. **Vitamin D supplementation** and **phosphate supplementation** prevent rickets.
2. **Pharmacologic treatment** is provided by **NTBC** (2-[2-nitro-4-trifluoromethylbenzoyl]-1,3-cyclohexanedione [Nitisinone]). NTBC inhibits 4-hydroxy phenylpyruvate dioxygenase, the second enzyme in tyrosine catabolic pathway proximal to the FAH block, and thus reduces production of the toxic products, such as succinylacetone. When NTBC treatment is started early in infancy, neurologic crises and liver failure are prevented and renal function is preserved. The effect on preventing HCC remains unknown.

3. **LT** reverses the hepatic metabolic disease, prevents neurologic disease, and stabilizes renal involvement. LT is indicated if NTBC therapy fails, disease is advanced at diagnosis, or HCC has developed or is likely to develop.

Gaucher Disease

GENETICS

1. This **most common lysosomal storage disease** is caused by a deficiency of the enzyme glucocerebrosidase. This deficiency results in accumulation of enzyme substrate (glucosyl-ceramide) in the lysosomes of macrophages throughout the body (primarily the spleen, liver, bone marrow, and bone and, less often, the lungs, skin, conjunctiva, kidney, and heart).
2. It is an autosomal recessive defect affecting 1 in 40,000 in the United States.
3. The affected gene is located on long arm of chromosome 1(1q2.1); >300 mutations have been identified.

CLINICAL FEATURES

1. A continuum of disease with variation even among persons with the same genotype
2. Three types of disease are recognized:
   - **Type I (nonneuropathic):** This type is most frequent, accounting for 95% of cases. The incidence in general population ranges from 1 in 20,000 to 1 in 200,000. The incidence in Ashkenazi Jews is 1 in 600. Patients present with hepatomegaly, splenomegaly (which may be profound), anemia, thrombocytopenia, osteopenia, and elevated serum aminotransferase levels. Progressive liver fibrosis and liver failure are rare.
   - **Type II and type III (neuropathic):** The incidence is <1 in 100,000. **Type II** causes progressive neurologic impairment at presentation and death by 2 years of age. **Type III** causes neurologic impairment varying from seizures to mild ataxia and dementia with associated hepatic dysfunction, but it is less severe than type II.
3. Liver involvement generally correlates with extrahepatic involvement. Storage cells are typically centrizonal. Patients may develop complications of portal hypertension.

DIAGNOSIS

1. Definitive diagnosis is made by an acid beta-glucosidase enzyme assay in leukocytes or fibroblasts or by genotyping.
2. Histopathologically, the disorder is characterized by lipid-laden histiocyte cells (Gaucher cells) in the spleen, hepatic sinusoids, bone marrow, and lymph nodes (Fig. 20.2).
3. The diagnosis should be considered in all adults and children with unexplained liver dysfunction, splenomegaly, hypersplenism, bleeding, and skeletal anomalies.
4. Prenatal diagnosis is possible with amniotic or chorionic villus sampling for genetic testing.

TREATMENT AND SCREENING

1. All patients (and siblings) with type III disease should be treated. Indications for treatment of type I disease include confirmation of the diagnosis (enzymatic or genetic) and at least two involved organ systems. Treatment is not effective for type II.
2. Enzyme replacement therapy: Imiglucerase is a recombinant acid beta-glucosidase.
3. Substrate reduction therapy is indicated for patients in whom enzyme replacement therapy is not an option.

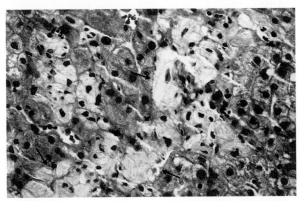

Fig. 20.2 Histopathology of liver involvement in Gaucher disease. Lipid-laden histiocytic cells *(arrows)* are seen in the hepatic sinusoids (PAS).

4. Bones should be monitored for disease with serial x-ray studies or magnetic resonance imaging (femur, spine, and symptomatic areas).
5. LT is generally not required except in rare cases of liver failure.
6. Gene therapy is under investigation.

Glycogen Storage Disease

GENETICS

Defects in enzymes involved in the degradation of glycogen to glucose result in excess hepatic glycogen accumulation. Liver disease is seen in types I, III, IV, VI, and IX glycogen storage disease (GSD).

1. **Type 1**
   - **Type Ia** is caused by glucose-6-phosphatase deficiency (autosomal recessive).
   - **Type Ib** is caused by abnormalities in endoplasmic reticulum translocase resulting in decreased glucose-6-phosphatase availability to substrate.
   - **Type Ic** is caused by phosphate-pyrophosphate translocase deficiency.
   - All type I defects result in decreased free glucose production. Excess glucose-6-phosphatase is shunted into pathways for synthesis of lactate, triglycerides, cholesterol, and uric acid, all of which are elevated in type I GSD.
2. **Type III** is caused by genetic deficiency of the debrancher enzyme (amylo-1,6-glucosidase) with autosomal recessive inheritance. The gene is located on chromosome 1p21.
3. **Type IV** is caused by an autosomal recessive deficiency of the glycogen debrancher enzyme (amylo-1,4 1,6-transglucosidase). The gene is located on chromosome 3p12.
4. **Types VI** and **IX** involve defects in phosphorylase or phosphorylase kinase.

CLINICAL FEATURES

Children present with nonspecific gastrointestinal symptoms, hepatomegaly, short stature, hypoglycemia, and failure to thrive. Without intervention, hepatomegaly (types I, VI, and IX), portal hypertension (types III and IV), or liver failure and death (type IV) ensue between 2 and 4 years of age.

1. **Type Ia:** Deficiency of glucose-6-phosphatase leads to profound hypoglycemia during fasting. In addition, patients present with lactic acidemia, hyperuricemia, hypertriglyceridemia,

hypercholesterolemia with accompanying massive hepatomegaly, short stature, and imma-turity. Characteristic "doll's facies" is the result of excessive facial fat deposits. Enlarged kidneys are also seen. In poorly treated patients, hepatic adenomas may develop after the first decade.

2. **Type Ib:** This disorder is similar to type Ia, with the addition of neutrophil dysfunction or neutropenia and occasionally inflammatory bowel disease. In poorly treated patients, hepatic adenomas may develop after the first decade.

3. **Type III:** This disorder has liver or muscle involvement. The presentation may be similar to, but milder than, type Ia, with hepatomegaly, hypoglycemia, hyperlipidemia, hyperuricemia, growth retardation, and similar laboratory test results. Hepatic fibrosis is more severe and may be progressive. Skeletal muscle weakness or cardiomyopathy may also be present.

4. **Type IV** (Andersen disease): The disease is heterogeneous, with three presentations: (1) progressive liver failure and cirrhosis leading to death in early childhood, (2) chronic liver disease without progressive fibrosis, and (3) abnormal neuromuscular development. Most patients have cirrhosis and possible brain and cardiac involvement leading to death by 5 years of age.

PATHOGENESIS AND DIAGNOSIS

1. GSD is characterized by abnormal accumulation of glycogen in tissues, including liver, heart, skeletal, muscle, kidney, and brain.
2. The diagnosis is made by liver or muscle analysis for specific enzyme activity or by genetic testing.
3. The diagnosis is suggested by abnormal structure of glycogen observed by electron microscopy of liver or muscle tissue.

TREATMENT AND SCREENING

1. For patients with GSD types I and III who have hypoglycemia, frequent feedings of a high-starch, low-simple-sugar diet or glucose polymers are used to maintain blood glucose levels. High-starch meals along with supplements of uncooked cornstarch are given throughout the day and at night.
2. Nocturnal nasogastric or gastrostomy tube drip feedings are also used to maintain normal serum glucose levels at night.
3. LT is the only effective treatment for patients with progressive liver failure and cirrhosis (types III and IV).
4. Patients with types VI and IX GSD usually do not require specific therapy but present with hepatomegaly and mildly elevated serum aminotransferase levels.
5. Vector-mediated gene therapy holds promise.

Cystic Fibrosis

GENETICS

1. This autosomal recessive disease affects 1 in 2000 to 1 in 3500 newborns; it is the **most com-mon potentially lethal inherited disease in the white population.**
2. Mutation occurs in the cystic fibrosis transmembrane conductance regulator (CFTR) gene, located on the long arm of chromosome 7; >1500 mutations have been identified, and ΔF508 is the most common.
3. CFTR functions as a chloride channel and may regulate other cellular transport pathways.

CLINICAL FEATURES

1. The clinical presentation of CF varies greatly, with epithelial cells of different organs affected by the CFTR defect. Airways, sweat glands, pancreas, intestine, and liver are the most commonly affected tissues.

2. The pathognomonic lesion of CF-associated liver disease is **focal biliary cirrhosis** (present in up to 70% of adults with CF). The patchy distribution of cirrhotic transformation spares many areas of the liver, thus preserving hepatic architecture and not causing significant symptoms. The focal nature explains the typically mild and insidious course of CF-associated liver disease.

3. Among patients with CF, 20% to 50% will develop clinical manifestations of liver disease.
   - Neonatal cholestasis in 3% to 5%
   - Isolated hepatomegaly in 6% to 30%
   - Hepatic steatosis in 23% to 67%
   - Gallstones in 12% to 27%
   - Portal hypertension and multilobular cirrhosis in 10% to 15%

4. Median life expectancy in all patients with CF has increased to 40 years. With advances in medical management and a longer duration of survival, the prevalence of recognized hepatobiliary involvement has increased.

PATHOGENESIS AND DIAGNOSIS

1. The pathophysiology of liver disease has not been fully elucidated. Proposed mechanisms include obstruction of intrahepatic bile ducts, altered bile acid metabolism, elevated cytokines, vitamin deficiencies, bacterial toxins, intestinal microbiota-initiated hepatic inflammation, and drug hepatotoxicity.

2. The diagnosis is made either by the gold standard **sweat chloride test** or by **CFTR genotype.**

3. Liver biopsy has a limited role in CF because of the patchy nature of disease. Serum aminotransferase and alkaline phosphatase levels may be elevated at some time in most patients with CF, and these values have little correlation with progressive liver disease.

TREATMENT AND SCREENING

1. Ursodeoxycholic acid, administered in a dose of 20 mg/kg per day (divided bid), has been shown to improve serum aspartate aminotransferase (AST), alanine aminotransferase (ALT), and GGTP levels, although long-term benefits are controversial.

2. Patients with severe steatosis and undernutrition may benefit from treatment of pancreatic insufficiency with enzyme replacement and assessment of the patient's carnitine status.

3. Taurine supplementation has been suggested to be beneficial in patients with CF who are receiving long-term ursodeoxycholic acid treatment and who have severe pancreatic insufficiency and poor nutritional status.

4. Surgical options for patients with end-stage liver disease and complications of portal hypertension include a transjugular portosystemic shunt, surgical portosystemic shunting, partial splenic embolization, splenectomy, and LT. Combined lung transplantation and LT may be performed.

5. Numerous novel therapies are under development, including small molecules that induce ribosomes to produce functional CFTR during mRNA translation and recombinant growth factor. An animal study has shown success with somatic gene transfer to correct CFTR defects. Newer therapies designed to increase trafficking and function of CFTR have demonstrated clinical benefit.

TABLE 20.2 ■ The Porphyrias

Affected Enzyme	Heme Metabolic Step	Resulting Disease[a]
	Glycine + succinyl CoA	
ALA synthase	↓	—
	ALA	
ALA dehydratase	↓	ALA dehydratase deficiency
	Porphobilinogen	
Porphobilinogen deaminase	↓	Acute intermittent porphyria
	Hydroxymethylbilane	
Uroporphyrinogen cosynthase	↓	Congenital erythropoietic porphyria
	Uroporphyrinogen III	
Uroporphyrinogen decarboxylase	↓	Porphyria cutanea tarda Hepatoerythropoietic porphyria
	Coprophyrinogen	
Coprophyrinogen oxidase	↓	Hereditary coproporphyria
	Protoporphyrinogen IX	
Protoporphyrinogen oxidase	↓	Variegate porphyria
	Protoporphyrin IX	
Ferrochelatase	↓	Erythropoietic protoporphyria
	Heme	

[a]The acute (neurovisceral) porphyrias are in red.

ALA, Aminolevulinic acid; *CoA,* coenzyme.

From Bloomer JR. The porphyrias. In: Schiff ER, Sorrell MF, Maddrey WC, eds. *Schiff's Diseases of the Liver,* 9th ed. Philadelphia: Lippincott Williams & Wilkins; 2003:1231–1260.

Porphyria

GENETICS

1. The porphyrias are a heterogeneous group of genetic and acquired disorders of the heme biosynthetic pathway (Table 20.2).
2. Three of the porphyrias are inherited in an autosomal recessive fashion, and five are inherited in an autosomal dominant fashion.

CLINICAL FEATURES

1. Porphyria consists of eight metabolic disorders classified according to the enzyme deficiency and tissue involvement (acute [neurovisceral], photocutaneous, and mixed forms). The presentation typically occurs during or after puberty; early childhood presentation has been reported.
2. **Acute porphyrias:** Acute intermittent porphyria, variegate porphyria, hereditary coproporphyria, and ALA dehydratase porphyria
   ■ They frequently begin in puberty and may diminish in the fifth decade.
   ■ Environmental agents and medications often precipitate attacks.
   ■ Symptoms include severe abdominal pain often associated with nausea, constipation, blood pressure derangements, hyponatremia, renal insufficiency, and neurologic complaints including peripheral neuropathy.

TABLE 20.3 ■ Precipitants of Acute Porphyria

Environmental	Pharmacologic
Alcohol	Anticonvulsants: Barbiturates, carbamazepine, phenytoin, valproic acid
Smoking	Antimicrobials: Dapsone, doxycycline, metronidazole, rifampin, sulfonamides
Infection	Cardiovascular agents: Amiodarone, nifedipine, verapamil
Stress	Diuretics: Furosemide, spironolactone, thiazides
Menstruation	Drugs of abuse: Cocaine, ecstasy, marijuana, amphetamines
Low-energy diets	

- Psychiatric symptoms may include depression, psychosis, and hysterical behavior.
- Hepatic abnormalities range from mild elevations in AST and ALT levels during attacks to liver failure.

3. **Photocutaneous porphyrias:** Erythropoietic protoporphyria, porphyria cutanea tarda (PCT), variegate porphyria, and hereditary coproporphyria
   - Porphyrin accumulation leads to photosensitization and skin damage following sunlight exposure. The characteristic lesions include skin fragility, subepidermal bullae, hyperpigmentation, and hypertrichosis. Cutaneous porphyrias are not associated with neurologic or psychiatric complaints; however, liver involvement is seen.
   - Spontaneous PCT is associated with alcoholic liver disease, HCV infection, iron overload states including hereditary hemochromatosis and Alagille syndrome. PCT is associated with a high rate of HCC.
4. **Mixed porphyrias** (combined acute and photocutaneous): Skin lesions occur in 50% of patients with variegate porphyria and in 30% of those with hereditary coproporphyria.

PATHOGENESIS AND DIAGNOSIS

1. Metabolite accumulation leads to diverse clinical manifestations. Acute porphyria results from the accumulation of one or both of the porphyrin precursors, ALA and porphobilinogen (PBG). In cutaneous porphyrias, the porphyrins accumulate.
2. The diagnosis can be challenging but is simplified by an improved understanding of the heme biosynthetic pathway, including metabolites.
3. Acute porphyrias are diagnosed by measurement of urinary ALA or PBG in a 24-hour urine collection. Levels 3 to 10 times the upper limit of normal (7 mg) are seen.
4. Erythrocyte porphobilinogen deaminase levels are reduced in acute intermittent porphyria.
5. Urine uroporphyrin levels are elevated in congenital erythropoietic porphyria, PCT, and hepatoerythropoietic porphyria.
6. Elevated water-insoluble fecal protoporphyrin levels are used to diagnose variegate porphyria and erythropoietic protoporphyria.

TREATMENT AND SCREENING

1. Treatment is aimed at reducing protoporphyrin levels in the liver.
2. Acute attacks
   - Identify precipitants and avoid or remove them (Table 20.3).
   - Manage fluid and electrolytes and manage pain; avoid oxycodone.
   - Adequate caloric intake can lead to resolution of an attack resulting from glucose inhibition of ALA synthase activity.

- Administer intravenous **hematin** for severe attacks. Hematin is a stable form of heme that inhibits ALA synthase and subsequent ALA and PBG accumulation.
- Chenodeoxycholic acid increases protoporphyrin excretion into the bile.
- LT has been used in severe cases, but the bone marrow continues to produce protoporphyrin, with resulting damage to the allograft. Therefore, bone marrow transplantation with or without LT has been suggested for patients with severe disease.

3. Photocutaneous porphyria
   - Ultraviolet exposure should be avoided (use sunscreen and protective clothing).
   - Patients with PCT respond to phlebotomy to reduce the iron burden; chloroquine is used to form complexes with uroporphyrin.
   - Treatment of erythropoietic protoporphyria includes administration of carotenoids for skin lesions.

Other Inborn Errors of Metabolism

HYPERAMMONEMIC SYNDROMES

1. **Multiple causes: Urea cycle enzyme deficiencies (e.g., ornithine transcarbamylase deficiency), transport defects of urea cycle intermediates, organic acidemias, fatty acid oxidation disorders, respiratory chain disorders, and disorders of pyruvate metabolism**
2. The presentation varies with the age of the patient. Neonates with hyperammonemia have poor suck, lethargy, and even seizures or coma. Older children present more insidiously with failure to thrive and persistent vomiting or irritability. Episodes may be precipitated by processes that cause endogenous protein catabolism (e.g., excessive protein intake, infection).
3. The diagnosis should be considered in any child with a family history of sudden infant death, Reye syndrome, cyclic vomiting, ataxia, or unexplained failure to thrive.
4. The diagnosis is made by blood ammonia levels, acid-base measurements, and serum glucose, lactate, pyruvate, ketone, and plasma amino acid levels. Determinations of urine organic and orotic acid excretion are essential in making the diagnosis and excluding other inborn errors of metabolism.
5. Treatment
   - Facilitation of ammonia removal: Dialysis, diversion of nitrogen from urea to other waste products with sodium benzoate
   - Decrease ammonia production: Adequate intravenous glucose administration and antibiotics
   - LT: May be lifesaving and corrects the metabolic abnormalities in urea cycle deficiencies
   - Gene therapy for urea cycle defects is a possible future therapy.

DISORDERS THAT CAUSE DAMAGE TO OTHER ORGANS (see also Chapter 25)

1. Crigler-Najjar syndrome type I
   - This autosomal recessive deficiency of hepatic uridine diphosphate–glucuronyl transferase results in the absence of bilirubin glucuronide conjugation in the liver and is characterized by unconjugated hyperbilirubinemia.
   - The diagnosis is suggested by failure of phenobarbital to induce enzymatic activity to decrease bilirubin levels, serum bilirubin values in excess of 15 to 20 mg/dL, the absence of bilirubin conjugates in bile, and genotyping.
   - Children who survive the neonatal period have an elevated risk of irreversible brain damage (kernicterus).

- Serum bilirubin levels increase with illness.
- Emergency treatment includes exchange transfusion and phototherapy (10 to 12 hours per day) to reduce serum bilirubin levels.
- Tin-protoporphyrin reduces serum bilirubin levels and may shorten the duration of daily phototherapy, but it increases photosensitivity.
- LT remains the only definitive treatment.

2. Primary hyperoxaluria (type I oxalosis)
   - This autosomal recessive inborn error of glyoxylate metabolism is caused by deficient or absent liver-specific peroxisomal alanine/glyoxylate aminotransferase.
   - Patients present with recurrent urolithiasis or nephrocalcinosis that leads to end-stage kidney disease and, if untreated, death. This disorder does not cause liver disease.
   - Treatment includes a large fluid intake, low intake of calcium and oxalate, and supplementation with pyridoxine, alkali citrate, or phosphate.
   - Early recurrence of renal disease is common following isolated renal transplantation because the underlying metabolic defect in the liver remains unchanged.
   - Combined LT and renal transplantation is now advocated. It is essential to maintain a high urinary output immediately after LT until the renal oxalate load is greatly reduced.

3. Primary hypercholesterolemia
   - A homozygous mutation in the gene for the low-density lipoprotein receptor results in increased serum cholesterol levels. The incidence is 1 per 1,000,000.
   - This disorder is a risk factor for myocardial ischemia and death within the first 3 decades of life.
   - The only effective treatment is LT; medications are not effective. Normalization of the metabolic defect before the development of atherosclerosis is the objective. Hepatocyte transplantation and gene therapy are being evaluated as definitive treatments.

FURTHER READING

Alwaili K, Alrasadi K, Awan Z, et al. Approach to the diagnosis and management of lipoprotein disorders. *Curr Opin Endocrinol Diabetes Obes.* 2009;16:132–140.

Chu AS, Perlmutter DH, Wang Y. Capitalizing on the autophagic response for treatment of liver disease caused by alpha-1-antitrypsin deficiency and other genetic diseases. *Biomed Res Int.* 2014:459823.

Colombo C. Liver disease in cystic fibrosis. *Curr Opin Pulm Med.* 2007;13:529–536.

Dhawan A, Mitry RR, Hughes RD. Hepatocyte transplantation for liver-based metabolic disorders. *J Inherit Metab Dis.* 2006;29:431–435.

Fairbanks KD, Tavill AS. Liver disease in alpha 1-antitrypsin deficiency: a review. *Am J Gastroenterol.* 2008;103:2136–2141.

Farrell PM, Rosenstein BJ, White TB, et al. Guidelines for diagnosis of cystic fibrosis in newborns through older adults: Cystic Fibrosis Foundation consensus report. *J Pediatr.* 2008;153:S4–S14.

Harmanci O, Bayraktar Y. Gaucher disease: new developments in treatment and etiology. *World J Gastroenterol.* 2008;14:3968–3973.

Hoppe B, Beck BB, Milliner DS. The primary hyperoxalurias. *Kidney Int.* 2009;75:1264–1271.

Junge N, Mingozzi F, Ott M, et al. Adeno-associated virus vector-based gene therapy for monogenetic metabolic diseases of the liver. *J Pediatr Gastroenterol Nutr.* 2015;60:433–440.

Koeberl DD, Kishnani PS, Chen YT. Glycogen storage disease types I and II: treatment updates. *J Inherit Metab Dis.* 2007;30:159–164.

Lim-Melia ER, Kronn DF. Current enzyme replacement therapy for the treatment of lysosomal storage diseases. *Pediatr Ann.* 2009;38:448–455.

Martins AM, Valadares ER, Porta G, et al. Recommendations on diagnosis, treatment, and monitoring for Gaucher disease. *J Pediatr.* 2009;155:S10–S18.

Moyer K, Balistreri W. Hepatobiliary disease in patients with cystic fibrosis. *Curr Opin Gastroenterol.* 2009;25:272–278.

Scott CR. The genetic tyrosinemias. *Am J Med Genet C Semin Med Genet.* 2006;142C:121–126.

Taddei T, Mistry P, Schilsky ML. Inherited metabolic disease of the liver. *Curr Opin Gastroenterol.* 2008;24:278–286.

CHAPTER 21

Budd-Chiari Syndrome and Other Vascular Disorders

Marlyn J. Mayo, MD ■ Mack C. Mitchell, MD

KEY POINTS

1 Hepatic vein occlusion, or Budd-Chiari syndrome (BCS), is an uncommon disorder characterized by hepatomegaly, ascites, and abdominal pain. The disorder most often occurs in patients with an underlying thrombotic diathesis including polycythemia vera, factor V Leiden mutation, protein C deficiency, antithrombin deficiency, paroxysmal nocturnal hemoglobinuria, tumors, and chronic inflammatory diseases.

2 The diagnosis is confirmed by visualization of thrombus or absent flow in hepatic veins by Doppler ultrasonography, computed tomography (CT), or magnetic resonance imaging (MRI).

3 BCS can be fatal without treatment. The approach to treatment should be stepwise beginning with anticoagulation, followed by angioplasty or transjugular intrahepatic portosystemic shunt (TIPS) placement for portal decompression. Liver transplantation (LT) should be reserved for patients with advanced disease who fail other treatments. Five-year survival rates are 85% to 90%.

4 Portal vein thrombosis (PVT) occurs in patients with an underlying thrombotic disorder, intraabdominal inflammation, injury to the portal vessels, or cirrhosis. Extension of hepatocellular carcinoma (HCC) into the portal vein can also result in thrombosis. In the acute phase, anticoagulation is recommended. Band ligation of varices and beta receptor antagonists are used to prevent variceal bleeding in patients with chronic PVT. TIPS may improve the rate of recanalization in patients with PVT who are awaiting transplantation.

5 Sinusoidal obstruction syndrome (SOS), previously known as venoocclusive disease, is an occlusive disorder of the small hepatic venules and is clinically similar to BCS. It develops as a result of toxic injury to the endothelial cells primarily in patients receiving cytoreductive therapy for allogeneic or autologous hematopoietic stem cell transplantation (HSCT). Unexpected weight gain and development of ascites are the hallmarks of SOS in this setting. Chronic hepatitis C infection appears to increase the risk of SOS. Treatment of mild-to-moderate SOS is largely supportive, but trials have suggested that defibrotide may improve survival in patients with severe SOS and multiorgan failure syndrome.

Budd-Chiari Syndrome

BCS results from obstruction to hepatic venous outflow and may result from either thrombotic or nonthrombotic occlusion.

CLASSIFICATION AND ETIOLOGY

1. BSC is classified according to
    a. Duration of symptoms and signs of liver disease

- **Acute:** Development of intractable ascites, abdominal pain, and hepatomegaly within 1 month
- **Subacute:** Insidious onset over 1 to 3 months with minimal to moderate ascites and evidence of collateral vessels around the hepatic veins
- **Chronic:** Typically discovered during evaluation of portal hypertension in patients without previous symptoms; progresses to congestive cirrhosis
  - b. **Site of obstruction**
    - Small hepatic veins, excluding terminal venules
    - Large hepatic veins
    - Hepatic inferior vena cava (IVC)
  - c. **Cause of obstruction**
    - Membranous webs
    - Direct infiltration by tumor or metastasis along veins
    - Thrombosis
2. The majority of patients with BCS present within 3 months of the onset of symptoms. Most have subacute or chronic disease at the time of presentation, suggesting that thrombosis of intrahepatic veins leads subsequently to occlusion of large collecting veins.
3. **Membranous occlusion of the hepatic veins (MOHV)** is a common cause of BCS in Asia but is rarely seen in the United States. The pathogenesis is the subject of controversy; many investigators have assumed that the webs are congenital, but the onset of symptoms in the fourth decade of life and the pathologic features are more suggestive of a postthrombotic event that may represent a complication of chronic BCS.
4. **The majority of patients with BCS have an underlying thrombotic diathesis. The disorder is idiopathic in <20% of cases. Disorders associated with BCS include the following:**
   - a. Hematologic disorders
     - Polycythemia rubra vera
     - Janus kinase 2 (*JAK2*) V617F gene mutation-associated myeloproliferative disorder
     - Paroxysmal nocturnal hemoglobinuria
     - Antiphospholipid antibody syndrome
   - b. Inherited thrombotic diathesis
     - Factor V Leiden mutation
     - Protein C deficiency
     - Prothrombin gene mutation (G20210A)
     - Protein S deficiency (rare)
     - Antithrombin deficiency (rare)
     - C677T methylenetetrahydrofolate reductase (MTHFR) mutation
   - c. Pregnancy or high-dose estrogen use (oral contraceptives)
   - d. Chronic infections of the liver
     - Amebic abscess
     - Aspergillosis
     - Hydatid cysts
     - Tuberculosis
   - e. Tumors
     - HCC
     - Renal cell carcinoma
     - Leiomyosarcoma
   - f. Chronic inflammatory diseases
     - Behçet's disease
     - Inflammatory bowel disease
     - Sarcoidosis

CLINICAL AND LABORATORY FEATURES

1. The classic triad of **hepatomegaly, ascites, and abdominal pain** is seen in the majority of patients but is nonspecific.
   - Splenomegaly may develop in almost one half of patients.
   - Peripheral edema suggests the possibility of thrombosis or compression of the IVC.
   - Jaundice is rare.
2. Persons with an acute presentation may progress rapidly and require urgent treatment, whereas those with a more insidious onset appear to progress slowly in developing complications of portal hypertension.
3. Routine biochemical and hematologic parameters
   - Little value in differential diagnosis
   - Abnormal but nonspecific
   - No distinctive pattern of abnormalities
4. Ascitic fluid characteristics are useful clues to diagnosis.
   - High protein concentration (>2.0 g/dL), particularly in acute presentation
   - Serum-ascites albumin gradient is usually >1.1.
   - White blood cell count is usually <500/mm^3.
5. Differential diagnosis includes the following:
   - Right-sided heart failure
   - Constrictive pericarditis
   - Metastatic disease involving the liver
   - HCC
   - Alcoholic liver disease
   - Granulomatous liver disease

DIAGNOSIS

1. A high index of suspicion is necessary for diagnosis because clinical manifestations and laboratory results are nonspecific.
2. Imaging techniques for visualizing hepatic veins
   a. **Ultrasonography**
      - Color-flow Doppler ultrasonography is better than duplex ultrasonography, which is superior to real-time ultrasonography.
      - Provides cost-effective confirmation of low or absent hepatic venous blood flow
      - Occasionally can visualize thrombus within hepatic veins
      - The sensitivity of color-flow Doppler ultrasonography is 85% to 90%, with similar specificity.
   b. **MRI with gadolinium contrast and/or pulsed sequencing**
      - Can visualize thrombus and detect absence of hepatic venous blood flow
      - Higher cost than Doppler ultrasonography
      - Sensitivity and specificity are approximately 90%.
   c. **Three-phase CT**
      - Provides 85% to 90% sensitivity and specificity (Fig. 21.1).
      - Can detect multifocal regenerative nodules (some of which are >2 cm) that develop in some patients
      - Perfusion abnormalities may result in a "nutmeg" appearance of the congested liver.
      - The caudate lobe is hypertrophied in 75% of patients due to the separate venous drainage of the caudate lobe.

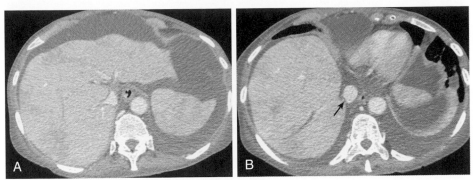

Fig. 21.1 Computed tomography in a patient with Budd-Chiari syndrome. The venous phase of vascular enhancement is shown. The liver is dysmorphic (better seen in A) and enhances in an inhomogeneous fashion. Ascites is present. The hepatic veins are visible as slender, unenhanced structures converging toward an enhanced patent inferior vena cava (most prominent in B) *(arrow)*. From Valla DC. Vascular diseases of the liver. In: Feldman M, Friedman LS, Brandt LJ, eds. *Sleisenger and Fordtran's Gastrointestinal and Liver Disease: Pathophysiology/Diagnosis/Management* 10th ed, Philadelphia: Saunders Elsevier; 2016:1393–1408.

3. Hepatic venography
   ■ Identifies thrombus within hepatic veins
   ■ "Spider-web" pattern of collateral vessels in chronic BCS
   ■ Inability to cannulate the hepatic vein orifices
   ■ Unnecessary if characteristic findings are noted on noninvasive imaging
   ■ Usually performed in conjunction with therapeutic intervention such as TIPS
4. Pathologic findings on liver biopsy specimens
   ■ Evidence of high-grade venous congestion
   ■ Centrilobular liver cell atrophy
   ■ Thrombi within terminal hepatic venules are rarely seen.
   ■ Heterogeneous involvement of the liver is occasionally problematic (i.e., sampling error).
5. **The diagnostic approach to a patient suspected of having hepatic vein occlusion should begin with color Doppler ultrasonography, followed by three-phase CT or MRI. If imaging is equivocal for BCS, then hepatic venography with inferior vena cavography should be performed to confirm the diagnosis. Liver biopsy may be of value to define the extent of fibrosis but is usually unnecessary.**

TREATMENT

1. **Medical therapy** provides short-term symptomatic benefit and is recommended as a first step.
   ■ Diuretics are useful for relieving ascites but do not alter the long-term outcome.
   ■ Anticoagulation with heparin followed by warfarin is recommended in all patients. It prevents repeat thromboses in patients with defined thrombotic disorders but may not relieve symptoms in the long term.
   ■ Thrombolytic therapy has been used successfully in a few reported cases, although the long-term benefit is unclear.
2. Minimally invasive approaches
   a. Rationale
      ■ Hepatocellular injury may result from microvascular ischemia due to congestion.

- Portosystemic shunting provides a low-pressure path to decompress the congested liver.

b. **Angioplasty** of short-segment obstructions such as webs or short hepatic vein stenoses; relief of obstruction is temporary, and repeated treatment is required for long-term management.
   - Placement of metal stents in the hepatic veins following angioplasty of short-segment stenoses has been used to improve long-term patency.
   - Placement of stents in the vena cava provides relief of compression from an enlarged caudate lobe and can be followed by a side-to-side portacaval or mesocaval shunt, if necessary.

c. **TIPS** can be performed in >90% of patients despite occlusion of hepatic veins.
   - The mortality rate is <2%; complication rates are 15% to 20%.
   - The liver transplant–free 5-year survival rate is approximately 85%.
   - Coated stents have better long-term patency rates.
   - Refractory encephalopathy develops in <10% of patients; it may require LT.

3. **LT**
   - Corrects some underlying clotting disorders and restores hepatocellular function
   - Actuarial 3-year survival rates are 80%, and 5-year survival rates are approximately 70%; survival rates have improved substantially since 2005.
   - Recommended in patients with hepatic decompensation who do not respond to minimally invasive procedures
   - BCS can recur in the posttransplant liver.

4. **Transcardiac membranotomy** has been used to relieve membranous obstruction of the IVC and rarely the hepatic veins. Other surgical procedures have been used in small numbers of patients with BCS from other causes. The results have been variable and are subject to the bias of reporting successes more often than failures.

5. **Surgical portosystemic shunting** was the mainstay of treatment for BCS before less invasive procedures such as TIPS were used widely; shunts remain an option but are **no longer the preferred approach** to management due to the high rate of complications.
   a. Options include the following:
      - Side-to-side portacaval shunt
      - Mesocaval shunt
      - Mesoatrial shunt
      - Side-to-side portacaval with cavoatrial shunt
   b. Success of portosystemic shunting depends on the following:
      - Experience of the surgeon with a particular shunt
      - The underlying disease
      - Host factors, including the extent of fibrosis or presence of cirrhosis
      - Overall hepatic function at the time of operation
   c. Patency rates of 65% to 95% depend on the following:
      - Duration of disease: The longer the duration, the lower the patency
      - Presence of fibrosis or cirrhosis: Lower patency rates
      - The type of shunt: Rates for mesoatrial shunts are slightly lower than those for mesocaval shunts.
      - Continued thrombotic diathesis from the underlying disease
   d. Survival rates of 38% to 87% at 5 years depend on the following:
      - Continued patency of the graft
      - Degree of fibrosis
      - Type of shunt

SUMMARY OF EVALUATION AND MANAGEMENT OF BUDD-CHIARI SYNDROME

1. The diagnosis of BCS should be suspected in any patient with ascites and hepatomegaly, particularly if there is evidence of a thrombotic diathesis. A high ascitic protein content or serum-ascites albumin gradient is a clue to the diagnosis. Anticoagulation should be considered in patients with an acute or subacute presentation and in those patients with a defined thrombotic disorder.
2. Color Doppler or duplex ultrasonography should be used to visualize the hepatic veins and determine the patency of the IVC. If there is doubt, a three-phase CT or MRI is indicated.
3. If there is evidence of hepatic vein outflow obstruction, angioplasty or TIPS should be considered to provide portal decompression. An IVC stent can be placed to relieve compression temporarily by an enlarged caudate lobe. **All patients with refractory ascites should undergo early portosystemic decompression.**
4. **If TIPS fails and cirrhosis is absent, surgical portosystemic shunting should be considered.** Hepatic venography and vena cavography are required to determine the need for a mesoatrial or a mesocaval shunt. Mesoatrial shunts are preferable in patients with a high pressure gradient across the hepatic cava, provided the surgeon is experienced in this operation. If the IVC is patent, mesocaval shunting with or without placement of an IVC stent is possible.
5. **If hepatic decompensation is present or if other interventions fail, LT is indicated.** Early portosystemic decompression with TIPS is desirable until a donor organ is available.

Portal Venous Thrombosis

CLASSIFICATION

1. **Acute PVT**
   - Symptoms <60 days before presentation
   - No evidence of underlying cirrhosis or portal hypertension by endoscopy or imaging
2. **Chronic PVT**
   - May develop in isolation or as a complication of cirrhosis
   - The presence of portal vein collaterals and portal hypertension distinguishes the chronic from the acute phase.
3. **Splenic vein thrombosis**
   - May develop in isolation from thrombosis within the main portal vein
   - Leads to splenomegaly and isolated gastric varices without esophageal varices

ETIOLOGY

1. **As many as 70% of patients with PVT have an underlying thrombotic disorder.**
   - PVT is associated with most of the same disorders that are associated with BCS (see discussion earlier in chapter).
   - Virchow triad (stasis, hypercoagulability, and endothelial dysfunction) are risk factors.
2. The following infections within the abdomen presumably result from pylephlebitis (septic phlebitis of the portal vein):
   - Acute appendicitis

- Acute cholecystitis or cholangitis
- Pancreatitis
- Neonatal omphalitis **(most common cause worldwide)**
3. Isolated thrombosis of the splenic vein may develop as a consequence of the following:
   - Chronic pancreatitis
   - Direct trauma to the abdomen
4. PVT in cirrhosis probably results from a combination of the following factors:
   - Diminished blood flow within the portal vein
   - Reduced levels of protein C, protein S, antithrombin, heparin cofactor, and plasminogen, all of which are synthesized by the liver, as well as increased levels of von Willebrand factor and factor VIII, both of which are cleared by the liver
   - HCC can lead to PVT either through a procoagulant pathway or by direct invasion into the portal vein.

CLINICAL FEATURES

1. Acute PVT
   - Abdominal pain and nausea
   - Intestinal ischemia may result particularly when thrombosis extends to the superior mesenteric vein.
   - Intestinal infarction is uncommon but can be fatal.
2. Chronic PVT
   - Esophageal varices
   - Splenomegaly
   - Thrombocytopenia
   - Variceal bleeding is often well tolerated in the absence of cirrhosis.
   - Ascites rarely develops in the absence of cirrhosis.
3. PVT in patients with cirrhosis
   - Frequency of up to 38%
   - More common in patients with decompensated than compensated cirrhosis
   - Likely related to low flow in the portal circulation and reduced levels of proteins C and S

DIAGNOSIS

1. **Doppler ultrasonography** has high sensitivity (>70%) and specificity (>80%) for diagnosing PVT. **CT** and **MRI** can identify thrombus within the portal vein and are helpful when the results of Doppler ultrasonography are equivocal. Sensitivity and specificity approach 98% (Fig. 21.2).
2. MR cholangiography can assess portal cholangiopathy, which increases the risk of biliary complications.
3. Proximal dilatation of the portal vein suggests acute thrombosis, whereas portal venous collaterals (including portal cavernoma) indicate chronic thrombosis.
4. Liver biochemical test levels are normal except in patients with underlying chronic liver disease.
5. A thorough evaluation for an underlying thrombotic disorder and HCC is warranted.

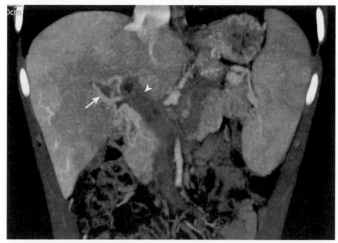

Fig. 21.2 Computed tomography in a patient with acute portal vein thrombosis. The portal venous phase is shown and demonstrates vascular enhancement. The portal and mesenteric veins are enlarged and lack enhancement *(arrowhead)*. Dilated veins are seen in the porta hepatis, particularly in the gallbladder wall *(arrow)*. From Valla DC. Vascular diseases of the liver. In: Feldman M, Friedman LS, Brandt LJ, eds. *Sleisenger and Fordtran's Gastrointestinal and Liver Disease: Pathophysiology/Diagnosis/Management* 10th ed, Philadelphia: Saunders Elsevier; 2016:1393–1408.

TREATMENT

1. **Acute PVT**
   a. **Anticoagulation** with heparin or low-molecular-weight heparin is indicated in the acute phase.
      ▪ It promotes recanalization if carried out within the first 30 days.
      ▪ It reduces the risk of complications such as bowel infarction.
      ▪ The need for long-term anticoagulation is based on the presence of an underlying thrombotic disorder.
   b. Thrombolysis is associated with a high rate of bleeding.
   c. Surgical thrombectomy is not recommended due to an unacceptable rate of complications, except possibly when resection of infarcted bowel is required.
2. **Chronic PVT**
   a. Long-term use of **beta receptor antagonists** has been reported to reduce the risk of variceal bleeding.
   b. **Band ligation of varices** is safe and is as effective in patients with other causes of varices.
   c. **TIPS** and **surgical portosystemic shunts** can be tried in patients who fail less invasive methods of treating varices.
   d. **Splenectomy** is effective in treating gastric varices due to isolated thrombosis of the splenic vein.
   e. **Long-term anticoagulation** is probably safe if patients are carefully selected, and indicated **in patients with prothrombotic state or with involvement of superior mesenteric vein.**

3. PVT in patients with cirrhosis
   a. Early anticoagulation achieves complete recanalization in 50% to 100%, but thrombosis may develop again in up to 40% when anticoagulation is discontinued.
   b. Anticoagulation with low-molecular-weight heparin may prevent development of PVT in cirrhosis.
   c. TIPS may improve chances for recanalization.
   d. Decompensation is more likely in the absence of recanalization; the outcome after LT is worse in those without than with recanalization pretransplantation.

Sinusoidal Obstruction Syndrome

DEFINITION AND ETIOLOGY

1. SOS was originally described by Chiari in 1899 and was further described as hepatic vein endophlebitis by Bras in 1954. Subsequently, it was recognized as a form of drug-induced liver injury. Histologic features include the following:
   - Subendothelial sclerosis of terminal hepatic venules
   - Thrombosis secondary to sclerosis
   - Perivenular and sinusoidal fibrosis, particularly in later stages and with chronic injury
   - Centrilobular hepatocyte necrosis (may be a primary event)
2. SOS (formerly **venoocclusive disease**) is most often seen as one of the following:
   - An **acute form** following HSCT. It is thought to be due to toxicity from the preparative regimen of high-dose cytoreductive therapy, with or without hepatic irradiation.
   - A **chronic, more indolent form** following toxicity of pyrrolizidine alkaloids from plants of the *Crotalaria*, *Senecio*, and *Heliotropium* genera. The alkaloids are ingested in the form of herbal teas, hence the term Jamaican bush tea disease.
3. Using a definition of SOS based on clinical manifestations (see discussion later in chapter), no single histologic feature is pathognomonic. A correlation exists between the number of histologic abnormalities and the clinical severity of SOS.

RISK FACTORS FOR ACUTE SOS FOLLOWING HSCT

- Pretransplant elevation in serum aminotransferase levels
- Past history of chronic hepatitis C infection or drug-induced hepatitis
- Past history of abdominal radiation
- Older or very young (<6.5 years) recipient age
- Poor pretransplant performance status and reduced lung diffusion capacity
  More intensive myeloablative cytoreductive regimens are associated with an increased incidence of SOS.
   - Radiation dose >12 Gy
   - Cyclophosphamide plus busulfan
   - Cyclophosphamide, carmustine (BCNU), and etoposide

PATHOGENESIS

1. Cytoreductive therapy is toxic primarily to endothelial cells, both sinusoidal and vascular. These cells are more susceptible to glutathione depletion in response to a variety of agents, including dacarbazine, azathioprine, and monocrotaline. Damaged endothelial cells slough into the sinusoid, causing obstruction, thereby sacrificing the integrity of the sinusoidal lining and inducing a localized inflammatory reaction.

2. Various cytokines including tumor necrosis factor α (TNF-α) are released in response to cytoreductive therapy. Patients with hepatic failure and multiorgan failure syndrome have also been shown to have high circulating levels of TNF-α and other cytokines. TNF-α in particular exerts procoagulant effects on protein C and may be involved in the pathogenesis of thrombosis in SOS; however, an understanding of the pathophysiology is speculative.

CLINICAL FEATURES AND DIAGNOSIS

1. SOS following HSCT has been defined as the **occurrence of two or more of the following characteristics appearing within 20 days after transplantation (Seattle criteria):**
   - Painful hepatomegaly
   - Sudden weight gain >2% of baseline body weight
   - Total serum bilirubin >2.0 mg/dL (34.2 μmol/L)

   The **Baltimore criteria** include total serum bilirubin >2.0 mg/dL and two of the following: Weight gain >5% of baseline, ascites, and hepatomegaly. These criteria are more stringent, and the prognosis is worse if the Baltimore criteria are used.
2. The development of **multiorgan failure syndrome** including renal insufficiency, cardiac failure, pulmonary infiltrates/acute respiratory distress syndrome, and bleeding indicates **severe SOS.**
3. CT may help to distinguish SOS from graft-versus-host disease (GVHD). Patients with SOS have periportal edema, ascites, and a narrow right hepatic vein, whereas those with GVHD often have thickening of the small bowel.
4. Using the Seattle criteria, SOS develops in up to 10% of patients who undergo HSCT. The overall survival rate for all patients with clinical evidence of SOS is 30%, but for those with severe SOS and multiorgan failure syndrome, it is only 15%.
5. The more chronic form of SOS develops in those who ingest pyrrolizidine alkaloids. Ingestion is most often inadvertent and can be due to contamination of foodstuffs with pyrrolizidine-containing plants. Clinical features of this condition are similar to those of hepatic vein occlusion and include tender hepatomegaly, abdominal pain, ascites, and fatigue. The absence of specific features and the lack of noninvasive methods for detecting this condition make diagnosis difficult. Liver biopsy specimens usually show sinusoidal and perivenular fibrosis as well as subendothelial sclerosis.

TREATMENT

1. Treatment of mild-to-moderate SOS following HSCT is largely supportive.
   - Attention should be paid to the patient's fluid status: Avoid excessive fluid administration that results in worsening of cardiac and pulmonary function.
   - Broad-spectrum antibiotics are used to treat presumptive infection, pending identification of a specific causative organism.
2. **Defibrotide,** a polydisperse mixture of single-stranded oligonucleotide, may be of benefit in treating **severe SOS.** A clinical trial of defibrotide improved survival of severe SOS with multiorgan failure syndrome to 38% compared with 25% in historic controls.
   - Support with platelets and red blood cell transfusions is often necessary because of the profound cytopenias that accompany HSCT.
   - Use of dopamine and other pressors may be necessary to maintain renal perfusion, particularly in the presence of a capillary leak syndrome.
   - Antithrombin may be of benefit in preventing progression of SOS if given early in the course of the illness.

- Prostaglandin E, ursodeoxycholic acid, pentoxifylline, and heparin all have had limited success in preventing SOS.
- TIPS is technically feasible and has been of benefit in a small number of patients with SOS.

3. Treatment of chronic SOS associated with ingestion of pyrrolizidine alkaloids often requires LT because of the extensive fibrosis that is usually present at the time of diagnosis. Early cases may be managed with a portosystemic shunt.

FURTHER READING

Berzigotti A, Garcia-Criado A, Darnell A, et al. Imaging in clinical decision-making for portal vein thrombosis. *Nat Rev Gastroenterol Hepatol*. 2014;11:308–316.

Chawla Y, Bodh V. Portal vein thrombosis. *J Clin Exp Hepatol*. 2015;5:22–40.

Chen H, Turon F, Hernandez-Gea V, et al. Nontumoral portal vein thrombosis in patients awaiting liver transplantation. *Liver Transpl*. 2016;22:352–365.

Coppell JA, Richardson PG, Soiffer R, et al. Hepatic veno-occlusive disease following stem cell transplantation: incidence, clinical course, and outcome. *Biol Blood Marrow Transplant*. 2010;16:157–168.

Garcia-Pagan JC, Heydtmann M, Raffa S, et al. TIPS for Budd-Chiari syndrome: long-term results and prognostics factors in 124 patients. *Gastroenterology*. 2008;135:808–815.

Mentha G, Giostra E, Majno PE, et al. Liver transplantation for Budd-Chiari syndrome: a European study on 248 patients from 51 centres. *J Hepatol*. 2006;44:520–528.

Mitchell MC, Boitnott JK, Kaufman S, et al. Budd-Chiari syndrome: etiology, diagnosis and management. *Medicine*. 1982;61:199–218.

Narayanan Menon KV, Shah V, Kamath PS. The Budd-Chiari syndrome. *N Engl J Med*. 2004;350:578–585.

Orloff MJ, Daily PO, Orloff SL, et al. A 27-year experience with surgical treatment of Budd-Chiari syndrome. *Ann Surg*. 2000;232:340–352.

Parikh S, Shah R, Kapoor P. Portal vein thrombosis. *Am J Med*. 2010;123:111–119.

Qi X, De Stefano V, Li H, et al. Anticoagulation for the treatment of portal vein thrombosis in liver cirrhosis: a systematic review and meta-analysis of observational studies. *Eur J Intern Med*. 2015;26:23–29.

Richardson PG, Riches ML, Kernan NA, et al. Phase 3 trial of defibrotide for the treatment of severe veno-occlusive disease and multi-organ failure. *Blood*. 2016;127:1656–1665.

Segev DL, Nguyen GC, Locke JE, et al. Twenty years of liver transplantation for Budd-Chiari syndrome: a National Registry analysis. *Liver Transpl*. 2007;13:1285–1294.

Valla DC. Primary Budd-Chiari syndrome. *J Hepatol*. 2009;50:195–203.

Villa E, Camma C, Marietta M, et al. Enoxaparin prevents portal vein thrombosis and liver decompensation in patients with advanced cirrhosis. *Gastroenterology*. 2012;143:1253–1260.

CHAPTER 22

The Liver in Heart Failure

Florence S. Wong, MD, FRACP, FRCP(C)

KEY POINTS

1 Liver involvement (cardiac hepatopathy) in either forward or backward heart failure is frequent, the extent of which depends on the severity of the heart failure.

2 Backward heart failure causes congestion of the liver with hepatomegaly with or without ascites and nonspecific liver biochemical test abnormalities.

3 Forward heart failure causes hypoxic damage to the liver if the circulatory failure is acute, severe, and prolonged. The pattern of a rapid rise and fall in serum aminotransferase levels is characteristic.

4 Alternative diagnoses should be considered if abnormal liver biochemical test results are unusually high in the absence of an acute presentation and, in particular, if the alkaline phosphatase level is more than twice normal or if the alanine aminotransferase (ALT) is much higher than the aspartate aminotransferase (AST) level.

5 Comorbid conditions such as diabetes mellitus that are independently associated with liver involvement such as steatosis or nonalcoholic steatohepatitis can increase the liver's susceptibility to damage when heart failure occurs.

6 No specific treatment is available for the liver dysfunction. Improvement in cardiac function results in return of liver biochemical test levels to normal, unless cardiac cirrhosis is already present.

7 Cardiac surgery, including heart transplantation, carries a high mortality rate in patients with cirrhosis.

Overview

1. Liver dysfunction (cardiac hepatopathy) has long been recognized as a complication of both severe acute and chronic heart failure.

2. Backward failure causes an increase in right ventricular pressure, which leads to perisinusoidal edema, and impaired oxygen diffusion to hepatocytes, especially around the central vein. Forward failure is usually related to profound hypotension, leading to hypoxia of hepatocytes. Frequently, both forward failure and backward failure occur in the same patient.

3. An understanding of the hepatic circulation and normal liver architecture is important to appreciate how the hemodynamic changes of heart failure affect the liver and lead to the associated clinical, biochemical, and histologic features.

Hepatic Circulation

HEPATIC BLOOD SUPPLY

1. The liver has a **dual blood supply.**
   - The portal vein supplies approximately 66% to 83% of the blood flow to the liver and brings nutrient-rich but relatively less well-oxygenated venous blood from the stomach, intestine, and spleen.
   - The hepatic artery, a branch of the celiac axis, provides the remaining 17% to 34% of the liver's blood supply; the arterial blood supplies approximately 50% of hepatic oxygen.
2. A reduction in portal inflow or hepatic sinusoidal pressure results in a reflex increase in hepatic arterial blood flow and thereby ensures a constant sinusoidal pressure.
3. Primary changes in hepatic arterial blood flow are not associated with changes in portal venous blood flow.
4. A decrease in cardiac output usually results in reduced hepatic blood flow. The percentage of cardiac output received by the liver, however, remains relatively stable at approximately 25%.
5. Decreased perfusion is usually compensated for by increased oxygen extraction, which can increase up to 95%.
6. Hypercapnia, if present, causes generalized vasodilatation that further increases blood flow to the liver.

HEPATIC VENOUS DRAINAGE

1. The liver is drained by the hepatic vein, which is formed by the right, middle, and left hepatic veins.
2. The hepatic vein, in turn, drains into the inferior vena cava and then into the right atrium.

HEPATIC MICROCIRCULATION

1. The portal vein and the hepatic artery divide into branches to the right and left lobes of the liver. These branches further subdivide five to six times until their terminal branches reach the portal tracts.
2. The portal vein tributaries open directly into hepatic sinusoids. The hepatic artery branches open into some, but not all, sinusoids. The sinusoids anastomose freely at all levels between the portal vein tributaries and the terminal hepatic venules.
3. Hepatic sinusoids have the following characteristics:
   - They form a rich vascular network that converges toward the terminal hepatic venule.
   - They are lined by both endothelial cells and specialized macrophages called Kupffer cells. No basement membrane underlies the endothelial cells.
   - The porous nature of the sinusoids allows for low hydrostatic pressure and free flow between the sinusoids and the interstitial space (the space of Disse).
4. The diameter of a sinusoid is less than that of erythrocytes, which have to squeeze through the lumen of the sinusoid. Therefore, narrowing of the sinusoidal lumen can seriously compromise oxygenation of hepatocytes.

Liver Histology

1. The **histologic unit** of the liver is the **lobule** (Fig. 22.1A).
   - Its boundaries are surrounded by connective tissue stroma and portal tracts.
   - The center of the lobule is the terminal hepatic vein.

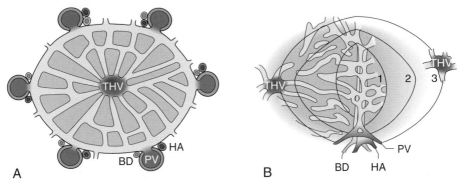

Fig. 22.1 A, The histologic unit of the liver: The lobule. B, The functional unit of the liver: The acinus. *BD,* Bile duct; *HA,* hepatic artery; *PV,* portal vein; *THV,* terminal hepatic vein; *1, 2, 3,* zones 1, 2, and 3 of Rappaport (see text).

2. The **functional unit** of the liver is the **acinus** (Fig. 22.1B).
   - Liver parenchymal cells are grouped into concentric zones (of Rappaport) centered around the portal tract; zone 1 is nearest, whereas zones 2 and 3 are more distal to the afferent blood vessels.
   - The oxygen tension and nutrient level of the blood decrease from zone 1 to zone 3.
   - Zone 1 hepatocytes are first to receive oxygenated blood and last to undergo necrosis.
   - Zones 2 and 3 receive blood of considerably less oxygen and nutrient content and are more vulnerable to hepatotoxic and hypoxic injury.

Pathophysiology

1. Hepatic ischemia develops when an imbalance occurs between hepatic oxygen supply and demand.
2. Forward failure of the heart leads to decreased cardiac output and hepatic blood flow.
3. Backward failure with venous engorgement causes hepatic congestion.
4. Both forward failure and backward failure of the heart lead to hepatocyte hypoxia and liver damage.
5. Decreased arterial oxygen saturation also contributes to liver damage (Fig. 22.2).

CHRONIC PASSIVE CONGESTION

1. The increased systemic venous pressure is reflected as hepatic venous hypertension, which can cause hepatic cell atrophy as a result of sinusoidal congestion and expansion.
2. The accompanying perisinusoidal edema can result in decreased diffusion of oxygen, nutrients, and other metabolites to hepatocytes.
3. Insufficient concentrations of substrates, accumulation of metabolites, and release of cytokines secondary to an inflammatory response all contribute to hypoxic damage, even in the presence of systemic circulatory support.
4. Collagenosis of the space of Disse from chronic congestion may play a minor role in impairing oxygen diffusion.

DECREASED HEPATIC BLOOD FLOW

1. In heart failure with low cardiac output, total hepatic blood flow falls by approximately one third.
2. Increased oxygen extraction by the liver in states of low hepatic blood flow ensures constant oxygen consumption within wide limits of hepatic blood flow. The liver, therefore, does not suffer adverse effects of hypoxia as a result of decreased hepatic blood flow under basal conditions.

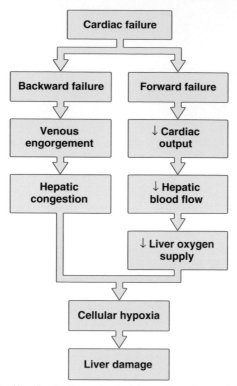

Fig. 22.2 Algorithm for the pathophysiology of liver damage in heart failure.

3. A >70% reduction in hepatic blood flow decreases oxygen uptake, galactose elimination capacity, and ATP concentrations and increases the lactate/pyruvate ratio (an index of tissue hypoxia).
4. Hepatic arterial vasoconstriction with intense selective splanchnic vasoconstriction in states of significant hypoperfusion and shock causes hypoxic damage to the liver.
5. Hypoxic damage characteristically occurs in the area adjacent to the terminal hepatic vein (zone 3 of the acinus), the area farthest away from the oxygen-carrying blood supply.
6. Loss of mitochondrial oxidative phosphorylation, as a result of hypoxia, leads to impaired membrane function, disrupted intracellular ion homeostasis, and reduced protein synthesis.
7. Low cardiac output and the consequent circulatory changes in the intestinal wall may also allow increased diffusion of endotoxin into the portal blood, thereby augmenting damage to the liver.
8. With reestablishment of the circulation, reperfusion injury can aggravate hepatic injury through the generation of reactive oxygen species when ischemic hepatocytes are reexposed to oxygen.
9. In acute heart failure, both reduced hepatic blood flow and increased central venous pressure contribute to the development of hypoxic (or ischemic) hepatitis.

Pathology

MACROSCOPIC

1. The liver is enlarged and purplish with rounded edges (Fig. 22.3).
2. Nodularity is inconspicuous, but if nodular regenerative hyperplasia (see discussion later in chapter) or cardiac cirrhosis is present, nodules may be seen.

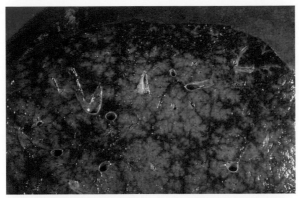

Fig. 22.3 Macroscopic appearance of the liver in heart failure.

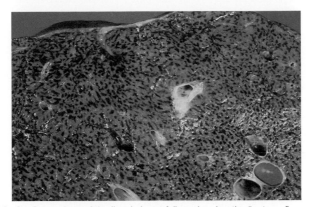

Fig. 22.4 Cut surface of the liver in heart failure showing the "nutmeg" appearance.

3. The cut surface shows prominent hepatic veins, which may be thickened.
4. A "nutmeg" appearance results from the contrasting combination of hemorrhagic central areas of the lobules and the normal paler portal and periportal areas (Fig. 22.4).
5. The portal areas may be more yellow than usual due to an increase in portal fat, making the contrast with the central hemorrhagic areas more obvious.

MICROSCOPIC

1. The severity of hepatic histopathologic changes generally correlates with the clinical or biochemical severity of heart failure and with cardiac weight and chamber size.
2. Early in heart failure, the terminal hepatic veins become engorged and dilated. Sinusoids adjacent to the terminal hepatic veins are also dilated and are filled with erythrocytes for a variable extent toward the portal areas. In severe cases, the appearance is that of peliosis hepatis (blood lakes).
3. Also evident are compression and variable atrophy of the liver cell plates and an apparent increase in the amount of lipofuscin in the cytoplasm of liver cells.
4. Moderately severe heart failure can result in zone 3 liver cell necrosis. The cellular infiltrate is inconspicuous.
5. In acute severe hypotension and shock, midzone necrosis can also occur.

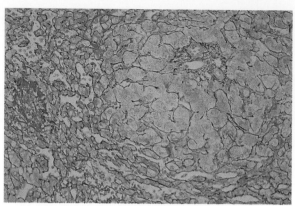

Fig. 22.5   Histopathology of the liver demonstrating collapse of the reticulin network around the terminal hepatic veins and nodular transformation in a patient with heart failure (Gordon and Sweet reticulin).

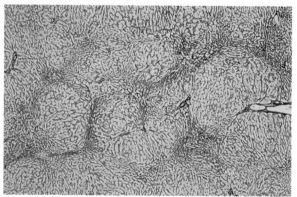

Fig. 22.6   Histopathology of the liver demonstrating nodular regenerative hyperplasia associated with heart failure (Gordon and Sweet reticulin).

6. The necrotic hepatocytes are often packed with a brownish pigment, likely related to bilirubin degradation.

7. Liver cell necrosis progresses from zone 3 to the portal areas as the heart disease progresses. In the most severe form of liver congestion from heart failure, only a small area of normal-appearing hepatocytes remains in the periportal area.

8. The reticulin network condenses and may collapse around the terminal hepatic vein following loss of liver cells (Fig. 22.5).
   - Bridging fibrosis can be seen extending from and joining adjacent terminal hepatic veins.
   - Ultimately, the unaffected portal areas are surrounded by rings of fibrous tissue, resulting in reverse lobulation.

9. True **cardiac cirrhosis** is rare and is associated with intimal fibrosis and thrombosis of small- and medium-sized hepatic veins. The resulting ischemia is responsible for hepatocellular necrosis, and the stasis augments fibroblast activation and collagen deposition.

10. Regeneration of hepatocytes around the periportal area can occur, leading to liver cell plates that are many cells thick. These regenerating hepatocytes can reorganize into rounded periportal masses abutting compressed central hepatocytes and congested and dilated sinusoids. Such changes are best described as **nodular regenerative hyperplasia** (Fig. 22.6).

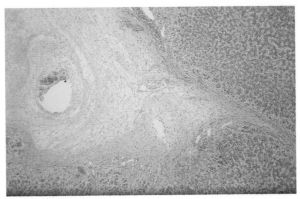

Fig. 22.7 Histopathology of the liver demonstrating phlebosclerosis in the wall of the terminal hepatic vein in a patient with heart failure (Masson trichrome).

11. The wall of the terminal hepatic vein can undergo varying degrees of fibrous thickening termed **phlebosclerosis** (Fig. 22.7).
12. Liver damage associated with heart failure is reversible once the heart failure is treated: Hepatocytes regenerate, fibrous bands become narrower and acellular, and near-normal hepatic architecture is restored.

Epidemiology

1. Liver involvement is common in severe heart failure.
2. The frequency is difficult to assess accurately because many cases of congestive hepatopathy are subclinical and undiagnosed.
3. The overall frequency of liver congestion in congestive cardiac failure depends on patient selection and the criteria used for defining liver involvement (clinical, biochemical, or histologic).
4. As the incidence of rheumatic valve disease has declined, coronary artery disease with associated congestive cardiomyopathy has become an important cause of liver congestion.
5. In patients with a cardiac index >2 L/min/m², only 20% to 30% of patients have minor elevations of serum liver enzyme levels. By contrast, in those with a cardiac index <1.5 L/min/m², up to 80% of patients have major liver biochemical abnormalities.

Etiology (Table 22.1)
CHRONIC CONGESTION

1. Left and right ventricular failure can often coexist, resulting in hepatic congestion.
2. In the past, rheumatic heart disease, with mitral stenosis and tricuspid regurgitation, was a common cause of left and right ventricular failure; and appears to produce the most severe hepatic congestion.
3. Other causes of hepatic congestion include constrictive pericarditis, severe pulmonary hypertension, tricuspid regurgitation, cor pulmonale, and cardiomyopathy.
4. Children with hypoplastic left heart syndrome and coarctation of the aorta are particularly prone to hepatic necrosis, possibly because of the combination of reduced systemic blood flow, a left-to-right shunt, and markedly elevated right ventricular pressure.

TABLE 22.1 ■ **Causes of Liver Disease in Patients With Heart Failure**

Chronic Congestion	Hypoxic Hepatitis	Coexisting Heart and Liver Diseases
Cardiomyopathy	Acute myocardial infarction with arrhythmia and shock	Congenital disorders: Alagille syndrome
Congenital cardiac abnormalities: Hypoplastic heart syndrome, coarctation of the aorta	Atrial fibrillation	Drugs: Amiodarone, statins
	Bacterial endocarditis	Hereditary disorders: Hereditary hemo-chromatosis, Wilson disease
Cor pulmonale	Chronic obstructive sleep apnea	Infiltrative diseases: Amyloidosis
Constrictive pericarditis	Exacerbation of heart failure	Liver conditions with cardiac involve-ment: Hepatitis C, excessive
Post-Fontan operation	Pulmonary embolism	alcohol intake, fatty liver, and
Rheumatologic heart disease	Respiratory failure	atherosclerosis
Severe pulmonary hypertension	Septic shock	Vascular tumors
Tricuspid regurgitation		

5. Adults who have survived a Fontan procedure performed in infancy have chronic elevation of the central venous pressure due to transfer of systemic venous return directly to the pulmonary artery without passing through the atrioventricular pumps. Often, cirrhosis is already present when liver involvement is recognized.

ACUTE HYPOXIC HEPATITIS

1. Acute myocardial infarction with arrhythmia and cardiogenic shock can complicate coronary artery disease, with resulting ischemia to the liver superimposed on the chronic hepatic congestion.
2. The abrupt onset of atrial fibrillation or the development of bacterial endocarditis can decrease left ventricular output and can aggravate hypoxic liver damage.
3. Other causes of hypoxic hepatitis include exacerbation of heart failure, pulmonary embolism, respiratory failure, chronic obstructive sleep apnea, and septic shock.

CONDITIONS THAT AFFECT BOTH THE HEART AND THE LIVER

- Congenital disorders: Alagille syndrome
- Drugs: Amiodarone can cause steatosis and fibrosis; statins can cause elevated serum aminotransferase levels.
- Hereditary disorders: Hereditary hemochromatosis, Wilson disease
- Infiltrative diseases: Amyloidosis
- Liver conditions with cardiac involvement: Hepatitis C, nonalcoholic fatty liver disease, atherosclerosis, excessive alcohol intake
- Vascular tumors: Hemangioendothelioma

Clinical Features

CONGESTIVE HEPATOPATHY

1. In most patients, the clinical picture is dominated by symptoms and signs of right-sided heart failure, rather than those of liver disease (Table 22.2).
2. Stigmata of liver disease, such as palmar erythema and spider telangiectasias, are rare, unless the liver disease and heart failure have a common cause, such as hemochromatosis.

TABLE 22.2 ■ **Findings in Patients With Cardiac Hepatopathy**

Finding	Acute Heart Failure (%)	Chronic Heart Failure (%)
Hepatomegaly	83	76
Jaundice	50	11
Ascites	42	68
Encephalopathy	25	2
Splenomegaly	8	15
Esophageal varices	0	8

Adapted from Myers RP, Cerini R, Sayegh R, et al. Cardiac hepatopathy: clinical, hemodynamic, and histologic characteristics and correlations. *Hepatology.* 2003;37:393–400.

3. Right upper quadrant discomfort or pain results from stretching of the liver capsule and is mediated by the phrenic nerve.
4. The liver can return to normal size as fibrosis develops during the course of severe hepatic congestion, but it is never reduced in size.
5. Jaundice
   ■ Mild jaundice is common, but deep icterus is rare.
   ■ Jaundice increases with prolonged and repeated bouts of heart failure.
   ■ Hyperbilirubinemia may be in part unconjugated, related to infarcts of tissues, especially pulmonary infarcts. Jaundice may then be prolonged, with conjugated hyperbilirubinemia, because of the inability of the hypoxic liver to handle the bilirubin load.
6. Patients with tricuspid regurgitation have a palpable systolic pulsation over the liver, related to the transmission of right atrial pressure to the hepatic vein.
7. Splenomegaly is frequent, but other features of portal hypertension are usually absent, except in severe cardiac cirrhosis associated with constrictive pericarditis.
8. Ascites is most likely related to increased sinusoidal pressure and permeability, and increased leakage of lymph, rather than cirrhosis. As a result, the ascitic protein content is high (≥2.5 g/dL), with a high serum-ascites albumin gradient (≥1.1 g/dL) (see Chapter 13).
9. Peripheral edema and pleural effusions probably reflect the cardiac disease rather than the concomitant hepatic congestion.

HYPOXIC HEPATITIS

1. Hypoxic hepatitis refers to diffuse hepatic injury as a result of acute hypoperfusion on a background of chronic congestion.
   ■ The term *ischemic hepatitis* is actually a misnomer, because it is now recognized that hypotension alone will not produce liver injury; however, the term is commonly used.
   ■ Patients with liver injury frequently have elevated jugular venous pressure in addition to the acute hypotension, suggesting underlying chronic congestion that predisposes these patients to the acute hypotensive insult.
   ■ The liver injury is characterized by centrilobular necrosis without inflammation.
2. Generally, no specific symptoms result from liver injury, but occasional patients have symptoms of acute hepatitis.
   ■ Some patients have changes in mental status that commonly reflect impaired cerebral perfusion rather than hepatic encephalopathy.

3. Hepatopulmonary syndrome develops in up to one half of patients but is reversible.
4. Occasionally, functional renal failure (increased serum creatinine and potassium, low urinary sodium, and a normal urinary sediment) occurs abruptly as a result of the systemic hypotension.
5. Acute liver failure with asterixis and coma as a complication of heart failure is rare. If it occurs, it usually develops 2 to 3 days after the circulatory failure.

CARDIAC CIRRHOSIS

1. Cardiac cirrhosis is rare, and the presentation is usually dominated by symptoms of right-sided heart failure.
2. Cardiac cirrhosis should be suspected in a patient with well-documented tricuspid regurgitation and absent hepatic pulsation.
3. Cardiac cirrhosis should also be considered in patients with the following conditions:
   - Severe mitral stenosis
   - Constrictive pericarditis
   - Prolonged or recurrent severe congestive heart failure
   - Clinically severe passive congestion of the liver, yet a nonenlarged liver, with splenomegaly and ascites

Laboratory Features

CONGESTIVE HEPATOPATHY

- The frequency of abnormal liver biochemical test levels in patients with heart failure varies widely in the published literature.
- In general, abnormalities in liver blood tests only occur in patients with a cardiac output of <1.5 L/min/m^2.
- Patients with higher right atrial pressures and more profound clinical manifestations of heart failure tend to have more abnormal laboratory results.
- A cholestatic pattern of liver biochemical abnormalities (elevated serum bilirubin and gamma-glutamyltranspeptidase levels) has been suggested to correlate independently with signs of right-sided heart failure.

1. Bilirubin
   - Serum bilirubin levels are increased in 15% to 50% of patients with heart failure.
   - Jaundice is usually mild in heart failure, with serum bilirubin levels generally <4.5 mg/dL (80 µmol/L).
   - Approximately 50% to 60% of the serum bilirubin is unconjugated, because of a combination of mild hemolysis, reduced uptake, and decreased conjugation by hepatocytes.
   - Markedly elevated serum bilirubin levels may be seen in acute right-sided heart failure. This hyperbilirubinemia appears to be related to hepatocellular dysfunction per se.
   - Serum bilirubin levels may fall rapidly after improvement in hepatic congestion, with levels normalizing in 3 to 7 days.
   - In patients with prolonged heart failure, serum bilirubin levels may not return to normal for months after relief of the hepatic congestion because of covalent bonding of conjugated bilirubin with albumin to form *delta bilirubin*, which has a prolonged half-life of 21 days.
   - **An elevated total bilirubin level is an independent predictor of adverse cardiac outcome and death in patients with heart failure.**
   - In patients who undergo heart transplantation, direct and indirect bilirubin levels more than three times the upper limit of normal are significant negative predictors of survival after discharge.

2. Aminotransferases
   - Serum levels are elevated in only 3% to 10% of patients with stable heart failure without decompensation. Levels are usually two to four times the upper limit of normal.
   - Serum AST levels tend to be higher than ALT levels, because cardiac myocytes are rich in AST; the increase in AST generally appears earlier than the increase in ALT.
   - Moderate increases in serum AST levels can also be caused by myocardial infarction; consequent myocardial dysfunction and heart failure can complicate the interpretation of the elevated AST level. Simultaneous measurement of a serum troponin level or the MB fraction of creatine kinase is helpful in diagnosing myocardial injury.
   - A significant, albeit weak, correlation exists between the aminotransferase levels and both the right atrial pressure and the cardiac index. Improvement in cardiac function results in a return of serum aminotransferase levels toward normal in 3 to 7 days.

3. Alkaline phosphatase
   - Elevated alkaline phosphatase (ALP) levels are uncommon in heart failure. When present, the elevation is mild, usually not exceeding twice the upper limit of normal, unless the liver disease and heart failure have a common cause.
   - The exact mechanism leading to an increased ALP level in patients with liver congestion is unknown. Both pressure-induced intrahepatic biliary obstruction and hepatic dysfunction may play a role.
   - When nodular regenerative hyperplasia complicates heart failure, the only abnormal liver biochemical test result may be an elevated serum ALP level.

4. International normalized ratio (INR)
   - The INR is increased in more than 80% of patients with heart failure.
   - Affected patients are therefore sensitive to the effects of warfarin.
   - With successful treatment of chronic heart failure, the prothrombin time takes 2 to 3 weeks to return to normal.
   - In acute congestion, the prothrombin time may increase rapidly to twice normal, is not responsive to vitamin K administration, and may return to normal rapidly with successful treatment of the congestion.

5. Serum albumin
   - Serum albumin levels are moderately decreased in 30% to 50% of patients with heart failure. Lower levels are seen in patients with ascites and edema.
   - Low serum albumin levels may result in part from decreased hepatic synthesis and in part from a dilutional effect secondary to fluid retention.
   - In general, the serum albumin level does not correlate with either the duration of heart failure or the extent of hepatic damage.
   - The serum albumin level may require more than 1 month to improve following resolution of heart failure.

HYPOXIC HEPATITIS

1. **Changes in serum liver biochemical test levels in hypoxic hepatitis are characteristic**, and the diagnosis can be made by observing the following evolution of these changes:
   - **Marked increases in serum aminotransferase levels (up to 100 times normal) with AST greater than ALT, occur within 24 to 48 hours of acute circulatory failure.**
   - A rapid return of the aminotransferase levels to normal occurs in 3 to 11 days after treatment of acute heart failure.
   - **A profound rise and fall in serum lactate dehydrogenase (LDH) levels, more so than the ALT, and an ALT/LDH ratio <1.5 are more typical of hypoxic hepatitis than of viral hepatitis.**

- Alkaline phosphatase levels generally remain normal.
- Serum bilirubin levels may rise but are rarely greater than four times the upper limit of normal.
- The INR is only mildly increased.

CARDIAC CIRRHOSIS

No biochemical test distinguishes a congested noncirrhotic liver from one with cardiac cirrhosis. Therefore, cardiac cirrhosis is a clinical and a histologic diagnosis.

LIVER DYSFUNCTION WITH THE USE OF A LEFT VENTRICULAR ASSIST DEVICE

- In patients with preexisting liver dysfunction, the insertion of a left ventricular assist device (LVAD) can improve serum liver biochemical test levels, likely related to a volume shift from the intrathoracic space to the systemic circulation, thereby improving liver blood flow.
- Liver dysfunction can also occur after implantation of an LVAD. This is usually multifactorial, related to prolonged cardiopulmonary bypass time, arterial hypotension, use of vasopressors, the presence of right ventricular failure, and the presence of a systemic inflammatory response syndrome.
- The course of the post-LVAD liver dysfunction can be monitored by a modified Model for End-stage Liver Disease (MELD) score that excludes the INR (MELD-XI score), due to the limitation imposed by concomitant anticoagulation (see also Chapter 32).

Imaging Features

DOPPLER ULTRASONOGRAPHY

- The first sign of hepatic congestion on ultrasonography is dilatation of the inferior vena cava and hepatic vein (>6 mm in diameter) and hepatomegaly with or without ascites.
- Loss of a normal triphasic flow pattern in the inferior vena cava and hepatic veins
- Increased pulsatility of the portal venous signal
- Biphasic waveforms in the presence of cirrhosis

CONTRAST-ENHANCED COMPUTED TOMOGRAPHY

- Lobulated, patchy, and inhomogeneous pattern in a large liver
- Irregular perivascular enhancement or delayed parenchymal enhancement
- Distended inferior vena cava and early reflux of contrast medium into the inferior vena cava and hepatic veins

MAGNETIC RESONANCE IMAGING

- The liver shows a reticular mosaic pattern of liver enhancement that becomes more homogeneous after 1 to 2 minutes.
- The hepatic veins and suprahepatic portion of the inferior vena cava show early enhancement due to reflux from the right atrium.
- The portal vein shows diminished, delayed, or absent enhancement.

ULTRASOUND ELASTOGRAPHY

- Ultrasound elastography is a rapid and noninvasive measure of liver stiffness; it is a surrogate for liver fibrosis and validated in alcoholic liver disease and viral hepatitis.
- It is less reliable in assessing liver stiffness in patients with heart failure because of the frequent presence of obesity and ascites, although several studies have reported a significant correlation between the central venous pressure and liver stiffness as measured by ultrasound elastography.
- Virtual touch quantification of transient elastography is a newer technique that uses a sound beam to gently compress deeper tissues and displays an elastogram of the tissue.
- Changes in liver stiffness as measured by elastography have been shown to correlate with changes in central venous pressure measurements and therefore can be used to assess the effectiveness of heart failure treatment.

Treatment

GENERAL MEASURES

1. **Treatment of liver congestion should be directed toward the primary problem—that is, the heart failure.**
2. Improvement in liver biochemical test levels usually follows clinical improvement unless cardiac cirrhosis is already present.
3. Management of established cardiac cirrhosis includes treatment of heart failure as well as paracentesis if ascites is refractory.
   - Routine intravenous replacement of albumin after paracentesis is unnecessary because synthetic hepatic function is relatively preserved.
   - Focal nodular hyperplasia nodules can also be found in patients with cardiac cirrhosis. The differential diagnosis includes macronodular regenerative nodules, dysplastic nodules, and hepatocellular carcinoma (HCC). Biopsy of a nodule may be required to establish the diagnosis definitively.
   - Once cardiac cirrhosis is established, screening for HCC, as in other causes of cirrhosis, is necessary, but cases of HCC arising in cardiac cirrhosis are uncommon.

DRUG TREATMENT OF HEART FAILURE WITH LIVER DYSFUNCTION

The liver plays a central role in drug metabolism; therefore, hepatic dysfunction due to liver congestion could potentially alter the pharmacokinetics of drugs used to treat heart failure.
1. Angiotensin converting enzyme inhibitors
   - These are usually prodrugs that require conversion into active metabolites in the liver, with the exception of lisinopril.
   - With liver dysfunction, transformation of the prodrug and inactivation of the active drug may be reduced. Therefore, frequent monitoring is required if usual doses of the drug are used.
2. Angiotensin receptor antagonists
   - The only drug in this class that undergoes extensive biotransformation is losartan. In patients with hepatic impairment, the bioavailability of losartan is doubled, and the elimination is halved; therefore, the starting dose used may need to be reduced.
   - This does not apply to valsartan or irbesartan.
3. Beta receptor antagonists
   - Propranolol undergoes extensive first-pass metabolism, and in liver dysfunction clearance is decreased significantly and the drug's half-life is increased. Therefore, a reduction in dose may be required.
   - No dose adjustments are needed for all the other beta blockers.

4. Digoxin
   ■ Digoxin is not metabolized by the liver; however, in patients with liver impairment, the volume of distribution is reduced and, therefore, a lower dose may be required.
5. Warfarin
   ■ Warfarin may be indicated in patients with heart failure because of thromboembolic events.
   ■ Warfarin is metabolized in the liver by the cytochrome P-450 system, and its metabolites are excreted in the bile.
   ■ Caution is required when warfarin is used because its metabolism is reduced in the setting of liver dysfunction, thereby predisposing patients to the risk of overanticoagulation.
   ■ Reduced hepatic synthesis of clotting factors will increase the likelihood of bleeding if anticoagulation is administered.
   ■ The INR should be monitored closely.
   ■ The use of direct-acting anticoagulants such as dabigatran, rivaroxaban, and apixaban is challenging in this setting because monitoring the degree of anticoagulation is difficult.
6. Statins
   ■ 3-Hydroxy-3-methylglutaryl-coenzyme A reductase inhibitors (statins) have been shown to reduce all-cause mortality in patients with heart failure.
   ■ They may also cause liver enzyme elevations, although hepatitis is rare.
   ■ The dose of a statin should be reduced in patients with known hepatic congestion to reduce the possibility of hepatitis.

CARDIAC SURGERY

1. **Clinical improvement in cardiac function can be dramatic following definitive treatment of heart failure,** such as valve replacement, pericardiectomy for constrictive pericarditis, or correction of a congenital anomaly.
2. Cardiac cirrhosis with or without hepatic failure, however, results in a substantial rise in the perioperative mortality rate and may therefore be a contraindication to surgery.
3. Patients with Child class A cirrhosis appear to tolerate cardiac surgery satisfactorily, whereas those with Child class B or C cirrhosis have high rates of major postoperative complications and death (see Chapter 32).
4. A Child-Turcotte-Pugh score >7 has a high sensitivity (86%) and specificity (92%) for predicting mortality after cardiac surgery with cardiopulmonary bypass and in one study performed better than the MELD score in this setting.
5. Cardiopulmonary bypass may aggravate preexisting coagulopathy, thereby leading to platelet dysfunction, fibrinolysis, and hypocalcemia. Limited evidence suggests that less invasive procedures such as angioplasty, valvuloplasty, and revascularization procedures without bypass are preferable in patients with cirrhosis.

CARDIAC TRANSPLANTATION

1. In patients without liver cirrhosis, cardiac transplantation can result in improvement in serum liver enzyme levels and liver function over the course of 3 to 12 months.
2. Cholestatic parameters tend to improve first, with the serum bilirubin level returning to normal within 3 months.
3. LDH and aminotransferase levels may take up to 12 months to normalize.
4. Cirrhosis has generally been considered a contraindication to heart transplantation. In the few cases of heart transplantation performed in patients with cirrhosis, a 50% in-hospital mortality rate was reported. Mortality is highest in patients with a MELD score >20.

5. The MELD score should be monitored serially in patients with heart failure, cirrhosis, and liver dysfunction.
6. In patients in whom liver function improves after cardiac transplantation, cirrhosis has been reported to reverse 10 years postcardiac transplant.
7. Mortality is highest in patients with a cardiac diagnosis other than cardiomyopathy and in those with a previous sternotomy and massive ascites.
8. Combined heart and liver transplantation is feasible at expert centers in carefully selected patients.

Prognosis

1. **The prognosis of liver dysfunction in the setting of cardiac disease is that of the underlying cardiac disease.**
2. In chronic heart failure, the outcome will be favorable if the underlying cardiac condition is treated and the hepatic congestion resolves.
3. In hypoxic hepatitis, the prognosis is often poor. Prolonged jaundice, especially if severe, is a poor prognostic sign.
4. An elevated serum total bilirubin level is the strongest predictor of all-cause mortality.
5. Death in hypoxic hepatitis is usually the result of heart failure. The hepatic disorder usually has little or no influence on the eventual outcome.
6. In general, the presence of cardiac cirrhosis in and of itself does not alter prognosis unless cardiac surgery is performed.

FURTHER READING

Allen LA, Felker GM, Pocock S, et al. Liver function abnormalities and outcome in patients with chronic heart failure: data from the Candesartan in heart failure. Assessment of reduction in mortality and morbidity (CHARM) program. *Eur J Heart Fail*. 2009;11:170–177.

Alvarez AM, Mukherjee D. Liver abnormalities in cardiac diseases and heart failure. *Int J Angiol*. 2011;20:135–142.

Bigeus J, Hillege HL, Postmus D, et al. Abnormal liver function tests in acute heart failure: relationship with clinical characteristics and outcome in the PROTECT study. *Eur J Heart Fail*. 2016;18:830–839.

Dichtl W, Vogel W, Dunst KM, et al. Cardiac hepatopathy before and after heart transplantation. *Transpl Int*. 2005;18:697–702.

Fouad YM, Yehia R. Hepato-cardiac disorders. *World J Hepatol*. 2014;6:41–54.

Hsu RB, Chang CI, Lin FY, et al. Heart transplantation in patients with liver cirrhosis. *Eur J Cardiothorac Surg*. 2008;34:307–312.

Millonig G, Friedrich S, Adolf S, et al. Liver stiffness is directly influenced by central venous pressure. *J Hepatol*. 2010;52:206–210.

Møller S, Bernardi M. Interactions of the heart and the liver. *Eur Heart J*. 2013;34:2804–2811.

Myers RP, Cerini R, Sayegh R, et al. Cardiac hepatopathy: clinical, hemodynamic, and histologic characteristics and correlations. *Hepatology*. 2003;37:393–400.

Raichlin E, Daly RC, Rosen CB, et al. Combined heart and liver transplantation: a single-center experience. *Transplantation*. 2009;88:219–225.

Samsky MD, Patel CB, deWald TA, et al. Cardiohepatic interactions in heart failure. *J Am Coll Cardiol*. 2013;61:2397–2405.

Shaheen AM, Kaplan GG, Hubbard JN, et al. Morbidity and mortality following coronary artery bypass graft surgery in patients with cirrhosis: a population-based study. *Liver Int*. 2009;29:1141–1151.

Shiffman ML. The liver in circulatory failure. In: Schiff ER, Sorrell MF, Maddrey WC, eds. *Schiff's Diseases of the Liver*. 10th ed. Philadelphia: Lippincott Williams & Wilkins; 2006:1185–1198.

Suman A, Barnes DS, Zein NN, et al. Predicting outcome after cardiac surgery in patients with cirrhosis: a comparison of Child-Pugh and MELD scores. *Clin Gastroenterol Hepatol*. 2004;2:719–723.

Vandeursen VM, Damman K, Hillege HL, et al. Abnormal liver function in relation to hemodynamic profile in heart failure patients. *J Card Failure*. 2010;16:84–90.

CHAPTER 23

The Liver in Pregnancy

Michelle Lai, MD, MPH ■ Jacqueline L. Wolf, MD

KEY POINTS

1. Liver diseases in pregnancy include those that occur exclusively in pregnancy and those that occur coincidentally in pregnancy or are present at the time of pregnancy.

2. Normal physiologic changes in pregnancy may alter the normal range for liver biochemical tests (Table 23.1).

3. Important clues to the diagnosis are found in the history and physical examination.

4. Laboratory findings with particular importance to diagnosing liver disease in pregnancy are proteinuria, hyperuricemia, elevated serum bile acid levels, thrombocytopenia, and anemia.

5. Abdominal ultrasonography may be helpful. Liver biopsy is rarely necessary, but it may be diagnostic for acute fatty liver of pregnancy.

6. Timely diagnosis and, hence, appropriate treatment are critical to outcome. Delivery of the infant is indicated for severe preeclampsia, eclampsia, acute fatty liver of pregnancy, and HELLP (hemolysis, elevated liver tests, low platelets) syndrome; and immunization is indicated in infants born to mothers with hepatitis B.

7. Although women with chronic liver disease may have more trouble conceiving, pregnancy has no adverse effect on the progression of liver disease.

Overview

1. Liver diseases in pregnancy consist of the following:
   - Those that occur exclusively during pregnancy
   - Those that occur coincidentally in pregnancy or are present at the time of pregnancy
2. The approach to the pregnant patient with abnormal liver biochemical test levels should include thorough history taking and physical examination.
3. Liver disorders unique to pregnancy include the following:
   - Hyperemesis gravidarum
   - Intrahepatic cholestasis of pregnancy (IHCP)
   - Acute fatty liver of pregnancy (AFLP)
   - Preeclampsia/eclampsia
   - HELLP syndrome
   - Hepatic rupture
4. Liver disorders that occur coincidentally with pregnancy include viral hepatitis, nonalcoholic fatty liver disease (NAFLD), Budd-Chiari syndrome, cholelithiasis, cholecystitis, Wilson disease, and autoimmune hepatitis (AIH).

TABLE 23.1 ■ **Changes in Liver Biochemical Test Levels in Normal Pregnancy**

Test	Change	Trimester of Maximum Change
ALT	None	—
AST	None	—
Alkaline phosphatase	↑ 2- to 4-fold	Third
Bilirubin	None	—
Albumin	↓ 10%–60%	Second
Cholesterol	↑ 2-fold	Third
Fibrinogen	↑ 50%	Second
Gamma globulins	None to slight ↓	Third
Transferrin	↑	Third

ALT, Alanine aminotransferase; *AST,* aspartate aminotransferase.

From Olans LB, Wolf JL. Liver disease in pregnancy. In: Carlson KJ, Eisenstat SA, eds. *The Primary Care of Women* 2nd ed. St. Louis: Mosby–Year Book; 2003:531–539.

Approach to the Pregnant Patient

HISTORY

1. Relation to time of gestation (Table 23.2)
2. Pruritus
   - Characteristic of IHCP
   - Affects palms of hands and soles of feet initially, then elsewhere
3. Nausea and vomiting
   - Occurs in 50% to 90% of all pregnancies ("morning sickness")
   - Key feature of hyperemesis gravidarum
   - When associated with headache and peripheral edema may indicate preeclampsia
   - When associated in late pregnancy with abdominal pain, with or without hypotension, may indicate hepatic rupture
4. Abdominal pain
   - The location, character, duration, and factors that induce or relieve pain should be noted.
   - Right upper quadrant or midabdominal pain in late pregnancy may have ominous implications. Consider cholelithiasis, AFLP, hepatic rupture, and preeclampsia.
5. Jaundice
   - Note the relation of jaundice to the onset of other symptoms.
   - Jaundice follows pruritus in IHCP.
6. Systemic symptoms
   - Headache, peripheral edema, foamy urine, oliguria, and neurologic symptoms may occur in preeclampsia.
   - Fever, malaise, and a change in stools may indicate infection such as hepatitis.
   - Easy bruisability may occur in HELLP syndrome.
   - Weight loss, weight gain, or dizziness may occur with liver disease in pregnancy.
7. History of past pregnancy and birth control use
   - Note the time of onset of symptoms in previous pregnancies.
   - Note the outcome of previous pregnancies.
   - A history of jaundice with previous birth control use is a risk factor for IHCP.

TABLE 23.2 ■ Differential Diagnosis of Elevated Serum Aminotransferase Levels and/or Jaundice According to Trimester of Pregnancy

Trimester	Differential Diagnosis
First	Hyperemesis gravidarum
	Gallstones
	Viral hepatitis
	Drug-induced hepatitis
	Intrahepatic cholestasis of pregnancy[a]
Second	Intrahepatic cholestasis of pregnancy
	Gallstones
	Viral hepatitis
	Drug-induced hepatitis
	Preeclampsia/eclampsia[a]
	HELLP syndrome[a]
Third	Intrahepatic cholestasis of pregnancy
	Preeclampsia/eclampsia
	HELLP syndrome
	Acute fatty liver of pregnancy
	Hepatic rupture
	Gallstones
	Viral hepatitis
	Drug-induced hepatitis

[a]Uncommon in this trimester.

HELLP, Hemolysis, elevated liver tests, low platelets.

From Olans LB, Wolf J. Liver disease in pregnancy. In: Carlson KJ, Eisenstat SA, eds. *The Primary Care of Women* 2nd ed. St. Louis: Mosby–Year Book; 2003:531–539.

8. Relevant pregnancy-related factors
   ■ Multiple versus single gestation (Table 23.3)
   ■ Primiparous versus multiparous
   ■ Medications
9. History of living in or travel to areas endemic for viral hepatitis

PHYSICAL EXAMINATION

■ Normal findings that occur in pregnancy include spider telangiectasias and palmar erythema.
■ Abnormal findings that may occur with liver disease in pregnancy are jaundice, hepatomegaly, hepatic tenderness, hepatic friction rub or bruit, splenomegaly, Murphy sign, and diffuse excoriations.
■ Systemic findings that may occur with liver disease in pregnancy are hypertension, orthostatic hypotension, peripheral edema, asterixis, hyperreflexia or other neurologic findings, ecchymoses, and petechiae.

TABLE 23.3 ■ **Rates of Recurrence of Pregnancy-Associated Liver Disease in Subsequent Pregnancies**

Disease	Rate of Recurrence (%)
Hyperemesis gravidarum	15.2
Intrahepatic cholestasis of pregnancy	0–70
Acute fatty liver of pregnancy	20–70 in carriers of LCHAD mutation
Preeclampsia	2–43
HELLP syndrome	4–27

HELLP, Hemolysis, elevated liver tests, low platelets; *LCHAD,* long-chain 3-hydroxyacyl-coenzyme A dehydrogenase.

DIAGNOSTIC TESTS

- The only major restrictions in diagnostic testing compared with the nongravid state are exposure to radiation or gadolinium.
- Routine blood chemistry tests and a blood count are helpful. Uric acid levels are often elevated in AFLP and may be elevated in preeclampsia.
- Hemolysis and a low platelet count occur in HELLP syndrome. Disseminated intravascular coagulation (DIC) with a low fibrinogen level, increased fibrin split products, and an elevated partial thromboplastin time may also occur in HELLP syndrome.
- Elevations in serum bile acid levels occur before or are concurrent with the onset of IHCP.
- Serum amylase and lipase levels should be checked in a patient with abdominal pain.
- If viral hepatitis is suspected, serologic tests should be checked for the following: Hepatitis A (immunoglobulin M [IgM] and IgG antibody to hepatitis A virus [anti-HAV]); hepatitis B (surface antigen [HBsAg] and antibody, core antibody, and, if HBsAg is positive, e antigen and antibody); hepatitis C (antibody to hepatitis C virus [anti-HCV] and possibly HCV RNA). If the patient has traveled to an endemic area, consider testing for hepatitis E (see Chapter 3).
- The benefits of endoscopy, including endoscopic retrograde cholangiopancreatography (ERCP), should be weighed against the risks in pregnancy. Risks include fetal hypoxia from sedative drugs or positioning. Sedative medications and radiation exposure should be minimized.
- Abdominal ultrasonography is safe and useful.
- Although abdominal computed tomography (CT) is more sensitive than abdominal ultrasonography for hepatic rupture and may yield more information, radiation exposure and the stability of the patient should be considered in decisions about the choice of imaging test.
- Angiography is rarely needed in cases of hepatic rupture.
- Magnetic resonance imaging (MRI) is probably safe, although this is not conclusively proven. Gadolinium should not be used in pregnancy.

Liver Disorders Unique to Pregnancy

Table 23.4 shows typical laboratory findings associated with these disorders.

HYPEREMESIS GRAVIDARUM

1. **Definition:** Intractable vomiting in pregnancy that leads to dehydration, electrolyte disturbances, weight loss of 5% or more, and nutritional deficiencies

TABLE 23.4 ■ **Results of Laboratory Tests in Pregnancy-Associated Liver Disease**

	Aminotrans-ferases[a]	Bile Acids[a]	Bilirubin	Alkaline Phosphatase[a]	Uric Acid	Platelets	PT/PTT	Urine Protein
Hyper-emesis gravidarum	1–20×	Normal	<5 mg/dL	1×		Normal	Normal	Normal	Normal
Intrahepatic cholestasis of preg-nancy	1–20×	30–100×	<5 mg/dL	1–3×		Normal	Normal	Normal	Normal
Acute fatty liver of pregnancy	5–10×	Normal	≤10 mg/dL	1–3×	↑	±↓	±↑	±↑
Preeclamp-sia/eclamp-sia	5–100×	Normal	≤5 mg/dL	1–3×	↑	±↓	±↑	↑
HELLP syndrome	1–100×	Normal	<5 mg/dL	1–3×	↑	↓	±↑	±↑
Hepatic rupture	2–100×	Normal	±↓	↓	Normal	±↓	±↑	Normal

[a]Results are indicated as times the upper limit of normal.

PT, Prothrombin time; *PTT*, partial thromboplastin time.

2. **Epidemiology**
   - Most common in first trimester
   - Incidence: 0.3% to 1% in northern European, Canadian, and American women but up to 3.9% in Asian women
   - Risk factors: Age <25 years, preexisting diabetes mellitus, hyperthyroidism, overweight, primiparity, multiple gestations, prior history of hyperemesis gravidarum, history of mother or sister with hyperemesis gravidarum, and molar pregnancy
3. **Etiology:** Thought to be multifactorial involving immunologic, hormonal, and psychological factors
4. **Clinical and laboratory features**
   - Liver biochemical test abnormalities in 50% of patients
   - Serum alanine aminotransferase (ALT) elevations generally 1- to 3-fold but may reach 20 times the upper limit of normal
   - Occasional serum alkaline phosphatase and bilirubin elevations
   - Concomitant hyperthyroidism in 50%
5. **Diagnosis:** Clinical
6. **Treatment:** Supportive with rehydration, vitamin supplementation, small and frequent low-fat meals, and antiemetics (e.g., metoclopramide 10 mg orally four times daily or 10 mg intramuscularly or intravenously every 4 to 6 hours or ondansetron 4 to 8 mg orally every 8 hours or 8 mg intravenously every 4 to 8 hours); nasojejunal tube feedings or total parenteral nutrition possibly needed in severe cases
7. **Outcome:** Observed lower rate of spontaneous abortion, but also lower birth weights and increased incidence of congenital hip dysplasia in infants. The recurrence rate is 15.2% in the second pregnancy (compared with a rate of 0.7% if hyperemesis gravidarum was not present in the first pregnancy).

Intrahepatic Cholestasis of Pregnancy

1. **Definition:** Reversible form of cholestasis characterized by intense pruritus in pregnancy, elevated serum ALT and fasting serum bile acid levels, and spontaneous relief of symptoms and signs within 4 to 6 weeks after delivery
2. **Epidemiology**
   - More common in late second or third trimester, but can occur in any trimester
   - Incidence: 0.1% to 2%, with higher incidence in South Asian, South American, and Scandinavian populations; highest incidence (up to 27%) in Chilean Araucanian Indians
   - Risk factors: Progesterone use in pregnancy; past medical or family history of IHCP; personal history of intrahepatic cholestasis resulting from oral contraceptive or estrogen ingestion; personal history of gallstone disease, chronic hepatitis C, or other types of chronic hepatitis
3. **Etiology:** Multifactorial, including genetic, hormonal, and environmental factors. Theories include the following:
   - Gene variants of hepatocanalicular transport proteins (ATP-binding cassette [ABC] transporter B4 = phosphatidylcholine floppase, ABC transporter B11 = bile salt export pump, ABC transporter C2 = conjugated organic anion transporter, ATP8B1 = FIC1, multidrug resistance [MDR]3 [hepatocellular phospholipid transporter ABCB4]) and their regulators (e.g., the bile acid sensor farnesoid X receptor [FXR]) are found in some patients; incidence of IHCP is increased in mothers of children with progressive familial intrahepatic cholestasis (PFIC) type 3
   - Mutations in ABCB4/MDR3 gene are found in 16% of women with ICP.
   - Inherited sensitivity to estrogens
   - Association with low serum selenium levels; decreasing incidence in Chilean population linked to increases in serum selenium levels
4. **Clinical and laboratory features**
   - Jaundice in 25% of patients following the onset of pruritus
   - Elevated serum aminotransferase levels (up to 4-fold), serum bile acid levels (30 to 100 times), levels of monosulfated or disulfated progesterone metabolites (particularly 3- and 5-alpha isomers), and occasionally serum cholesterol and triglyceride levels
   - Liver biopsy (not usually indicated) specimens reveal cholestasis with minimal hepatocellular necrosis.
5. **Diagnosis:** Clinical
6. **Treatment**
   - Symptom management: Sleeping in a cold room, topical alcohol and camphor menthol lotion, cholestyramine, and ursodeoxycholic acid (UDCA) 10 to 15 mg/kg body weight
   - Close monitoring and early delivery of fetus
7. **Outcome**
   - In mothers, increased risk (<8%) of future gallstone disease, chronic hepatitis C, cirrhosis, and other hepatobiliary diseases
   - Increased risk of preterm delivery (19% to 60%); meconium staining of amniotic fluid (9% to 24%); fetal bradycardia (14%); fetal distress (22% to 33%); fetal loss (0.4% on average, 4.1% in severe cases), particularly when fasting serum bile acid levels are >40 μmol/L

ACUTE FATTY LIVER OF PREGNANCY

1. **Definition:** A rare, life-threatening complication of pregnancy manifested by microvesicular fatty infiltration of the liver and progressive liver failure
2. **Epidemiology**
   - Onset in third trimester (usually after 35 weeks but as early as 26 weeks; can occur in the immediate postpartum period)

- Incidence: 1 in 10,000 to 15,000 deliveries
- Risk factors: Primigravida, multiple gestations, and male fetuses

3. **Etiology:** Defects in mitochondrial fatty acid beta-oxidation in the mother: Most commonly caused by fetal deficiency in the long-chain 3-hydroxyacyl-coenzyme A dehydrogenase (LCHAD) enzyme. LCHAD is part of mitochondrial trifunctional protein (MTP) and catalyzes the third step in β-oxidation of long-chain fatty acids. Up to 70% of cases result from homozygous LCHAD deficiency in the fetus, with a heterozygous mother.
   - Abnormal concentrations of fetal long-chain fatty acids enter the maternal circulation and have toxic effects in the mother
   - G1528C (E474Q mutation) in the MTP causes LCHAD deficiency.
   - Other defects that cause AFLP: Fetal hepatic carnitine palmitoyl transferase I deficiency, fetal short-chain acyl-CoA dehydrogenase deficiency, maternal only or fetal fatty acid oxidation defect in medium-chain acyl-CoA dehydrogenase
   - Nutritional factors, alterations in lipoprotein synthesis, and enzyme deficiencies in the mitochondrial urea cycle are other proposed pathogenic factors.
   - Oxidative stress in mitochondria and peroxisomes of placenta in mothers with AFLP

4. **Clinical and laboratory features**
   - Symptoms include headache, fatigue, malaise, nausea, vomiting, and abdominal pain.
   - Jaundice may follow a prodrome.
   - Progressive liver failure, with coagulopathy, encephalopathy, or renal failure, may occur.
   - 20% to 40% of patients have signs of preeclampsia.
   - Serum aminotransferase levels are elevated (usually <500 U/L).
   - Serum alkaline phosphatase and bilirubin levels are mildly to moderately elevated.
   - Hyperuricemia occurs in 80%.

5. **Diagnosis**
   - Abdominal ultrasonography and CT are inconsistent in detecting fatty infiltration.
   - Swansea criteria (Box 23.1): 85% positive predictive value and 100% negative predictive value
   - If the disorder and a risk of delivering a premature infant are clinically suspected, then emergency liver biopsy should be done. Frozen liver biopsy specimen shows a microvesicular fatty infiltrate of liver detectable by Oil-Red-O stain.

BOX 23.1 ■ Swansea Criteria for Diagnosing Acute Fatty Liver of Pregnancy

Six or more of the following features in the absence of another explanation:
   Vomiting
   Abdominal pain
   Polydipsia/polyuria
   Encephalopathy
   Elevated serum bilirubin level
   Hypoglycemia
   Elevated serum uric acid level
   Leukocytosis
   Elevated serum aminotransferase levels
   Elevated plasma ammonia level
   Renal impairment
   Coagulopathy
   Ascites or bright liver on ultrasonography
   Microvesicular steatosis on liver biopsy specimen

6. **Treatment**
   - **Rapid delivery of the infant is critical.** Most women improve, but fulminant hepatic failure may occur and treatment with liver transplantation has been reported.
   - Screening for a fatty acid oxidation defect is indicated in affected patients.
7. **Outcome**
   - Maternal mortality rate: 8% to 18%
   - Fetal mortality rate: 9% to 23%
   - Recurrence in mother: 20% to 70% if she is an LCHAD mutation carrier

PREECLAMPSIA/ECLAMPSIA

1. **Definition: Preeclampsia** is the **triad of hypertension, proteinuria, and edema.** Preeclampsia is a multisystem disease with renal, hematologic, hepatic, central nervous system, and fetal-placental involvement. **Eclampsia** is the presence of **convulsions or coma in addition to the symptoms and signs of preeclampsia.**
2. **Epidemiology**
   - More common in late second or third trimester, but may occur postpartum
   - Incidence: Preeclampsia in 2% to 8% of pregnancies, eclampsia in 0.1% to 0.2%
   - Risk factors: Insulin resistance, obesity, extremes of maternal age (age <20 years or >45 years), primigravida, infection, family history of preeclampsia/eclampsia, multiple gestations, hydatidiform mole, fetal hydrops, polyhydramnios, and inadequate prenatal care
3. **Etiology:** Unknown. Thought to be a two-stage model with abnormal placentation followed by endothelial activation in the third trimester. Proposed mechanisms include vasospasm, abnormal placental development, abnormal endothelial reactivity, activation of coagulation, and decreased nitric oxide synthesis. Levels of fms-like tyrosine kinase 1 (sFlt1, also known as soluble vascular endothelial growth factor) are high, and upregulation of placental endoglin occurs. Elevation of circulating soluble endoglin begins 2 to 3 months before preeclampsia. A mutation in the gene encoding STOX1 transcription factor has been proposed to cause susceptibility, but data are still unclear.
4. **Clinical and laboratory features**
   a. Hypertension
      - Mild preeclampsia: Blood pressure ≥140/90 mm Hg but <160/110 mm Hg
      - Severe preeclampsia: Blood pressure ≥160/110 mm Hg
   b. Convulsions or coma in eclampsia
   c. Headaches, visual changes, abdominal pain, heart failure, respiratory distress, and oliguria are possible in severe disease.
5. **Diagnosis**
   - Clinical features suggest the diagnosis.
   - Serum aminotransferase levels are elevated in 90% of patients with eclampsia, 50% with severe preeclampsia, and 24% with mild preeclampsia.
   - Serum aminotransferase levels are elevated 5 to 100 times, with modest increases in serum bilirubin levels (up to 5 mg/dL).
   - Thrombocytopenia and microangiopathic hemolytic anemia may occur.
   - Liver biopsy specimens, if available, may demonstrate periportal deposition of fibrin and fibrinogen associated with hemorrhage, with or without necrosis. In some cases, microvesicular fatty infiltration is seen, suggesting overlap with AFLP.
6. **Treatment**
   - **Delivery of the infant is the preferred treatment of eclampsia and near-term preeclampsia.** Management remote from term is controversial but may include bed rest, antihypertensive therapy, and intravenous magnesium sulfate.

- The incidence of preeclampsia is **not** reduced with nutritional supplementation, including calcium, or with low-dose aspirin.

7. **Outcome**
   - Morbidity and mortality rates correlate with severity.
   - The most common cause of death is cerebral involvement.
   - The risk of hepatic rupture and HELLP syndrome is increased.
   - Risks to the fetus include prematurity, fetal growth retardation, abruptio placentae, and low birth weight.
   - Increased perinatal morbidity and mortality in the mother and fetus correlate with the severity of preeclampsia, preterm delivery, multiple gestations, and preexisting maternal medical conditions.
   - Postdelivery liver biochemical test abnormalities generally resolve.
   - Women subsequently have an increased risk of hypertension, type 2 diabetes mellitus, and stroke.
   - Offspring have an increased risk of hypertension and double the risk of stroke later in life.

HELLP SYNDROME

1. **Definition:** Hemolysis, elevated liver tests, and low platelets
2. **Epidemiology**
   - More common in the third trimester (usually at or after 32 weeks but as early as 25 weeks); 15% to 25% of cases occur postpartum (most within 2 days of delivery) but can be later
   - Incidence: 0.2% to 0.6% of all pregnancies; 4% to 15% in women with preeclampsia/eclampsia
   - May occur in patients with AFLP or de novo
   - Risk factors: Caucasian, multiparity, age >25 years
3. **Etiology:** Unknown. Pathogenic factors may include abnormal vascular tone, vasospasm, activation of coagulation, increased levels of soluble endoglin, and LCHAD deficiency in the infant.
4. **Clinical and laboratory features**
   a. Epigastric pain (65%), nausea or vomiting (30%), headache (31%), hypertension (85%), visual changes, weight gain, edema
   b. Microangiopathic hemolytic anemia with increased serum lactate dehydrogenase and indirect bilirubin levels and decreased haptoglobin levels
   c. Elevated serum aminotransferase levels (from mild to 10 to 100 times)
   d. Decreased platelet count (may be <10,000/mm^3)
   e. Proteinuria
   f. Positive D-dimer test is possibly predictive of HELLP syndrome in preeclamptic patients.
   g. Postpartum resolution of the following:
      - Thrombocytopenia, usually within the first 5 days
      - Hypertension or proteinuria, if present, up to 3 months
5. **Diagnosis:** Presence of hemolytic anemia, elevated serum aminotransferase levels, and low platelets
6. **Treatment**
   - **Delivery of the infant is indicated in the presence of maternal or fetal distress or a rapidly dropping platelet count.** Coexisting preeclampsia or AFLP may dictate early delivery.
   - Hospitalization is indicated for treatment of hypertension, stabilization of disseminated intravascular coagulation (DIC), seizure prophylaxis, and fetal monitoring.
   - Glucocorticoids are recommended if gestation is <34 weeks, to improve fetal lung maturity, but the use of glucocorticoids to improve postpartum maternal outcome remains experimental.
7. **Outcome**
   - Maternal mortality rate: 1%
   - Perinatal infant mortality rate: 7% to 22%

■ Complications: Maternal DIC, abruptio placentae, eclampsia, ascites, subcapsular hematoma, hepatic rupture, wound hematoma, and renal, cardiopulmonary, or hepatic failure

■ Increased risk of infant prematurity, intrauterine growth retardation, DIC, and thrombocytopenia

■ Recurrence rate in mother: Up to 27%

HEPATIC RUPTURE

1. **Definition:** Rupture of the hepatic capsule
2. **Epidemiology**
   ■ Occurs in 1 in 45,000 to 1 in 250,0000 deliveries
   ■ Incidence: 0.9% to 2% in patients with HELLP syndrome
   ■ Most cases are associated with preeclampsia, eclampsia, AFLP, or HELLP.
   ■ Also occurs with hepatocellular carcinoma, adenoma, hemangioma, and hepatic abscess
   ■ Recurrence is rare.
3. **Etiology**: In HELLP and preeclampsia/eclampsia, hepatic rupture is usually preceded by severe intraparenchymal hepatic hemorrhage that progresses to subcapsular hematoma in patients with severe thrombocytopenia.
4. **Clinical and laboratory features**
   ■ Usually occurs in third trimester or occasionally within 24 hours of delivery
   ■ Typical symptoms: Sudden onset of abdominal pain, nausea, and vomiting followed by abdominal distention and hypovolemic shock
   ■ Usually involves the right lobe of liver but may occur in either or both lobes
   ■ Serum aminotransferase levels are increased 2 to 100 times and associated with anemia and consumptive thrombocytopenia, with or without DIC.
5. **Diagnosis:** Abdominal ultrasonography, CT, MRI, and angiography are useful.
6. **Treatment**
   ■ Early recognition leads to **prompt delivery and surgical or radiologic intervention.**
   ■ Surgical therapies include application of direct pressure, evacuation, packing or hemostatic wrapping, topical hemostatic agents, oversewing lacerations, hepatic artery ligation, partial hepatectomy, and liver transplantation.
   ■ Angiographic embolization is an alternative option.
7. **Outcome**
   ■ Maternal mortality rate: 10% to 30% (caused by hemorrhagic shock, hepatic failure, cerebral hemorrhage)
   ■ Fetal mortality rate: 10% to 80% (caused by placental rupture, prematurity, intrauterine asphyxia)

Pregnancy in Patients With Chronic Liver Disease

OVERVIEW

■ Patients have more difficulty conceiving.
■ Pregnancy has no adverse effect on the progression of liver disease.

CIRRHOSIS (see also Chapters 11 and 12)

1. **The risk of bleeding esophageal varices is increased** (more commonly in the second and third trimesters).
   a. Etiology: Expanded maternal blood volume and fetal compression of maternal inferior vena cava and collateral vasculature

   b. Risk of esophageal bleeding in patients with:
   - Cirrhosis: 18% to 32%
   - Known portal hypertension: 50%
   - Preexisting varices: 78%

   c. Treatment
   - Treatment of variceal bleeding is the same as in a nongravid patient and includes band ligation or sclerotherapy and, if necessary, transjugular intrahepatic portosystemic shunt placement or portosystemic shunt surgery.
   - Screening endoscopy is recommended in patients with cirrhosis before pregnancy or early in the second trimester.
   - Areas of controversy include the delivery method (elective caesarian section to avoid Valsalva maneuver during vaginal birth) and whether to initiate primary prophylaxis to prevent variceal bleeding with banding or a beta receptor antagonist.

   d. Outcome: Maternal mortality rate of 18% to 50%

2. Other complications that occur in pregnant patients with cirrhosis are hepatic decompensation (24%), splenic artery aneurysm rupture (2.6%), postpartum uterine hemorrhage (7% to 10%), spontaneous abortion (30% to 40%), prematurity (25%), fetal stillbirth (13%), and neonatal mortality (4.8%).

3. Medications prescribed to manage the complications of cirrhosis should be reviewed carefully for safety in pregnancy (e.g., furosemide, spironolactone, beta receptor antagonists, fluoroquinolones, and rifaximin are pregnancy category C drugs according to the U.S. Food and Drug Administration [FDA]; octreotide and lactulose are FDA category B drugs [old classification]).

WILSON DISEASE (see also Chapter 19)

1. Impact on pregnancy: The disease may decrease fertility and increases the rate of recurrent spontaneous abortions.

2. Treatment: Pregnant patients should continue anticopper therapy (penicillamine, trientine, zinc) during pregnancy because serious adverse maternal outcomes, including death, can result if anticopper therapy is stopped.
   - Data in pregnancy are limited for all three anticopper drugs.
   - Penicillamine is potentially teratogenic in animals and humans. Trientine is teratogenic in animals.
   - Penicillamine is considered safe during pregnancy at relatively low doses (0.25 to 0.5 g/day). Trientine has appeared safe and effective based on limited data; however, due to issues with impaired wound healing, the dose should be decreased as early in pregnancy as possible. Because of the potential teratogenic effects of penicillamine and trientine, zinc is recommended during pregnancy by some authorities.

3. Special considerations: Genetic counseling should be offered.

AUTOIMMUNE HEPATITIS (see also Chapter 7)

1. Impact on pregnancy
   - The natural history of AIH is variable during pregnancy.
   - Successful pregnancies can occur in women with well-controlled AIH.
   - The rate of fetal loss is 19% to 24% (no different from that for other chronic diseases).

2. Treatment
   - Cessation of therapy during pregnancy is associated with relapse of disease.
   - The use of azathioprine is controversial, but reports of experience in patients taking azathioprine following organ transplantation or for inflammatory bowel disease have described good outcomes for mothers and infants.

- Patients should be monitored closely for flare-ups of AIH during pregnancy and in the early postpartum period.
3. Special consideration: Women of childbearing age with AIH should be counseled to consider pregnancy only if the disease is well controlled.

PRIMARY BILIARY CHOLANGITIS (see also Chapter 16)

1. Impact on pregnancy
   - Some data suggest that women with primary biliary cholangitis may be able to have normal pregnancies.
   - Antimitochondrial antibody titers and serum alkaline phosphatase, ALT, bile acid, bilirubin, IgG, and IgM levels improve during pregnancy.
   - The risk of a postpartum flare-up exists.
2. Treatment: Continue UDCA, which is safe in pregnancy.

PRIMARY SCLEROSING CHOLANGITIS (see also Chapter 17)

1. Impact on pregnancy: The natural history in pregnancy is unknown.
2. Treatment: Continue UDCA, which is safe in pregnancy, may improve maternal symptoms, and appears to decrease the risk of fetal complications.

NONALCOHOLIC FATTY LIVER DISEASE (see also Chapter 9)

1. Impact on pregnancy: Associated with higher risks of gestational diabetes, preeclampsia, cesarean section, preterm birth, and low birth weight
2. Treatment: Close monitoring of weight and complications of metabolic syndrome

Viral Hepatitis and Herpes Simplex Virus Infections in Pregnant Women (see also Chapters 3–6)

OVERVIEW

- Of all the viral hepatitides, only the course of hepatitis E is affected by pregnancy (see Chapter 3).
- Viral hepatitis may occur throughout pregnancy.

HEPATITIS A (see also Chapter 3)

1. Epidemiology
   - Acute infection only (no chronic disease)
   - Acute infection during pregnancy in the United States is rare.
   - Perinatal transmission is rare.
2. Treatment
   - The course and management are unaffected by pregnancy.
   - Prevention with immunoglobulin in an exposed mother is safe for mother and fetus.
   - Infection in the second or third trimester has been reported to be associated with preterm labor.
   - For infants of mothers who are infectious at or soon after delivery, the dose of immunoglobulin is 0.02 mL/kg intramuscularly (vaccination against HAV can be considered at age 2 years).

TABLE 23.5 ■ **Treatment of Neonates Born to Mothers With Hepatitis B**

Treatment	Age of Administration to Infant Based on Hepatitis B Surface Antigen Status of Mother		
	+	Unknown	–
Hepatitis B immunoglobulin 100 IU (0.5 mL IM)	≤12 hr	≤12 hr	Not administered
Hepatitis B vaccine, first dose 5.0–10 µg (0.5–1 mL IM)	≤12 hr	≤12 hr	≤1 wk
Subsequent hepatitis B vaccine dose:			
Recombivax HB 5 µg (0.5 mL)	1 mo	1–2 mo	1–2 mo
Engerix-B 10 µg (0.5 mL)	6 mo	6 mo	6–18 mo

IM, Intramuscularly.

Adapted from American College of Obstetricians and Gynecologists. ACOG practice bulletin no. 86: viral hepatitis in pregnancy. *Obstet Gynecol.* 2007;110:941–956.

HEPATITIS B (see also Chapter 4)

1. Epidemiology
   ■ Prevalence of 0.7% to 0.9% among pregnant women in the United States
2. Transmission to the infant may occur without immunoprophylaxis.
   ■ When the mother is HBsAg and HBeAg positive, the chronic infection rate is 90%.
   ■ When the mother is HBsAg positive and HBeAg negative, the chronic infection rate is 40%.
   ■ The risk of transmission to the infant correlates with the mother's serum HBV DNA level.
   ■ Following infection of the mother in the first trimester, 10% of neonates become HBsAg positive.
   ■ Following infection of the mother in the third trimester, 80% to 90% of neonates become HBsAg positive.
   ■ Transmission to the neonate is usually perinatal.
3. Treatment: A combination of active (HBV vaccine) and passive (hepatitis B immunoglobulin) immunotherapy of the newborn is 85% to 95% effective in decreasing perinatal transmission to <10% (Table 23.5). Antiviral treatment should be prescribed to the mother in the third trimester if the maternal HBV DNA level is >6 to 8 log10 copies/mL.

HEPATITIS C (see also Chapter 5)

1. Epidemiology
   ■ The overall rate of mother-to-infant transmission is generally low (2.4%). Risk factors for vertical transmission are maternal serum viral level, intrapartum invasive procedures, and human immunodeficiency virus coinfection.
   ■ HCV infection does not adversely affect pregnancy.
   ■ The course of HCV infection is not affected by pregnancy.
2. Treatment
   ■ No effective prevention is available for infants.
   ■ Treatment of chronic hepatitis C with ribavirin-containing regimens is **contraindicated** in pregnancy because ribavirin is teratogenic. There are no safety data for the new direct-acting antiviral therapies in pregnancy. Postpone treatment until after delivery and breastfeeding.

HEPATITIS D (see also Chapter 4)

- Rare instances of vertical transmission have been reported.
- HBV infection should be controlled to prevent the spread of hepatitis D virus.

HEPATITIS E (see also Chapter 3)

- Jaundice is nine times more common in pregnant than nonpregnant women with hepatitis E.
- Hepatitis E is the leading cause of fulminant hepatic failure in pregnancy.
- The disease is more severe in the third trimester than at other times, with a maternal mortality rate of up to 27%, compared with 0.5% to 4% in nonpregnant patients. In patients with acute liver failure (see Chapter 2), the mortality rate is 65% in pregnant women compared with 23% in nonpregnant women.
- The risk of abortion and intrauterine death is 12%.
- Vertical transmission occurs in up to 33% at any point during pregnancy.
- No specific therapy during pregnancy exists.
- No FDA-approved vaccines are available. Two vaccines are available in other countries but have not been well studied in pregnancy.

HERPES SIMPLEX VIRUS INFECTIONS (see Chapter 6)

- Disseminated herpes simplex virus (HSV) infection during pregnancy is rare, but it has been reported, usually in the late second or third trimester.
- The clinical presentation can include acute hepatitis (see Chapter 2).
- Fever, nausea, vomiting, abdominal pain, leukopenia, thrombocytopenia, coagulopathy, and markedly elevated serum aminotransferase levels are often present.
- Liver biopsy specimens show extensive necrosis, often hemorrhagic, with typical intranuclear viral inclusion particles.
- Hepatic necrosis, DIC, hypotension, and death can occur rapidly if antiviral therapy is not initiated promptly.

Budd-Chiari Syndrome (see also Chapter 21)

1. Definition: Thrombosis of one or more of the three hepatic veins
2. Epidemiology
   - 20% of cases are associated with pregnancy and oral contraceptive use.
   - Postpartum onset is rare and is associated with a poor prognosis.
3. Etiology
   - A hypercoagulable state (e.g., factor V Leiden mutation) may play a role.
   - It may be associated with antiphospholipid antibodies, preeclampsia, and ingestion of herbal teas.
4. Clinical features
   - Symptoms are usually acute in pregnancy.
   - Features include abdominal pain, hepatomegaly, and ascites.
5. Diagnosis
   - MRI, ultrasonography, and liver biopsy are used.
   - If possible, venography or angiography should be avoided until after pregnancy.
6. Treatment: Same as in nonpregnant patients
7. Outcome: With acute onset in pregnancy, the maternal mortality rate is as high as 70%.

Cholelithiasis and Cholecystitis in Pregnant Women (see also Chapter 34)

1. **Epidemiology**
   - Symptomatic onset is most common in the second and third trimesters.
   - The frequency in pregnancy is 18% to 19% in multiparous women and 7% to 8% in primiparous women. Symptomatic gallstones occur only in 0.1% to 0.3% of pregnancies.
   - Risk factors include increasing age, increasing frequency and number of pregnancies, obesity, high serum leptin levels, insulin resistance, and low high-density lipoprotein levels.
   - Frequency rates of new biliary sludge and gallstones in pregnancy are 3.2% and 1.9%, respectively, with 2% progressing from sludge to stones, at the end of the second trimester and, similarly, new biliary sludge 5.1%, new gallstones 2.8%, and progression of sludge to stones 2.3%, respectively, 2 to 4 weeks postpartum.
   - Sludge disappears in 96% by 12 months after delivery; gallbladder stones disappear in 20% of women by 1 year. Cholecystectomy occurs in 0.8% of women within 1 year of pregnancy.
2. **Etiology**
   - Increased estrogen levels lead to increased lithogenicity of bile in the second and third trimesters (increased cholesterol secretion and supersaturation of bile).
   - Increased progesterone levels lead to larger gallbladder volume and decreased emptying time.
3. **Clinical features**
   - Vomiting occurs in 32%, dyspepsia in 28%, and pruritus in 10%.
   - Biliary pain occurs in 29% with preexisting stones and in 4.7% with sludge but generally does not occur in patients with new sludge or new stones.
4. **Treatment**
   a. Conservative medical management with intravenous fluids, correction of electrolytes, bowel rest, and broad-spectrum antibiotics is considered safe in pregnancy.
   b. Laparoscopic cholecystectomy should be performed in the second trimester if medical management fails or the patient has a relapse. Surgery should be avoided in the first trimester if possible.
      - A questionable increase in spontaneous abortions occurs when surgery is performed in the first trimester.
      - Surgery in the third trimester is associated with premature labor in 40% of cases.
   c. ERCP should be done for choledocholithiasis; it can be performed safely by shielding the fetus from radiation exposure and minimizing fluoroscopy time.

FURTHER READING

Aggarwal R, Naik S. Epidemiology of hepatitis E: current status. *J Gastroenterol Hepatol.* 2009;24:1484–1493.

Badizadegan K, Wolf JL. Liver pathology in pregnancy. In: Odze RD, Goldblum JR, eds. *Surgical Pathology of the GI Tract, Liver, Biliary Tract, and Pancreas.* Philadelphia: Saunders Elsevier; 2015:1462–1474.

Date RS, Kaushal M, Ramesh A. A review of the management of gallstone disease and its complications in pregnancy. *Am J Surg.* 2008;196:599–608.

Floreani A, Gervasi MT. New insights on intrahepatic cholestasis of pregnancy. *Clin Liver Dis.* 2016;20:177–189.

Garcia-Tejedor A, Maiques-Montesinos V, Diago-Almela VJ, et al. Risk factors for vertical transmission of hepatitis C virus: a single center experience with 710 HCV-infected mothers. *Eur J Obstet Gynecol Reprod Biol.* 2015;194:173–177.

Hagström H, Höijer J, Ludvigsson JF, et al. Adverse outcomes of pregnancy in women with non-alcoholic fatty liver disease. *Liver Int.* 2016;36:268–274.

Knight M, Nelson-Piercy C, Kurinczuk JJ, et al. A prospective national study of acute fatty liver of pregnancy in the UK. *Gut*. 2008;57:951–956.

Ko CW, Beresford SA, Schulte SJ, et al. Incidence, natural history, and risk factors for biliary sludge and stones during pregnancy. *Hepatology*. 2005;41:359–365.

Marschall HU, Wikström Shemer E, Ludvigsson JF, et al. Intrahepatic cholestasis of pregnancy and associated hepatobiliary disease: a population-based cohort study. *Hepatology*. 2013;58:1385–1391.

Rac MW, Sheffield JS. Prevention and management of viral hepatitis in pregnancy. *Obstet Gynecol Clin North Am*. 2014;41:573–592.

Society for Maternal-Fetal Medicine (SMFM). Hepatitis B in pregnancy screening, treatment, and prevention of vertical transmission. *Am J Obstet Gynecol*. 2016;214:6–14.

Tan J, Surti B, Saab S. Pregnancy and cirrhosis. *Liver Transpl*. 2008;14:1081–1091.

United States Preventive Services Task Force. Screening for hepatitis B virus infection in pregnancy: U.S. Preventive Services Task Force reaffirmation recommendation statement. *Ann Intern Med*. 2009;150:869–873.

Westbrook RH, Yeoman AD, Kriese S, et al. Outcome of pregnancy in women with autoimmune hepatitis. *J Autoimmun*. 2012;38:J239–J244.

Wilson SG, White AD, Young AL, et al. The management of the surgical complications of HELLP syndrome. *Ann R Coll Surg Engl*. 2014;96:512–516.

CHAPTER 24

The Liver in Systemic Disease

Jeremy F.L. Cobbold, PhD, MRCP ■ John A. Summerfield, MD, FRCP, FAASLD

KEY POINTS

1 Abnormal liver biochemical test levels are associated with many different systemic diseases. These abnormalities are generally incidental, but in some systemic diseases the liver may be severely compromised (Table 24.1).

2 In evaluating patients with systemic disease and liver dysfunction, the challenge for the clinician is to distinguish among hepatic manifestations of the systemic disease, liver toxicity from drugs used to treat that disease, and a coexisting primary liver disorder.

3 Liver involvement can occur in heart failure, connective tissue diseases, endocrine disorders, granulomatous diseases, lymphoma, hematologic diseases, systemic infections, gastrointestinal disorders including celiac disease and inflammatory bowel disease (IBD), and amyloidosis.

Cardiac Disease (see Chapter 22)

HEART FAILURE

The liver may become congested secondary to right-sided heart failure; the following clinical, laboratory, and pathologic features related to the liver may be seen:

1. A dull ache in the right upper quadrant
2. Hepatomegaly is noted in 50% of cases and is associated with splenomegaly or ascites in 10% to 20%. Other signs of right-sided heart failure include raised jugular venous pressure and peripheral edema (Table 24.2).
3. Abnormal liver biochemical test results include a raised bilirubin level in 25% to 75% of patients and normal or mildly elevated serum aminotransferase levels. The serum alkaline phosphatase (ALP) level is usually (but not always) normal. Up to 75% of patients have a prolonged prothrombin time (PT).
4. Histopathologic examination shows an enlarged purplish liver with the cut surface having alternating patches of congested centrilobular regions and pale, less involved areas, the so-called **nutmeg** appearance.
5. Microscopically, the central veins and centrilobular sinusoids are dilated and engorged with blood; inflammation is not observed. Longstanding hepatic congestion can result in extensive fibrosis, so-called **cardiac cirrhosis.** Treatment of the underlying heart failure normally leads to improvement in both clinical and laboratory parameters of liver function.

TABLE 24.1 ■ The Liver in Systemic Disease

Disorder(s)	Hepatic Manifestations	Liver Biochemical Test Levels (Most Common Abnormalities)
Cardiovascular		
Heart failure	Vascular congestion; hepatomegaly	↑Bili; ↑ALT; ↑PT
Ischemic (hypoxic) hepatitis	Hepatocellular necrosis	↑↑↑ALT; ↑Bili
Autoimmune		
Immunoglobulin G4–related disease	Sclerosing cholangitis, pancreatitis; IgG4-positive plasma cells on immunostaining	↑↑Bili, ↑↑ALP
Polymyalgia rheumatica and giant cell arteritis	Hepatocellular necrosis; portal inflammation	↑ALP; ↑ALT
Rheumatoid arthritis; Felty syndrome; adult Still disease	Nonspecific: Portal inflammatory infiltrates and fibrosis; drug hepatotoxicity	↑ALP; ↑ALT
Systemic lupus erythematosus	Autoimmune hepatitis; autoimmune cholangiopathy; nodular regenerative hyperplasia; drug hepatotoxicity	↑↑ALP; ↑Bili; ↑↑ALT
Systemic sclerosis; Sjögren syndrome	Budd-Chiari syndrome; antimitochondrial antibodies; primary biliary cholangitis	↑↑ALP; ↑Bili; (±↑)ALT
Endocrine and Metabolic		
Hyperthyroidism	Nonspecific inflammation and cholestasis	↑ALP; ↑ALT; ↑GGTP
Type 2 diabetes mellitus	Steatosis; steatohepatitis	↑ALT; ↑GGTP
Granulomatous		
Sarcoidosis	Epithelioid granulomas	↑↑ALP; ↑ALT
Hematologic		
Lymphomas, acute and chronic leukemias, myeloproliferative disorders (including myelofibrosis)	Hepatomegaly; infiltration; extrahepatic biliary obstruction	↑ALP; ↑Bili
Sickle cell disease	Hemolysis; ischemia; pigment cholelithiasis	↑↑Bili; ↑ALP; ↑ALT
Infectious		
Pneumonia	Nonspecific inflammatory changes	↑↑Bili; ↑ALP
Sepsis	Intrahepatic cholestasis; ischemic hepatitis; drug hepatotoxicity	↑Bili; ↑ALP; ↑ALT
HIV infection	Hepatomegaly; coinfection with hepatitis B or C	↑ALT
Tuberculosis	Caseating granulomas; drug hepatotoxicity	↑ALT; ↑↑Bili; ↑ALP
Gastrointestinal and Nutritional		
Celiac disease	Elevated aminotransferase levels; association with primary biliary cholangitis, autoimmune hepatitis, and PSC; jaundice	↑ALT
Inflammatory bowel disease	Association with primary sclerosing cholangitis, cholangiocarcinoma; hepatic steatosis; immunosuppressant medication hepatotoxicity; jaundice	↑ALT
Obesity	Steatosis; steatohepatitis	↑ALT; ↑GGTP
Anorexia	Steatosis; liver failure	↑ALT
Amyloidosis		
	Infiltration; vascular congestion	↑↑ALP; ↑ALT

ALT, Alanine aminotransferase; *ALP,* alkaline phosphatase; *Bili,* bilirubin; *GGTP,* gamma-glutamyltranspeptidase; *PT,* prothrombin time.

TABLE 24.2 ■ Symptoms and Signs of Hepatic Congestion in 175 Patients With Acute or Chronic Right-Sided Heart Failure

	Acute Heart Failure (%)	Chronic Heart Failure (%)
Any hepatomegaly (>11 cm span)	99	95
Marked hepatomegaly (>5 cm below right costal margin)	57	49
Peripheral edema	77	71
Pleural effusion	25	17
Splenomegaly	20	22
Ascites	7	20

Adapted from Richman SM, Delman AJ, Grob D. Alterations in indices of liver function in congestive heart failure with particular reference to serum enzymes. *Am J Med.* 1961;30:211–225.

ISCHEMIC HEPATITIS AND LEFT-SIDED HEART FAILURE

Hepatic damage associated with acute left ventricular failure is frequently termed **ischemic (or hypoxic) hepatitis.** It usually occurs in the setting of an acute myocardial infarction or cardiogenic shock but can result from an abrupt, severe decrease in cardiac output from any cause, vasoactive drugs (e.g., cocaine, ergotamine overdose), or severe hypoxemia.

1. The major manifestations are biochemical: Elevated serum levels of aspartate and alanine aminotransferase (AST, ALT) and lactate dehydrogenase (LDH) (predominantly hepatic fraction) to 25 or more times the upper limits. Values peak within 1 to 3 days of the inciting event and rapidly return to near normal, usually within 7 to 10 days. Serum bilirubin and ALP levels are generally normal or only mildly elevated. Liver failure and hepatic encephalopathy can occur.

2. Mortality rates in patients with ischemic hepatitis are high (40% to 50% in some series) but do not correlate with the degree of liver biochemical test abnormalities. The cause of death is related to the cause of the ischemic injury to the liver and not to liver failure. Treatment should be directed to correcting the underlying disease process.

Systemic Autoimmune Diseases

IMMUNOGLOBULIN G4-RELATED DISEASE

1. Immunoglobulin G4–related disease (IgG4-RD) is a multisystem fibroinflammatory condition associated with type 1 autoimmune pancreatitis, which affects 60% of patients with IgG4-RD and is also associated with sialadenitis, tubulointerstitial nephritis, dacryoadenitis, and periaortitis.

2. Sclerosing cholangitis occurs in 13% of patients with IgG4-RD, usually in association with autoimmune pancreatitis, and typically presents with obstructive jaundice.

3. Imaging appearances resemble other pancreaticobiliary diseases such as primary sclerosing cholangitis (PSC), cholangiocarcinoma, or pancreatic cancer. Elevated serum IgG4 values (or an IgG4 to IgG1 ratio of >0.24) can discriminate IgG4-RD from other pancreaticobiliary diseases.

4. The disorder is typically responsive to high-dose oral glucocorticoids. Relapse may be treated with immunomodulators and consideration of the monoclonal CD20 antibody rituximab.

POLYMYALGIA RHEUMATICA AND GIANT CELL ARTERITIS

1. Abnormalities in liver biochemical tests may be seen in both polymyalgia rheumatica and giant cell arteritis. Elevation of serum ALP levels occurs in approximately 30% of patients; elevated serum aminotransferase levels may also be observed.
2. Liver biopsy specimens demonstrate focal hepatocellular necrosis, portal inflammation, and scattered small epithelioid granulomas.
3. The liver abnormalities usually do not cause clinical problems and resolve within a few weeks of the initiation of glucocorticoid therapy.

RHEUMATOID ARTHRITIS

1. Liver disease in rheumatoid arthritis (RA) is most commonly seen in patients with **Felty syndrome** (splenomegaly and neutropenia in the setting of RA). These patients frequently have hepatomegaly, and approximately 25% have elevated serum aminotransferase and ALP levels. Liver biopsy findings are usually nonspecific: Infiltration of portal areas with lymphocytes and plasma cells and mild portal fibrosis.
2. Some patients with RA develop **nodular regenerative hyperplasia** with atrophy and formation of regenerative nodules that may result in portal hypertension, ascites, and variceal hemorrhage (see Chapter 22). The pathogenesis of nodular regenerative hyperplasia has been proposed to be drug-induced or immune complex–induced obliteration of the portal venules.
3. Hepatotoxicity can be associated with salicylates, gold, and methotrexate.

ADULT STILL DISEASE

1. This multisystem inflammatory disorder of unknown origin is characterized by spiking fever, evanescent rash, arthritis, and multiorgan involvement.
2. Liver abnormalities, including hepatomegaly and elevated liver enzyme levels, are seen in 50% to 75% of patients; nonsteroidal antiinflammatory drug use may be a cofactor.
3. After consideration of the possible contribution of medications to hepatic dysfunction, treatment of the underlying disorder with antiinflammatory drugs, immunosuppressant medications, or biologic agents is indicated.

SYSTEMIC LUPUS ERYTHEMATOSUS

1. Liver biochemical test abnormalities are common in systemic lupus erythematosus (SLE), but clinically significant liver disease is uncommon.
2. Frequent abnormalities include elevated ALT and ALP levels, normally less than four times the upper limit of normal. In a few patients (approximately 5%), jaundice develops.
3. Causes of liver biochemical abnormalities in SLE are as follows:
   - Steatosis (most common finding on liver biopsy specimens)
   - Autoimmune hepatitis, as a result of either SLE itself or coexistent classic autoimmune hepatitis (see Chapter 7)
   - Autoimmune cholangiopathy, with a greater increase in the ALP level than the ALT level
   - Nodular regenerative hyperplasia (may be seen in all connective tissue diseases)
   - Coexistent viral hepatitis (In one study, 11% of patients with SLE were positive for hepatitis C viral RNA.)
   - Budd-Chiari syndrome, particularly in patients with antiphospholipid syndrome (see Chapter 21)
   - Drugs, especially methotrexate and salicylates

4. Drugs suspected of causing abnormal liver biochemical test levels, particularly salicylates, should be withdrawn. Otherwise, the treatment of liver dysfunction in SLE depends on the cause. Most abnormal liver biochemical test results do not represent clinically significant liver disease.

SYSTEMIC SCLEROSIS (SCLERODERMA)

1. From 8% to 15% of patients with systemic sclerosis have **antimitochondrial antibodies;** these patients often have evidence of **primary biliary cholangitis (PBC, previously termed primary biliary cirrhosis)** on liver biopsy specimens (see Chapter 16). These changes are more frequent in patients with limited rather than diffuse forms of systemic sclerosis.
2. Nearly 5% of patients with PBC have symptoms of systemic sclerosis, which may antedate the diagnosis of PBC by many years.

SJÖGREN SYNDROME

1. Between 5% and 10% of patients with Sjögren syndrome and approximately 40% with both Sjögren syndrome and RA have **antimitochondrial antibodies;** most of these patients also have elevated serum ALP levels.
2. Liver biopsy specimens in these patients frequently demonstrate changes of stage 1 PBC, even in the absence of liver biochemical test abnormalities.
3. The risk of clinical PBC in these patients is uncertain. Whether any early therapeutic intervention is of value is also unclear.

OTHER CAUSES OF VASCULITIS

1. Persons with **polyarteritis nodosa** often have chronic hepatitis B virus infection (see Chapter 4).
2. Persons with **cryoglobulinemia** often have chronic hepatitis C virus infection (see Chapter 5).

Endocrine and Metabolic Disorders

HYPERTHYROIDISM

1. Untreated hyperthyroidism is associated with abnormalities of liver biochemical test values, usually with a cholestatic picture. In severe cases the ischemic consequences of high-output heart failure may be observed (see discussion earlier in chapter).
2. Treatment with propylthiouracil may also lead to hepatotoxicity (see Chapter 10).

TYPE 2 DIABETES MELLITUS AND THE METABOLIC SYNDROME

1. **Nonalcoholic fatty liver disease** (NAFLD) may be considered the liver manifestation of the metabolic syndrome of obesity, insulin resistance, hypertension, and dyslipidemia (see Chapter 9). Approximately 60% of patients with type 2 diabetes mellitus have evidence of NAFLD and the frequency increases to more than 90% in obese persons with type 2 diabetes mellitus.
2. A subset of patients will develop progressive disease, with an increased risk of the complications of cirrhosis, including hepatocellular carcinoma.
3. The most common cause of death in such patients remains cardiovascular disease.

Granulomatous Disease and Sarcoidosis (see Chapter 28)

1. Granulomatous diseases of the liver have numerous causes.
   - Systemic infections (e.g., tuberculosis [TB])
   - Malignant disease (e.g., Hodgkin lymphoma)
   - Drugs
   - Autoimmune disorders (e.g., autoimmune hepatitis)
   - Idiopathic conditions (e.g., sarcoidosis)
2. Abnormalities of liver biochemical test values are common in sarcoidosis but rarely require treatment. Typically, minor elevations of both aminotransferases and ALP levels are seen.
3. Rarer clinical manifestations include chronic intrahepatic cholestasis, portal hypertension, and Budd-Chiari syndrome.
4. Liver biopsy specimens demonstrate granulomas in the portal and periportal regions; cholestatic and necroinflammatory features may also be seen.
5. No treatment is required for patients with asymptomatic disease; ursodeoxycholic acid, glucocorticoids, or methotrexate may be considered in patients with symptomatic disease.

Lymphoma and Hematologic Diseases

LYMPHOMA

1. The liver may be involved in 5% of patients with **Hodgkin lymphoma** at presentation but in up to 50% of patients at autopsy. In addition, nonspecific inflammatory infiltrates or noncaseating granulomas are seen in the absence of direct hepatic involvement with lymphomas.
   - An elevated serum ALP level of up to two times the upper limit of normal is common even in the absence of direct liver involvement.
   - Jaundice is uncommon in Hodgkin lymphoma and usually reflects hepatic infiltration with lymphoma, rather than extrahepatic biliary obstruction.
2. Hepatic involvement is observed in 25% to 50% of patients with **non-Hodgkin lymphoma;** rarely, the liver may be the primary site of involvement. Typically, the lymphoma produces a nodular infiltrate of the portal areas. The clinical and laboratory presentation is similar to that of Hodgkin lymphoma, except that extrahepatic biliary obstruction, usually at the level of the porta hepatis, is much more common.

MALIGNANT HEMATOLOGIC CONDITIONS

1. **Systemic mastocytosis** may manifest with hepatosplenomegaly as well as with lymphadenopathy and skin lesions. Liver biopsy specimens show polygonal cells containing eosinophilic granules, predominantly in the portal tracts. Giemsa and toluidine blue staining allows detection of the characteristic metachromatic cytoplasmic granules. Periportal fibrosis may also be present. Cirrhosis develops in approximately 5% of patients.
2. Hepatomegaly is common in **acute lymphoblastic leukemia** and **acute myeloid leukemia** at diagnosis and is present in 95% and 75%, respectively, of cases postmortem. Liver biopsy is seldom performed because of the high risk of hemorrhage.
3. Most patients with chronic leukemias (e.g., **chronic lymphocytic leukemia, hairy cell leukemia)** also demonstrate evidence of liver infiltration at autopsy.
4. **Multiple myeloma** is rarely associated with clinically significant liver disease; hepatic manifestations may include diffuse sinusoidal or portal infiltration, nodular regenerative hyperplasia, jaundice, and complications of portal hypertension. Multiple myeloma is also associated with **amyloidosis** (see discussion later in chapter).

5. Massive hepatomegaly is seen in **primary myelofibrosis** and other myeloproliferative disorders and is associated with extramedullary hematopoiesis and increased hepatic blood flow. The most common biochemical abnormality is an elevated serum ALP level, which may be associated with the severity of sinusoidal dilatation.

SICKLE CELL DISEASE

1. Although liver biochemical test abnormalities are common in patients with sickle cell disease, these abnormal values are frequently caused by other factors such as chronic viral hepatitis or heart failure.
2. **Hepatic crisis** usually occurs in the setting of sickle cell crisis and is marked by right upper quadrant pain, jaundice, and tender hepatomegaly.
   - Serum bilirubin levels are frequently as high as 10 to 15 mg/dL and may be as high as 40 to 50 mg/dL.
   - Serum AST and ALT levels are also elevated, usually up to 10 times normal.
   - The LDH level may be increased markedly, reflecting both liver dysfunction and hemolysis.
   - Hemolysis may contribute to rises in bilirubin and aminotransferase levels, whereas a raised ALP level is often of bone origin.
   - Liver biopsy specimens in hepatic crisis demonstrate sinusoidal distention, erythrocyte sickling, and phagocytosis of erythrocytes by Kupffer cells.
   - The differential diagnosis includes acute cholecystitis and cholangitis.
   - Treatment is supportive and usually results in clinical improvement in a few days, although fatal liver failure has been described.
3. **Pigment gallstones** have been reported in 40% to 80% of patients with sickle cell disease; choledocholithiasis has been described in 20% to 65% of patients at the time of cholecystectomy.
   - Abdominal ultrasonography or computed tomography (CT) may be helpful in establishing the diagnosis of cholecystitis.
   - Endoscopic retrograde cholangiopancreatography (ERCP) may be necessary to identify and treat stones in the bile duct.

Infections (see Chapter 31)

Many systemic infections may cause abnormalities in liver biochemical test results, either directly or indirectly. The abnormalities usually resolve on resolution of the underlying infection. Pneumonia is often accompanied by elevated liver enzymes. In particular, *Legionella pneumophila* (causing Legionnaires' disease), *Mycoplasma pneumoniae,* and *Pneumococcus* spp. infections may be associated with markedly raised serum aminotransferase levels and cholestasis.

SYSTEMIC INFECTION, SEPSIS, AND THE CRITICALLY ILL PATIENT

Elevated liver enzyme levels are often seen in patients with systemic sepsis. The causes and possible mechanisms are multiple; in most cases, the effect is multifactorial.
1. **Intrahepatic cholestasis** is common in sepsis, independent of the causative organism. Canalicular excretion of conjugated bilirubin is thought to be inhibited by high levels of proinflammatory cytokines, such as tumor necrosis factor alpha and interleukin-6. Usually, no evidence of cholangitis is seen on liver biopsy specimens.
2. Biochemical findings include mildly raised serum ALP levels (one to three times the upper limit of normal) and increased serum bilirubin levels, although these levels may be discordant.
3. Antibiotics such as amoxicillin-clavulanic acid and flucloxacillin are associated with a cholestatic drug reaction (see Chapter 10).

4. Ischemic hepatitis (see discussion earlier in chapter) may occur in a septic patient as a result of hemodynamic instability.
5. Parenteral nutrition is associated with hepatotoxicity and nonalcoholic steatohepatitis (see Chapters 9 and 10), which may be ameliorated by the addition of choline to the formula.

HUMAN IMMUNODEFICIENCY VIRUS INFECTION (see Chapter 27)

1. Approximately 70% of patients with the acquired immunodeficiency syndrome (AIDS) have clinical hepatomegaly, often with abnormal liver biochemical test levels.
2. The picture is usually hepatitic, with elevation of serum aminotransferases predominating, often related to coinfection with hepatitis B virus (HBV) or hepatitis C virus (HCV).

TUBERCULOSIS (see Chapters 28 and 31)

1. Miliary TB may affect the liver and may cause hepatitis and rarely jaundice. Liver biopsy specimens reveal multiple caseating granulomas.
2. Drug therapy, particularly with isoniazid and rifampin, may cause hepatitis with elevated serum aminotransferase levels and jaundice.
3. Coinfection with human immunodeficiency virus (HIV) or HCV is thought to be an independent risk factor for the development of antituberculosis drug-induced hepatitis.

Gastrointestinal and Nutritional Disorders

CELIAC DISEASE

1. Serum aminotransferase levels are elevated (less than five times the upper limit of normal) in 40% of adults with celiac disease at the time of diagnosis. Histologic findings in the liver are seen in 66% of these patients but are usually mild and nonspecific.
2. Adherence to a gluten-free diet leads to normalization of serum aminotransferase levels in 75% to 95% of patients with celiac disease, usually within 1 year.
3. Autoimmune liver diseases are more prevalent in patients with celiac disease compared with the general population, including PBC, autoimmune hepatitis, and PSC. The pathogenesis of these associations is unclear, but certain human leukocyte antigen (HLA) associations have been postulated. Adherence to a gluten-free diet has generally not been shown to provide benefit.
4. Other liver diseases associated with celiac disease are listed in Box 24.1.
5. Celiac disease may be associated with an increased risk of death from liver cirrhosis.

INFLAMMATORY BOWEL DISEASE

1. Liver abnormalities
   - Abnormal liver biochemical values (mild elevations of serum aminotransferase and ALP levels) are common in patients with IBD, with a frequency of approximately 30%.
   - In a large series, abnormal liver biochemical values were associated with increased mortality, but not with IBD activity, although the reason for the increased mortality was unclear.
   - **Steatosis** is the most commonly observed abnormality on liver biopsy specimens. In addition, **chronic hepatitis** characterized by either portal or lobular infiltrates of mononuclear inflammatory cells may be found. It is not clear whether hepatitis is a direct consequence of IBD or a manifestation of **PSC** or another cause of liver disease such as **hepatitis C** or drugs. The frequency of **autoimmune hepatitis** is increased in patients with IBD.
   - Patients with Crohn disease infrequently develop hepatic **granulomas** or **amyloidosis**.

BOX 24.1 ■ Liver Diseases Associated With Celiac Disease

Isolated elevation of the aminotransferase levels ("celiac hepatitis"), reversible on gluten-free diet
Cryptogenic cirrhosis
Autoimmune liver disorders
   Primary biliary cholangitis
   Autoimmune hepatitis
   Autoimmune cholangitis
   Primary sclerosing cholangitis
Chronic hepatitis C
Hemochromatosis
Nonalcoholic fatty liver disease
Acute liver failure
Regenerative nodular hyperplasia
Hepatocellular carcinoma

Adapted from Rubio-Tapia A, Murray JA. The liver in celiac disease. *Hepatology.* 2007;46:1650–1165.

---

2. Biliary abnormalities
   - **PSC** is the most important hepatobiliary complication of IBD; it occurs in 5% to 10% of patients with ulcerative colitis but in fewer than 1% of those with Crohn disease (see Chapters 17 and 35).
   - The only sign of early PSC may be an elevated serum ALP level. Patients with more advanced disease may present with pruritus or jaundice.
   - Progression varies widely among affected persons, possibly related to an individual's HLA status.
   - Most patients ultimately develop biliary cirrhosis with increasing serum levels of bilirubin and ALP and portal hypertension with ascites and variceal bleeding. Bacterial cholangitis may also be observed, particularly in patients who have undergone surgical or endoscopic intervention of the bile ducts.
   - Up to 20% of patients with PSC develop **cholangiocarcinoma.**
   - The diagnosis of PSC is made by visualization of the biliary tree by magnetic resonance cholangiopancreatography (MRCP) or ERCP. The typical pattern is of multiple bile duct strictures with areas of beaded dilatation. Distinguishing benign strictures from cholangiocarcinoma by radiographic criteria is often difficult. Brush cytology and biopsy obtained at ERCP may be helpful (see Chapters 35 and 36).
   - Neither medical nor surgical treatment of the underlying IBD alters the course of PSC. Treatment with ursodeoxycholic acid may result in some improvement in symptoms and liver biochemical test values. Patients with advanced liver disease secondary to PSC may be candidates for liver transplantation if they have not already developed cholangiocarcinoma, although PSC may recur in the graft.

OBESITY

1. The worldwide prevalence of obesity continues to rise and is closely associated with insulin resistance and NAFLD (see Chapter 9).
2. The mainstay of treatment is weight loss by dietary restriction. Bariatric surgery (gastric bypass or banding) reduces the severity of nonalcoholic steatohepatitis in obese patients.

ANOREXIA NERVOSA

1. Patients with anorexia nervosa may have elevated levels of liver biochemical test values, predominantly the aminotransferases.
2. Up to 30% of patients with moderately severe (body mass index 12 to 16) and 75% of those with severe (body mass index <12) anorexia nervosa have raised aminotransferase levels; marked increases are often a marker of impending multiorgan failure.
3. Transient increases in liver enzyme levels may occur during refeeding in patients with anorexia nervosa and other causes of starvation; generally, the abnormalities resolve completely when refeeding is completed.

Amyloidosis

Systemic amyloidosis is characterized by the extracellular deposition of fibrillar protein in many tissues. It may be classified as **AL (primary amyloid)** and **AA (secondary amyloid)**, accounting for approximately 90% of cases. The amyloid protein is seen as green birefringent extracellular material when stained with Congo red dye and viewed under polarized light.

- In **primary amyloidosis** (approximately 80% of all cases), the amyloid consists of kappa or lambda immunoglobulin light chains produced by a monoclonal population of plasma cells. Bence Jones proteinuria may also be present, and approximately one third of patients have multiple myeloma.
- In **secondary amyloidosis,** the amyloid is derived from serum amyloid A, secreted by the liver as an acute phase reactant in response to chronic infections or inflammatory processes such as TB, lepromatous leprosy, osteomyelitis, RA, Crohn disease, or lymphoma.
- The clinical presentation is usually nonspecific, and patients may present with symptoms related to deposition of amyloid in other organs: Heart failure, nephrotic syndrome, intestinal malabsorption, peripheral or autonomic neuropathy, and carpal tunnel syndrome.
- **Hepatic amyloidosis** should be suspected in patients with hepatomegaly in the setting of a chronic infectious or inflammatory process, particularly if it is associated with proteinuria or monoclonal gammopathy.
- Hepatomegaly (due to passive congestion or infiltration) is found in up to 60% of affected patients; splenomegaly is much less common (approximately 5%).
- Abnormalities of liver biochemical test values include a marked increase in serum ALP levels, with aminotransferases less than twice normal. The serum albumin level may be low, often secondary to proteinuria, which may be in the nephrotic range in 30% of patients.
- Liver biopsy should be avoided because of an increased risk of bleeding after biopsy.
- The prognosis of patients with systemic amyloidosis is generally poor, with a median survival of <2 years. Mortality is usually the result of cardiac or renal disease and only rarely hepatic involvement. Treatment of predisposing chronic inflammatory conditions may improve the outcome.

FURTHER READING

Berry PA, Cross TJ, Thein SL, et al. Hepatic dysfunction in sickle cell disease: a new system of classification based on global assessment. *Clin Gastroenterol Hepatol.* 2007;5:1469–1476.

Chowdhary VR, Crowson CS, Poterucha JJ, et al. Liver involvement in systemic lupus erythematosus: case review of 40 patients. *J Rheumatol.* 2008;35:2159–2164.

Csepregi A, Szodoray P, Zeher M. Do autoantibodies predict autoimmune liver disease in primary Sjögren's syndrome? Data of 180 patients upon a 5 year follow-up. *Scand J Immunol.* 2002;56:623–629.

Ebert EC, Hagspiel KD. Gastrointestinal and hepatic manifestations of systemic lupus erythematosus. *J Clin Gastroenterol.* 2011;45:436–441.

Ebert EC, Kierson M, Hagspiel KD. Gastrointestinal and hepatic manifestations of sarcoidosis. *Am J Gastro-enterol.* 2008;103:3184–3192.

Ebert EC, Nagar M. Gastrointestinal manifestations of amyloidosis. *Am J Gastroenterol.* 2008;103:776–787.

Gertz MA, Kyle RA. Hepatic amyloidosis: clinical appraisal in 77 patients. *Hepatology.* 1997;25:118–121.

Giallourakis CC, Rosenberg PM, Friedman LS. The liver in heart failure. *Clin Liver Dis.* 2002;6:947–967.

Kyle V. Laboratory investigations including liver in polymyalgia rheumatica and giant cell arteritis. *Baillieres Clin Rheum.* 1991;5:475–484.

Mendes FD, Levy C, Enders FB, et al. Abnormal hepatic biochemistries in patients with inflammatory bowel disease. *Am J Gastroenterol.* 2007;102:344–350.

Pope JE, Thompson A. Antimitochondrial antibodies and their significance in diffuse and limited sclero-derma. *J Clin Rheumatol.* 1999;5:206–209.

Rubio-Tapia A, Murray JA. The liver in celiac disease. *Hepatology.* 2007;46:1650–1658.

Smit WL, Culver EL, Chapman RW. New thoughts on immunoglobulin G4-related sclerosing cholangitis. *Clin Liver Dis.* 2016;20:47–65.

Walker NJ, Zurier RB. Liver abnormalities in rheumatic diseases. *Clin Liver Dis.* 2002;6:933–946.

Youssef WI, Tavill AS. Connective tissue diseases and the liver. *J Clin Gastroenterol.* 2002;35:345–349.

CHAPTER 25

Pediatric Liver Disease

Chatmanee Lertudomphonwanit, MD ■ William F. Balistreri, MD

KEY POINTS

1 The liver is physiologically immature during the perinatal period, and significant maturational changes in hepatic metabolic processes occur in early life. These metabolic processes affect the presentation of and reaction to viral and toxin exposures.

2 Inherited and metabolic liver diseases commonly present in infants and young children; the etiologies of liver disease in adolescents are more similar to those in adults (Table 25.1).

3 Liver diseases in children may manifest as hyperbilirubinemia, hepatomegaly, liver failure, acute or chronic hepatitis, portal hypertension, or systemic disease resulting from the secondary effects of liver disease.

4 The secondary effects of liver disease may be life threatening and include the following:

- Metabolic derangements, such as hypoglycemia
- Coagulopathy secondary to low levels of vitamin K–dependent clotting factors that may result in intracranial hemorrhage in the infant
- Persistent endogenous "toxin" exposure, as may be seen in diseases such as galactosemia or fructosemia
- Portal hypertension with hypersplenism and gastrointestinal bleeding

Consequences of Physiologic Immaturity of the Liver

1. **Low postnatal blood glucose concentration:** Significant hypoglycemia is uncommon in full-term infants with regular feeding practices; however, there is a potential for hypoglycemia because the process of gluconeogenesis and glycogenolysis rapidly matures after birth. Premature infants are at greatest risk of hypoglycemia because of reduced glycogen reserves and inadequate hepatic ketogenic response to hypoglycemia, which may continue through 8 weeks of postnatal life.

2. **Altered metabolism and clearance of potentially toxic endogenous and exogenous toxic compounds**
   - Hepatic concentrations of cytochrome P-450 are low in infants. Similarly, activities of aminopyrine N-demethylase and aniline p-hydroxylase are low. Hepatic processes, such as clearance of certain drugs or bilirubin that depend on these systems, are inefficient. Therefore, potentially toxic serum levels of these compounds may be reached.
   - Lower levels of glutathione peroxidase and glutathione S-transferase (GST) are present in infants, thus making the infant liver potentially prone to oxidant injury.

3. **Altered bile acid pool size and composition:** This may lead to inefficient micelle solubilization or to the accumulation of harmful atypical bile acids, which may exacerbate cholestasis and liver injury.

335

TABLE 25.1 ■ Clues to a Diagnosis of Metabolic Liver Disease in Neonates, Infants, and Children

History	Physical Examination	Laboratory Findings
Symptoms provoked by illness or fasting	Marked hepatomegaly	Hypoglycemia (without severe liver dysfunction)
Consanguinity in family	Cataracts	Severe coagulopathy (without severe liver dysfunction)
Maternal liver disease during pregnancy	Unusual odors	Hyperammonemia (without severe liver dysfunction)
History of miscarriage in previous gestation	Developmental delay, psychomotor retardation, hypotonia, seizures	Retractable organic acidemia, lactic acidemia

BOX 25.1 ■ Warning Signs of Pathologic Jaundice in Neonates

Elevated serum bilirubin level occurring before 36 hours of age or lasting longer than 14 days of age
Total serum bilirubin level >12 mg/dL at any time
Conjugated serum bilirubin level >1 to 2 mg/dL, or 20% of total bilirubin, at any time

4. **Physiologic jaundice**
   ■ **Up to one third of newborns develop unconjugated hyperbilirubinemia within the first week of life;** this spontaneously resolves with no complications.
   ■ Breast-fed infants have a higher risk of developing jaundice than do formula-fed infants.
   ■ Jaundice in preterm infants may present earlier, last longer, and be greater in severity than in term infants.
   ■ Physiologic jaundice reflects the transition of clearance and metabolism of unconjugated bilirubin from the maternal system to the infant. The pathogenesis is likely multifactorial:
     – Increased production of bilirubin: The newborn has a large red cell mass, and the cells have a shorter half-life than adult red cells.
     – Reduced intracellular conjugation due to low expression of hepatic uridine diphosphate (UDP)–glucuronyl transferase
     – Increased reabsorption of unconjugated bilirubin via the enterohepatic circulation due to altered intestinal microflora and more endogenous or exogenous beta-glucuronidase
   ■ Treatment is usually not required for physiologic jaundice. Interruption of breastfeeding is not necessary.
   ■ Although **pathologic jaundice** is not common, it is important to recognize and obtain further investigations. Warning signs of pathologic jaundice are shown in Box 25.1.

Hyperbilirubinemia

PATHOPHYSIOLOGY

Alterations in any step in bilirubin metabolism may cause jaundice (Fig. 25.1; the numbers in the figure correspond to the numbers [1 to 8] in the following outline).

1. **Increased bilirubin production:** This can result from an increase in the release of heme from red blood cells, for the following reasons.
   ■ *Hemolytic diseases* due to blood group incompatibility (ABO, Rh, and other minor blood groups), red cell enzyme defects (glucose-6-phosphate dehydrogenase [G6PD]; or pyruvate kinase [PK], hexokinase [HK]), and structural/red cell membrane defects (congenital spherocytosis, hereditary elliptocytosis)
   ■ *Reabsorption* of hemolyzed blood from a hematoma

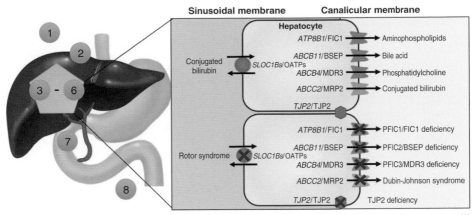

Fig. 25.1 Steps in bilirubin metabolism. (1) Bilirubin production; (2) uptake of bilirubin into hepatocytes; (3) intracellular binding; (4) conjugation; (5) excretion of conjugated bilirubin; (6) excretion of bile component via hepatocyte membrane transporters to intrahepatic bile ducts; (7) extrahepatic biliary tract; (8) enterohepatic circulation. The numbers correspond to the steps described in the text. The inset shows the genes and corresponding proteins (with their transport products shown outside the upper hepatocyte) mutated in disorders (shown outside the lower hepatocyte) affecting steps 3 through 6. The full names of the genes and proteins are given in the text.

2. **Decreased bilirubin uptake into the hepatocyte**
   - This may be caused by hypothyroidism or gestational hormones that may inhibit the uptake of bilirubin across the hepatocyte membrane.
   - A decrease in the amount of bilirubin bound to serum proteins also results in decreased uptake by hepatocytes. The reduction in bilirubin binding may be the result of hypoalbuminemia, generalized hypoproteinemia, or displacement of bilirubin from these proteins by certain drugs.
3. **Abnormalities of intracellular binding or storage of bilirubin within the hepatocyte:** These are rare disorders and include deficiencies or alteration in GST, the primary intracellular binding protein for bilirubin. Treatment is not indicated, because there is no associated morbidity or mortality.
4. **Inefficient conjugation of bilirubin:** Within the hepatocyte, bilirubin is conjugated with glucuronic acid by (UDP)–glucuronyl transferase to form bilirubin monoglucuronide or diglucuronide.
   a. **Gilbert syndrome**
      - The most common hereditary hyperbilirubinemia syndrome; caused by mutations in the promotor region of the *UGT1* gene, resulting in decrease in (UDP)–glucuronyl transferase activity
      - The main clinical features are intermittent benign elevations of serum unconjugated bilirubin levels in otherwise asymptomatic subjects; this is especially prominent during periods of stress such as a viral illness. Gilbert syndrome can also contribute to neonatal hyperbilirubinemia and lead to higher serum bilirubin levels.
      - The diagnosis is based on exclusion of hemolysis or liver cell injury; genetic testing is available.
      - No treatment is required; the only long-term consequence is an increased risk of gallstones.
   b. **Crigler-Najjar syndrome** (autosomal recessive diseases caused by various types of mutations in *UGT1* gene)
      - Crigler-Najjar syndrome **type I** is characterized by an absence of bilirubin (UDP)-glucuronyl transferase and leads to severe hyperbilirubinemia (usually >20 mg/dL). This is associated with neurologic effects secondary to **kernicterus.**

- Crigler-Najjar syndrome **type II** is caused by a reduction of (UDP)–glucuronyl transferase and has a milder phenotype (total bilirubin usually <20 mg/dL).
- Treatment includes exchange transfusion and aggressive phototherapy to keep bilirubin levels below the threshold for kernicterus. Phenobarbital therapy can be used in Crigler-Najjar syndrome type II, which generally has better prognosis than type I. Liver transplantation is the definitive treatment for Crigler-Najjar type I.

5. **Alterations in the excretion of conjugated bilirubin from the hepatocyte:** In normal circumstances, bilirubin diglucuronide is predominantly excreted into the canaliculus by a carrier protein localized to the multidrug resistance–associated protein (MRP2) on the canalicular membrane. A fraction of bilirubin glucuronide is secreted into sinusoidal blood; reuptake into hepatocyte occurs via transporters (*gene*/protein) *ABCC3*/MRP3 or *SLCO1B1*/OATP1B1 and *SLCO1B3*/OATP1B3 (OATP stands for organic anion-transporting polypeptide). Diseases that cause alterations of these steps can result in hyperbilirubinemia (both unconjugated and conjugated bilirubin) and include the following:

   a. **Dubin-Johnson syndrome:**
      - An autosomal recessive disease caused by a mutation in ABCC2 on chromosome 10q24 that results in alterations in bilirubin excretion via MRP2
      - Characterized by elevated serum levels of conjugated and unconjugated bilirubin and otherwise normal liver biochemical test levels; commonly presents in young adulthood
      - Hyperbilirubinemia can be accentuated during pregnancy or with use of oral contraceptives.
      - The diagnosis is based on normal total coproporphyrin levels in urine but an increase in the percentage of coproporphyrin I. Liver biopsy specimens, if obtained, show a characteristic melanin-like pigment deposited in hepatocytes in an otherwise histologically normal liver.
      - Because of the benign nature of this syndrome, no treatment is required.

   b. **Rotor syndrome:**
      - An autosomal recessive disease caused by mutations in *SLCO1B1* and *SLCO1B3* on chromosome 12 that results in an absence of OATP1B1 and OATP1B3 on the basolateral surface of hepatocytes
      - Clinically indistinguishable from Dubin-Johnson syndrome
      - Urine test is definitive: There is an increase in total coproporphyrin levels.
      - Like Dubin-Johnson syndrome, Rotor syndrome is benign, and no treatment is required.

6. **Abnormalities of hepatocyte excretory function or intrahepatic bile ducts (intrahepatic cholestasis [or both]);** impairment of canalicular membrane transporters or obstruction of bile flow at the level intrahepatic bile duct. May be the result of a genetic abnormality in a hepatocyte transport protein (a to d, *following*), hepatocellular excretory function (e, *following*), or intrahepatic bile ducts (f, *following*):

   a. **Progressive familial intrahepatic cholestasis, type I (PFIC-1; FIC1 deficiency)**, previously known as **Byler disease,** is an autosomal recessive disease caused by defects in the *ATP8B1* gene on chromosome 18q21–22 that encodes the FIC1 protein.
      - FIC1 is a P-type adenosine triphosphatase (ATPase) that functions in the transport of aminophospholipids across the hepatocyte canalicular plasma membrane.
      - Patients characteristically have a low serum gamma-glutamyltranspeptidase (GGTP) level in the setting of cholestasis.
      - Severe pruritus is noted at an average age of onset of 3 months.
      - Because the *ATP8B1* gene is distributed in various tissues, extrahepatic features can include growth failure, chronic diarrhea, pancreatitis, and sensorineural hearing loss.
      - FIC1 deficiency exhibits a variable clinical course with the potential for progression to cirrhosis and end-stage liver disease.

- Treatment is aimed at ameliorating pruritus. Liver transplantation is curative of the liver disease and typically is required in the first decade of life; however, liver steatosis and chronic diarrhea may be aggravated following liver transplantation.
- A milder form of *ATP8B1* mutation is called **benign recurrent intrahepatic cholestasis (BRIC)** and is characterized by recurrent episodes of jaundice and pruritus without progression to end-stage liver disease.

b. **Progressive familial intrahepatic cholestasis, type II (PFIC-2; BSEP deficiency),** is clinically similar to PFIC-1 but without extrahepatic features. Both are associated with low serum GGTP levels. The disease results from defects in the hepatocyte bile salt export pump (BSEP) caused by mutations in the *ABCB11* gene on chromosome 2q24 leading to accumulation of bile salts within hepatocytes and an eventual effect on hepatocellular function.
  - BSEP deficiency can also vary from a mild phenotype (BRIC) to a more severe form requiring liver transplantation.
  - A liver biopsy specimen will reveal neonatal hepatitis with giant cell transformation of hepatocytes.
  - Patients who are BSEP deficient, especially those with biallelic truncating mutations, are at high risk for the development of hepatocellular carcinoma (HCC). Therefore, surveillance is justified.

c. **Progressive familial intrahepatic cholestasis, type III (PFIC-3; MDR3 deficiency)** progresses rapidly to cirrhosis and liver failure.
  - Unlike other types of PFIC, this syndrome is characterized by elevated serum levels of GGTP.
  - PFIC-3 is caused by mutations in the *ABCB4* gene on chromosome 7q21-36, which encodes an active export pump involved with the translocation of phosphatidylcholine across the canalicular hepatocyte membrane.

d. **TJP2 deficiency** is caused by protein-truncating mutations in *TJP2*, resulting in failure of protein localization and disruption of tight junction structure. These mutations have been found to be associated with a low-GGTP cholestatic phenotype in infants.

e. **Hepatocellular damage** caused by various etiologies, such as metabolic disorders, sepsis, urinary tract infection, and drug or toxin toxicity, can also present with hyperbilirubinemia, particularly cholestasis, presumably secondary to hepatocyte damage or altered bile flow (or both).

f. **Intrahepatic bile duct paucity,** defined as a reduced ratio of interlobular bile ducts to portal tracts (normal is 0.9 to 1.8; paucity is <0.5), may be **nonsyndromic or syndromic,** as in **Alagille syndrome,** which is associated with peripheral pulmonic stenosis, butterfly vertebrae, posterior embryotoxon, and characteristic facies.

7. **Structural abnormalities of the extrahepatic biliary tract** prevent drainage of bile from the canaliculus into the intestine and can cause accumulation of bile and reflux of bilirubin into the systemic circulation.

a. **Biliary atresia** is a progressive disease characterized by inflammation and fibrosis of the extrahepatic biliary tract resulting in partial or complete obliteration of the extrahepatic bile ducts.
  - Biliary atresia typically manifests as cholestasis (conjugated hyperbilirubinemia) with acholic stools between 2 and 6 weeks of age.
  - Phenotypically, there are at least two forms: (1) The majority of patients (85%) present as isolated biliary atresia (also known as the postnatal form); (2) another group is associated with major anomalies with or without laterality defects. Associated anomalies in the latter group included anomalies of spleen (asplenia, polysplenia) and of the cardiovascular, gastrointestinal (intestinal malrotation, atresia), and genitourinary systems; <10% of cases may have cystic dilatation of extrahepatic bile duct in addition to fibrosing obstruction.

- Diagnosis is based on clinical, biochemical, and histologic data. Liver biopsy specimens show portal fibrosis and bile duct proliferation; if extrahepatic bile duct obstruction cannot be ruled out, intraoperative cholangiography should be performed.
- This anomaly is treated initially by surgical creation of a **Kasai portoenterostomy,** which allows drainage of bile directly from the liver into the intestine. Although the procedure is not curative, it may delay the progression of disease.
- **End-stage liver disease secondary to biliary atresia is the most common reason for liver transplantation in children.**

    b. **Choledochal cyst,** a cystic dilatation of the biliary tract, may be exclusively extrahepatic or include dilatations of the intrahepatic biliary tract.

- The clinical presentation with abdominal pain and jaundice, with or without a palpable abdominal mass, may occur at any age.
- The diagnosis can be made by ultrasonography, computed tomography (CT), or endoscopic retrograde or magnetic cholangiopancreatography (ERCP, MRCP).
- Treatment is with surgical excision of the dilated segment, rather than bypass or drainage, because of the increased frequency of malignancy in the epithelium of the cyst.

8. **Alterations in the enterohepatic circulation** can produce an increase in reabsorption of bilirubin from the intestine. The cause may be intestinal obstruction, as in intestinal atresia or Hirschsprung disease, or alterations in the bacterial flora because of the use of antibiotics.

COMPLICATIONS

1. **Unconjugated hyperbilirubinemia**
   - Kernicterus (bilirubin encephalopathy) may result from elevated levels of unconjugated bilirubin. Populations at risk include neonates and individuals with Crigler-Najjar syndrome, type I.
   - Unconjugated bilirubin levels >30 mg/dL are associated with development of encephalopathy.
   - Factors that increase the risk of kernicterus include hypoalbuminemia and bilirubin displacement from albumin by drugs or organic anions.
2. **Cholestasis**
   - Malnutrition secondary to intestinal fat malabsorption can lead to failure to thrive and fat-soluble vitamin deficiencies.
   - Intractable pruritus
   - Xanthomatosis secondary to alterations in cholesterol metabolism
   - HCC can occur in many diseases associated with intrahepatic cholestasis, such as FIC1, BSEP, and MDR3 deficiency; surveillance for HCC is required.

TREATMENT

1. Unconjugated hyperbilirubinemia
   - Double-volume exchange transfusion lowers the risk of kernicterus in the newborn by rapidly reducing the serum bilirubin concentration.
   - Phototherapy: Photoisomerization of bilirubin to a more polar compound allows excretion of bilirubin in the urine.
   - Bilirubin metabolism can be accomplished by administration of phenobarbital, which induces microsomal enzymes that facilitate bilirubin metabolism.
2. Cholestasis
   - Treatment of all forms of intrahepatic cholestasis is symptomatic, with special consideration given to management of malnutrition and pruritus.
   - Ursodeoxycholic acid, a choleretic bile acid, 15 mg/kg per day in divided doses, can be used to augment bile flow in patients with cholestasis.

- Supplementation with fat-soluble vitamins is also necessary because intestinal absorption is poor without normal bile flow.
- Liver transplantation may be required in some cases.

Liver Failure (see Chapter 2)

- Encephalopathy is difficult to assess in young children and may not be clinically apparent until later stages of disease; it is not a required diagnostic criterion for pediatric acute liver failure.
- **Diagnostic criteria for acute liver failure in children:** No known evidence of chronic liver disease, biochemical evidence of acute liver injury, and coagulopathy not corrected by vitamin K (prothrombin time [PT] >15 seconds or international normalized ratio [INR] >1.5 with hepatic encephalopathy and PT ≥20 or INR ≥2 without hepatic encephalopathy)
- Specific etiologies vary widely in each age group, and the cause may not be identified in 50% of cases. Acetaminophen toxicity is the most common identifiable cause in older children and adolescents, whereas infectious causes (e.g., hepatitis A virus) are more common in developing countries. Metabolic diseases, including tyrosinemia type I (see Chapter 20) and viral hepatitis (e.g., herpes simplex virus [see Chapter 6]) are common identifiable causes of acute liver failure in infants and neonates (Table 25.2).
- Early recognition of acute liver failure and timely investigations (Table 25.3) along with supportive treatment and monitoring in an intensive care unit are recommended.
- The outcome of pediatric liver failure varies according to the etiology. **Because liver transplantation is often lifesaving, a transplant center should be contacted early in the course.**

GALACTOSEMIA

Galactosemia resulting from deficiency of galactose-1-phosphate uridyltransferase (GALT) usually manifests within the first few days of life.

- GALT deficiency leads to accumulation of galactose-1-phosphate and galactitol.
- The initial presentation may be with *Escherichia coli* sepsis in a neonate.
- Hypoglycemia can occur while an infant is being fed breast milk or a lactose-containing formula. Urine-reducing substances could be found.
- The diagnosis is based on absence of GALT activity in red blood cells. Newborn screening programs are also available in many states in the United States.

TABLE 25.2 ■ **Causes of Acute Liver Failure in Neonates and Infants**

Category	Cause
Infection	Herpesvirus, enterovirus, hepatitis B virus
Metabolic disease	Galactosemia, tyrosinemia, hereditary fructose intolerance (after introduction of fructose and/or sucrose), citrin deficiency, glycosylation defect, Niemann-Pick disease type C, mitochondrial hepatopathies
Ischemia	Congenital heart disease, severe asphyxia
Immune dysregulation	Hemophagocytic lymphohistiocytosis, gestational alloimmune liver disease
Drugs and toxins	Valproic acid, acetaminophen
Other	Reye syndrome, malignancy

- If the disorder is not treated, the affected infant will succumb to hepatic failure.
- Treatment is by removal of lactose (and galactose) from the diet, because lactose is broken down to glucose and galactose.

PRIMARY MITOCHONDRIAL HEPATOPATHIES

Mitochondrial defects commonly present as neonatal liver failure, progressive liver disease with sudden deterioration in early childhood (often associated with neuromuscular symptoms), or progression to chronic fibrosing liver disease. Typical features that may suggest a mitochondrial liver disease include neurologic involvement, episodes of hypoglycemia, hyperammonemia, and lactic acidosis.

1. **Fatty acid oxidation defects** such as medium-chain acyl-coenzyme A (CoA) dehydrogenase deficiency (MCAD) and long-chain 3-hydroxyacyl-CoA dehydrogenase (LCHAD) deficiency manifest with hepatomegaly, hypoglycemia, and increased serum aminotransferase levels. These defects result in an inability to use fat, which builds up in the liver. In decompensated patients, hypoketosis is manifest in the setting of hypoglycemia.
   - Decompensation is often precipitated by common childhood illnesses such as otitis media or acute gastroenteritis and is characterized by lethargy and severe hypoglycemia. These episodes respond rapidly to fluid and glucose replacement.
   - The diagnosis is suggested by an abnormal urine organic acid profile. The ratio of ketone bodies to dicarboxylic acid is low, signifying an inability to metabolize stored fats. Total serum carnitine levels are low, whereas the fraction of acylcarnitine is usually high.
2. **Respiratory chain defects,** as in **Alpers syndrome** (*POLG*-related disorders), usually manifest with neurologic disease (refractory seizures and psychomotor regression) and

---

TABLE 25.3 ■ **Diagnostic Investigation and Specific Treatment in Acute Liver Failure in Neonates and Infants**

Disease	Diagnostic Investigation	Specific Treatment
Galactosemia	Red blood cell galactose-1-phosphate uridyltransferase (GALT)	Lactose-free formula
Hereditary fructose intolerance	Quantitative enzyme assay for fructose-1-phosphate aldolase (aldolase B)	Fructose-free diet
Tyrosinemia type I (see Chapter 20)	Urine succinylacetone	NTBC (0.5–1 mg/kg/day), elimination diet
Gestational alloimmune liver disease	Oral mucosal biopsy or abdominal MRI (extrahepatic iron deposition)	Double-volume exchange transfusion followed by IV immunoglobulin (1 g/kg)
Citrin deficiency	Plasma amino acid, genetic testing	Low-carbohydrate (lactose free), high-protein, and high-fat diet, MCT supplement
Herpesvirus infection	Viral serology and PCR	Acyclovir (60 mg/kg/day IV)
Hemophagocytic lymphohistiocytosis (HLH)	Diagnostic criteria (see text)	HLH-2004 treatment protocol: Etoposide, dexamethasone, cyclosporine, intrathecal methotrexate (if neurologic involvement)

IV, Intravenously; *MCT,* medium-chain triglycerides; *MRI,* magnetic resonance imaging; *NTBC,* 2 (2-nitro-4-trifluoromethylbenzoyl)-1, 3-cyclohexenedione; *PCR,* polymerase chain reaction.

progressive hepatic failure. In some cases, liver involvement can be accelerated by valproic acid exposure. Initially, it is frequently difficult to differentiate the disorders from the side effects of seizure medications. Typical liver biochemistry reveals mild ALT and AST elevations with impaired synthetic function (hypoglycemia, hypoalbuminemia, and coagulopathy).

3. **Mitochondrial DNA depletion syndrome,** which resembles Alpers syndrome, is characterized by a tissue-specific reduction in mitochondrial DNA copy number. Affected patients with the hepatocerebral form of this disorder usually present within the first few weeks or months of life with progressive liver failure and neurologic symptoms including hypotonia and seizure. Unremitting lactic acidosis and hypoglycemia are common laboratory findings.

GESTATIONAL ALLOIMMUNE LIVER DISEASE

Gestational alloimmune liver disease results from an intrauterine alloimmune liver injury and is the **most common cause of neonatal liver failure.** It is characterized by a combination of severe liver disease in newborns and extrahepatic siderosis.

- An affected infant usually presents shortly after birth with hypoglycemia, marked coagulopathy, and jaundice (both conjugated and unconjugated hyperbilirubinemia); serum aminotransferase levels are disproportionately low. The serum alpha fetoprotein (AFP) level is characteristically high (100,000 to 600,000 ng/mL).
- Iron studies reveal high iron saturation with low transferrin levels. Elevated serum ferritin can be found but is nonspecific.
- Demonstration of extrahepatic siderosis, either by oral mucosal biopsy or abdominal MRI, is required for diagnosis.
- Treatment with double-volume exchange transfusion and intravenous immunoglobulin has been shown to improve outcome.
- The risk of recurrence in subsequent pregnancies is high; therefore preventive treatment with intravenous immunoglobulin, 1 g/kg body weight starting at 14 and 16 weeks of gestation then weekly from week 18 until the end of gestation, is recommended for high-risk women.

CITRIN DEFICIENCY

Citrin deficiency is an autosomal recessive disorder that results from a deficiency of the glutamate-aspartate transporter in the mitochondrial membrane caused by mutations in *SLC25A13*. The disease is more prevalent in Japan and East Asian countries. Two forms are recognized:

1. **Neonatal intrahepatic cholestasis associated with citrin deficiency (NICCD)** presents during the neonatal period. Symptoms vary from transient neonatal intrahepatic cholestasis to acute liver failure.
    - Hypoglycemia and the detection of urine-reducing substance are common, as in galactosemia. Other characteristic laboratory findings include high levels of AFP and an increased branched-chain aromatic amino acid ratio in plasma.
    - Treatment consists of a lactose-free formula with medium-chain triglyceride supplementation in infants. Liver dysfunction usually resolves in the first year of life. Affected children may subsequently develop a preference for a protein-rich diet and aversion to high-carbohydrate food.
2. **Citrullinemia type 2** presents in older children or adulthood with the acute onset of neuropsychiatric problems and hyperammonemia. Treatment consists of arginine supplementation and a high-protein, low-carbohydrate diet.

REYE SYNDROME

Reye syndrome is a rare cause of fulminant hepatic failure in children.

■ It typically manifests following a prodromal febrile illness such as an upper respiratory tract or varicella infection and is associated with aspirin treatment.

■ Protracted vomiting occurs 5 to 7 days after the onset of the initial illness, usually as the inciting illness is improving. Progression to hepatic failure with associated neurologic deterioration, seizures, and coma may occur rapidly.

■ Serum aminotransferase levels are typically more than three to four times the upper limit of normal. The ammonia level is markedly elevated, with mild-to-moderate prolongation of the PT and a normal serum bilirubin level. Hypoglycemia is also common.

■ Liver histology demonstrates hepatocytes with foamy accumulation of triglyceride. Electron microscopy demonstrates alterations in mitochondrial structure; similar alterations are seen in mitochondria in the brain.

■ Treatment is supportive and focuses on controlling intracranial pressure and glucose levels. Survival depends on early diagnosis; patients treated before severe neurologic involvement occurs have a greater chance of complete recovery.

Hepatomegaly

The liver may increase in size because of cell hyperplasia or hypertrophy, fibrosis, venous congestion, infiltration with fat or the accumulation of substances not normally present in the liver, and tumor infiltration.

INFLAMMATORY CELL INFILTRATION AND KUPFFER CELL PROLIFERATION

Involves various etiologies such as viral hepatitis and autoimmune hepatitis (see Chapters 3 to 7).

FIBROSIS

Fibrocystic liver disease results from lack of normal embryonic development of the biliary tract. A spectrum of diseases is seen, depending on the size of the bile duct involved. Many variants are associated with cystic disorders of the kidneys (see also Chapter 30).

1. **Congenital hepatic fibrosis** is characterized by hepatic fibrosis and portal hypertension, and is typically associated with autosomal recessive polycystic kidney disease (ARPKD). Patients with more severe liver manifestations usually present at an older age or during adolescence. Hepatomegaly and splenomegaly, secondary to portal hypertension, are common physical findings.

2. **Caroli disease and Caroli syndrome:** Cystic liver disease involving the large intrahepatic bile ducts. Because of bile stasis in the cysts, affected patients are predisposed to recurrent cholangitis. Ductal plate malformation, as in congenital hepatic fibrosis, is also found in Caroli syndrome. Portal hypertension is a common presentation and usually precedes cholangitis.

VENOUS CONGESTION

Cardiac dysfunction or **hepatic outflow obstruction (Budd-Chiari syndrome)** can result in passive congestion of the liver, which may manifest as hepatomegaly together with ascites and abdominal pain (see Chapters 21 and 22).

ACCUMULATION OF METABOLIC SUBSTANCES

1. **Fat**
   - Hepatomegaly due to fat accumulation is seen in many disorders, the most common of which are obesity, rapid weight change, diabetes mellitus, and malnutrition. **Obesity as well as rapid weight gain** can lead to hepatomegaly, which is associated with steatosis, mild inflammation, and Kupffer cell hyperplasia. **Nonalcoholic fatty liver disease (NAFLD)** is estimated to affect 3% to 10% of the general pediatric population and up to 40% to 80% in the obese pediatric population (see Chapter 9).
   - Progression from steatosis to steatohepatitis to advanced fibrosis and cirrhosis has been documented in children as in the adult population, even in children with normal or mild elevations of the serum ALT (evidence-based standards for normal ALT levels proposed in children are ≤25 U/L for boys and ≤22 U/L for girls).
   - The presence of the metabolic syndrome (visceral obesity, hypertension, insulin resistance/diabetes mellitus, and dyslipidemia) appears to be more important than obesity alone in the development of steatosis and steatohepatitis.
   - Ethnic background is also a risk factor; Hispanics and Native Americans are at highest risk, and African Americans are at lowest risk.
   - Because NAFLD is rare in children 3 to 10 years of age, patients in this age group require a detailed diagnostic workup to exclude other etiologies, especially other metabolic liver diseases.
   - **Treatment consists primarily of weight loss and control of hyperglycemia and hyperlipidemia.** Weight loss should not be rapid, because of the potential to aggravate hepatic inflammation; weight loss of 500 g/week has been advocated in children.
   - A randomized, placebo-controlled trial in children has shown histologic benefit to vitamin E treatment in patients with NASH or borderline NASH as well as improvement in serum aminotransferase levels.

2. **Cholesterol**
   Lysosomal acid lipase deficiency (LAL-D) is an autosomal recessive disorder characterized by a decrease in the lysosomal acid lipase enzyme. This results in decreased degradation of cholesterol.
   - LAL-D is caused by mutation in the *LIPA* gene on chromosome 10q23.2-q23.3 resulting in different degrees of lysosomal acid lipase activity.
   - Common hepatic features include hepatomegaly (from cholesteryl ester and triglyceride accumulation), elevated serum aminotransferase levels, progressive liver fibrosis, and cirrhosis.
     a. **Cholesteryl ester storage disease (CESD),** a milder disease with residual enzyme activity, presents with unexplained hepatomegaly and dyslipidemia (typically type IIb hyperlipoproteinemia). The onset of disease may be noted at any age. Progressive liver disease with steatosis, fibrosis, and cirrhosis can occur in more than half of patients.
     b. **Wolman disease,** a severe form of LAL-D, is due to nearly complete deficiency of LAL enzyme activity.
        - The disease usually presents in the neonatal period with persistent vomiting, diarrhea, malabsorption (secondary to accumulation of lipid in the intestinal epithelium), failure to thrive, and hepatosplenomegaly. Adrenal calcification is a striking feature.
        - Neurologic deterioration and death occur by 6 to 12 months of age.
   - Enzyme replacement therapy with recombinant human lysosomal acid lipase has been approved to treat children and adults with LAL-D. Intravenous administration of this drug has been shown the improve survival outcome in infants with Wolman disease, with improvement in serum ALT and lipid levels and hepatic fat content in patients with CESD after 20 weeks of treatment.

3. **Glycogen**
    a. **Glycogen storage disease (GSD)** manifests as hepatomegaly, usually without splenomegaly, secondary to accumulated glycogen in hepatocytes (see also Chapter 20).
        ■ In **GSD I,** activity of glucose-6-phosphatase is absent or abnormal; therefore, gluconeogenesis cannot proceed. Profound hypoglycemia develops after short periods of fasting with lactic acidosis, hyperuricemia, hypophosphatemia, and hyperlipidemia. Treatment includes a high-starch diet often in the form of cornstarch or continuous feedings to provide a continuous source of glucose. Patients are at an increased risk of hepatic adenomas.
        ■ **GSD IV** is rare and manifests in infancy with hepatosplenomegaly and poor weight; it is caused by a debranching enzyme deficiency. Like GSD I, GSD IV results in defective gluconeogenesis and accumulation of glycogen. Because this type of disease can progress to cirrhosis with hepatic failure, liver transplantation is considered an effective treatment; however, cardiac and neurologic features have been reported to become apparent after transplantation.
    b. **Mauriac syndrome,** found in patients with type 1 diabetes mellitus, is characterized by the triad of poorly controlled diabetes mellitus, growth retardation, and hepatomegaly.
        ■ Liver histology demonstrates diffused enlarged hepatocytes with glycogen accumulation, as in GSD.
        ■ Different degrees of fatty infiltration and fibrosis may present.
        ■ The disorder resolves with improvement in glycemic control.
4. **Sphingolipid**
    a. **Gaucher's disease** results from an autosomal recessive deficiency of glucocerebrosidase, the lysosomal enzyme responsible for degrading sphingolipids (see also Chapter 20). Three forms are recognized:
        ■ Type I typically manifests with hepatosplenomegaly and is a chronic nonneuropathic form of the disease. This type is the most common variant and account for 90% of cases.
        ■ Type II also manifests with hepatosplenomegaly but has neuropathic features and is often fatal by 2 years of age.
        ■ Type III is associated with hepatosplenomegaly and the later onset of neuropathic features.
    b. **Niemann-Pick diseases**
        ■ **Niemann-Pick disease types A and B** are autosomal recessive diseases caused by *SMPD1* mutations that result in decreased sphingomyelinase activity, which causes accumulation of sphingomyelin in the reticuloendothelial system in many organs including the liver. Cherry-red maculae are seen on eye examination. Liver biopsy specimens are characterized by lipid-laden "foam cells" and stored sphingomyelin in macrophages.
        ■ **Niemann-Pick disease type C,** unlike types A and B, results from lipid-trafficking defects that causes accumulation of unesterified cholesterol and sphingolipid in affected cells. The onset of neurocognitive dysfunction and visceral disease is variable but more common in childhood than in infancy and adulthood.
5. **Abnormal alpha-1 antitrypsin**
    Alpha-1 antitrypsin deficiency, specifically the PiZZ and PiSZ phenotypes, are associated with liver disease due to accumulation of abnormal alpha-1 antitrypsin in the endoplasmic reticulum. Affected patients may present with neonatal cholestasis or features of liver disease later in infancy or childhood. Liver transplantation has been undertaken to treat liver disease associated with this disorder (see Chapter 20).
6. **Copper storage diseases** (see also Chapter 19)
    Wilson disease is a genetic disease caused by copper overload; the abnormal gene is located on chromosome 13.

- The carrier rate is 1 in 90; expression of the disease appears to be variable. Defective copper excretion results in excess accumulation in the liver with subsequent accumulation in the central nervous system and other organs.
- Liver disease manifests in the second to fourth decades of life. Later presentation tends to be neurologic or psychiatric.
- Diagnosis is by a serum ceruloplasmin level <20 mg/dL, liver copper >250 µg/g dry weight, and urinary copper excretion >100 µg/day.
- Liver biopsy specimens show steatosis early in the course; the disease progresses to inflammation and fibrosis with cirrhosis. A copper stain of the liver may be helpful in the diagnosis but is not specific, and the absence of stainable copper does not exclude Wilson disease.
- Without treatment, the disease can be progressive and fatal as a result of hepatic failure. It is controllable with copper chelation therapy. D-penicillamine and trientine are chelators that increase urinary excretion of copper. Zinc, which blocks intestinal absorption of copper, has also been used.
- Some patients present with acute liver failure; the only effective treatment option in this situation is liver transplantation, which is curative.

TUMOR INFILTRATION

Tumor infiltration of the liver can contribute to hepatomegaly.

- Primary tumors include embryonal rhabdomyosarcoma of the biliary tract, teratoma, hepatoblastoma, hemangioendothelioma, and HCC.
- Tumors that may infiltrate the liver secondarily include neuroblastoma, Wilms tumor, and lymphoma.
- CT can identify tumors initially as focal abnormalities rather than as diffuse infiltration. Diagnosis is by biopsy.
- Treatment depends on the tumor type.

Viral Hepatitis (see Chapters 3 to 5)

- Hepatitis A and hepatitis B are the most common causes of viral hepatitis in children.
- Although both hepatitis A and hepatitis B may manifest as an acute febrile illness with jaundice and hepatomegaly, the courses may differ.
- In addition, the presentations and courses differ from those in adults.
1. **Hepatitis A**
   - Hepatitis A virus is transmitted by the fecal-oral route, and outbreaks can often be traced to daycare centers where hygiene may be suboptimal. Adults who work with children in daycare centers are at an increased risk of contracting this disease.
   - The disease is often mildly symptomatic (75% to 95%) in children without visible jaundice, whereas adults are more commonly symptomatic (75% to 95%).
   - Because the disease is self-limited, no specific therapy is required, but follow-up is needed to exclude progression to acute liver failure.
   - Hepatitis A vaccination is highly effective in preventing clinical disease (94%) for children and adults at high risk.
2. **Hepatitis B**
   - Perinatal transmission of hepatitis B virus from a highly infectious mother is an important route of infection in endemic areas. Acute symptoms are uncommon, particularly in infants and young children. Older children exhibit a clinical course similar to that of adults.

- Rarely, an associated immune complex–mediated extrahepatic disease, such as membranous glomerulonephritis or papular acrodermatitis of childhood (Gianotti-Crosti syndrome), occurs.
- Infants born to mothers who are positive for hepatitis B surface antigen (HBsAg) (especially those positive for hepatitis B e antigen [HBeAg]) are at high risk of chronic hepatitis B, usually remain in the immune tolerant phase during childhood, and are at risk of developing HCC later in life.
- For infants born to HBsAg-positive mothers, administration of hepatitis B immune globulin within 4 to 6 hours of birth followed by the first dose of the hepatitis B vaccine and subsequent completion of the series can prevent the disease in the infant.
- Antiviral therapy should be considered for women who are also HBeAg positive and have high serum levels of hepatitis B viral DNA.

3. **Hepatitis C**
   - Maternal-to-infant transmission is a common route for childhood infection, with perinatal transmission rate of 5%; intravenous drug abuse is a common route of transmission in adolescents.
   - Acute hepatitis C is not commonly detected in children; the disease progresses slowly during the childhood period, and advanced liver disease and serious complications are rare.
   - In the United States, approved treatment for children includes peginterferon-alfa2b in combination with ribavirin. Response rates are low, and side effects are frequent. In 2017, the combination of oral direct-acting antiviral agents ledipasvir and sofosbuvir was approved for children aged 12 to 17 with infection caused by genotypes 1, 4, 5, or 6. Because these agents are highly effective and less toxic than interferon-based regimens, treatment may be deferred until these new agents are approved for children under age 12 or other regimens are approved for children with genotype-2 or genotype-3 infection.

Systemic Conditions Affecting the Liver (see Chapter 24)

1. **Cystic fibrosis (CF)**
   - CF is a disease of altered chloride secretion, most commonly affecting the lungs and pancreas. Many patients with CF have associated **focal and multilobular biliary cirrhosis,** with complications such as portal hypertension.
   - The presence of liver disease does not appear to depend on the genotype of CF, nor is it related to the severity of pulmonary disease.
   - Patients present with hepatomegaly, which may be erroneously attributed to hyperinflation of the lungs.
   - Patients with CF are known to have a high frequency of biliary sludge, cholelithiasis, bile duct strictures, microgallbladder, and prolonged neonatal cholestasis.
   - Treatment with ursodeoxycholic acid has been shown to improve the abnormal laboratory findings associated with liver disease in CF; however, it is unclear whether prophylactic therapy with ursodeoxycholic acid is beneficial for all patients with CF.

2. **Sickle cell disease**
   - Patients with sickle cell disease commonly have hepatomegaly, apparently secondary to sinusoidal dilatation and Kupffer cell hyperplasia.
   - An increased frequency of cholelithiasis secondary to rapid hemoglobin turnover is seen in this population.

3. **Total parenteral nutrition (TPN)**
   - In children, especially neonates, prolonged TPN can be associated with cholestasis, which may progress to cirrhosis and liver failure.
   - The precise pathogenesis of liver disease resulting from TPN is unknown. It is likely multifactorial, including toxic substrates in the TPN solution, nutrient and micronutrient

deficiency, and toxic bacterial by-products (proinflammatory lipopolysaccharides) that cross the atrophic intestinal mucosal barrier.

■ Neonates are at high risk for TPN-induced cholestasis because of hepatic immaturity and a high requirement for energy to ensure adequate growth. An upper limit of 3.5 g/kg per day of lipid has been recommended in infants; however, lower infusion rates have been associated with a reduced rate of cholestasis.

■ Risk factors include prematurity, abdominal surgery, necrotizing enterocolitis, and infections, particularly catheter-related bloodstream infections.

■ The most effective treatment is administration of enteral feedings and cessation of TPN. Fish oils or multisource lipid emulsions as the lipid component are associated with resolution of jaundice and may reduce hepatobiliary disease.

4. **Celiac disease**
   ■ Patients with celiac disease may present with serum aminotransferase elevations, a prolonged prothrombin time, or nonspecific liver histologic changes even in the absence of gastrointestinal symptoms.
   ■ Celiac disease has also been associated with autoimmune hepatitis, primary sclerosing cholangitis (PSC), and primary biliary cholangitis.
   ■ A gluten-free diet typically normalizes both laboratory and liver histologic abnormalities.

5. **PSC and inflammatory bowel disease (IBD)** (see Chapter 17)
   ■ Patients with IBD, especially ulcerative colitis, may develop PSC. A significant proportion have autoimmune features (autoimmune sclerosing cholangitis).
   ■ The progression of PSC is unrelated to the duration or severity of the IBD and may precede intestinal symptoms.
   ■ Treatment of IBD with immunosuppression does not ameliorate the symptoms or evolution of PSC.

6. **Childhood histiocytic syndromes:** Abnormal activation of the reticuloendothelial system may result in liver disease.
   a. **Langerhans cell histiocytosis (LCH)**
      ■ The incidence of LCH is four to five cases per 100,000, with a median age at diagnosis of ~30 months.
      ■ Abnormally activated Langerhans cells can infiltrate the liver, thereby resulting in elevated serum aminotransferase levels, hypoalbuminemia, prolongation of the prothrombin time, and hepatomegaly.
      ■ Liver histology commonly demonstrates a portal tract inflammatory infiltrate composed of lymphocytes, neutrophils, and eosinophils. LCH may be apparent if liver tissue is immunostained for S-100 protein.
      ■ Sclerosing cholangitis is the classic process ascribed to LCH. Patients who require liver transplantation may be at increased risk of acute cellular rejection and posttransplantation lymphoproliferative disease.
   b. **Hemophagocytic lymphohistiocytosis (HLH)**
      ■ The incidence of HLH is 1.2 cases per 100,000 per year, with a median age at diagnosis of 2.9 months.
      ■ This multiorgan disease is caused by abnormal activation of nonmalignant macrophages.
      ■ Clinical presentation is variable and includes acute liver failure in infancy.
      ■ Liver histology reveals portal infiltrates (with lymphocytes) of varying size.
      ■ Diagnostic criteria include five of the following eight features: Fever, splenomegaly, cytopenia ($\geq$2 cell lines): Hemoglobin <9 g/dL; platelets <100 × 10^9/L; neutrophils <1.0 × 10^9/L, hypertriglyceridemia ($\geq$265 mg/dL) and/or hypofibrinogenemia ($\leq$150 mg/dL), hemophagocytosis in bone marrow or spleen or lymph nodes (no evidence of malignancy), low or absent NK cell activity, serum ferritin $\geq$500 µg/L, and soluble IL-2R alpha level $\geq$2400 U/mL.
      ■ Treatment is with bone marrow transplantation.

7. **Muscular dystrophies:** Not associated with liver disease but often with an elevated serum aspartate aminotransferase (AST) level that leads the clinician to believe that the liver is involved. Further evaluation reveals an elevated creatine kinase and/or aldolase level, thus confirming that the origin of the AST is muscle.

8. **Inborn errors of glycosylation:** Carbohydrate-deficient glycoprotein syndromes comprise a group of multisystem disorders with defects in *N*-linked oligosaccharide assembly.
   - Type Ia, the most common and best described, is caused by defects in the *phosphomanno-mutase 2 (PMM2)* gene and has an incidence of 1 in 80,000.
   - Infants have a high mortality risk from multisystem disease. Those surviving infancy often have profound psychomotor and mental retardation. Patients can present in infancy with variable degrees of liver dysfunction secondary to steatosis or fibrosis.
   - The diagnosis is made by abnormal isoelectric focusing of serum transferrin.
   - Treatment with D-mannose may ameliorate hepatic and gastrointestinal symptoms in patients with type Ib (phosphomannose isomerase deficiency, a primarily liver and intestinal disorder with mild neurologic involvement).

FURTHER READING

Beath SV, Kelly DA. Total parenteral nutrition-induced cholestasis: prevention and management. *Clin Liver Dis.* 2016;20:159–176.

Feldman AG, Mack CL. Biliary atresia: clinical lessons learned. *J Pediatr Gastroenterol Nutr.* 2015;61:167–175.

Fretzayas A, Moustaki M, Liapi O, et al. Gilbert syndrome. *Eur J Pediatr.* 2012;171:11–15.

Grijalva J, Vakili K. Neonatal liver physiology. *Semin Pediatr Surg.* 2013;22:185–189.

Jacquemin E. Progressive familial intrahepatic cholestasis. *Clin Res Hepatol Gastroenterol.* 2012;36:S26–S35.

Memon N, Weinberger BI, Hegyi T, et al. Inherited disorders of bilirubin clearance. *Pediatr Res.* 2016;79:378–386.

Mieli-Vergani G, Vergani D. Paediatric autoimmune liver disease. *Arch Dis Child.* 2013;98:1012–1017.

Mieli-Vergani G, Vergani D. Sclerosing cholangitis in children and adolescents. *Clin Liver Dis.* 2016;20:99–111.

Mitchel EB, Lavine JE. Review article: the management of paediatric nonalcoholic fatty liver disease. *Aliment Pharmacol Ther.* 2014;40:1155–1170.

Molleston JP, Schwimmer JB, Yates KP, et al. Histological abnormalities in children with nonalcoholic fatty liver disease and normal or mildly elevated alanine aminotransferase levels. *J Pediatr.* 2014;164:707–713.

Pan X, Kelly S, Melin-Aldana H, et al. Novel mechanism of fetal hepatocyte injury in congenital alloimmune hepatitis involves the terminal complement cascade. *Hepatology.* 2010;51:2061–2068.

Santos JL, Choquette M, Bezerra JA. Cholestatic liver disease in children. *Curr Gastroenterol Rep.* 2010;12:30–39.

Stender S, Frikke-Schmidt R, Nordestgaard BG, et al. Extreme bilirubin levels as a causal risk factor for symptomatic gallstone disease. *JAMA Intern Med.* 2013;173:1222–1228.

Suchy FJ, Sokol RJ, Balistreri WF, eds. *Liver Disease in Children.* 4th ed. Cambridge: Cambridge University Press; 2014.

CHAPTER 26

Liver Disease in the Elderly

Teresita Gomez de Castro, MD ■ Hanisha Manickavasagan, MD ■
Santiago J. Muñoz, MD

KEY POINTS

1 The clinical presentation, prognosis, and management of several liver disorders can be different in older adults than in younger persons.

2 Hepatic blood flow, liver size, and hepatic regenerative capacity decrease with age; these changes result in decreased metabolism of certain medications and a reduced ability of the liver to recover promptly from diseases such as acute viral hepatitis or drug-induced liver injury (DILI).

3 Certain disorders, such as acute liver failure and DILI, are more severe and have a worse prognosis in elderly patients than in younger patients.

4 The development of hepatocellular carcinoma (HCC) is directly related to the duration of cirrhosis; therefore, older patients with cirrhosis should be diligently screened for HCC.

5 Advanced age is not a contraindication to liver transplantation (LT), which should be considered in selected older patients with irreversible end-stage liver disease. Conversely, livers from older donors can be successfully transplanted, albeit with some risk of poor graft function.

Cellular and Biochemical Aspects

OVERVIEW

1. The aging process affects the liver, but to a lesser degree than other organs.
2. Hepatic size decreases by 20% to 40% in the elderly, and hepatic blood flow decreases by one third with advancing age; these changes may reflect alterations in cellular function and biochemical pathways in the liver.
3. These age-related alterations are of considerable importance, given the aging of our population and the fact that older adults use approximately one third of all prescribed medications, many of which are metabolized by the liver.

CELLULAR AND BIOCHEMICAL CHANGES IN THE AGING LIVER

1. Senescence of liver cells is characterized primarily by decreased production of hepatic proteins; some abnormal proteins accumulate in aging liver cells (Box 26.1).
2. Histopathologic changes seen in aging livers include increases in cell size, the number of abnormal nuclei, and the frequency of chromosomal abnormalities. Often, the number and size of lysosomes also increase. Mitochondria increase in volume but decrease in number, and, together with decreased hepatic blood flow, these changes may contribute to reduced

---

BOX 26.1 ■ Proteins That Accumulate in Aging Livers

Aminoacyl-tRNA synthetases
Cathepsin D
Glucose-6-phosphate dehydrogenase
Phosphoglycerate kinase
NADP cytochrome c reductase
Superoxide dismutase

NADP, Nicotinamide adenine dinucleotide phosphate.

---

metabolism of certain drugs. The observed decrease in telomeric length of hepatic stellate cells (HSCs) in the aged liver may lead to an increased tendency to fibrogenesis.
3. The thickness of hepatic sinusoidal cells and their number and the size of their fenestrae are reduced in aging, thereby causing disturbance of the exchange of molecules between hepatocytes and plasma that flows within the sinusoids.
4. Lipofuscin, the "wear-and-tear" pigment, is a common finding on liver biopsy specimens from elderly persons. Lipofuscin has been thought to represent extensive nonenzymatic glycosylation and cross-linking of heterogeneous cellular components, including nucleic acids, proteins, and lipids. Evidence suggests that lipofuscin may represent, at least in part, accumulation of retinyl palmitate. Lipofuscin was previously thought to be biologically inert, but there is increasing evidence that lipofuscin interferes with hepatocyte gene transcription processes, thereby diminishing cell survival.
5. As individuals age, hepatocytes become less sensitive to insulin and corticosteroids. Protein breakdown and both transcriptional and translational processes decrease. The altered breakdown of cellular protein may have important consequences for the cell life cycle and may be a major feature of the aging process.

Pathophysiology of the Aging Liver

OVERVIEW

1. Serum levels of routine liver biochemical tests, such as albumin, aminotransferases, and bilirubin, do not change significantly as persons age.
2. Age-related changes include decreases in liver weight, hepatic blood flow, metabolism of drugs, responsiveness to hormonal and growth factors, and delayed regeneration.

CHANGES IN DRUG METABOLISM

1. **The systemic clearance of many drugs that are metabolized by the hepatic cytochrome P-450 (CYP) system (e.g., midazolam, phenytoin, propranolol, acetaminophen) is decreased in older adults.** However, the enzymatic activities of CYP3A and CYP2E1 do not change with aging; this finding suggests that older persons may be just as susceptible as younger persons to DILI, caused by agents such as acetaminophen and ethanol.
2. Other mechanisms must be present to explain the reduced hepatic clearance of the previously mentioned drugs. **A 40% decrease in hepatic volume and a 50% reduction in liver blood flow in older persons** account for the reduction in systemic clearance of drugs, such as propranolol, that have a high first-pass hepatic uptake. The decrease in liver volume is most likely responsible for impaired clearance of medications that do not undergo significant first-pass hepatic uptake.

3. The volume of distribution of water-soluble drugs is generally reduced in older adults because of an increase in the ratio of body fat to body water. Although the metabolism of ethanol is essentially unaltered by aging, elevated blood ethanol levels can be observed in elderly subjects after the acute intake of ethanol as a result of a reduction in the volume of distribution.

4. The age-related reduction in hepatic blood results mostly from a decrease in portal blood flow. Sensitive Doppler techniques have shown that portal blood flow decreases from 740 ± 150 mL/min in persons <40 years of age to 595 ± 106 mL/min in healthy persons who are >71 years of age. The reduction in portal vein blood flow may relate to atherosclerosis, with a resulting decrease in mesenteric arterial blood flow.

ALTERATIONS IN CHOLESTEROL METABOLISM

1. The cholesterol content of bile increases with advancing age, as does the lithogenic index, because of the combination of increased hepatic secretion of cholesterol and decreased bile acid production. The elderly gallbladder also may be less responsive to endogenous cholecystokinin (CCK), with a resulting decrease in postprandial contraction of the gallbladder. Supersaturated bile is four times as frequent in elderly women as in younger women.

2. The frequency of gallstones increases with age. Approximately 40% to 60% of persons in their eighth decade of life have gallstones. Complications of gallstone disease are more severe in older adults.

Hepatic Diseases in Older Adults

ACUTE VIRAL HEPATITIS (see Chapters 3–6)

In older adults, the course of acute viral hepatitis may be more prolonged, severe, and indolent than in younger patients, probably because of an increased likelihood of comorbid conditions, an aged-related decline in immune function, and the decreased regenerative ability of the aging liver.

1. **Hepatitis A**
   - Hepatitis A is relatively uncommon in older adults because of a high rate of preexisting immunity. However, increasing proportions of older persons in Western countries are not immune to hepatitis A (e.g., 30% in the U.S. population who are >50 years of age).
   - Acute hepatitis A in older patients is associated with high hospitalization and complication rates, severe hepatocellular dysfunction, coagulopathy, and a mortality rate of 4% (nearly 10 times that of young patients).
   - Older persons who plan to travel to areas where hepatitis A is endemic should be tested for antibody to hepatitis A virus. If seronegative, they should receive the first dose of the hepatitis A virus vaccine at least 4 weeks before travel; other indications for hepatitis A vaccination, as recommended by the Advisory Committee on Immunizations Practices, apply to older persons as well.

2. **Hepatitis B**
   - Acute hepatitis B is less common in older persons than in younger persons.
   - The presentation is generally more cholestatic in older adults, with less hepatocellular necrosis. However, patients are frequently symptomatic and sicker and have a longer recovery time.
   - Although the clearance of the hepatitis B surface antigen (HBsAg) takes somewhat longer in older than younger persons, the overall prognosis is similar in the two groups; however, older adults are more likely to remain chronically infected with hepatitis B virus (HBV).

- The prevalence rates of hepatitis B e antigen (HBeAg) and antibody to HBeAg (anti-HBe) are inversely related to a patient's age during the natural history of chronic HBV infection.
- Older adults do not respond as well as younger persons to hepatitis B vaccination, probably because of a decrease in the number of antibody-producing B cells. Higher vaccine doses or booster immunization may be necessary for successful hepatitis B vaccination of older persons.

3. **Hepatitis C**
   - The incidence of acute HCV is lower in older adults than in young persons.
   - As with acute hepatitis A and B viral infections, a cholestatic component may be prominent in older persons with acute HCV infection.
   - The probability of progression to chronicity is related to age at initial infection with HCV.

4. **Hepatitis E**
   - The majority of patients with acute HEV infection are >60 years of age. In the United States, 3% of patients with acute liver injury suspected to be DILI are actually found to be positive for immunoglobulin M antibody to HEV.

5. Other causes of hepatitis
   - In immunosuppressed and debilitated patients with hepatitis, the possibilities of herpesvirus or cytomegalovirus infection should be considered and appropriately investigated.
   - In the older person who presents with apparent acute viral hepatitis, the differential diagnosis should include ischemic (hypoxic) hepatitis, sepsis, hepatic metastases, drug-induced hepatitis, sporadic acute hepatitis E, and obstructive jaundice (see Chapter 1).
   - Conversely, older patients with jaundice and elevated liver enzyme levels presumed to result from extrahepatic biliary obstruction require evaluation for acute viral hepatitis.

CHRONIC VIRAL HEPATITIS (see Chapters 4 and 5)

1. **Chronic hepatitis B**
   - The clinical presentation of chronic hepatitis B in older persons is generally similar to that of younger patients. However, many older patients with chronic hepatitis B are HBeAg negative and have lower levels of serum HBV DNA compared with younger patients—findings that indicate a lesser degree of viral replication and infectivity. This serologic profile generally indicates a long duration of the disease and is termed the *low replicative state.*
   - Persons in a low replication state generally do not require antiviral therapy unless they have cirrhosis. Older patients may progress to cirrhosis at an annual rate of 4%.
   - The main antiviral agents for treatment of chronic HBV infection include entecavir, tenofovir, and peginterferon alpha-2a; lamivudine, adefovir, and telbivudine are no longer considered first-line agents. Treatment with tenofovir and entecavir have been showed to be equally effective in younger and older persons.
   - The dose of entecavir, tenofovir, and other nucleoside or nucleotide analogues must be reduced when the creatinine clearance is <50 mL/min, as occurs frequently in older patients.
   - Advanced age is associated with an increased risk of HCC and requires vigilant surveillance in older patients.

2. **Chronic hepatitis C**
   - The clinical presentation of chronic hepatitis C is similar in both young and older patients.
     a. The majority (about 70%) of patients with chronic HCV infection are part of the baby boom generation (persons born within the years 1945 and 1965).
     b. The high frequency of chronic HCV infection in this cohort is the basis for the recommendation by the Centers for Disease Control and Prevention and U.S. Public Health Service to test for HCV all persons born in those years.

> **BOX 26.2 ■ Examples of Therapeutic Agents for Which the Risk of Hepatotoxicity Increases With Age**
>
> Dantrolene
> Floxacillin
> Halothane
> Isoniazid
> Methyldopa
> Sulindac
>
> ---
>
> Adapted from Dice JF. Aging and the uncertain role of sirtuins. In: Arias IM, Wolkoff A, Boyer J, et al, eds. *The Liver: Biology and Pathobiology,* Singapore: Wiley-Blackwell; 2009:955–960.

    c. Normal serum alanine aminotransferase (ALT) levels are observed more often in older than in younger chronically HCV-infected persons.

    d. Spontaneous clearance of newly acquired HCV infection is less likely in older than younger patients.

    e. Therapy with the direct-acting antiviral agents (DAAs) is equally efficacious in older as in younger patients.

    f. Older age at infection is associated with progression of hepatic fibrosis and increasing risk of HCC.

3. An important complication of chronic hepatitis B and C is the development of HCC. **Because the development of HCC correlates with the duration of chronic hepatitis, older patients with cirrhosis resulting from chronic hepatitis B or C should be screened twice yearly with ultrasonography of the liver and serum alpha fetoprotein testing** (see Chapters 11 and 29).

DRUG-INDUCED LIVER INJURY (see Chapter 10)

1. **The risk of DILI increases with advancing age.** Approximately 20% of cases of jaundice in older adults are secondary to medications and supplements, compared with 2% to 5% of patients of all ages who require hospitalization for jaundice.

2. Increased drug toxicity is caused by altered volumes of distribution, decreased clearance secondary to reduced hepatic blood flow and volume, depressed enzyme systems (in particular CYPs), decreased hepatic response to injury, decreased hepatic regeneration, and decreased renal clearance.

3. Older persons are more likely to be taking multiple medications. A 3-fold higher frequency of adverse drug reactions has been reported in patients taking six medications compared with those taking a single agent. Such polypharmacy increases the chance that CYP activity will increase or decrease, thereby leading to drug-drug interactions and associated toxicity.

4. **Drug-induced hepatotoxicity should be a major diagnostic consideration in older adults who present with elevated serum liver enzyme levels or jaundice.** The most common classes of drugs that cause toxicity in older persons include antibiotics (e.g., amoxicillin-clavulanic acid), cardiovascular drugs (e.g., amiodarone), and analgesics/antipyretics (e.g., acetaminophen). Box 26.2 lists examples of drugs for which hepatotoxicity increases with age.

5. All unnecessary medications should be discontinued in older persons. If hepatoxicity is suspected, a drug in a different class must be substituted for an essential agent.

NONALCOHOLIC FATTY LIVER DISEASE AND NONALCOHOLIC STEATOHEPATITIS (see Chapter 9)

1. Nonalcoholic fatty liver disease (NAFLD) is present in 20% to 30% of the general population. The prevalence of NAFLD and its progressive variant (nonalcoholic steatohepatitis [NASH]) is higher in the older population, in whom the frequency of NASH-related hepatic fibrosis is also increased.

2. The prevalence of metabolic syndrome, which includes insulin resistance, obesity, diabetes mellitus, hypertriglyceridemia, and hypertension, increases with age and is almost universally present in persons with NAFLD.
3. Bariatric surgery may be a therapeutic option in morbidly obese older patients with NASH in whom cirrhosis has not yet occurred.
4. HCC may develop in occasional patients with NASH in the absence of cirrhosis.

AUTOIMMUNE LIVER DISEASES

1. **Autoimmune hepatitis** (see Chapter 7)
   - **17% to 56% of patients present after age 65;** the male to female ratio in this group is 1 to 9.
   - Older patients commonly present with jaundice, fatigue, or drowsiness and are more likely than younger patients to present with ascites.
   - The management strategy is identical in all adults but, in older persons, is associated with lower failure rates for therapy and need for LT. However, older patients are at higher risk of treatment-related complications such as osteoporosis, compression fractures, glaucoma, arterial hypertension, and obesity.
2. **Primary biliary cholangitis** (PBC; formerly known as primary biliary cirrhosis) (see Chapter 16)
   - PBC affects middle-aged women primarily, but up to 50% of patients in some populations present for the first time after age 65.
   - The most common phenotypic expression of PBC in older persons is the asymptomatic variant, with no or few symptoms (pruritus, weight loss, fatigue) compared with patients who are <65 years of age.
   - An increasing number of patients with PBC have been on therapy with ursodeoxycholic acid for >20 years and are now considered older adults.
   - In the registration trials for obeticholic acid (approved for use in PBC in 2016), nearly 1 in 4 enrolled patients were >65 years of age.
   - It is particularly important to screen older patients for decreased bone density and to treat those with low density appropriately.
3. **Primary sclerosing cholangitis** (see Chapter 17)
   - This usually occurs in the third or fourth decade; therefore, the diagnosis is unusual in an elderly patient. Increased age is an independent risk factor for a poor outcome.
   - In elderly patients presenting with cholestatic jaundice and a cholangiogram suggestive of primary sclerosing cholangitis, carcinoma of the biliary tract should be excluded (see Chapter 36).

ALCOHOLIC LIVER DISEASE (see Chapter 8)

1. **A substantial proportion of patients with alcoholic liver disease present at or beyond the fifth and sixth decades of life.**
2. An age-related decrease in ethanol metabolism leads to increased acetaldehyde levels in the liver, which underlies the steatosis that occurs in the older liver in which mitochondrial fatty acid oxidation is decreased.
3. Older patients are more likely than younger patients to have histologically advanced liver disease and exhibit the classic signs of hepatic decompensation: Ascites, jaundice, and lower extremity edema.
4. Overall mortality from alcoholic liver disease is higher in patients who are >60 years of age: 34% at 1 year, compared with 5% in younger patients. In patients >70 years of age, the 1-year mortality rate increases dramatically to 75%.

METABOLIC LIVER DISEASES

1. **Hereditary hemochromatosis** (HH) (see Chapter 18)
   - Most persons with HH present by middle age, but some present at an advanced age with HCC or other complications of end-stage liver disease.
   - Men with the *HFE* gene mutation C282Y may live long lives without biochemical or histologic abnormalities; only a minority of C282Y homozygous persons phenotypically express HH.
   - Female patients typically become symptomatic approximately 10 years after their male counterparts, because of the iron-depleting effects of regular menses and childbirth.
   - Common symptoms may include fatigue, diabetes mellitus, impotence, and arthritis, all of which are common in the older population. HH should also be considered in an older person presenting with a neurologic disorder, because iron overload can manifest as a cerebellar syndrome.
   - A major cause of death in patients with cirrhosis due to HH is HCC; screening with ultrasonography and serum alpha fetoprotein testing should be performed every 6 months (see Chapter 29).
   - Older patients may not tolerate intensive phlebotomy therapy and may require less frequent phlebotomies of smaller volumes than younger patients.
2. **Alpha-1 antitrypsin deficiency (α-1 ATD)** (see Chapter 20)
   - Patients with homozygous α-1 ATD usually present before age 65.
   - Heterozygous α-1 ATD has been thought to be the cause of cirrhosis in approximately 5% of patients with cirrhosis >65 years of age; however, heterozygous α-1 ATD is frequent in the overall population. No evidence indicates that intracellular α-1 ATD globular inclusions are hepatotoxic in heterozygotes.
   - Although no specific effective treatment for α-1 ATD–related liver disease exists, diagnosis is important so that heterozygous or affected family members can be advised to avoid behaviors, such as alcohol intake, smoking, and intravenous drug use, that may jeopardize their hepatic and pulmonary function.
3. **Wilson disease** (see Chapter 19): De novo diagnosis of Wilson disease is rare in older persons, although reports exist of patients with Wilson disease who have been diagnosed after age 70.

LIVER ABSCESS (see Chapter 30)

1. Most patients with a pyogenic liver abscess in the Northern Hemisphere are >60 years of age, with a reported mean age of 47 to 65 years of age.
2. The diagnosis is more difficult to make in older than in younger persons, because the typical presentation of fever, jaundice, and right upper quadrant pain may be absent. Older patients are more likely to have nonspecific symptoms, such as epigastric pain, weakness, fatigue, and shortness of breath.
3. Although the source of approximately one half of hepatic abscesses is the biliary tract (most often as a result of ascending cholangitis), other intraabdominal and gastrointestinal sources should be investigated, including the following:
   - Penetrating gastric or duodenal ulcers
   - Pancreatitis
   - Perihepatic abscess
   - Portal vein thrombosis
   - Peritonitis (of any cause)
   - Inflammatory bowel disease
   - Colon cancer

TABLE 26.1 ■ **Management of Biliary Disease in Older Patients**

Condition	Treatment
Acute or chronic cholecystitis	Early cholecystectomy (preferably laparoscopic); if cholecystectomy is not possible, a percutaneous cholecystostomy tube should be placed, followed by cholecystectomy when possible
Cholangitis with choledocholithiasis	ERCP with sphincterotomy and stone extraction
Choledocholithiasis with gallstones in the gallbladder	ERCP with sphincterotomy; if symptoms persist, cholecystectomy or percutaneous cholecystostomy with laparoscopic bile duct exploration should be performed
Asymptomatic gallstones	Observation generally preferred over prophylactic intervention

ERCP, Endoscopic retrograde cholangiopancreatography.

- Diverticulitis or diverticular abscess
- Cryptogenic conditions (in some cases resulting from poor dentition)
4. Older patients are more likely to have gallstone-related disease or a malignant tumor and more often have polymicrobial infection than younger patients.
5. **Almost one third of older persons with a hepatic abscess at autopsy may be misdiagnosed in life as having a hepatic malignant disease.** A diagnosis of tumor should be confirmed by needle biopsy, especially if an alternative primary site of malignancy is not identified.
6. As in younger persons, pyogenic abscesses can be treated successfully by percutaneous aspiration and drainage in conjunction with systemic intravenous antibiotics.

GALLSTONES AND BILIARY DISEASE (see Chapter 34)

1. **Gallstones** are an age-related phenomenon. The mortality of untreated biliary tract disease also increases with age. Cancer of the gallbladder is more likely to occur in older persons than in younger persons (see Chapter 36).
   - Age-related changes including increased lithogenicity of bile, deconjugation of bile pigments, increased bactobilia, and altered gallbladder motility all may contribute to increased gallstone formation.
   - The frequency of bile duct stones reaches 50% in patients with cholelithiasis who are >80 years of age.
2. The management of **biliary disease** with respect to age is summarized in Table 26.1.
   - With the advent of laparoscopic cholecystectomy, early operative intervention has brought the mortality and morbidity rates for younger and older patients closer together.
   - Morbidity and mortality rates for endoscopic retrograde cholangiopancreatography (ERCP) with sphincterotomy do not differ significantly between older and younger persons, despite a longer duration of hospitalization in older patients.
   - Incidental appendectomy during cholecystectomy should not be performed in older patients because of the risk of wound infection and the relatively low lifetime risk of acute appendicitis.

HEPATIC TUMORS (see Chapter 29)

1. HCC
   - Older patients with cirrhosis are at increased risk of HCC; a clear association exists between the development of HCC and the duration of cirrhosis. In the Western world, 50% of patients with cirrhosis in whom HCC develops are >60 years of age and 40% are >70 years of age.

TABLE 26.2 ■ **Survival Rates in Acute Liver Failure**

	Age <60 yr (%)	Age ≥60 yr (%)
Acetaminophen Related		
Native liver	65	60
Liver graft	83	NA
Overall	73	60
Nonacetaminophen Related		
Native liver	31	25
Liver graft	91	80
Overall	68	48

Adapted from Schiødt FV, Chung RT, Schilsky ML, et al. Acute liver failure in the elderly. *Liver Transplant.* 2009;15: 1481–1487.

- Because of its long natural history, HCV-related cirrhosis is the leading cause of HCC in the elderly (with a frequency of 5% per year). Increasingly, NAFLD has been found to be a cause of HCC in the elderly, including, in some cases, those without cirrhosis.
- Screening for HCC should be performed as described previously; early detection of small HCCs may allow the use of curative therapies (resection, transplantation) and prolong survival.
- Nonsurgical treatments of HCC in the elderly include radiofrequency ablation, transcatheter arterial chemoembolization (TACE), yttrium-90 radioembolization, and microwave ablation, with outcomes similar to those in younger patients. For unresectable late-stage HCC, chemotherapy with sorafenib prolongs survival.
- Hepatic resection for HCC can be done safely in well-compensated cirrhotic patients ≥70 years of age with mild or no portal hypertension, depending on the location and size of the tumor (see Chapter 32). The overall prognosis, however, is worse than for patients <70 years of age, even when curative resection is achieved.
- Older age correlates with recurrence of HCC and worse outcomes.
- LT may be a treatment option in select older patients (see discussion later in chapter).
2. Metastatic tumors
- Metastasis is the most common malignant tumor found in the liver in older persons.
- The frequency of hepatic metastases is greatest for tumors of the colon, pancreas, and stomach arising within the drainage area of the portal vein, but other tumors, such as lung and breast cancer, can also metastasize to the liver.
- Survival is directly correlated with the extent of hepatic involvement.
- Therapy may prolong survival; 20% of patients who undergo surgical resection of a solitary hepatic metastasis may be alive 5 years after resection.

ACUTE LIVER FAILURE (see Chapter 2)

1. **Regardless of the cause, acute liver failure (ALF) has a higher mortality rate in older persons than in the young** (Table 26.2).
2. ALF resulting from hepatitis A is particularly devastating in older adults, with a mortality rate much higher than that in young persons (see earlier discussion).
3. Age >40 years is a negative prognostic indicator for non–acetaminophen-induced ALF.
4. **The best treatment for ALF in older persons is to prevent its occurrence,** as follows:

- Vaccination against HAV and HBV should be considered in all susceptible older persons.
- Isoniazid and other drugs with high hepatotoxicity potential should not be used in older adults unless absolutely necessary.
- Unintentional overdose of acetaminophen should be avoided by carefully reviewing an older patient's medication list (including use of supplements) at each office visit.
- Periodic monitoring of liver enzyme levels should be performed in older patients who require treatment with medications known to have hepatotoxic potential.

PORTAL HYPERTENSION (see Chapter 12)

1. Older adults admitted to the hospital with bleeding esophageal varices have short-term mortality rates similar to those of younger patients; however, their 1-year survival rate is less than that of their younger counterparts.
2. Continuous infusion of octreotide is preferable to vasopressin or terlipressin in the medical treatment of bleeding varices in older persons.
3. Variceal band ligation and beta receptor antagonist blocker therapy can be used to prevent recurrent variceal bleeding. Some older patients may be unable to tolerate the adverse effects (e.g., fatigue, dizziness, depression) of beta blockers.
4. A transjugular intrahepatic portosystemic shunt (TIPS) or portacaval shunt can be used to treat recurrent variceal bleeding; however, the usefulness of a shunt is limited by the relatively high frequency of postshunt hepatic encephalopathy.
    - A small-caliber stent of 7 to 8 mm should be used in patients who are >60 years of age, to decrease the risk of hepatic encephalopathy.
    - Lowering the hepatic venous pressure gradient to just below 12 mm Hg may also minimize the risk of post-TIPS hepatic encephalopathy in older cirrhotic patients.
5. Older patients with refractory ascites or recurrent variceal bleeding, who are otherwise in good physiologic condition, should be considered for LT evaluation (see discussion later in chapter).

LIVER TRANSPLANTATION (see Chapter 33)

1. Advanced age is not a contraindication to LT. Some studies, but not all, have shown that in patients >60 years of age, 10-year survival after LT is comparable to that for younger patients. In 1999, 16% of liver transplant recipients in Europe were >60 years of age, and in 2000, >10.7% of liver transplant recipients in the United States were >65 years of age. **The decision to proceed with LT should be based on the overall health of the patient, not on chronologic age.**
2. Factors contributing to worse mortality in older patients include pre-LT hospitalization and a higher Model for End-stage Liver Disease (MELD) score (see Chapter 33). The most common causes of death in long-term liver transplant recipients ≥60 years of age are cardiovascular events, whereas for those <60 years of age, it is infection.
3. Donor livers from persons >60 years of age can be used safely. The increasing demand for donor livers has led to the more frequent use of livers from older donors.
    - Several groups have reported that patient and graft outcomes are identical regardless of the age of the donor liver. Older livers often have more steatosis and fall within the categories of marginal or extended donors. Nevertheless, they can be offered to waitlisted patients with lower MELD scores but a high need for LT.
    - The function of an older liver may be slightly worse in the early postoperative period, as evidenced by higher peak serum ALT and bilirubin levels and slightly lower bile outputs.

4. A significant increase in the frequency of delayed function is observed in livers from donors who are >50 years of age compared with donors who are <30 years of age. Recipients who experience delayed function are three times as likely to require repeat LT. Early recognition of delayed function and subsequent repeat LT lead to similar 1-year patient survival rates in both groups.

5. In general, livers from donors >65 years of age are offered preferentially to patients who have HCC or have a high MELD score. The graft ischemic time should be kept to a minimum when an older donor liver is used, to lessen preservation injury and postoperative hepatic graft dysfunction.

6. The fact that livers from older donors are able to withstand the often extreme physiologic conditions imposed by LT (harvesting, implantation, reperfusion, rejection, toxic effects of drugs, infection) and ultimately provide excellent function is a clear demonstration that the human liver is highly resilient to the aging process.

7. LT using older liver donors can now be performed successfully in patients with HCV infection due to the availability of multiple DAAs, with safe cure of the HCV infection in the liver allograft in the majority of recipients.

8. Livers from HCV-infected donors are increasingly being used for patients with HCC or high MELD score, due also to the easy cure of HCV after LT with DAA-based antiviral regimens.

FURTHER READING

Bertolotti M, Lonardo A, Mussi C, et al. Nonalcoholic fatty liver disease and aging: epidemiology to management. *World J Gastroenterol*. 2014;20:14185–14204.

Carrion A, Martin P. Viral hepatitis in the elderly. *Am J Gastroenterol*. 2012;107:691–697.

Czaja AJ. Clinical features, differential diagnosis and treatment of autoimmune hepatitis in the elderly. *Drugs Aging*. 2008;25:219–239.

Frith J, Jones D, Newton JL. Chronic liver disease in an ageing population. *Age Ageing*. 2009;38:11–18.

Junaidi O, Di Bisceglie AM. Aging liver and hepatitis. *Clin Geriatr Med*. 2007;23:889–903.

Kim I, Kisseleva T, Brenner D. Aging and liver disease. *Curr Opin Gastroenterol*. 2015;31:184–191.

Koehler E, Sanna D, Hansen B. Serum liver enzymes are associated with all-cause mortality in an elderly population. *Liver Int*. 2013;34:296–304.

Mindikoglu AL, Miller RR. Hepatitis C in the elderly: epidemiology, natural history, and treatment. *Clin Gastroenterol Hepatol*. 2009;7:128–134.

Oishi K, Itamoto T, Kobayashi T, et al. Hepatectomy for hepatocellular carcinoma in elderly patients aged 75 years or more. *J Gastrointest Surg*. 2009;13:695–701.

Onji M, Fujioka S, Takeuchi Y, et al. Clinical characteristics of drug-induced liver injury in the elderly. *Hepatol Res*. 2009;39:546–552.

Saab S, Rheem J, Sundaram V. Hepatitis C infection in the elderly. *Dig Dis Sci*. 2015;60:3170–3180.

Saneto H, Kobayashi M, Kawamura Y, et al. Clinicopathological features, background liver disease, and survival analysis of HCV-positive patients with hepatocellular carcinoma: differences between young and elderly patients. *J Gastroenterol*. 2008;43:975–981.

Seitz HK, Stickel F. Alcoholic liver disease in the elderly. *Clin Geriatr Med*. 2007;23:905–921.

Sheedfar F, Di Biase S, Koonen D, et al. Liver diseases and aging: friends or foes? *Aging Cell*. 2013;12:950–954.

Tajiri K, Shimizu Y. Liver physiology and liver diseases in the elderly. *World J Gastroenterol*. 2013;19:8459–8467.

CHAPTER 27

Hepatobiliary Complications of HIV

Vincent Lo Re III, MD, MSCE ■ K. Rajender Reddy, MD, FACP

KEY POINTS

1 Approximately 10% of human immunodeficiency virus (HIV)–infected persons worldwide are chronically infected with hepatitis B virus. The choice of antiviral therapy depends on the need for HIV treatment.

2 Approximately 30% of HIV-infected persons are chronically coinfected with hepatitis C virus (HCV). Antiretroviral therapy may improve hepatic outcomes and survival among coinfected patients. Direct-acting antiviral agents (DAAs) have revolutionized HCV therapy to the extent that HIV-coinfected patients are no longer considered to be a "special" population.

3 The pathogenesis of liver disease in HIV-infected persons with HCV infection includes dysregulation of T cells, increased replication of HCV, intestinal villous effacement, and CD4+ cell depletion, which in turn leads to increased intestinal microbial product translocation into the portal venous system. The liver is then exposed to lipopolysaccharide (LPS), which binds to Kupffer cells and interacts with LPS-binding protein, and other cytokines leading to upregulation of proinflammatory and profibrogenic cytokines and thereby cause liver disease. In addition, there is accelerated hepatocyte apoptosis, which leads to more inflammation and fibrosis. Furthermore, an increase in steatohepatitis and direct infection of hepatic stellate cells promote inflammation and hepatic fibrosis.

4 Infiltrative infections (mainly disseminated bacterial and fungal processes) may lead to hepatocellular necrosis or granulomatous inflammation in HIV-infected patients with advanced immunosuppression. *Mycobacterium avium* complex (MAC) infection is most common.

5 Macrovesicular hepatic steatosis is identified in 40% to 69% of liver biopsy specimens in patients coinfected with HIV and HCV, and steatosis is associated with more advanced hepatic fibrosis.

6 Virtually every antiretroviral medication has been associated with hepatotoxicity. In the setting of suspected hepatotoxicity, discontinuation of antiretroviral therapy (ART) should be considered if (1) serum aminotransferase levels exceed 10 times the upper limit of normal, (2) overt jaundice is identified, (3) symptomatic hepatitis develops, or (4) findings consistent with drug hypersensitivity (e.g., rash, fever, eosinophilia) are observed.

7 Acquired immunodeficiency syndrome (AIDS) cholangiopathy is a syndrome of biliary obstruction resulting from infection-associated strictures of the biliary tract, typically seen in patients with a CD4+ cell count <100/mm³. *Cryptosporidium parvum* is the most commonly associated pathogen.

Viral Hepatitis and Other Viral Infections

HEPATITIS A VIRUS (see Chapter 3)

1. The seroprevalence of antibody to hepatitis A virus (HAV) is high among HIV-infected persons, with a range of 40% to 70%.
2. The annual cumulative frequency of HAV infection is reported to be 5.8% per year among HIV-positive persons.
3. HAV viremia is prolonged in HIV-infected persons, and the level of HAV viremia is higher compared with those without HIV infection, even with relatively high CD4+ T lymphocyte counts.
4. No evidence indicates that ART has a detrimental effect on the course of HAV infection.
5. **Hepatitis A vaccination is recommended for all HIV-positive/HAV-seronegative persons,** with standard doses given 6 to 12 months apart. Immune response is excellent (overall response rate, 78% to 94%), even in persons with CD4+ cell counts <200/mm^3 (response rate 64%).

HEPATITIS B AND D VIRUSES (see Chapter 4)

1. **Worldwide, 10% of HIV-infected persons are chronically infected with hepatitis B virus (HBV).**
2. HIV adversely affects the natural history of HBV infection. Compared with those infected with HBV alone, HIV-coinfected persons have a higher rate of progression from acute to chronic HBV infection, higher serum HBV DNA levels, lower rates of spontaneous hepatitis B e antigen (HBeAg) to antibody to HBeAg (anti-HBe) seroconversion, increased frequency of reactivation episodes, faster progression to hepatic cirrhosis, and earlier development of, and more aggressive, hepatocellular carcinoma (HCC).
3. HIV coinfection may accelerate progression of hepatitis D virus (HDV)–associated liver disease.
4. All HIV/HBV-coinfected patients with active HBV replication should be considered for HBV antiviral therapy, which can potentially prevent the development of liver-related complications and reduce HBV transmission.
5. The goals of HBV treatment in HIV-infected persons are suppression of HBV DNA to an undetectable level (as for persons without HIV infection), return of serum aminotransferase levels to normal, HBeAg seroconversion (not applicable to HBeAg-negative chronic hepatitis B), and improvement in liver histology.
6. Several antiviral medications have been approved in the United States for chronic HBV treatment, and some of these have also been approved for HIV treatment (Box 27.1).

BOX 27.1 ■ Antiviral Medications for Chronic Hepatitis B

Interferon alfa
Peginterferon alfa
Lamivudine[a]
Adefovir
Entecavir
Telbivudine
Tenofovir disoproxil fumarate[a,b]
Tenofovir alafenamide[a,b]
Emtricitabine[a]

---

[a]Also approved to treat HIV infection.
[b]Tenofovir is also available in combination with emtricitabine (Truvada).

7. **Combination oral nucleoside or nucleotide therapy (tenofovir disoproxil fumarate 300 mg daily or tenofovir alafenamide 25 mg daily plus either emtricitabine 200 mg daily or lamivudine 300 mg daily) is the regimen of choice.** The preferred form of tenofovir is tenofovir alafenamide, which is not known to have the renal toxicity or decrease in bone mineral density associated with tenofovir. Because replication of both viruses depends on reverse transcription, dual HIV/HBV therapy can include the same reverse transcriptase-inhibiting agents to treat both viruses.

8. In the absence of ART, entecavir can reduce HIV RNA levels and select for HIV-resistance mutations; therefore, it should not be used in an HIV-infected person without ART.
   - Telbivudine does not have intrinsic activity against HIV in vitro, but it has been associated with declines in HIV RNA levels and can select for lamivudine-resistance mutations. It is not a recommended treatment for the HIV/HBV-coinfected patient.

9. Frequent toxicities and low rates of therapeutic success have limited peginterferon alfa-2a use as HBV therapy in HIV-infected persons.

10. Because lamivudine resistance occurs at a rate of 15% to 25% per year, lamivudine resistance may be present in HIV-infected patients who previously received lamivudine as part of an ART regimen. Tenofovir remains active in patients with lamivudine-resistant HBV infection and can suppress HBV DNA to undetectable levels, because of the potency of tenofovir and the lack of cross-resistance between lamivudine and tenofovir.

11. For patients receiving combination tenofovir plus emtricitabine (or lamivudine) who fail to suppress HBV DNA by 96 weeks, entecavir 1 mg daily may be added.

12. Because HCC can occur at any stage of chronic HBV infection, screening with abdominal ultrasonography and alpha fetoprotein testing is recommended every 6 to 12 months (see Chapter 29).

13. HBV vaccination is recommended in all HIV-positive hepatitis B surface antibody (anti-HBs)–negative persons. The presence in serum of isolated hepatitis B core antibody (anti-HBc) with no other HBV markers most likely reflects previous exposure and recovery, rather than a false-positive result, but not necessarily.

14. Anti-HBs titers should be assessed after HBV vaccination in HIV-infected persons. Immune reactivity to the HBV vaccine is frequently suboptimal in these persons in terms of rate of response, antibody titers, and durability. A CD4+ cell count >500/mm^3 and an HIV viral load <1000 copies/mL promote optimal vaccine responses. Revaccination should be instituted if the anti-HBs titer is <10 mIU/mL.

HEPATITIS C VIRUS (see Chapter 5)

1. **30% of HIV-infected persons are chronically coinfected with HCV.**

2. The natural history of HCV infection is adversely influenced by HIV coinfection. Compared with persons infected with HCV alone, HIV-coinfected persons more commonly progress to chronic HCV infection; have higher HCV RNA levels; are at higher risk of cirrhosis, hepatic decompensation, and liver-related death; and have a shorter survival once end-stage liver disease develops.

3. **HCV-related liver disease is now a leading cause of death in the HIV-infected population.**

4. HIV/HCV coinfection increases the risk of HCC compared with HIV monoinfection but not with HCV monoinfection.

5. Available data suggest that ART favorably affects the course of HIV disease in HIV-infected patients, decreases mortality from liver disease, and should not be withheld from HIV/HCV-coinfected persons on account of potential toxicity.

6. The stage of hepatic fibrosis can help guide HCV treatment decisions in HIV/HCV patients. The incidence rate of hepatic decompensation events or death is higher in coinfected patients with more advanced fibrosis at the time of staging.

7. The timing of HCV therapy depends on the need for HIV treatment. HCV treatment should be considered first if liver disease is advanced and HIV infection is at an early stage. If HIV infection requires treatment, ART should be initiated first, and once the HIV infection is controlled, HCV therapy can be considered.

8. Given accelerated progression to end-stage liver disease among HIV/HCV-infected patients, **treatment of chronic HCV infection should be considered in all coinfected patients who do not have decompensated cirrhosis or other contraindications.** DAAs are currently the standard of care. Options include PRoD (paritaprevir [that is ritonavir-boosted], ombitasvir, and dasabuvir); ledipasvir and sofosbuvir; daclatasvir and sofosbuvir ± ribavirin; grazoprevir and elbasvir plus ribavirin; and velpatasvir and sofosbuvir. The main goals of treatment are viral eradication (i.e., sustained virologic response) and reduction in the risk of liver-related complications.

9. Drug-drug interaction is common in persons on DAAs. Therefore careful attention to drug-drug interactions is necessary before consideration of HCV therapy in persons with HCV/HIV coinfection (see Chapter 10).

OTHER VIRUSES (see Chapters 3 and 6)

1. **Acute infection with HIV** may manifest with hepatitis as part of a mononucleosis-like illness with fever, malaise, and myalgia; hepatosplenomegaly on physical examination; and elevations of serum aminotransferase and alkaline phosphatase (ALP) levels. This presentation is referred to as the **acute retroviral syndrome.**

2. Several other common viral infections can secondarily affect the liver and cause acute hepatitis. **Adenovirus, Epstein-Barr virus, cytomegalovirus, herpes simplex virus, and varicella-zoster virus** are rare causes of acute viral hepatitis in HIV-infected persons.

3. **Hepatitis E virus** (HEV) infection has been described in HIV-infected persons. HEV genotype 3–related chronic infection can lead to cirrhosis. The seroprevalence of HEV antibodies in those with HIV infection ranges from 1.5% to 29%. HEV infection needs to be excluded in patients with an acute hepatitis-like illness. HEV infection may also mimic drug-induced liver injury.

Other Infections (see also Chapter 31 and Box 27.2)

DISSEMINATED *MYCOBACTERIUM AVIUM* COMPLEX INFECTION

1. The designation MAC refers to infections caused by one of two nontuberculous mycobacterial species, either *Mycobacterium avium* or *M. intracellulare.*

2. In patients with AIDS, MAC infection usually presents as disseminated disease and may involve the liver.

3. Symptoms of disseminated MAC infection include fever, night sweats, abdominal pain (especially right upper quadrant), diarrhea, and weight loss. Hepatosplenomegaly may be identified on physical examination.

4. Laboratory abnormalities frequently include anemia and elevated serum ALP and lactate dehydrogenase levels.

5. The diagnosis may be confirmed by the following:
   - Isolation of MAC from cultures of blood, lymph node, or bone marrow
   - Histopathologic findings on a liver biopsy specimen showing granulomas with positive acid-fast bacilli stains
   - Mycobacterial growth from culture of liver tissue obtained by biopsy

---

BOX 27.2 ■ Selected Causes of Liver Disease in HIV-Infected Patients

Infections

Bacteria

Mycobacterium avium complex
Mycobacterium tuberculosis
Bartonella henselae (peliosis hepatis)

Viruses

Hepatitis A virus
Hepatitis B virus
Hepatitis C virus
Hepatitis D virus (with hepatitis B)
Other: Adenovirus, Epstein-Barr virus, cytomegalovirus, human immunodeficiency virus, herpes simplex virus, varicella-zoster virus, hepatitis E virus

Fungi

Candida albicans
Coccidioides immitis
Cryptococcus neoformans
Histoplasma capsulatum
Penicillium marneffei
Pneumocystis jirovecii
Sporothrix schenckii

Protozoa

Microsporidia spp.
Schistosoma spp.
Toxoplasma gondii

Malignant Diseases

Lymphoma
Kaposi sarcoma
Hepatocellular carcinoma
Nonalcoholic fatty liver disease

Medications and Toxins

Acetaminophen
Alcohol
Antimicrobials: Macrolides, trimethoprim-sulfamethoxazole
Antituberculosis drugs: Isoniazid, rifampin
Nucleoside analogs: Didanosine, stavudine, zidovudine
Non-nucleoside reverse transcriptase inhibitors: Nevirapine

PELIOSIS HEPATIS

1. *Bartonella henselae* can cause peliosis hepatis, a vascular proliferative hepatic infection in HIV-infected persons with advanced immunosuppression characterized by multiple blood-filled cystic spaces.
2. Patients may report fever, abdominal pain, nausea, vomiting, anorexia, and weight loss. Hepatosplenomegaly may be detected on physical examination. Increased serum ALP levels and thrombocytopenia or pancytopenia may be identified.
3. Computed tomography (CT) typically shows hepatosplenomegaly and hypodense lesions scattered throughout the hepatic parenchyma.

4. Positive *Bartonella* serology can be used to support the diagnosis in the appropriate clinical setting, but the diagnosis is confirmed by isolation of *Bartonella* from cultures of blood or liver tissue or by Warthin-Starry staining of a biopsy specimen.
5. Oral erythromycin 500 mg four times daily or doxycycline 100 mg twice daily for 4 months is the recommended therapy for peliosis hepatitis. Oral azithromycin 500 mg daily or clarithromycin 500 mg twice daily for 4 months may be an option for patients who cannot tolerate erythromycin or doxycycline.

FUNGAL AND PROTOZOAL INFECTIONS

A number of fungi and protozoa may infiltrate the liver in patients with AIDS, usually as part of disseminated disease (see Box 27.2).

Malignant Diseases

LYMPHOMA (see also Chapter 24)

1. Non-Hodgkin lymphoma accounts for most systemic AIDS-related lymphomas, and the liver is involved in approximately one third of cases.
2. Hepatic involvement may be clinically silent or associated with pain and "B" symptoms, including fever, weight loss, and night sweats. Jaundice may occur with intrahepatic or extrahepatic bile duct obstruction.
3. Imaging usually reveals solitary or multiple hepatic lesions and involvement of abdominal lymph nodes.
4. The diagnosis can be established by biopsy of the hepatic lesions or an involved lymph node.

KAPOSI SARCOMA

1. This is observed predominantly in men who have sex with men.
2. Typically, it involves the liver in the setting of cutaneous disease. Abdominal pain, hepatomegaly, and elevations of serum ALP levels may be observed.
3. Abdominal ultrasonography may reveal nonspecific, small (5- to 12-mm) hyperechoic nodules. CT of the liver may show enhancing lesions in capsular, hilar, and portal areas with invasion into liver parenchyma.

HEPATOCELLULAR CARCINOMA (see also Chapter 29)

1. HCC is increasingly recognized in HIV-infected patients with cirrhosis.
2. It may occur in the setting of chronic HBV infection in the absence of cirrhosis.
3. Patients typically have evidence of advanced liver disease and may have an elevated serum alpha fetoprotein level and one or more liver masses on abdominal imaging studies.

Nonalcoholic Fatty Liver Disease (see Chapter 9)

1. Macrovesicular hepatic steatosis is a common histologic finding in patients coinfected with HIV and HCV and is identified in 40% to 69% of liver biopsy specimens.
2. Risk factors for hepatic steatosis among HIV/HCV-coinfected patients include white race, increased body mass index, hyperglycemia, use of dideoxynucleoside analogs (i.e., didanosine and stavudine), and lower plasma levels of high-density lipoprotein cholesterol.

3. Steatosis and steatohepatitis have been associated with more advanced HCV-related hepatic fibrosis in HIV-infected persons.
4. The frequency of hepatic steatosis among HIV/HBV-coinfected persons and HIV-monoinfected persons remains unclear.
5. Most patients are asymptomatic.
6. Hepatomegaly is a frequent finding.
7. Elevated serum aminotransferase or ALP levels may be identified. Evidence of fatty liver may be noted on abdominal ultrasonography or CT.

Antiretroviral-Induced Hepatotoxicity

1. **Virtually every ART has been associated with elevations in liver biochemical test levels** (see Box 27.2).
2. Four main mechanisms of ART-related hepatotoxicity occur in HIV-infected persons, as follows:
   - Mitochondrial toxicity
   - Hypersensitivity reactions involving the liver
   - Direct drug toxicity
   - Immune reconstitution following initiation of ART in the presence of hepatitis virus coinfection
3. No clinical finding is specific for ART-induced hepatotoxicity. Symptoms may be absent or may consist of abdominal discomfort, nausea, rash, anorexia, jaundice, or fever.
4. Hepatotoxicity is usually suggested by elevations in serum aminotransferase levels. Cholestasis is less frequent, and some cases are characterized by mixed hepatitis and cholestasis (Table 27.1).
5. Based on the AIDS Clinical Trial Group liver toxicity scale, severe hepatotoxicity is defined as either a grade 3 (5.1 to 10 times the upper limit of normal) or grade 4 (>10 times the upper limit of normal) change in serum aminotransferase levels during ART or a >3.5-fold increase in these levels above baseline if aminotransferase levels are elevated at the time ART is initiated.
6. HBV infection and HCV infection increase the risk of ART-associated hepatotoxicity, and the risk among HIV/HCV-coinfected patients with advanced fibrosis or cirrhosis is increased further. Eradication of HCV with antiviral therapy has been shown to improve tolerance to ART.
7. Patients with aminotransferase elevations before the initiation of ART have an increased risk of hepatotoxicity. Alcohol and cocaine use can exacerbate ART-induced hepatotoxicity.
8. In the setting of suspected hepatotoxicity, discontinuation of ART medications should be considered in the following circumstances:
   - Serum aminotransferase levels >10 times the upper limit of normal
   - Overt jaundice with elevated direct bilirubin levels
   - Symptomatic hepatitis (increased risk of severe liver injury)
   - Findings consistent with drug hypersensitivity (e.g., rash, fever, eosinophilia)
9. Hepatotoxicity may be caused by various non-ART drugs used in patients with HIV infection (see Table 27.1; see also Chapter 10).

AIDS-Related Biliary Tract Diseases

AIDS CHOLANGIOPATHY

1. This syndrome of biliary obstruction resulting from infection-associated strictures of the biliary tract is typically seen in patients with a CD4+ cell count <100/mm^3.
2. The incidence of AIDS cholangiopathy has declined substantially with the use of ART.

TABLE 27.1 ■ **Nonantiretroviral Therapy Drugs Related to Hepatotoxicity**

Drugs	Typical Pattern of Hepatotoxicity
Antituberculosis Therapy	
Isoniazid, rifampin, pyrazinamide Ethambutol	Hepatocellular and cholestatic
Antifungals	
Amphotericin B, fluconazole, ketoconazole	Hepatocellular
Antivirals	
Acyclovir, ganciclovir	Hepatocellular
Antibiotics	
Azithromycin	Cholestatic
Ciprofloxacin	Hepatocellular
Trimethoprim/sulfamethoxazole	Hepatocellular or cholestatic
Anabolic Steroids	
Nandrolone, testosterone	Cholestatic; also tumors, peliosis hepatis

3. *Cryptosporidium parvum* is the most common pathogen associated with AIDS cholangiopathy; MAC, cytomegalovirus, *Microsporidia* spp., and *Cyclospora cayetanensis* have also been identified. Noninfectious causes include lymphoma or Kaposi sarcoma infiltrating the biliary tract. No specific cause is found in 20% to 40% of cases.
4. This condition should be suspected in patients with advanced immunosuppression (CD4+ cell count <100/mm^3) who present with fever, right upper quadrant or epigastric abdominal pain, nausea, vomiting, diarrhea, jaundice, and hepatomegaly.
5. The severity of abdominal pain varies with the biliary tract lesion. Severe abdominal pain usually suggests papillary stenosis, whereas milder abdominal pain is often associated with intrahepatic and extrahepatic sclerosing cholangitis without papillary stenosis.
6. Serum aminotransferase, ALP, and total bilirubin levels are typically mildly elevated, but 20% of patients may have normal liver biochemical test levels.
7. Imaging may demonstrate intrahepatic or extrahepatic biliary tract dilatation or thickening of the bile duct.
8. Endoscopic retrograde cholangiopancreatography (ERCP) is the preferred approach because it may be diagnostic (ampullary biopsy) and therapeutic (sphincterotomy). Cholangiography reveals one of four patterns:
    ■ Sclerosing cholangitis and papillary stenosis (most common)
    ■ Sclerosing cholangitis alone
    ■ Papillary stenosis alone
    ■ Long extrahepatic bile duct strictures with or without sclerosing cholangitis
9. Treatment is primarily endoscopic; the approach varies with the anatomic abnormality.
    ■ Papillary stenosis: Consider sphincterotomy
    ■ Isolated or dominant bile duct stricture: Consider endoscopic stenting
    ■ Isolated intrahepatic sclerosing cholangitis: Consider ursodeoxycholic acid 300 mg three times daily
10. Empiric antimicrobial therapy directed against typical pathogens (e.g., *C. parvum*) does not affect symptoms or cholangiographic abnormalities.

ACALCULOUS CHOLECYSTITIS

1. This may occur in patients with AIDS cholangiopathy.
2. Typical causes include cytomegalovirus, *C. parvum, Microsporidia* spp., and *Isospora belli*. Less common causes are *Candida albicans, Klebsiella pneumoniae, Salmonella typhimurium,* and *Pseudomonas aeruginosa.*
3. The presentation may be similar to that of calculous cholecystitis, with severe right upper quadrant pain, fever, and Murphy sign. Critically ill patients may present with unexplained fever or vague abdominal discomfort (see Chapter 34).
4. Physical examination may reveal a palpable right upper quadrant mass and jaundice (20%).
5. Leukocytosis, hyperbilirubinemia, and elevations in serum ALP and aminotransferase levels may be observed.
6. Abdominal ultrasonography may demonstrate a thickened (>3- to 4-mm) gallbladder wall, pericholecystic fluid, stones, or ductal abnormalities. In stable patients in whom the diagnosis is unclear after ultrasonography, cholescintigraphy with a hepatobiliary iminodiacetic acid (HIDA) scan may be useful. The diagnosis is confirmed by demonstrating failure of the gallbladder to opacify.
7. Once acalculous cholecystitis is established, secondary infection with enteric pathogens is common. After blood cultures are obtained, broad-spectrum antibiotics (e.g., piperacillin-tazobactam, ampicillin-sulbactam, third-generation cephalosporin with metronidazole, imipenem) should be initiated. Antibiotic therapy can be narrowed after microbiologic diagnosis.
8. Definitive therapy is cholecystectomy. If surgical intervention is contraindicated, drainage of the gallbladder through percutaneous cholecystostomy should be considered.

NONCIRRHOTIC PORTAL HYPERTENSION

Portal hypertension has been described in persons with HIV infection.
1. Portal hypertension is presinusoidal and is secondary to conditions such as noncirrhotic portal fibrosis, nodular regenerative hyperplasia, portal vein thrombosis, or a combination of these conditions.
2. Liver function is often well preserved, and the clinical picture is dominated by cytopenias, splenomegaly, and variceal hemorrhage.
3. Didanosine has been implicated in the pathogenesis of portal hypertension.
4. The long-term prognosis is generally good; liver failure is rare.

FURTHER READING

Achary C, Dharel N, Sterling RK. Chronic liver disease in the human immunodeficiency virus patient. *Clin Liver Dis.* 2015;19:1–22.

Amorosa VK, Slim J, Mounzer K, et al. The influence of abacavir and other antiretroviral agents on virologic response to hepatitis C virus therapy among antiretroviral-treated HIV-infected patients. *Antivir Ther.* 2010;15:91–99.

Gandhi RT, Wurcel A, Lee H, et al. Response to hepatitis B vaccine in HIV-1–positive subjects who test positive for isolated antibody to hepatitis B core antigen: implications for hepatitis B vaccine strategies. *J Infect Dis.* 2005;191:1435–1441.

Laurence J. Hepatitis A and B immunizations of individuals infected with human immunodeficiency virus. *Am J Med.* 2005;118:S75–S83.

Lo Re III V, Kostman JR, Amorosa VK. Management complexities of HIV/hepatitis C virus coinfection in the twenty-first century. *Clin Liver Dis.* 2008;12:587–609.

Lo Re III V, Kostman JR, Gross R, et al. Incidence and risk factors for weight loss during dual HIV/hepatitis C virus therapy. *J Acquir Immune Defic Syndr.* 2007;44:344–350.

McGovern BH, Ditelberg JS, Taylor LE, et al. Hepatic steatosis is associated with nucleoside analogue use and hepatitis C genotype 3 infection in HIV-seropositive patients. *Clin Infect Dis.* 2006;43:365–372.

Mendizabal M, Craviotto S, Chen T, et al. Noncirrhotic portal hypertension: another cause of liver disease in HIV patients. *Ann Hepatol.* 2009;8:390–395.

Nunez M. Hepatotoxicity of antiretrovirals: incidence, mechanisms and management. *J Hepatol.* 2006; 44:S132–S139.

Pineda JA, Romero-Gomez M, Diaz-Garcia F, et al. HIV coinfection shortens the survival of patients with hepatitis C virus–related decompensated cirrhosis. *Hepatology.* 2005;41:779–789.

Puri P, Kumar S. Liver involvement in human immunodeficiency virus infection. *Indian J Gastroenterol.* 2016;35:113–116.

Soriano V, Puoti M, Garcia-Gasco P, et al. Antiretroviral drugs and liver injury. *AIDS.* 2008;22:1–13.

Soriano V, Puoti M, Peters M, et al. Care of HIV patients with chronic hepatitis B: updated recommendation from the HIV-Hepatitis B Virus International Panel. *AIDS.* 2008;2:1399–1410.

Sulkowski MS, Mehta SH, Torbenson M, et al. Hepatic steatosis and antiretroviral drug use among adults coinfected with HIV and hepatitis C virus. *AIDS.* 2005;19:585–592.

Weber R, Sabin CA, Friis-Moller N, et al. Liver-related deaths in persons infected with the human immunodeficiency virus: the D: A:D study. *Arch Intern Med.* 2006;166:1632–1641.

CHAPTER 28

Granulomatous Liver Disease

Jay H. Lefkowitch, MD

KEY POINTS

1 Granulomas consist of activated macrophages (epithelioid macrophages) accompanied by T lymphocytes and other immune cells, which infiltrate liver tissue as nodular lesions in reaction to indigestible or foreign antigen or are due to triggering of an untoward immunologic reaction (e.g., drug-induced liver injury [DILI]).

2 The major causes of hepatic granulomas include infectious agents (especially tuberculosis), sarcoidosis, primary biliary cholangitis (PBC), drugs, systemic diseases (e.g., Crohn disease), and neoplasms (e.g., Hodgkin lymphoma).

3 An elevated serum alkaline phosphatase level is the chief abnormality in serum liver biochemical tests.

4 The cause of hepatic granulomas may remain unknown in up to 50% of cases.

5 The workup for hepatic granulomas includes a complete history of therapeutic drugs, tests for antimitochondrial antibodies and angiotensin converting enzyme (ACE), and staining liver specimens with acid-fast and silver stains for mycobacteria and fungi, respectively.

Overview of Granulomas

DEFINITION AND PATHOGENESIS

1. Granulomas are rounded 1- to 2-mm nodular collections of activated macrophages, T lymphocytes, and other immune cells that can infiltrate many tissues, including the liver, in response to an indigestible or foreign antigen or as a manifestation of an untoward immunologic response to a drug, bile duct injury (e.g., PBC), or other factors (Fig. 28.1).
2. The principal immune cells in granulomas are activated macrophages resembling epithelial cells (epithelioid macrophages); CD4+ T cells (T helper [Th] lymphocytes); and sometimes multinucleated giant cells that develop from macrophage fusion.
3. The cause of the granuloma influences the constituent immune cells and secreted products: type 1 T helper (Th1) cells and cytokines predominate in mycobacterial granulomas, whereas type 2 T helper (Th2) cells and cytokines predominate in schistosomal granulomas (Fig. 28.2).
4. Granulomas evolve by the elaboration of secretory products (cytokines and chemokines) by their constituent cells (interferon-gamma and interleukin-2 from Th lymphocytes), expansion of macrophage and T-cell pools, and specialization of macrophages for antigen digestion (Fig. 28.3).
5. Granulomas ultimately may persist, resolve, or undergo fibrosis or calcification.

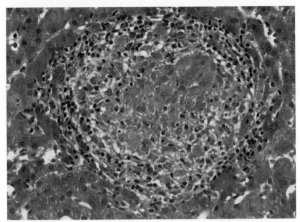

Fig. 28.1 Histopathology of a noncaseating hepatic granuloma (sarcoidosis). Epithelioid macrophages occupy the center of the granulomas with peripherally dispersed lymphocytes (hematoxylin and eosin [H&E]).

MORPHOLOGIC TYPES

Several types of granulomas are described in liver disease and are based on their histologic features and constituents (Table 28.1). The presence of abundant eosinophils within granulomas warrants exclusion of DILI and parasite infestation.

INCIDENCE AND LOCATION

1. **Granulomas are found in 2.4% to 14.6% of liver biopsy specimens,** according to surveys by McCluggage and Sloan (1994) and Martin-Blondel et al. (2010), although the figure of 10% is often quoted.
2. Granulomas are found in any of the following microscopic sites in the liver, alone or in combination:
   - Lobular (tuberculosis, sarcoidosis, drugs)
   - Portal/periportal (sarcoidosis)
   - Periductal (PBC)
   - Perivenous (mineral oil lipogranulomas)
   - Periarterial and intraarterial (phenytoin)

Causes of Hepatic Granulomas

The etiology is multifactorial; the major causes and examples are shown in Table 28.2.

Clinical and Biochemical Features

SYMPTOMS AND SIGNS

They often include the following:
- Abdominal pain
- Weight loss
- Fatigue
- Chills

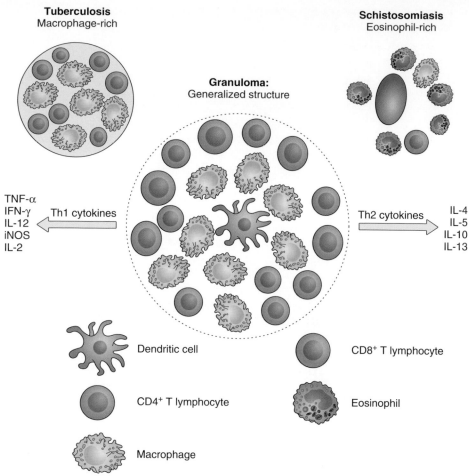

Fig. 28.2 Generalized and specialized structural and functional characteristics of hepatic granulomas. The cellular constituents of hepatic granulomas are diagrammed at the bottom. Note that tuberculosis macrophage-rich granulomas show a type 1 T helper (Th1)–predominant lymphocytic response, with release of Th1 cytokines. In schistosomiasis, in contrast, enhanced numbers of eosinophils are present within the granulomas (mediated by secretion of interleukin 5 [IL-5]). In addition, release of IL-13 in schistosomiasis is an important factor resulting in portal fibrosis in the disease. *IFN-γ,* Interferon-gamma; *iNOS,* inducible nitric oxide synthetase; *TNF-α,* tumor necrosis factor alpha.

- Hepatomegaly
- Splenomegaly
- Lymphadenopathy
- Fever of unknown origin

LIVER BIOCHEMICAL FEATURES

1. The liver biochemical test pattern is that of **infiltrative disease.**
    - An elevated alkaline phosphatase is typical: 3 to 10 times normal.
    - Serum aminotransferase levels are usually normal or only mildly raised.
2. Liver biochemical test levels may be normal.

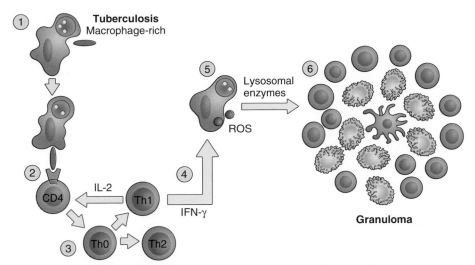

Fig. 28.3 Development of a granuloma (red rods represent mycobacteria). Step 1: A macrophage engulfs mycobacterium. Step 2: Macrophage presentation of mycobacterial protein product(s) to a receptor on CD4+ lymphocytes. Step 3: CD4+ lymphocytes differentiate to precursor T helper lymphocytes (Th0), later differentiating into Th1 lymphocytes. Step 4: Th1 lymphocytes secrete interleukin 2 (IL-2), a clonal expander of CD4+ cells, as well as interferon gamma (IFN-γ), which upregulates lysosomal enzymes and reactive oxygen species (ROS) in macrophages in step 5. Step 6: Further recruitment of macrophages and lymphocytes with ongoing digestion of mycobacteria.

TABLE 28.1 ■ **Types of Granuloma**

Type	Histologic Features	Cause(s)
Caseating	Peripheral macrophages ± giant cells; central necrosis	Tuberculosis
Noncaseating	Cluster of macrophages ± giant cells	Sarcoidosis Drugs
Lipogranuloma	Lipid vacuole(s) surrounded by macrophages and lymphocytes	Fatty liver Mineral oil
Fibrin-ring (doughnut granuloma)	Central lipid vacuole or empty space Macrophages and lymphocytes Ring of fibrin	Q fever Allopurinol Hodgkin lymphoma

OTHER LABORATORY FEATURES

1. The serum ACE level is elevated in sarcoidosis, PBC, silicosis, and asbestosis.
2. Serum globulin levels are elevated in sarcoidosis, berylliosis, and chronic granulomatous disease of childhood.
3. Peripheral blood eosinophilia may be present with drug- or parasite-related granulomas.

Specific Types of Granulomatous Liver Disease

SARCOIDOSIS (see also Chapter 24)

1. Sarcoid granulomas preferentially cluster in portal and periportal regions and are associated with hyaline fibrosis (Fig. 28.4).

TABLE 28.2 ■ Causes of Hepatic Granulomas

Etiology	Specific Cause(s)
Infection	Viral: Cytomegalovirus, infectious mononucleosis, hepatitis C virus infection Bacterial: Brucellosis, tuberculosis Rickettsial: Q fever Spirochetal: *Treponema pallidum* infection Fungal: Histoplasmosis Parasitic: Schistosomiasis
Primary biliary cholangitis	Early stages most commonly
Foreign body	Suture, talc
Systemic disease	Sarcoidosis, Crohn disease
Drug	Allopurinol, phenytoin, penicillin
Neoplasia	Hodgkin lymphoma

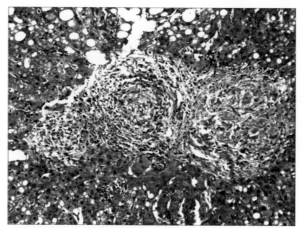

Fig. 28.4 Histopathology of clustered portal and periportal granulomas in a liver biopsy specimen from a patient with sarcoidosis. Sarcoid granulomas often result in hyaline fibrosis (shown as increased blue-staining collagen fibers surrounding the granulomas) (trichrome).

2. Granulomas are noncaseating, may contain inclusions (asteroid and Schaumann bodies), and can be located within lobular parenchyma as well as in or near portal tracts.
3. Other pathologic features may be seen, as described by Devaney et al. (1993):
   ■ Chronic intrahepatic cholestasis due to bile duct destruction
   ■ Bile duct damage resembling that seen in PBC
   ■ Periductal fibrosis resembling that seen in primary sclerosing cholangitis
   ■ Suppurative cholangitis
   ■ Granulomatous phlebitis
   ■ Hepatitis, including portal and lobular lymphocyte and plasma cell infiltrates with liver-cell necrosis
   ■ Cirrhosis rarely

TUBERCULOSIS (see also Chapter 31)

1. Caseation is seen in 29% of liver biopsy specimens and 78% of autopsy specimens in *Mycobacteria tuberculosis* infection (Fig. 28.5).

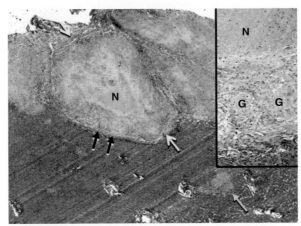

Fig. 28.5 Histopathology of hepatic tuberculosis. This wedge liver biopsy specimen shows several tuberculomas (the yellow arrows demarcate tuberculomas). Note the caseating necrosis (N) at the center of the tuberculoma, and several intact granulomas (G) at the periphery *(black arrows)*. The necrosis and granulomas are shown at higher magnification in the inset (H&E).

2. An acid-fast stain is infrequently positive (<10% of proven cases).
3. Tuberculous granulomas may be found throughout the liver parenchyma.
4. Rupture into bile ducts may result in tuberculous cholangitis.

SCHISTOSOMIASIS (see also Chapter 31)

1. The dense portal fibrosis seen grossly in advanced schistosomiasis is known as *Symmers clay pipestem fibrosis.*
2. Schistosome eggs arrive in portal vein radicles where granulomas are formed, with a peripheral rim of eosinophils (Fig. 28.6).
3. Fine black hemozoin pigment (derived from breakdown of hemoglobin by adult worms) may be seen microscopically in macrophages within granulomas, portal tracts, and sinusoids.
4. Patients with schistosomiasis should be tested for hepatitis B and C virus infections because of common endemicity and contributions of viral infection to comorbidity.

ACQUIRED IMMUNODEFICIENCY SYNDROME (see also Chapter 27)

1. Acid-fast and silver stains should be performed when granulomas are found in liver specimens from patients with acquired immunodeficiency syndrome (AIDS).
2. Granulomas due to *Mycobacterium avium* complex in AIDS characteristically show pale staining epithelioid macrophages containing linear structures (mycobacteria) on a routine hematoxylin and eosin stain, with abundant, packed organisms in each macrophage on an acid-fast stain.
3. Cytomegalovirus hepatic infection occasionally results in small noncaseating granulomas.
4. Other infections identified in hepatic granulomas in patients with AIDS include histoplasmosis, cryptococcosis, and toxoplasmosis.
5. Treatment with antibiotics (e.g., sulfonamides, isoniazid) may cause hepatic granulomas.

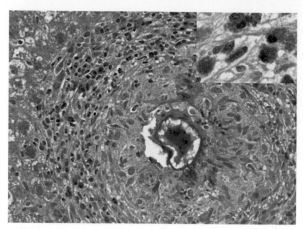

Fig. 28.6   Histopathology of a schistosomal granuloma. The center of the granuloma contains an ovum with miracidium, surrounded by abundant macrophages. The periphery of the granuloma shows lymphocytes and eosinophils. The eosinophil component is highlighted in the inset, upper right (H&E).

PRIMARY BILIARY CHOLANGITIS (see also Chapter 16)

1. Granulomas may be seen in approximately 25% of patients with PBC.
2. Granulomas are usually seen in earlier stages of PBC, in portal tracts near or surrounding damaged bile ducts (Fig. 28.7).
3. Occasionally small, ill-defined histiocytic granulomas may be found within the lobular parenchyma (reported in 22.8% of PBC liver biopsy specimens by Drebber et al. [2009]).

LIPOGRANULOMAS

1. These are due to fatty liver or dietary mineral oil ingestion (in laxative or food products).
2. They consist of fat vacuoles, scattered lymphocytes and macrophages, and strands of connective tissue.
3. Mineral oil lipogranulomas are seen in portal tracts or near central veins (Fig. 28.8), or both.
4. This type of granuloma usually has no major clinical consequences, although two rare cases of lipogranulomas associated with venous outflow obstruction have been described, as cited by Quaglia et al. (2012).

FIBRIN-RING ("DOUGHNUT") GRANULOMAS

1. These granulomas consist of a central vacuole or empty space, a surrounding pink ring of fibrin, epithelioid macrophages, and lymphocytes (Fig. 28.9).
2. Fibrin strands in these granulomas can be stained with the phosphotungstic acid-hematoxylin (PTAH) (see Fig. 28.9) or Lendrum methods.
3. Fibrin-ring granulomas were first described in Q fever.
4. These granulomas have been considered to be nonspecific because of their association with diverse conditions.
   - Q fever
   - Hodgkin lymphoma
   - Allopurinol

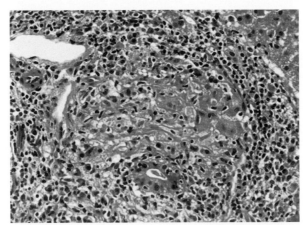

Fig. 28.7 Histopathology of a granuloma in primary biliary cholangitis. The portal tract shown here contains a granuloma in the center of the field. Note that at the 6 o'clock position, a damaged interlobular bile duct ("florid bile duct lesion") infiltrated by mononuclear cells is visible. Granulomas arise near damaged bile ducts presumably because of release of antigenic material following duct injury (H&E).

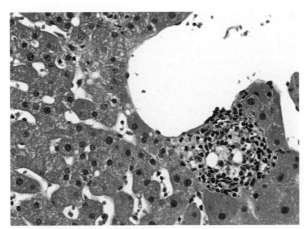

Fig. 28.8 Histopathology of a lipogranuloma that appears attached to a central vein. Lipid vacuoles are surrounded by a mixture of macrophages and lymphocytes. Similar lesions may appear within portal tracts and are often related to exposure to mineral oil (H&E).

- Cytomegalovirus
- Epstein-Barr virus
- Leishmaniasis
- Toxoplasmosis
- Hepatitis A virus
- Systemic lupus erythematosus
- Giant-cell arteritis
- Staphylococcal infection
- Boutonneuse fever (*Rickettsia conorii*)

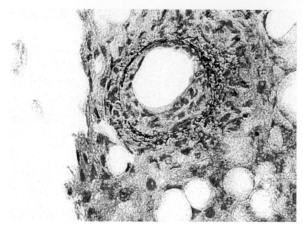

Fig. 28.9   Histopathology of a fibrin-ring granuloma. This lesion (at the center of the field) is also called a "doughnut" granuloma because of the empty-appearing hole or lipid vacuole in the center, surrounded by a ring of fibrin (appearing here as filamentous, magenta strands) and mononuclear cells (phosphotungstic acid-hematoxylin).

DRUG-RELATED GRANULOMAS

1. Approximately one third of hepatic granulomas may be due to drugs, according to McMaster and Hennigar (1981).
2. Drug-related granulomas may be found throughout the hepatic parenchyma, may contain eosinophils, and may be accompanied by other evidence of drug hepatitis (cholestasis, fat, hepatocyte ballooning, and apoptosis).
3. The list of causative drugs is extensive (see also Chapter 10).
4. Drug-related granulomas usually heal without sequelae.

MISCELLANEOUS CONDITIONS

1. Granulomas can be seen in *primary sclerosing cholangitis*, but only rarely (3% to 4%), as described by Ludwig and colleagues (1995).
2. *Idiopathic granulomatous hepatitis,* described by Simon and Wolff (1973), is seen in patients with fever of unknown origin and no established cause for the granulomas found on liver biopsy specimens (Fig. 28.10).
3. Patients with *chronic hepatitis C* may have small, noncaseating granulomas in their liver biopsy specimens; these may recur after liver transplantation, as described by Vakiani et al. (2007).
4. The presence of multiple granulomas with abundant eosinophils, sometimes with central necrosis (Fig. 28.11), warrants exclusion of *parasitic infestations*, including visceral larva migrans (*toxocariasis*) and *Capillariasis*.

Therapy

1. Therapy should be directed toward the causative agent, when known, including antibiotics for microbial infection, removal of the implicated drug in drug-related cases, and glucocorticoids in sarcoidosis.
2. In *idiopathic granulomatous hepatitis*, the disease may resolve spontaneously, with glucocorticoid treatment, or with methotrexate.

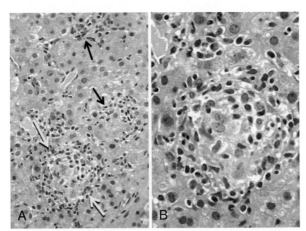

Fig. 28.10 Histopathology of idiopathic granulomatous hepatitis. A full hematologic, immunologic, and infectious workup and complete drug history failed to reveal an etiology in a middle-aged woman with fever of unknown origin. A, A needle liver biopsy specimen shows lobular nonnecrotizing granulomas *(between yellow arrows)* and numerous necroinflammatory foci *(black arrows).* B, A high-power view of one of the lobular granulomas shows macrophages with ample pink cytoplasm admixed with lymphocytes (H&E).

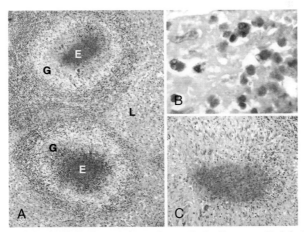

Fig. 28.11 Histopathology of hepatic granulomas in a patient with a parasitic infection. A, Miliary-type hepatic granulomas (G) with central eosinophilic necrosis (E), a reaction to intrahepatic migration of *Toxocara* larvae, are present in this case of presumed visceral larva migrans (toxocariasis). *Capillaria* infestation may produce similar lesions. B, Abundant eosinophils are present in these granulomas. C, Higher magnification of a granuloma shows peripherally arranged macrophages, lymphocytes, and eosinophils, with central eosinophilic necrosis (H&E).

FURTHER READING

Denk H, Scheuer PJ, Baptista A, et al. Guidelines for the diagnosis and interpretation of hepatic granulomas. *Histopathology.* 1994;25:209–218.

Devaney K, Goodman ZD, Epstein MS, et al. Hepatic sarcoidosis. Clinicopathologic features in 100 patients. *Am J Surg Pathol.* 1993;17:1272–1280.

Drebber U, Mueller JJM, Klein E, et al. Liver biopsy in primary biliary cirrhosis: clinicopathological data and stage. *Pathol Int.* 2009;59:546–554.

Ishak KG. Granulomas of the liver. In: Ioachim HL, ed. *Pathology of Granulomas*. New York: Raven; 1983:307–370.

Knox TA, Kaplan MM, Gelfand JA, et al. Methotrexate treatment of idiopathic granulomatous hepatitis. *Ann Intern Med*. 1995;122:595.

Lamps LW. Hepatic granulomas: a review with emphasis on infectious causes. *Arch Pathol Lab Med*. 2015;139:867–875.

Ludwig J, Colina F, Poterucha JJ. Granulomas in primary sclerosing cholangitis. *Liver*. 1995;15:307–312.

Martin-Blondel G, Camara B, Selves J, et al. Etiology and outcome of liver granulomatosis: a retrospective study of 21 cases. *Rev Med Interne*. 2010;31:97–106.

McCluggage WG, Sloan JM. Hepatic granulomas in Northern Ireland: a thirteen year review. *Histopathology*. 1994;25:219–228.

McMaster KR, Kennigar GR. Drug-induced granulomatous hepatitis. *Lab Invest*. 1981;44:61–73.

Musso C, Castelo JS, Tsanaclis AMC, et al. Prevalence of Toxocara-induced liver granulomas, detected by immunohistochemistry, in a series of autopsies at a Children's Reference Hospital in Vitoria, ES, Brazil. *Virchows Arch*. 2007;450:411–417.

Quaglia A, Burt AD, Ferrell LD, et al. Systemic disease. In: Burt AD, Portmann BC, Ferrell L, eds. *MacSween's Pathology of the Liver*. 6th ed. Edinburgh: Elsevier Churchill Livingstone; 2012:935–987.

Simon HB, Wolff SM. Granulomatous hepatitis and fever of unknown origin: a study of 13 patients. *Medicine*. 1973;52:1–21.

Tjwa M, De Hertogh G, Neuville B, et al. Hepatic fibrin-ring granulomas in granulomatous hepatitis: report of four cases and review of the literature. *Acta Clin Belg*. 2001;56:341–348.

Vakiani E, Hunt KK, Mazziotta RM, et al. Hepatitis C-associated granulomas after liver transplantation: morphologic spectrum and clinical implications. *Am J Clin Pathol*. 2007;127:128–134.

CHAPTER 29

Hepatic Tumors

Wei Zhang, MD, PhD ■ Adrian M. Di Bisceglie, MD, FACP

KEY POINTS

1 Hemangioma of the liver is found in up to 20% of the normal population and is rarely of clinical consequence.

2 Other benign tumors of the liver are rare, including hepatic adenoma, which usually requires surgical resection because of the risks of rupture and the possible development of malignancy.

3 In the presence of cirrhosis, hepatocellular carcinoma (HCC) accounts for approximately 75% of all liver tumors. The most important risk factors for development of HCC are cirrhosis of any cause, hepatitis B virus (HBV) infection, and hepatitis C virus (HCV) infection with advanced fibrosis.

4 Liver transplantation seems to offer the best chance of cure in HCC, but is resource intensive and can only be used in a limited proportion of patients; few patients are suitable candidates for potentially curative surgery.

5 Cholangiocarcinoma (CC) is rising in incidence in the United States, probably in association with cirrhosis and HBV and HCV infection. Liver transplantation for early-stage perihilar-type CCs after neoadjuvant chemoradiation has become an appealing option.

Benign Tumors of the Liver

HEPATIC ADENOMA

■ This is a benign proliferation of hepatocytes. It is a rare tumor that occurs largely in female patients. Its incidence has increased since the 1960s, probably related to the introduction and increased use of oral contraceptives.

■ Hepatic adenoma is a multifactorial disease. Although oral contraceptive (OCP) use, female sex, anabolic androgens, and age are major risk factors, hepatic adenoma can still occur in males and females who are not taking OCPs.

■ There are **four major molecular subgroups** according to their genetic and phenotype characteristics: **Hepatocyte nuclear factor (HNF)–1α mutated, β-catenin activated, inflammatory, and unclassified hepatic adenoma.**

■ Hepatic adenoma with β-catenin activated mutation has a high risk of malignant transformation.

■ Inflammatory hepatic adenoma includes telangiectatic hepatic adenoma (THA), previously classified as "telangiectatic focal nodular hyperplasia." Risk factors for THA include OCP use, hormonal therapy, and obesity. Some inflammatory hepatic adenomas may also have β-catenin activation, making them at increased risk of malignant transformation.

- Adenomas are usually single but may be multiple, rarely with more than five lesions. The size is variable but typically greater than 5 cm in diameter at diagnosis and sometimes massive.
- **Hepatic adenomatosis** is a rare condition characterized by large numbers of adenomas (>10) in the liver with a high rate of recurrence. Patients with metabolic syndrome may also have associated hemangioma and focal nodular hyperplasia (FNH) in addition to adenomatosis.
- Patients typically present with pain or discomfort in the right upper quadrant, although occasional tumors are found incidentally. Adenomas, especially telangiectatic hepatic adenomas, may rupture, resulting in hemoperitoneum.
- Complications include hemorrhage and malignant transformation. Risk factors for malignant transformation include male sex, large size (>10 cm), and β-catenin activated mutation. Malignancy associated with hepatic adenoma carries a good prognosis after surgery.
- The presence of a mass in the liver may be confirmed by computed tomography (CT), ultrasonography, or magnetic resonance imaging (MRI). Technetium (^{99m}Tc) radioisotope scan may show a defect within the liver. The diagnosis may be confirmed by liver biopsy. Histologic examination of hepatic adenoma shows benign hepatocytes organized in cords but with no portal tracts.
- Treatment includes discontinuing the use of estrogens. Surgical resection is usually recommended for adenomas >5 cm in diameter, in men, and for telangiectatic and unclassified adenomas because of an increased risk of complications. Liver transplantation may be considered for adenomas found in association with type I glycogen storage disease.

TUMORLIKE LESIONS OF HEPATOCYTES

1. **Focal nodular hyperplasia (FNH)** represents an abnormal proliferation of hepatocytes around an abnormal hepatic artery. The artery is usually embedded in a **characteristic "spoke-wheel" central stellate scar.**
   - FNH is usually clinically silent and is typically found incidentally, often at the time of imaging or abdominal surgery for another reason.
   - In comparison with adenoma, FNH tends to be smaller and carries little risk of rupture. Multiple lesions are found in approximately 20% of patients.
   - The gold standard diagnosis is contrast-enhanced CT or MRI. However, some FNH may not have typical radiographic features, and a biopsy may be required to confirm the diagnosis. A hepatic arteriogram may suggest the diagnosis if a tumor is found surrounding a large hepatic artery.
   - The diagnosis may be difficult to make on needle biopsy. Excisional biopsy may be required and is usually curative.
   - Asymptomatic cases do not need intervention. For symptomatic patients, other diagnoses need to be ruled out before treatment is started. Embolization and radiofrequency ablation seem to have fewer complications and lower morbidity compared with surgical resection.
2. **Nodular regenerative hyperplasia (NRH)** is characterized by the formation of small regenerative nodules composed of hepatocytes throughout the liver. The pattern is similar to cirrhosis, except that these nodules do not have a surrounding rim of fibrosis.
   - NRH is **often associated with identifiable systemic diseases** such as autoimmune disorders, rheumatoid arthritis (including Felty syndrome), and myeloproliferative disorders (see Chapter 24).
   - The pathogenesis is believed to be related to obliterative portal venopathy associated with thrombosis or phlebitis causing ischemia.
   - The incidence of NRH increases with age and is found most commonly in persons >60 years old.

- Symptomatic NRH is often complicated by the development of presinusoidal portal hypertension. Patients may present with splenomegaly and hypersplenism or bleeding esophageal varices.
- In general, patients with NRH tolerate variceal bleeding better than those with cirrhosis, presumably because they have relatively well-preserved hepatic synthetic function.
- Liver biopsy is required for the definitive diagnosis of NRH.
- Asymptomatic NRH does not require intervention. For symptomatic patients, treat portal hypertension. Beta receptor antagonist therapy, endoscopic therapy, or rarely, portal decompression can be used to prevent rebleeding from varices.

3. **Adenomatous hyperplasia** (macroregenerative nodule, dysplastic nodule)
   - This term is used for regenerative nodules of hepatocytes >1 cm in diameter found in association with cirrhosis or, rarely, submassive hepatic necrosis. Adenomatous hyperplasia **represents a form of dysplastic nodule.**
   - In the context of cirrhosis, adenomatous hyperplasia is considered to be premalignant and is strongly associated with the development of HCC.
   - No specific therapy is needed, but percutaneous ablation therapy may be considered. In patients with cirrhosis, the presence of adenomatous hyperplasia should signal the need for intensive surveillance for the development of HCC (see discussion later in chapter).

4. **Partial nodular transformation:** This rare condition is characterized by the presence of nodules of hepatocytes located in the perihilar region and associated with portal hypertension.

HEMANGIOMA

- Hemangiomas of the liver are the **most common benign hepatic tumors**, identified in as many as 20% of autopsies. They are found more frequently in women but are not related to OCP use.
- They are composed of an endothelial lining on a thin fibrous stroma making up cavernous, blood-filled spaces.
- The tumor is usually small; they are referred to as *giant or cavernous hemangiomas* if >10 cm in diameter.
- Patients are usually asymptomatic and are found incidentally during imaging studies but, if large enough, may cause some abdominal discomfort. Occasionally, thrombosis within a giant hemangioma may result in consumption of platelets and thrombocytopenia, particularly in children (*Kasabach-Merritt syndrome*). Hemangiomas have been documented to increase in size over time but have no potential to become malignant.
- Percutaneous needle biopsy should be avoided because of the risk of bleeding.
- Hemangiomas usually do not require any specific therapy. They may be resected if they are associated with significant symptoms or the tumor size is >10 cm.

BENIGN HEPATIC TUMORS OF CHOLANGIOCELLULAR ORIGIN

1. **Bile duct adenoma:** This is typically a solitary subcapsular tumor, composed of a proliferation of small, round, normal-appearing bile ducts with cuboidal epithelium.
2. **Biliary microhamartoma** (von Meyenburg complex): This is part of the spectrum of adult polycystic disease but may also be found together with polycystic disease (adult or childhood type), congenital hepatic fibrosis, or Caroli disease (see Chapters 25, 30, and 35).
3. **Biliary cystadenoma:** This multiloculated cyst is analogous to mucinous cystadenomas of the pancreas. It is thought to be the precursor to the development of biliary cystadenocarcinoma. Complete surgical resection is highly recommended because of its high risk of recurrence and malignant transformation.

TABLE 29.1 ■ **Benign Hepatic Tumors of Mesenchymal Origin**

Tumor	Comment
Angiomyolipoma	Distinct radiographic appearance
Fibroma	Solid fibrous tumor of the liver
Infantile hemangioendothelioma	Tumor of infancy; may be complicated by thrombocytopenia, high-output heart failure; may require resection or ablation
Inflammatory pseudotumor	Chronic inflammation and fibrosis; may cause pain, fever
Leiomyoma	Extremely rare
Lipoma	Collection of lipocytes; distinct from focal fatty change within hepatocytes
Lymphangiomatosis	Masses of prominent, dilated lymphatic channels
Mesenchymal hamartoma	Childhood tumor with a mixture of elements (bile ducts, vessels, and mesenchyma)
Myxoma	Myxomatous connective tissue

4. **Biliary papillomatosis:** This rare condition consists of multicentric biliary tract adenomatous polypoid tumors that have an increased risk of transforming to adenocarcinoma (analogous to familial adenomatous polyposis).

BENIGN HEPATIC TUMORS OF MESENCHYMAL ORIGIN

These tumors are listed in Table 29.1.

Malignant Tumors of the Liver

METASTATIC DISEASE

The liver is a common site of metastasis. **Metastases are by far the most common form of hepatic malignancy.** The most frequent sites of origin for hepatic metastases are lung, breast, and gastrointestinal and genitourinary tracts.

HEPATOCELLULAR CARCINOMA

HCC is a malignant tumor of hepatocytes.
1. **Epidemiology**
   - HCC is one of the most common malignant diseases worldwide. The incidence varies considerably around the world. High-incidence areas include China, Taiwan, Korea, and other parts of Southeast Asia, as well as most of sub-Saharan Africa, where the incidence may be as high as 120 per 100,000 population per year. Areas of intermediate incidence include Japan, the countries of southern Europe (particularly Italy and Spain), and the Middle East. Regions of low incidence include northern countries of Europe, the United States, and South America, where the rate may be as low as 5 per 100,000 population. The incidence of HCC is rising in many developed Western countries.
   - The median age at diagnosis is in the fourth decade of life in high-incidence areas; it manifests at an older age in other regions, and it is more common in men than in women.

TABLE 29.2 ■ **Known and Possible Risk Factors in Hepatocellular Carcinoma**

Known	Possible
Cirrhosis (of any cause)	Alcohol (in absence of cirrhosis)
Chronic hepatitis B	Anabolic or estrogenic steroids
Chronic hepatitis C with cirrhosis	Nonalcoholic steatohepatitis without cirrhosis
Nonalcoholic steatohepatitis with cirrhosis	Smoking

Inherited metabolic disorders:
  Alpha-1 antitrypsin deficiency
  Hemochromatosis
  Hereditary tyrosinemia	

Carcinogens:
  Aflatoxin
  Thorotrast[a]	

[a]Thorotrast is a contrast agent that was used for arteriography for a period after World War II. It contains thorium dioxide, a low-level emitter of alpha particles, which is retained in Kupffer cells.

2. **Risk factors**
   a. HCC is one of the few human cancers for which an etiologic factor can be identified in most cases. Known and possible risk factors are shown in Table 29.2.
   b. **Chronic HBV infection is the most common etiologic factor in high-incidence areas**, whereas chronic HCV infection plays the most important etiologic role in areas of intermediate incidence.
      ■ The precise mechanism by which chronic viral hepatitis results in HCC is not known but may be through liver regeneration and injury characteristic of cirrhosis.
      ■ In addition, HBV is a DNA virus whose genome may become integrated within the genome of hepatocytes, thereby possibly influencing actions of oncogenes or tumor suppressor genes. The X protein of HBV is known to be a transactivator (i.e., it is capable of initiating gene transcription, thereby possibly activating growth factors or oncogenes). Carboxyterminally truncated pre-S or S polypeptides may also contribute to development of HCC (see Chapter 4).
      ■ HCV is an RNA virus that does not become integrated into the host genome. **Almost all cases of HCV-related HCC are associated with cirrhosis or advanced hepatic fibrosis.** Alcohol may be an important cofactor with HCV in the development of HCC.
   c. Certain metabolic diseases may be associated with the development of HCC, but virtually always in the presence of cirrhosis (e.g., hemochromatosis, alpha-1 antitrypsin deficiency). Hereditary tyrosinemia is a rare inborn error of metabolism associated with severe liver injury and regeneration and development of HCC in childhood.
   d. Environmental toxins play a role in the pathogenesis of HCC in some parts of the world. Aflatoxin is formed as a product of fungal contamination of stored foodstuffs. It is directly hepatocarcinogenic in rodents and, in humans, interacts with HBV, often in association with a characteristic mutation in codon 249 of the *TP53* tumor suppressor gene, to cause HCC.
   e. Nonalcoholic fatty liver disease (NAFLD) with advanced fibrosis and cirrhosis is increasingly recognized as a risk factor for HCC. HCC may also occur in NAFLD without cirrhosis.
   f. Diabetes mellitus, obesity, and cigarette smoking are emerging risk factors for HCC.

3. **Clinical features**
   - Abdominal pain or discomfort and weight loss are the most frequent presenting symptoms. HCC may occasionally rupture, manifesting as an acute abdomen. Many patients diagnosed with HCC are asymptomatic, with the tumor detected incidentally or during screening of an at-risk person.
   - HCC may also be associated with various paraneoplastic manifestations, including hypoglycemia, erythrocytosis, hypercholesterolemia, and feminization.
4. **Diagnosis**
   a. The use of **imaging studies** is critical. **Ultrasonography, CT, and MRI** are the mainstays of diagnosis.
      - Small HCCs are seen on ultrasonography as hypodense lesions. Tumors as small as 0.5 to 1 cm may be detected.
      - CT is useful in confirming the presence of tumors >1 cm in diameter and in assessing the extent of tumor within the abdomen.
   b. The use of multiphasic CT or MRI with multiphase images has greatly enhanced the sensitivity of detection.
      - The diagnosis of HCC can be made with confidence if a lesion is at least 10 mm and has a characteristic appearance with arterial enhancement and venous washout on multiphasic imaging.
   c. Serologic markers may be useful in diagnosis. Approximately 80% to 90% of patients with HCC have an elevated serum level of **alpha fetoprotein (AFP)**, although most patients with a small tumor (<5 cm in diameter) have normal or minimally elevated levels.
      - AFP values may be raised in patients with chronic viral hepatitis and cirrhosis without HCC, thus causing diagnostic confusion.
      - AFP-L3 represents a lectin-bound fraction of AFP that may be more specific than AFP for HCC.
   d. **Liver biopsy** may be required to confirm a diagnosis of HCC. The risk of bleeding after liver biopsy for HCC and other forms of malignancy is slightly higher than after liver biopsy for benign disease. Biopsy of the nontumorous portion of the liver is advisable to evaluate the severity of underlying liver disease, particularly if resection is contemplated.
   e. **Fibrolamellar HCC** is a variant of HCC usually not associated with cirrhosis or any of the other known etiologic factors. It has a better prognosis than other forms of HCC.
   f. Steatohepatitic hepatocellular carcinoma (SH-HCC) is another histologic variant of HCC associated with steatohepatitis and the metabolic syndrome. The prognosis is similar to that of typical HCC.
5. **Treatment**
   - **The overall outlook is poor.** In Africa and Asia, where the diagnosis is often made when the tumor is at an advanced stage, HCC is associated with mean survival times measured in weeks to months.
   - Fig. 29.1 offers an approach to the management of patients with HCC based on the stage of the tumor and degree of liver dysfunction.
   - **Surgery:** Large resections of the liver are possible if cirrhosis is not present. However, only small resections, segmentectomy, or enucleation may be possible in a cirrhotic liver, so most patients are not amenable to surgery at the time of diagnosis because of the extent of the tumor or severity of the underlying liver disease. Rates of recurrence and development of new tumors after resection are high.
   - **Liver transplantation** appears to result in a survival rate similar to that of resection in patients with cirrhosis, but with a lower recurrence rate. It is considered in patients who meet the **Milan criteria: One lesion <5 cm or up to three lesions each <3 cm, with no extrahepatic spread or vascular invasion.** HCC now represents an important indication

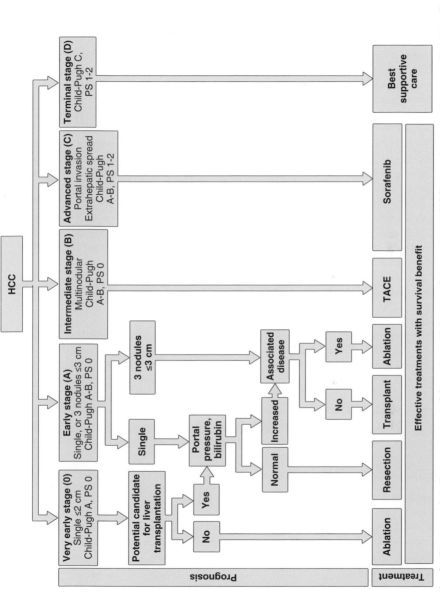

Fig. 29.1 Algorithm for the approach to the management of the patient with hepatocellular carcinoma (HCC) according to the Barcelona Clinic Liver Cancer staging classification. The Child-Pugh classification is not sensitive to accurately identify those patients with advanced liver failure that would deserve consideration of liver transplantation. Patients with end-stage cirrhosis due to impaired liver function (Child-Pugh class C or earlier stages with predictors of poor prognosis such as a high Model for End-stage Liver Disease [MELD] score) should be considered for liver transplantation. In these patients, HCC may become a contraindication to transplantation if the enlistment criteria are exceeded. *PS*, Performance status; *TACE*, transarterial chemoembolization.

for liver transplantation in developed Western countries. Unfortunately, liver transplantation is not available in all countries, and limitations of the supply of donor organs prevent widespread applicability of this form of treatment.

- **Radiofrequency ablation (RFA)** is a technique that can be performed percutaneously and allows complete ablation of liver tumors with only one or two sessions. RFA is noninferior and is more cost effective than surgery for patients with early-stage HCCs. Newer ablation techniques include microwave ablation.
- **Injection of absolute ethanol** is associated with tumor necrosis and is easy to perform, with few side effects. Its use should be confined to tumors <4 cm in diameter. It may be most useful in patients with decompensated cirrhosis who will not tolerate surgery or in cases of recurrent HCC after surgery.
- **Transcatheter arterial chemoembolization (TACE),** in which chemotherapeutic agents are injected into the hepatic artery, which is subsequently occluded, is effective in shrinking tumors and improves survival in selected patients. TACE is used for patients with intermediate-stage HCC and preserved liver function and for downstaging to Milan criteria for liver transplantation. A newer approach using drug-eluting beads (DEB-TACE) has shown similar response with fewer systemic adverse events compared with conventional TACE using lipiodol particles.
- **Targeted molecular therapies** appear promising in the treatment of HCC. **Sorafenib,** a multikinase inhibitor, has become the standard systemic therapy in patients with advanced HCC. Regorafenib is a multikinase inhibitor that may be used in patients who have stopped responding to sorafenib.
- **Systemic chemotherapy** has not been as effective as regional chemotherapy (administered through the hepatic artery) or sorafenib. Cisplatin, in combination with other agents, appears to be the most effective chemotherapeutic agent.

6. **Prevention**
   - **HCC is potentially a preventable form of cancer.** The widespread use of HBV vaccination is expected to decrease the rate of HCC in many high-incidence areas of the world. The incidence of HCV infection may also decline because of increased awareness and screening of donated blood.
   - At present, an effective vaccine is not available against HCV. Newer antiviral treatment regimens with a high cure rate may help decrease the risk of HCC. Antiviral therapy of HBV infection with nucleos(t)ide analogues appears to decrease the risk of HBV-related HCC (see Chapters 4 and 5).

CHOLANGIOCARCINOMA (see also Chapter 36)

1. **Epidemiology**
   - CC is much less common than HCC and is distributed more evenly around the world. CC tends to occur at an older age than HCC and has a more even sex distribution.
   - The risk of CC appears to be increasing in the United States, probably in association with the increased prevalence of cirrhosis.
2. **Risk factors** (Table 29.3)
3. **Clinical features**
   - CC is divided into three types: Intrahepatic, perihilar, and distal extrahepatic. The epidemiology, pathogenesis, and management differ somewhat among the three types.
   - The **intrahepatic** type is located proximally to the second-degree bile ducts and is rarely associated with primary sclerosing cholangitis. The incidence seems to be increasing globally for unclear reasons. This type often manifests with abdominal pain, malaise, and weight loss.

TABLE 29.3 ■ Risk Factors for Cholangiocarcinoma

Primary sclerosing cholangitis

Chronic hepatitis B and C with cirrhosis

Liver fluke infection (*Clonorchis sinensis* or *Opisthorchis viverrini*)

Intrahepatic lithiasis, cholelithiasis

Congenital anomalies (e.g., Caroli disease, choledochal cysts)

Exposure to Thorotrast (see Table 29.2)

Benign cysts, von Meyenburg complex

Inflammatory bowel disease

- The **perihilar** type **(Klatskin tumor)** is the most common subtype, accounting for >50% of all CCs. It originates from the secondary branches of the right and left bile ducts to above the junction of cystic duct and is often associated with chronic inflammation in bile ducts, as in primary sclerosing cholangitis. Perihilar CC often manifests with features of biliary obstruction (pruritus, jaundice, pale stool, and dark urine).
- The **distal** type originates from the cystic duct to the ampulla of Vater. The clinical manifestations are similar to those of the perihilar type.
- **Mixed hepatocellular-cholangiocellular carcinomas** (mixed HCC/CC), also called combined hepatocellular-cholangiocellular carcinomas, have been acknowledged as a distinct subtype of CC. It has features of both HCC and CC and is associated with a worse prognosis compared with hepatocellular carcinoma.

4. **Diagnosis**
   - The definitive diagnosis of all three types of CCs is by biopsy. However, this approach is controversial because of concern for tumor seeding by percutaneous or endoluminal biopsy.
   - Fluorescence in situ hybridization improves the performance of cytology for the diagnosis of perihilar and distal CCs. Elevated serum levels of carbohydrate antigen (CA) 19-9 may also be useful in establishing the diagnosis.
   - CC may be difficult to distinguish from other forms of adenocarcinoma, and in some cases the diagnosis may be confirmed only at laparotomy or autopsy. Mixed HCC/CC may be found in association with cirrhosis.

5. **Treatment**
   - **Surgery** is the treatment of choice for resectable CCs. Distal CC may need to be treated by the Whipple procedure. **Liver transplantation for early-stage perihilar CCs** after neoadjuvant chemotherapy and/or chemoradiation has become an appealing option, but patients must be very carefully selected.
   - Chemotherapy with gemcitabine and cisplatin is recommended for patients with locally advanced or metastatic CC.

PEDIATRIC TUMORS OF THE LIVER (see also Chapter 25)

- Some tumors of the liver occur specifically in children. Furthermore, they often occur at specific ages, as shown in Fig. 29.2.
- **Hepatoblastoma** is the most common primary pediatric liver tumor that occurs in children <3 years of age. It is an embryonal tumor originated from a hepatocyte precursor cell (hepatoblast). The most common presentation is with abdominal distention or an abdominal mass. There are two types: Epithelial and mixed epithelial/mesenchymal

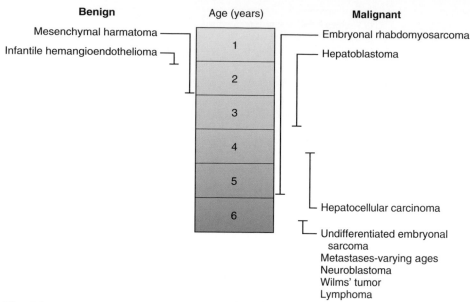

Fig. 29.2 Tumors that occur in children at specific ages. (From Di Bisceglie AM. Tumors of the liver. In: Feldman M, ed. *Atlas of the Liver,* 4th ed. Philadelphia: Springer; 2007. ©A. M. Di Bisceglie.)

hepatoblastoma. The tumor is not associated with cirrhosis. Patients usually have elevated serum AFP levels, but in small-cell undifferentiated hepatoblastoma, the AFP level is normal or low. Hepatoblastoma is considered potentially curable with a combination of surgery and chemotherapy.

■ Although **HCC** is typically a disease of adults, it has been recorded in children as young as 4 years of age in association with HBV infection.

■ Other less common liver malignancies include embryonal sarcoma, angiosarcoma, and embryonal rhabdomyosarcoma.

OTHER TUMORS OF THE LIVER

1. **Epithelioid hemangioendothelioma**
   ■ This is a rare soft tissue tumor of vascular origin that may arise in organs other than the liver, particularly the lung. Histology shows intermediate malignant potential, between that of benign hemangioma and the highly aggressive angiosarcoma.
   ■ Vascular invasion is a prominent feature. Malignant cells in this tumor stain positively for factor VIII. The tumor must be distinguished histologically from angiosarcoma and CC.
   ■ Approximately one third of patients have metastases. Nevertheless, examples of prolonged survival with this tumor are common.
   ■ Surgical resection is the mainstay of treatment, but many patients have malignancy in both lobes, thereby making the tumor unresectable. This tumor is important to recognize because of its malignant behavior and because it is potentially curable with extensive resection or even liver transplantation.
2. **Primary hepatic lymphoma**
   ■ Although secondary involvement of the liver by lymphoma is common, primary lymphoma may also arise in the liver.

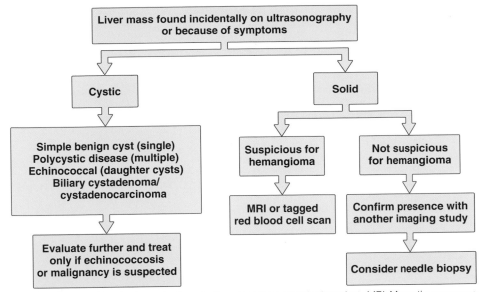

Fig. 29.3 Algorithm for the evaluation of a liver mass in a noncirrhotic patient. *MRI*, Magnetic resonance imaging. (From Di Bisceglie AM. Tumors of the liver. In: Feldman M, ed. *Atlas of the Liver,* 4th ed. Philadelphia: Springer; 2007. ©A. M. Di Bisceglie.)

- These tumors are often of B-cell origin and occur with increased frequency in patients with human immunodeficiency virus infection and acquired immunodeficiency syndrome.
- These tumors respond poorly to chemotherapy and are associated with a poor prognosis.

3. **Angiosarcoma**
    - This is a high-grade malignant tumor of blood vessels arising within the liver.
    - Predisposing factors are exposure to vinyl chloride monomers and exposure to the intravenous contrast agent thorotrast (no longer in use).
    - The tumor grows rapidly, responds poorly to radiation or chemotherapy, and has a poor prognosis.

Diagnostic Approach to Liver Masses or Tumors

The approach is different depending on whether the patient has cirrhosis. An algorithm for evaluating the noncirrhotic patient is shown in Fig. 29.3.

FURTHER READING

Arzumanyan A, Reis HM, Feitelson MA. Pathogenic mechanisms in HBV- and HCV-associated hepatocellular carcinoma. *Nat Rev Cancer.* 2013;13:123–135.

Bridgewater J, Galle PR, Khan SA, et al. Guidelines for the diagnosis and management of intrahepatic cholangiocarcinoma. *J Hepatol.* 2014;60:1268–1289.

Bruix J, Han KH, Gores G, et al. Liver cancer: approaching a personalized care. *J Hepatol.* 2015;62:S144–S156.

Bruix J, Reig M, Sherman M. Evidence-based diagnosis, staging, and treatment of patients with hepatocellular carcinoma. *Gastroenterology.* 2016;150:835–853.

El-Serag HB. Epidemiology of viral hepatitis and hepatocellular carcinoma. *Gastroenterology.* 2012; 142:1264–1273.

Forner A, Llovet JM, Bruix J. Hepatocellular carcinoma. *Lancet.* 2012;379:1245–1255.

Lencioni R, de Baere T, Soulen MC, et al. Lipiodol transarterial chemoembolization for hepatocellular carcinoma: a systematic review of efficacy and safety data. *Hepatology*. 2016;64:106–116.

Lopez-Terrada D, Alaggio R, de Davila MT, et al. Towards an international pediatric liver tumor consensus classification: proceedings of the Los Angeles COG liver tumors symposium. *Mod Pathol*. 2014;27:472–491.

Marrero JA, Ahn J, Reddy RK, et al. ACG clinical guideline: the diagnosis and management of focal liver lesions. *Am J Gastroenterol*. 2014;109:1328–1347.

Mittal S, El-Serag HB, Sada YH, et al. Hepatocellular carcinoma in the absence of cirrhosis in United States veterans is associated with nonalcoholic fatty liver disease. *Clin Gastroenterol Hepatol*. 2016;14:124–131.

Morgan RL, Baack B, Smith BD, et al. Eradication of hepatitis C virus infection and the development of hepatocellular carcinoma: a meta-analysis of observational studies. *Ann Intern Med*. 2013;158:329–337.

Nault JC, Bioulac-Sage P, Zucman-Rossi J. Hepatocellular benign tumors-from molecular classification to personalized clinical care. *Gastroenterology*. 2013;144:888–902.

Razumilava N, Gores GJ. Cholangiocarcinoma. *Lancet*. 2014;383:2168–2179.

Rizvi S, Gores GJ. Pathogenesis, diagnosis, and management of cholangiocarcinoma. *Gastroenterology*. 2013;145:1215–1229.

Siegel RL, Miller KD, Jemal A. Cancer statistics. *CA Cancer J Clin*. 2016;66:7–30.

CHAPTER 30

Hepatic Abscesses and Cysts

Helen M. Ayles, MBBS, MRCP, DTM&H, PhD ■
Sarah Lou Bailey, BSc, MBChB, MRCP

KEY POINTS

1. Hepatic abscesses are most commonly pyogenic in Western countries, but amebic abscesses are common in areas of the world where *Entamoeba histolytica* is endemic. Less frequent causes include fungal and tuberculous abscesses.

2. Diagnosis of hepatic abscess relies on good history taking and simple imaging.

3. The differentiation between amebic and pyogenic hepatic abscess (as well as fungal or tubercular abscess) relies on an adequate history (including travel history), imaging pattern, culture results, and serologic testing.

4. A history of dysentery or diarrhea is present in only 20% of patients with an amebic liver abscess (ALA). Amebic liver abscess is readily treated by antibiotics and luminal amebicides.

5. Pyogenic liver abscess is a life-threatening condition, resulting from infected blood or bile. Abscesses are frequently polymicrobial and include anaerobic organisms. Treatment is with appropriate antibiotics and drainage.

6. The most common infective cause of hepatic cysts worldwide is *Echinococcus granulosus*, the agent of hydatid disease; other noninfective causes include simple cysts, tumors, congenital biliary diseases, and polycystic disease.

Amebic Liver Abscess

OVERVIEW

1. Worldwide, 480 million people are infected with *Entamoeba histolytica.*
2. Amebic infection may be asymptomatic or may manifest as dysentery, ALA, or other (rarer) manifestations.
3. The diagnosis and management of ALA have been revolutionized by advances in imaging and interventional radiology.
4. Treatment now relies almost entirely on drug therapy.

PARASITOLOGY

1. Amebic liver abscess is caused by the protozoan *E. histolytica.* The reservoir of infection is human (Fig. 30.1).
2. The infective form is the cyst (12 μm in diameter), which is ingested. Excystation occurs in the small intestine. The trophozoite (10 to 60 μm) infects the colon and may cause inflammation and dysentery. Amebae spread to the liver through the portal circulation.

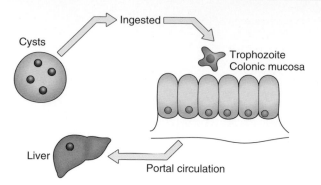

Fig. 30.1 Life cycle of *Entamoeba histolytica*.

3. The cyst is able to survive outside the body for weeks or months, whereas the trophozoite degenerates in minutes.
4. Amebae may be pathogenic or nonpathogenic. The nonpathogenic form has been reclassified as *Entamoeba dispar*. Pathogenic species can be differentiated from nonpathogenic species by the following:
   - Zymodeme analysis: 22 distinct isoenzyme patterns (zymodemes) on electrophoresis have been isolated.
   - RNA and DNA probes

EPIDEMIOLOGY

1. **Infection with *E. histolytica* affects 10% of the world's population**; 40 to 50 million people develop amebic colitis or ALA, and 40,000 to 100,000 deaths occur each year.
2. The prevalence of infection varies from <1% in industrialized countries to 50% to 80% in some tropical regions.
3. Spread is by the fecal-oral route and is increased by the following:
   - Poor sanitation
   - Contamination of food by flies
   - Unhygienic food handling
   - Unclean water
   - Use of human feces as fertilizer
4. **High-risk groups:**
   - Persons of lower socioeconomic status in endemic areas
   - Immigrants from endemic areas
   - Institutionalized populations (e.g., inpatients of psychiatric hospitals)
   - Men who have sex with men
   - Travelers
   - Persons who are immunosuppressed, including those with human immunodeficiency virus (HIV) infection

PATHOGENESIS

1. In the liver, *E. histolytica* lyses the host's tissue with proteolytic enzymes contained in cytoplasmic vacuoles.
2. The hepatic lesion is a well-demarcated abscess consisting of necrotic liver and usually affecting the right lobe. The initial host response to the ameba is neutrophil migration, but the

ameba can also lyse neutrophils, thus releasing their enzymes and assisting in the process of tissue destruction.

3. The abscess contains acellular debris; amebic trophozoites are found only at the periphery of the lesion, where they can invade further.

4. The following host factors contribute to the severity of disease:
   - Age (children more than adults)
   - Pregnancy
   - Malnutrition and alcoholism
   - Glucocorticoid use
   - Malignant disease

CLINICAL FEATURES

- ALA manifests with amebic colitis in fewer than 10% of cases.
- Patients may have a past history of diarrhea or dysentery.
- *E. histolytica* can be isolated from the stool in approximately 50% of cases.

1. Socioeconomic and demographic features
   - Emigrant from or resident in an endemic area
   - Traveler to an endemic area
   - Men more than women (3 to 10 times)
   - Young adults more than children or elderly persons
2. Symptoms
   - Fever, rigors, night sweats
   - Nausea, anorexia, malaise
   - Right upper quadrant abdominal discomfort
   - Weight loss
   - Chest symptoms: Dry cough, pleuritic pain
   - Diaphragmatic irritation: Shoulder tip pain, hiccups
3. Physical examination
   - Fever
   - Tender hepatomegaly
   - Chest signs: Dull right base (usually from raised hemidiaphragm); crackles at right base; pleural rub
   - Jaundice and peritonitis or pericardial rub are rare and poor prognostic signs.

DIAGNOSIS

1. Laboratory findings (Table 30.1)
   - An increased serum bilirubin level is uncommon.
2. Diagnostic imaging
   a. Chest film
      - Elevation of right hemidiaphragm
      - Blunting of right costophrenic angle
      - Atelectasis
   b. Ultrasonography
      - Round or oval single lesion (sometimes multiple)
      - Lack of significant wall echoes, so the transition from abscess to normal liver is abrupt
      - Hypoechoic appearance compared with normal liver; diffuse echoes throughout abscess
      - Peripheral location, close to liver capsule
      - Distal enhancement

TABLE 30.1 ■ **Laboratory Findings in Amebic Liver Abscess**

Laboratory Finding	Frequency (%) or Comment
Leukocytosis	80
Elevated serum alkaline phosphatase level	80
Anemia	>50
Increased erythrocyte sedimentation rate	Common
Proteinuria	Common
Elevated serum aminotransferase levels	Poor prognostic sign

   c. Computed tomography (CT)
      ■ Well-defined lesions, round or oval, mostly single (sometimes multiple)
      ■ Low density compared with surrounding liver tissue
      ■ Nonhomogeneous internal structure
   d. Magnetic resonance imaging (MRI)
      ■ Abscess characterized by low signal intensity on T1-weighted images and high signal intensity on T2-weighted images
   e. Radionuclide imaging
      ■ ALA appears as a cold spot, apparently distinguishing it from a pyogenic abscess; this modality has not been researched extensively for this use.
3. Serologic tests: **The detection of antibodies is the mainstay of diagnosis of invasive amoebiasis. Positive serologic tests are found in 95% to 100% of patients with ALA,** even if they have received some antiamebic therapy.
      ■ Commercial enzyme-linked immunosorbent assay (ELISA) is most commonly used and has a sensitivity and specificity as high as 97.9% and 94.8%, respectively.
      ■ The ELISA is positive in *all* forms of invasive amebic disease (including dysentery). Serologic tests may remain positive for a prolonged period even after treatment of ALA. Combined testing may be necessary for accurate diagnosis.
      ■ The cellulose acetate precipitation (CAP) test is highly sensitive and specific; it becomes negative quickly after successful treatment and is regarded as a reference test for amebic serology.
4. **Aspiration of abscess** (when the diagnosis is uncertain or rupture is imminent)
      ■ Yellow to dark brown "anchovy sauce"
      ■ Odorless
      ■ "Pus" consisting mainly of acellular debris; most amebae are found in the abscess wall.
      ■ Absence of bacteria on culture (mixed amebic and pyogenic abscesses more commonly reported especially with nucleic acid diagnostic techniques)
      ■ Polymerase chain reaction (PCR) testing for *E. histolytica* confirms the diagnosis.

COMPLICATIONS

1. Rupture of abscess into the following:
   a. Chest, causing
      ■ Hepatobronchial fistula (± expectoration of "anchovy" pus)
      ■ Lung abscess
      ■ Amebic empyema
   b. Pericardium, causing
      ■ Heart failure

- ■ Pericarditis
- ■ Cardiac tamponade (often fatal; may be followed by constrictive pericarditis)
  c. Peritoneum, causing
- ■ Peritonitis
- ■ Ascites
2. Secondary infection is usually iatrogenic following aspiration.
3. Other complications (rare)
   - ■ Acute liver failure
   - ■ Hemobilia
   - ■ Inferior vena cava obstruction
   - ■ Budd-Chiari syndrome
   - ■ Hematogenous spread causing cerebral abscess
4. Factors predisposing to complications
   - ■ Age >40 years
   - ■ Concomitant glucocorticoid use
   - ■ Multiple abscesses
   - ■ Large abscess (>10 cm in diameter)
   - ■ Erythrocyte sedimentation rate (ESR) and C-reactive protein levels are reported to be high in patients who present with or develop systemic complications.

TREATMENT AND PROGNOSIS

Treatment of amebic liver abscess is usually with drugs alone.
1. **Commonly used regimens** (administered orally)
   - ■ Metronidazole 750 mg three times daily for 5 to 10 days (pediatric, 35 to 50 mg/kg per day in three divided doses for 5 days), or
   - ■ Tinidazole 2 g/day for 3 days (pediatric, 50 to 60 mg/kg daily for 5 days), or
   - ■ Chloroquine 1 g loading dose for 1 to 2 days, then 500 mg/day for 20 days (pediatric, 10 mg/kg base).
   - ■ **Luminal amebicides** must **always** be used following the aforementioned regimens.
     - – Diloxanide furoate 500 mg three times daily (pediatric, 20 mg/kg per day in three divided doses) for 10 days, or
     - – Diiodohydroxyquin 650 mg three times daily (pediatric, 30 to 40 mg/kg per day in three divided doses; maximum 2 g/day) for 20 days, or
     - – Paromomycin sulfate 25 to 35 mg/kg/day in three divided doses (pediatric, 25 to 35 mg/kg per day in three divided doses) for 5 to 10 days
2. Optimal management
   - ■ **Patients with suspected ALA should be started on therapy while awaiting serologic confirmation.** Response is usually rapid, with defervescence occurring in 48 to 72 hours.
   - ■ In uncomplicated ALA, such as those with small solitary right lobe abscesses, there is no evidence that therapeutic aspiration, in combination with drug therapy, improves time to resolution of symptoms or reduces hospitalization.
   - ■ Critically ill patients, those with left lobe abscess, or those who do not respond to initial drug therapy may require radiologically guided fine-needle aspiration to avoid rupture and to exclude a pyogenic abscess.
   - ■ Complications such as rupture of the abscess may be managed medically but often require percutaneous drainage (Fig. 30.2). Surgical drainage is seldom required.
3. Prognosis
   a. Amebic liver abscess is an **eminently treatable** condition.

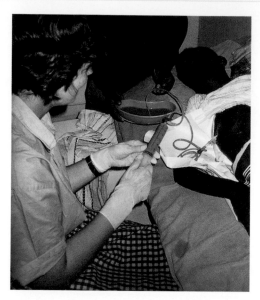

Fig. 30.2   Drainage of an amebic liver abscess in rural Africa.

  b. The mortality rate is <1% in uncomplicated disease.
  c. Delay in diagnosis may result in abscess rupture, with a higher mortality rate.
  ■ Rupture into chest or peritoneum: 20% mortality rate
  ■ Rupture into pericardium: 32% to 100% mortality rate

Pyogenic Liver Abscess

OVERVIEW

1. **Pyogenic liver abscess is a life-threatening condition.**
2. The incidence varies but is estimated to be 8 to 20 per 100,000 hospital admissions in the United States.
3. Improvements in prognosis have resulted from better imaging and microbiologic analysis, but delays in diagnosis or failure to recognize this condition can result in high morbidity and mortality rates.
4. Pyogenic liver abscess is most frequently secondary to bile duct obstruction but is often associated with other medical conditions such as diabetes mellitus, immunosuppressive therapies, systemic infection, diverticular disease, and colorectal carcinoma.

MICROBIOLOGY

Cultures of blood or abscess contents are positive in most cases.
■ Abscesses are **often polymicrobial.**
■ *Klebsiella* species (particularly *K. pneumonia*e) have overtaken *Escherichia coli* as the most commonly reported causative bacteria.
■ Microaerophilic organisms, particularly *Streptococcus anginosus (S. milleri),* are increasingly common causes but need careful cultivation to isolate.

TABLE 30.2 ■ **Comparisons Between Two Retrospective Population-Based Studies of Patients with Pyogenic Liver Abscess**

	North America N = 17,787 1994–2005		Taiwan N = 1522 2000–2011	

Demographics and Underlying Conditions

Age (% of total)

Age	%	Age	%
18–34	8.5	20–29	2.8
35–49	18.5	30–39	6.5
50–64	30.1	40–49	13.9
65–85	42.9	50–59	24.0
		60–69	21.0
		>70	31.8

Gender (%)

Male	Female	Male	Female
59.9	40.1	63.6	36.4

Comorbidities (%)

Biliary disease	21.9	Diabetes mellitus	35.3
Diabetes mellitus	20.1	Cholelithiasis	13.1
History of cancer	16.2	Hepatocellular carcinoma	9.8
History of liver transplant	3.3	Cirrhosis	6.5
Cirrhosis	2.7	Viral hepatitis	6.1
Chronic renal failure	1.4	Other malignancies	5.5
		Renal disease	1.7

Incidence

Overall	3.59/100,000	13.52/100,000
Trend	Increasing from 2.7 to 4.1/100,000	Increasing from 10.8 to 15.5/100,000

Management and outcome

Mortality (%)	5.6	8.2
Complications (%)	N/A	10.8%

N/A, Not available.

From Meddings L, Myers RP, Hubbard J, et al. A population-based study of pyogenic liver abscesses in the United States: incidence, mortality, and temporal trends. *Am J Gastroenterol.* 2010;105:117–124; Chen YC, Lin CH, Chang SN, et al. Epidemiology and clinical outcome of pyogenic liver abscess: an analysis from the National Health Insurance Research Database of Taiwan, 2000-2011. *J Microbiol Immunol Infect.* 2016;49:646-653.

■ Anaerobic organisms are commonly isolated from polymicrobial abscesses.
■ Unusual organisms include *Salmonella, Haemophilus,* and *Yersinia* spp. Tuberculosis, actinomycosis, and melioidosis also occur, especially in patients with defective immunity (e.g., HIV infection, posttransplantation status).

EPIDEMIOLOGY

1. Pyogenic liver abscess is rare; population-based studies report an incidence of 3.6/100,000 in the United States, with increasing incidence being seen in some parts of Asia such as Taiwan, where an incidence of 17.6/100,000 is reported. Table 30.2 shows data from two population-based studies—one in the United States and one in Taiwan.

2. Compared to ALA, pyogenic liver abscess occurs more commonly in middle-aged and older people. It is seen equally in men and women.
3. Pyogenic liver abscess often occurs in patients with a **predisposing medical condition.**
   - Biliary disease
   - Hypertension
   - Malignant disease
   - Previous abdominal surgery or endoscopic procedure
   - Diabetes mellitus
   - Cardiovascular disease
   - Crohn disease
   - Diverticulitis
   - History of trauma
4. No geographic or racial differences are noted.

PATHOGENESIS

1. Pyogenic infection is carried to the liver through the blood or bile. Frequently, no infective source is found (cryptogenic liver abscess); however, when one can be identified, **common sources** include the following:
   - Cholangitis, secondary to biliary stricture, stones, or endoscopic intervention
   - Intraabdominal sepsis (e.g., diverticulitis, peritonitis)
   - Generalized septicemia
   - Dental infection
   - Trauma, including liver biopsy or surgery
   - Secondary infection of a preexisting liver cyst, neoplasm (including after ablative therapy), or rarely an amebic abscess
2. The right lobe of the liver is the most frequently involved.
3. Abscesses may be single or multiple; those caused by hematogenous spread are frequently multiple.
4. The abscess contains polymorphonuclear neutrophils and necrotic liver cells surrounded by a fibrous capsule.

CLINICAL FEATURES

1. History
Table 30.2 shows the results of two retrospective hospital-based studies showing frequencies of presenting symptoms and a history of comorbidities.
2. Physical examination
   - Fever
   - Finger clubbing (rare)
   - Jaundice
   - Tender hepatomegaly
   - **The classic triad of fever, jaundice, and tender hepatomegaly is found in <10% of patients.**

DIAGNOSIS

1. Laboratory findings (Table 30.3)
2. Diagnostic imaging
   a. Chest film abnormal in 50%

TABLE 30.3 ■ **Clinical Features from Two Hospital-Based Retrospective Studies of Pyogenic Liver Abscess**

	United Kingdom N = 73 1993–2008	Australia N = 63 1998–2008
Demographics		
Age	Mean 64.7 (21–93)	Mean 64 (31–97)
Gender (%)	Male 53 (73%) Female 20 (27%)	Male 42 (67%) Female 21 (33%)
Duration	17.3 days (range 1–168)	7 days
Symptoms and Signs (%)		
Anorexia	62	–
Abdominal pain	60	RUQ tenderness 39
Fever	58	59
Nausea/vomiting	50	–
Weight loss	45	–
Hepatomegaly	32	–
Jaundice	25	–
Shock	18	13
Ascites	10	–
Abnormal Laboratory Values (%)		
Hemoglobin <10 g/dL	19	24
White blood cell count >10 × 10⁹/L	93	74
C-reactive protein >10 mg/L	100	100
Serum bilirubin	38 (>22 µmol/L)	54 (>18 µmol/L)
Alanine aminotransferase elevation	63	73
Alkaline phosphatase elevation	85	71
Albumin <35 g/L	95	73
Microbiology Results (%)		
Streptococcus anginosus	12	25
Escherichia coli	24	16
Klebsiella spp.	10	21

RUQ, Right upper quadrant.

From Bosanko NC, Chauhan A, Brookes M, et al. Presentations of pyogenic liver abscess in one UK centre over a 15-year period. *J R Coll Physicians Edinb.* 2011;41:13–17; Pang TC, Fung T, Samra J, et al. Pyogenic liver abscess: an audit of 10 years' experience. *World J Gastroenterol.* 2011;17:1622–1630.

■ Elevation of right hemidiaphragm
■ Blunting of right costophrenic angle
■ Atelectasis
■ If a gas-forming organism is the cause of abscess, fluid levels may be visible below the diaphragm.
b. Ultrasonography
■ Round, oval, or elliptoid lesion
■ Irregular margin
■ Hypoechoic with variable internal echoes

   c. CT
- Highly sensitive; detects up to 94% of lesions
- Lesions show reduced attenuation and possibly enhance with contrast.

   d. MRI
- More sensitive than CT for detecting small lesions
- Lesions have low signal intensity on T1-weighted images and very high signal intensity on T2-weighted images; lesions enhance with gadolinium.

   e. Radioisotope study
- Gallium is avidly taken up by abscesses.

3. Microbiology
- Blood cultures should be taken before initiation of antibiotic therapy.
- Positive blood cultures occur in 50% to 100%.
- Aspiration of the abscess increases the yield of a positive microbiologic diagnosis.
- In polymicrobial abscesses, all the causative organisms may not be present in the blood.

COMPLICATIONS

- Sepsis and associated complications including shock, acute respiratory distress syndrome, renal failure
- Metastatic infection, especially common with *Klebsiella,* including endophthalmitis, meningitis, brain abscess, and pneumonia
- Rupture with local infection such as empyema or peritonitis

TREATMENT

1. In the past, standard treatment involved open surgical drainage of the abscess in combination with broad-spectrum antibiotics. Studies since the 1990s have shown improved results with either **percutaneous drainage or aspiration in combination with antibiotics.** Some patients can be managed medically without surgery or aspiration.
2. It is usually possible to combine diagnostic and therapeutic aspiration in these patients.
3. Complications of drainage include hemorrhage, perforation of a viscus, infection from the drain, and catheter displacement.
4. **Antibiotic therapy should include coverage against gram-negative organisms as well as microaerophilic and anaerobic organisms.** Empiric first-line regimens are as follows:
   - Suspected biliary source: Ampicillin + gentamicin + metronidazole
   - Suspected colonic source: Third-generation cephalosporin + metronidazole
5. Antibiotic therapy is usually administered intravenously initially. The duration of intravenous antibiotic therapy and the decision to change to oral therapy are governed by the individual clinical response. Antibiotic use for a **total duration of 2 to 3 weeks** is recommended.
6. Surgical intervention may be required if the patient fails to respond rapidly to therapy; a flexible approach must be adopted.

PROGNOSIS

1. Untreated pyogenic liver abscess has a mortality rate approaching 100%.
2. Mortality rates have decreased to as low as 2.5%, but are usually 10% to 30%, depending on the underlying cause of the abscess and associated medical conditions. Improved mortality rates are thought to result from advanced imaging and diagnostic techniques and the use of percutaneous drainage.

3. Increased mortality has been associated with older age, bacteremia, and the presence of multiple comorbidities and malignancy.
4. Decreased mortality has been seen in patients who undergo percutaneous aspiration compared with those who do not, presumably because of a greater ability to tailor the choice of antibiotics.

Hepatic Cysts

OVERVIEW

Causes of cystic lesions in the liver are diverse.

1. **Congenital**
   a. **Polycystic disease**
      - **Infantile polycystic disease** is a rare autosomal recessive condition that results in cyst formation in the liver and kidneys. Hepatomegaly is often present at birth. Renal damage is usually the cause of reduced life span.
      - **Adult polycystic disease** is most commonly an autosomal dominant condition predominantly affecting the kidneys but with hepatic cysts in 33% of patients.
         - It is rarely associated with liver dysfunction.
         - Genes responsible for autosomal dominant polycystic kidney disease are *PKD-1* and *PKD-2*, which express polycystin-1 and -2, respectively. Isolated polycystic liver disease has been linked to two genes, *PRKCSH* and *SEC63*, which express hepatocystin and SEC63p, respectively. The gene responsible for autosomal recessive polycystic kidney disease is *PKHD1*, which expresses fibrocystin.
         - Treatment should be considered only in the presence of symptoms. The optimal management is debated but depends on cyst morphology, severity of cystic disease, comorbidity, and recurrence rates; options include cyst unroofing (fenestration), liver resection, and, for those with end-stage disease, liver transplantation.
   b. Choledochal cysts (see also Chapter 35)
      - Many disease entities manifest with cystic dilatation of the biliary tract. **Caroli disease** is one of these conditions in which nonobstructive dilatation of intrahepatic bile ducts occurs.
2. **Acquired**
   a. **Benign tumors** (e.g., hamartomas)
   b. **Simple cysts**
      - Most are small and incidental.
      - Treatment is indicated only for symptomatic cysts: Aspiration combined with sclerosis, open surgery, or laparoscopic cyst unroofing, which is considered to be the optimal standard of care.
   c. **Infective**, most commonly hydatid disease (caused by *Echinococcus granulosus;* see the discussion that follows)

Hydatid Disease of the Liver (Fig. 30.3)

OVERVIEW

- Hydatid cystic disease has a worldwide distribution and is endemic in many sheep- and cattle-rearing regions of the world.
- Hydatid disease is a chronic and potentially dangerous condition that is often overlooked as a cause of abdominal pain and hepatic disease.

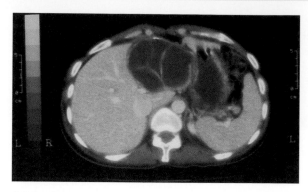

Fig. 30.3   Computed tomography of a multilocular hydatid cyst of the liver.

PARASITOLOGY

Hydatid cystic disease is caused by *Echinococcus granulosus*.

- *E. granulosus* is a 3- to 6-mm tapeworm.
- A carnivorous host, usually a dog, becomes infected by eating the viscera of infected sheep that contain hydatid cysts.
- Scolices from the cysts adhere to the small intestine of the dog and develop into the tapeworm.
- The tapeworm produces up to 500 ova in the host bowel.
- Infected dogs excrete *Echinococcus* eggs in feces. Eggs are viable in the environment for several weeks.
- Eggs are ingested by humans, either from contamination of soil and foodstuffs or from the dog's coat, and they hatch in the intestine to form oncospheres that invade tissue to enter the portal circulation.
- Each oncosphere matures into a vesicle and subsequently a cyst, the metacestode.
- Cysts can form in any organ, most commonly the liver (50% to 70%). Cysts consist of a germinal layer that buds asexually to form daughter cysts, which contain protoscolices, the infective forms that are ingested by the definitive host (Fig. 30.4).

EPIDEMIOLOGY

1. Infections with *E. granulosus* occur worldwide. The scale of human disease is not fully documented, but rural communities face a significant health problem from infection.
   Areas with a documented high prevalence of disease include the following sheep farming areas:
   - Mediterranean countries
   - Northern Kenya (Turkana district)
   - Areas of South America
   - Wales
   - New Zealand
2. A case-control study conducted in Spain found that **long-term coexistence with dogs is a major risk factor** for the development of *E. granulosus* infection, especially coexistence with dogs with the opportunity to eat potentially infected offal.

PATHOGENESIS

1. Spread of oncospheres is through the bloodstream, usually the portal circulation, and results in hepatic disease in 50% to 70% of cases. Other sites of disease are as follows:
   - Lung (20% to 30%)
   - Bone (<10%)

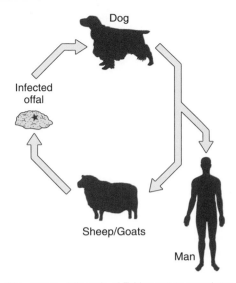

Fig. 30.4 Life cycle of *Echinococcus granulosus*.

- Brain
- Heart
2. Cysts enlarge slowly and cause tissue damage directly or by compromising the blood supply. The parasite causes a host response to form a collagenous capsule around the germinal layer. This capsule may calcify. Often, no host inflammatory response occurs.

CLINICAL FEATURES

1. Symptoms
   - Cysts may be asymptomatic and often become symptomatic only after decades, because of their slow growth. Symptoms are caused by pressure effects.
   - Symptoms may follow cyst rupture or leakage.
   - The presentation of a secondary infection of a hydatid cyst resembles the presentation of a pyogenic abscess.
2. Physical examination
   - Tender mass
   - Chest signs, especially at the right base
   - Fever
   - Jaundice

DIAGNOSIS

1. Laboratory findings
   - Elevated serum alkaline phosphatase level
   - Peripheral eosinophilia (>7%) in 30% of patients, usually indicating leakage or rupture of cyst
   - Elevated serum bilirubin level (uncommon)
2. Diagnostic imaging
   a. Chest film
      - Elevation of the right hemidiaphragm
      - Cysts may be visible in the lung.
      - Calcification of hepatic cyst may be visible below the diaphragm.

  b. Ultrasonography
     ■ Cysts may be anechoic.
     ■ Cysts are typically round.
     ■ Septate or daughter cysts are often visible.
     ■ Separation of germinal membrane may be seen: "Water-lily sign."
     ■ Collapsed cysts may be visible.
     ■ Calcification of cyst wall
     ■ Hydatid "sand"
  c. CT (see Fig. 30.3)
     ■ Germinal layer seen clearly
     ■ Daughter cysts readily visualized
     ■ Lesion is of low attenuation: 3 to 30 Hounsfield units.
  d. MRI
     ■ Characteristic low-intensity rim 4 to 5 mm thick, best seen on T2-weighted images
     ■ Lesion center nonhomogeneous
     ■ Lesion is hypointense on T1-weighted images, hyperintense on T2-weighted images.
3. Serologic tests: Indirect hemagglutination (IHA) and ELISA are 75% to 94% sensitive. Specificity is lower, necessitating a confirmatory test (e.g., molecular biologic methods, immunoblotting).
4. Molecular biologic tests: PCR-derived probes allow diagnosis and species differentiation.

COMPLICATIONS

1. Leakage or rupture of cyst (sometimes iatrogenic from aspiration of undiagnosed hydatid cyst) may result in the following:
   ■ Allergic reaction, including anaphylaxis (may be fatal)
   ■ Dissemination of disease
   ■ Cholangitis if cyst ruptures into the biliary tract
   ■ Hemoptysis and secondary infection if bronchial rupture
2. Secondary infection of cyst behaves like a pyogenic abscess.

TREATMENT

1. Limited evidence exists for the best management of hydatid cysts. The World Health Organization Informal Working Group on Echinococcosis (WHO-IWGE) have provided expert opinion based on many cases that relies on an image-based classification and stage-specific approach to therapy. Fig. 30.5 shows the categorization of cysts.
2. **Therapeutic options depend on the classification of the cyst, available surgical and medical expertise, and ability of the patient to adhere to long-term monitoring.** Table 30.4 shows the consensus view from the WHO-IWGE.
3. **Surgery** is the treatment of choice for complex cysts, such as larger cysts with daughter cysts, peripheral cysts at risk of rupture, infected cysts, and larger class CE2 and CE3a cysts. Surgical options include the following:
   ■ Radical surgery: Pericystectomy or hepatic resection
   ■ Conservative surgical treatment through unroofing and management of the residual cavity
   ■ Laparoscopic procedures
The technique chosen depends on the condition of the patient, characteristics of the cyst, and experience of the surgeon. The complication rate of surgery may be high. For example, in a series of 59 patients, 57% had dissemination of infection, secondary infection, fistula formation, or complications from seepage of scolicidal agents into the biliary tract (causing a syndrome resembling sclerosing cholangitis).

CL CE1 CE2 CE3 CE4 CE5

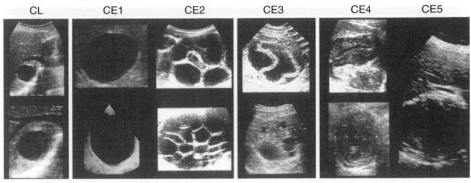

Fig. 30.5 World Health Organization Informal Working Group on Echinococcus classification of hydatid cysts. *CE*, Cystic echinococcus; *CL*, cystic lesions. *CE1* is unilocular; *CE2* is multilocular with daughter cysts or septae; *CE3* has a detached membrane or daughter cysts in a solid matrix; *CE4* has a heterogenous matrix; and *CE5* has a solid cyst wall. (From Brunetti E, Kern P, Vuitton DA. Writing panel for the W-I. Expert consensus for the diagnosis and treatment of cystic and alveolar echinococcosis in humans. *Acta Trop.* 2010;114:1–16.)

TABLE 30.4 ■ Therapeutic Options for Treatment of Hydatid Liver Cysts

WHO Classification[a]	Cyst Size	Therapeutic Option
CE1	≤5 cm	Drug therapy
	>5 cm	PAIR plus drug therapy
CE2	—	Non-PAIR percutaneous therapy
CE3a	≤5 cm	Drug therapy
	>5 cm	PAIR plus drug therapy
CE3b	—	Non-PAIR percutaneous therapy plus drug therapy
CE4	—	Watch and wait
CE5	—	Watch and wait

[a]See Fig. 30.5.

CE, Cystic echinococcus; *PAIR*, puncture, aspiration installation of protoscolicide for 5 to 10 minutes and re-aspiration; *WHO*, World Health Organization.

- Regardless of the type of surgical technique used, **the combination of surgery with drug therapy is the safest and most effective approach.**
- Hydatid cysts manifesting with secondary infection should be treated as pyogenic abscesses; however, aspiration of an infected hydatid cyst is more hazardous than is aspiration of a pyogenic abscess.
4. **Drug therapy** includes the following:
   a. **Albendazole is the drug of choice:** 10 to 14 mg/kg/day orally for 3 months initially (may continue for 1 year) or
   b. Mebendazole: 30 to 70 mg/kg/day orally for 3 months (may require up to 200 mg/kg per day)
      - Benzimidazole agents act on the germinal layer.
   c. Praziquantel: 40 mg/kg orally per day for 14 days; has been used as a protoscolicide and, as such, has an important role preoperatively.

TABLE 30.5 ■ **Comparison of Amebic and Pyogenic Liver Abscess and Hydatid Cyst**

Parameter	Amebic Liver Abscess	Pyogenic Liver Abscess	Hydatid Cyst
Age	Any, mostly younger	Any, mostly older	Any, mostly older
Sex	Male > female	Equal	Equal
Epidemiologic features	Residence or travel in endemic area; poverty, poor hygiene	None; occasional association with helminth infection	Residence in endemic area; farm animal exposure
Associated medical conditions	Rare	Common (e.g., surgery; biliary tract disease; diverticulitis)	Rare
Significant jaundice	Rare	Common	Rare
Multiple lesions	Infrequent	Common	Septate and daughter cysts
Liver biochemical test levels	Mildly abnormal	More markedly abnormal	Mildly abnormal
Amebic serology	Positive	Negative	Negative
Hydatid serology	Negative	Negative	Positive
Blood cultures	Negative; positive result indicates superinfection	Frequently positive	Negative; positive result indicates superinfection
Abscess contents	Thick fluid; variable color, yellow-brown, odorless	Pus; creamy yellow, foul smelling	Aspiration not recommended; thin fluid
Effectiveness of medical therapy	Almost always	Often	Sometimes but often used in combination with surgery
Surgery required	Rarely	Sometimes	Often

5. Percutaneous techniques are minimally invasive procedures and are the procedures of choice in patients in whom surgery is not an option.
   ■ **PAIR** (*p*uncture, *a*spiration *i*nstallation of protoscolicide for 5 to 10 minutes and *r*e-aspiration) is recommended for class CE1 and CE3a cysts.
   ■ Other percutaneous techniques are used when PAIR would not be safe because of the location or complexity of the cyst (class CE2, CE3b) and combine resection and aspiration.
   ■ Large cysts (>10 cm) may require continuous percutaneous drainage.
   ■ Drug therapy starting before aspiration and continuing for 1 month after percutaneous therapy is required.

PROGNOSIS

1. Hydatid cysts may remain asymptomatic throughout a person's life.
2. Cyst rupture or infection is associated with considerable mortality.
3. Watchful waiting may be warranted in the case of uncomplicated, inactive cysts. This involves regular ultrasonography scans to observe the cysts.

Diagnostic Approach to Hepatic Abscesses and Cysts

Clinical, diagnostic, and therapeutic ccomparisons of ALA, pyogenic liver abscess, and hydatid cysts are summarized in Table 30.5. A diagnostic approach to distinguishing liver abscesses from cysts is summarized in Fig. 30.6. Key features include the following:
■ Important clues to the diagnosis are found in a carefully taken history from the patient.
■ The geographic history is of vital importance.

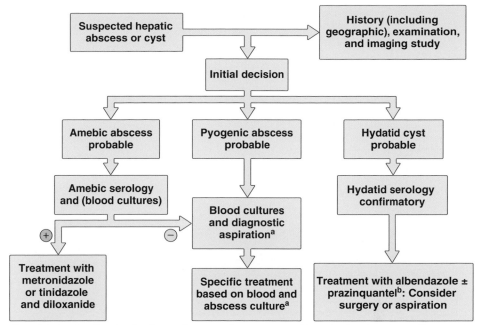

Fig. 30.6 Algorithm for the diagnostic approach to a suspected hepatic abscess or cyst. [a]Presumptive treatment is usually begun on the basis of clinical suspicion pending test results. [b]Indications for diagnostic aspiration: Diagnosis of pyogenic abscess, critically ill patient requiring urgent diagnosis, failure of initial therapy.

SEROLOGIC TESTS AND BLOOD CULTURES

- Serologic tests are positive in 90% to 100% of cases of amebic liver abscess.
- Serologic tests are positive in 75% to 95% of cases of hepatic hydatid disease.
- Blood cultures should be performed on all febrile patients; amebic and hydatid cavities may become superinfected.
- Blood cultures alone are positive in at least 50% of patients with a pyogenic liver abscess.

IMAGING

- Imaging confirms the diagnosis of a cyst or abscess.
- **Ultrasonography is the investigation of choice** because of high sensitivity, lack of radiation, low cost, and ready availability.
- CT may provide further information, especially in pyogenic liver abscess (contrast enhanced) and hydatid disease.
- MRI may be more sensitive than ultrasonography and CT for detecting small lesions.

ASPIRATION

- Required for diagnosis and treatment in cases of suspected pyogenic abscess
- Gives a microbiologic diagnosis in more than 80% of patients with pyogenic abscess. Combined aspiration and blood cultures positively identify the causative organism in more than 85% of cases.
- May be performed in cases of suspected amebic abscess if the abscess is large and rupture is imminent or if the diagnosis is in doubt. Usually, aspiration is *not* required for diagnosis.

- In the case of suspected hydatid disease, aspiration should only be performed by an experienced operator under imaging guidance through as thick a rim of normal liver as possible and preferably as part of a planned PAIR procedure. It may be indicated if the cyst appears to be infected. In the event of aspiration of a hydatid cyst, efforts should be taken to prevent leakage of cyst contents, which has potentially serious sequelae.

FURTHER READING

Alam F, Salam MA, Hassan P, et al. Amebic liver abscess in northern region of Bangladesh: sociodemographic determinants and clinical outcomes. *BMC Res Notes.* 2014;7:625.

Bammigatti C, Ramasubramanian NS, Kadhiravan T, et al. Percutaneous needle aspiration in uncomplicated amebic liver abscess: a randomized trial. *Trop Doct.* 2013;43:19–22.

Bosanko NC, Chauhan A, Brookes M, et al. Presentations of pyogenic liver abscess in one UK centre over a 15-year period. *J R Coll Physicians Edinb.* 2011;41:13–17.

Brunetti E, Kern P, Vuitton DA, et al. Expert consensus for the diagnosis and treatment of cystic and alveolar echinococcosis in humans. *Acta Trop.* 2010;114:1–16.

Chavez-Tapia NC, Hernandez-Calleros J, Tellez-Avila FI, et al. Image-guided percutaneous procedure plus metronidazole versus metronidazole alone for uncomplicated amoebic liver abscess. *Cochrane Database Syst Rev.* 2009;(1): CD004886.

Chen YC, Lin CH, Chang SN, et al. Epidemiology and clinical outcome of pyogenic liver abscess: an analysis from the National Health Insurance Research Database of Taiwan, 2000-2011. *J Microbiol Immunol Infect.* 2016;49:646–653.

Congly SE, Shaheen AA, Meddings L, et al. Amoebic liver abscess in USA: a population-based study of incidence, temporal trends and mortality. *Liver Int.* 2011;31:1191–1198.

Heneghan HM, Healy NA, Martin ST, et al. Modern management of pyogenic hepatic abscess: a case series and review of the literature. *BMC Res Notes.* 2011;4:80.

Jaiswal V, Ghoshal U, Baijal SS, et al. Evaluation of antigen detection and polymerase chain reaction for diagnosis of amoebic liver abscess in patients on anti-amoebic treatment. *BMC Res Notes.* 2012;5:416.

Meddings L, Myers RP, Hubbard J, et al. A population-based study of pyogenic liver abscesses in the United States: incidence, mortality, and temporal trends. *Am J Gastroenterol.* 2010;105:117–124.

Nunnari G, Pinzone MR, Gruttadauria S, et al. Hepatic echinococcosis: clinical and therapeutic aspects. *World J Gastroenterol.* 2012;18:1448–1458.

Pang TC, Fung T, Samra J, et al. Pyogenic liver abscess: an audit of 10 years' experience. *World J Gastroenterol.* 2011;17:1622–1630.

Reyna-Fabian ME, Zermeno V, Ximenez C, et al. Analysis of the bacterial diversity in liver abscess: differences between pyogenic and amebic abscesses. *Am J Trop Med Hyg.* 2016;94:147–155.

Rinaldi F, De Silvestri A, Tamarozzi F, et al. Medical treatment versus "watch and wait" in the clinical management of CE3b echinococcal cysts of the liver. *BMC Infect Dis.* 2014;14:492.

CHAPTER 31

Other Infections Involving the Liver

Patricia Pringle, MD ■ Raymond T. Chung, MD

KEY POINTS

1 Primary bacterial infection of the liver is rare. Systemic infections can cause hepatic derangements, ranging from mild liver biochemical test abnormalities to frank jaundice and, rarely, hepatic failure.

2 Many different spirochetal, protozoal, helminthic, and fungal organisms can involve the liver.

3 Schistosomiasis, capillariasis, toxocariasis, and strongyloidosis evoke strong host inflammatory responses and hepatic fibrosis that contribute to the hepatic manifestations.

4 Leishmaniasis and malaria lead to disease primarily through disruption of reticuloendothelial system function.

5 Liver flukes and ascariasis cause cholangitis and biliary hyperplasia; liver fluke infection is associated with cholangiocarcinoma.

6 Echinococcosis causes cystic disease (see Chapter 30).

7 Advances in drug therapy have rendered nearly all nonviral infections of the liver readily treatable; therefore, prompt diagnosis in the appropriate clinical context is essential.

Bacterial Infections Involving the Liver

Bacterial infections can affect the liver directly and often give a clinical picture of acute hepatitis.

LEGIONELLA PNEUMOPHILA

■ Pneumonia is the predominant clinical manifestation; abnormal liver biochemical test levels are frequent, usually without jaundice and without affecting the clinical outcome.

■ Liver histologic features are nonspecific, with portal infiltration, microvesicular steatosis, and focal necrosis; occasional organisms are seen.

■ Initial treatment is with a **fluoroquinolone or macrolide antibiotic.**

STAPHYLOCOCCUS AUREUS AND STREPTOCOCCUS PYOGENES (TOXIC SHOCK SYNDROME)

■ Multisystem disease caused by massive immune activation by superantigens: Staphylococcal toxic shock syndrome toxin (TSST-1), streptococcal toxic shock syndrome toxin (STSS), and other enterotoxins. *S. aureus* cases were described originally in association with tampon use and are now more frequently a complication of surgical wound infections, most commonly in the postpartum period. The case-fatality rate is 1.8% in menstrual cases and 5% in nonmenstrual cases. *S. pyogenes* cases are typically caused by invasive infections.

- Typical findings include fever, a scarlatiniform rash (coarse rash with punctate dark papules on a diffuse erythematous base), mucosal hyperemia, vomiting, diarrhea, and hypotension, with rapid development of multiorgan failure. Hepatic involvement is almost always present, results from hypoperfusion and circulating toxins, and is marked by deep jaundice and high serum aminotransferase levels.
- Liver histologic findings include microvesicular steatosis, necrosis, and centrilobular cholestasis.
- The diagnosis is primarily clinical and infrequently confirmed by culture of toxigenic *S. aureus* or *S. pyogenes* or by demonstration of superantigens.
- Treatment of **S. aureus infection** is with **intravenous clindamycin plus nafcillin for methicillin-sensitive isolates or vancomycin or linezolid for methicillin-resistant isolates; S. pyogenes infection** is treated with **clindamycin and penicillin.** Intravenous immune globulin may be beneficial in cases of *Staphylococcus* toxic shock syndrome, but data are more convincing for its use in cases caused by *S. pyogenes.*

CLOSTRIDIUM PERFRINGENS

- Usually seen in association with a mixed anaerobic infection that results in rapid development of local wound pain, abdominal pain, and diarrhea, *Clostridium perfringens* infection is associated with myonecrosis or gas gangrene.
- Jaundice may develop in up to 20% of patients with gas gangrene and is predominantly a consequence of massive intravascular hemolysis caused by the bacterial exotoxin, with resulting unconjugated hyperbilirubinemia.
- Liver involvement may include abscess formation and gas in the portal vein.
- The case survival rate is approximately 80%.
- Treatment is with **intravenous penicillin and clindamycin.**

LISTERIA MONOCYTOGENES

- Infection caused by *L. monocytogenes* is characterized by meningoencephalitis and pneumonitis; hepatic involvement in adult human infection is rare.
- Neonates, older adults, pregnant women, and patients with immune deficiency are most commonly affected.
- Serum aminotransferase levels are typically high with liver involvement.
- Patients may present with a single abscess, multiple microabscesses, or diffuse or granulomatous hepatitis; the outcome is worse with multiple abscesses.
- Treatment is with **ampicillin and gentamycin,** typically for 3 to 4 weeks.

NEISSERIA GONORRHOEAE

- Half of all patients with disseminated gonococcal infection have abnormal liver biochemical test levels, mainly elevated serum alkaline phosphatase levels, and elevated aspartate aminotransferase (AST) levels. Jaundice is uncommon.
- Perihepatitis **(Fitz-Hugh–Curtis syndrome)** is a common complication of gonococcal infection that affects women almost exclusively. It is believed to result from direct spread of infection from the pelvis and does not affect overall outcome. It can also be caused by infection with *Chlamydia trachomatis.*
- Sudden onset of sharp right upper quadrant pain, often following lower abdominal pain as an indicator of long-standing pelvic inflammatory disease, is typical.
- Fitz-Hugh–Curtis syndrome can be distinguished from gonococcal bacteremia by a characteristic friction rub over the liver and negative blood cultures. The diagnosis is made by nucleic

acid amplification testing or culture. Laparoscopy may show characteristic "violin-string" adhesions between the liver capsule and the anterior abdominal wall.

- Treatment is with **intravenous ceftriaxone.**

BURKHOLDERIA PSEUDOMALLEI (MELIOIDOSIS)

- *B. pseudomallei* is a soil- and waterborne gram-negative bacterium that causes melioidosis; it is found predominantly in Southeast Asia and India. The clinical spectrum ranges from asymptomatic infection to fulminant septicemia.
- Severe disease involves the lung, gastrointestinal tract, and liver, with hepatomegaly and jaundice; liver histologic changes include inflammatory infiltrates, multiple small and large abscesses, and focal necrosis.
- Chronic disease is characterized by granulomas with central necrosis resembling tuberculous lesions. Organisms are rarely seen on Giemsa stains of liver biopsy specimens. The diagnosis can be made by serologic testing using an indirect hemagglutination assay, although this test remains positive after acute illness.
- Initial antibiotic therapy consists of **intravenous ceftazidime, imipenem, or meropenem.**

SHIGELLA AND *SALMONELLA* SPECIES

- Cholestatic hepatitis can be attributable to enteric infection with *Shigella* species; liver histologic findings include portal and periportal polymorphonuclear infiltration, focal necrosis, and cholestasis.
- **Typhoid fever**, caused by *Salmonella typhi*, frequently involves the liver. Some patients may present with acute hepatitis, characterized by fever and tender hepatomegaly. Cholangitis, cholecystitis, and liver abscesses may occur.
- Mild-to-moderate elevations of serum bilirubin and aminotransferase levels are common in typhoid fever.
- Hepatic damage appears to be mediated by bacterial endotoxin, which can produce nonspecific reactions, such as sinusoidal and portal inflammation, necrosis, hypertrophy of Kupffer cells, and nonnecrotizing granulomas.
- The diagnosis is made by culture of *S. typhi* from blood, stool, urine, or "rose spots" on the skin. First-line treatment is with a **fluoroquinolone,** although resistance is increasing in some areas.

YERSINIA ENTEROCOLITICA

- Infection caused by *Y. enterocolitica* manifests as ileocolitis in children and terminal ileitis and mesenteric adenitis in adults.
- Patients with hepatic involvement have underlying comorbidities such as diabetes mellitus, cirrhosis, or hemochromatosis; excess tissue iron appears to be a predisposing factor.
- The subacute septicemic form of the disease resembles typhoid fever or malaria. Multiple abscesses are diffusely distributed in the liver and spleen. The mortality rate approaches 50%.
- **Aminoglycosides or tetracyclines** are first-line treatment, although **fluoroquinolones** may also be effective.

COXIELLA BURNETII (Q FEVER)

- Q fever is characterized by relapsing fevers, headache, myalgias, malaise, pneumonitis, and culture-negative endocarditis; the liver is commonly affected. The predominant abnormality is elevated aminotransferase levels.

- The hepatic histologic hallmark is the intraacinar granuloma with a central fat vacuole surrounded by a fibrin ring and macrophages ("fibrin-ring granuloma" or "doughnut" lesion).
- The diagnosis is confirmed by serologic testing for complement-fixing antibodies.
- **Doxycycline** is the treatment of choice.

RICKETTSIA RICKETTSII (ROCKY MOUNTAIN SPOTTED FEVER)

- Mortality caused by this systemic tickborne illness has decreased considerably as a result of early recognition; a few patients present with multiorgan manifestations and have a high mortality rate.
- Hepatic involvement, predominantly as jaundice, is frequent in multiorgan Rocky Mountain spotted fever; pathologic examination reveals portal perivascular inflammation and vasculitis.
- **Doxycycline** is the preferred treatment.

ACTINOMYCES ISRAELII (ACTINOMYCOSIS)

- *A. israelii* is found worldwide in soil.
- Cervicofacial infection is the most frequent manifestation of actinomycosis, and gastrointestinal involvement is common (13% to 60% of cases).
- Hepatic involvement is present in 15% of abdominal actinomycosis cases, most often as abscesses and is thought to result from metastatic spread from other abdominal sites through the portal vein. The course is more indolent than that of other causes of pyogenic hepatic abscess (see Chapter 30). Abscesses may be multiple and in both lobes of the liver.
- The diagnosis is based on aspiration of an abscess cavity and visualization of characteristic "sulfur granules" or a positive anaerobic culture.
- The treatment of choice is a prolonged course of **intravenous penicillin;** alternative options include **tetracycline or clindamycin.**

BARTONELLA BACILLIFORMIS (BARTONELLOSIS, OROYA FEVER)

- *B. bacilliformis* is endemic to Colombia, Ecuador, and Peru and is transmitted by infected sandflies.
- An acute febrile illness is accompanied by jaundice, hemolysis, hepatosplenomegaly, and lymphadenopathy.
- Centrilobular necrosis of the liver and splenic infarction may occur.
- Mortality rates resulting from sepsis or hemolysis approach 40%, but prompt treatment with **chloramphenicol, fluoroquinolones, or tetracycline** prevents fatal complications.

BRUCELLA SPECIES (BRUCELLOSIS)

- Brucellosis may be acquired from infected pigs (*Brucella suis*), cattle (*B. abortus*), goats (*B. melitensis*), or sheep (*B. ovis*).
- The infection manifests as an acute febrile illness with arthralgias, headaches, and malaise or as a subacute or chronic disease.
- Hepatomegaly and abnormal liver biochemical test levels are common; jaundice may be present in severe cases. Typically, liver histologic examination shows multiple noncaseating granulomas and, less often, focal portal tract infiltration or fibrosis.
- The diagnosis is confirmed by serologic testing in combination with an animal exposure history.
- Imaging reveals lesions with central calcification and a necrotic rim.

- Treatment is with a prolonged course of combination antimicrobial therapy with **doxycycline plus streptomycin, rifampin, or gentamycin.**

Spirochetal Infections of the Liver

LEPTOSPIRA SPECIES (LEPTOSPIROSIS)

1. Leptospirosis is among the most common zoonoses in the world, with a wide range of domestic and wild animal reservoirs. Human-to-human transmission is uncommon; rather, transmission occurs via contaminated urine, soil, water, or animal tissue. Up to 80% of the population has been exposed in some tropical countries; it is uncommon in the United States. Human disease can occur as one of two syndromes: Anicteric leptospirosis and Weil disease.
2. **Anicteric leptospirosis** accounts for more than 90% of cases and is characterized by a self-limited biphasic course. A few patients have elevated serum aminotransferase and bilirubin levels with hepatomegaly.
   - The first phase begins abruptly, with viral illness–like symptoms associated with fever, leptospiremia, and characteristic conjunctival suffusion (an important diagnostic clue) and lasts 4 to 7 days; leptospires are present in the blood or cerebrospinal fluid (CSF).
   - The second, or immune, phase, lasting 4 to 30 days, follows 1 to 3 days of improvement and is characterized by myalgias, nausea, vomiting, abdominal tenderness, and aseptic meningitis in up to 80% of patients.
3. **Weil disease** is a severe icteric form of leptospirosis and constitutes 5% to 10% of all cases. Complications are mainly the result of direct vascular damage by the *Leptospira*. The two phases of disease are less distinct.
   - The first phase is often marked by jaundice, which may last for weeks.
   - During the second phase, fever may be high, and hepatic and renal manifestations predominate. Jaundice is marked, with serum bilirubin levels approaching 30 mg/dL. Aminotransferase levels usually do not exceed five times the upper limit of normal, and thrombocytopenia is common. Acute tubular necrosis, which can lead to renal failure, cardiac arrhythmias, and hemorrhagic pneumonitis, are common. Mortality rates range from 5% to 40%.
4. The diagnosis is made on clinical grounds in conjunction with positive cultures of blood or CSF in the first phase or urine in the second phase. Isolation of the organism is difficult and may require many weeks. Microagglutination testing and serologic testing by enzyme-linked immunosorbent assay (ELISA) may confirm the diagnosis in the second phase.
5. Liver histologic examination reveals individual hepatocyte damage and canalicular cholestasis with mild portal inflammation.
6. **Doxycycline** 200 mg per day is given in mild cases (effective only if given early) and as prophylaxis. Severe cases require **intravenous penicillin,** with the risk of a Jarisch-Herxheimer reaction. Most patients recover without residual organ impairment.

TREPONEMA PALLIDUM (SYPHILIS)

1. **Congenital syphilis**
   - Liver involvement may result from immunologic mechanisms and is worsened by penicillin treatment.
   - Newborns have characteristic mucocutaneous lesions and osteochondritis, as well as hepatosplenomegaly and jaundice.
   - Liver histologic examination reveals diffuse hepatitis with spirochetes seen mostly in the spaces of Disse.

- Treatment is with **aqueous crystalline penicillin G or procaine penicillin G.**
2. **Secondary syphilis**
   - Liver involvement is characteristic (up to 50% of cases) and usually manifests with non-specific symptoms. Jaundice, hepatomegaly, and right upper quadrant tenderness are less common. Nearly all patients exhibit generalized lymphadenopathy.
   - Biochemical testing generally reveals low-grade elevations of serum aminotransferase and bilirubin levels, with a disproportionate elevation of the serum alkaline phosphatase level.
   - Liver histologic examination reveals focal necrosis, especially in the periportal and centrilobular regions, or granulomas and portal vasculitis. Spirochetes may be demonstrated by silver staining in up to one half of patients.
   - Liver dysfunction may be worsened by the Jarisch-Herxheimer reaction as a response to treatment, which can occur with treatment of all spirochete infections.
   - Treatment is with **benzathine penicillin.**
3. **Tertiary (late) syphilis**
   - Hepatic lesions are common but typically silent. Occasionally, tender hepatomegaly and nodularity may raise the suspicion of metastatic cancer (hepar lobatum).
   - If hepatic involvement is unrecognized, hepatocellular dysfunction and complications of portal hypertension can ensue.
   - Characteristic lesions are single or multiple gummas with central necrosis, often surrounded by granulation tissue consisting of a lymphoplasmacytic infiltrate with endarteritis obliterans. Exuberant deposition of scar tissue can ensue. Treponemes are rarely found.
   - Treatment is with **benzathine penicillin.**

BORRELIA BURGDORFERI (LYME DISEASE)

- Lyme disease is a multisystem disease caused by the tickborne spirochete *B. burgdorferi*. Predominant manifestations are dermatologic, cardiac, neurologic, and musculoskeletal. Hepatic involvement occurs in 20% to 40% of affected patients and usually manifests as hepatomegaly with increased serum aminotransferase and lactate dehydrogenase levels.
- In early stages, spirochetes disseminate hematogenously from the skin and multiply in the organs of the reticuloendothelial system, including the liver. The clinical picture is suggestive of acute hepatitis and often accompanies erythema chronicum migrans, the sentinel rash.
- Liver histologic examination reveals hepatocyte ballooning, marked mitotic activity, microvesicular fat, hyperplasia of Kupffer cells, a mixed sinusoidal infiltrate, and intraparenchymal and sinusoidal spirochetes on Warthin-Starry stain.
- The diagnosis is confirmed by serologic testing in a patient with a typical clinical history.
- Hepatic involvement does not appear to affect the overall outcome, which is excellent in primary disease after antibiotic treatment with **doxycycline or penicillin.**

Parasitic Diseases that Involve the Liver (Table 31.1)

PROTOZOAL INFECTIONS

1. **Amebic liver abscess** (see Chapter 30)
2. **Malaria**
   Malaria is one of the most important public health problems worldwide, annually infecting about 200 million persons and causing at least half a million deaths according to a 2014 World Health Organization (WHO) report.

TABLE 31.1 ■ **Parasitic Infections of the Liver and Biliary Tract**

Disease	Endemic Areas	Predisposing Factors	Pathophysiology	Manifestations	Diagnosis	Treatment[a]
Protozoans						
Amebiasis (*Entamoeba histolytica*)	Worldwide, especially Africa, Asia, Mexico, South America	Poor sanitation, sexual exposure	Hematogenous spread and tissue invasion, abscess formation	Fever, RUQ pain, peritonitis, elevated right hemidiaphragm, rupture	Cysts in stool, serology (e.g., ELISA, CIE, IHA), hepatic imaging	Metronidazole 750 mg [PO or IV] tid × 7–10 d or tinidazole 2 g × 3 d, followed by iodoquinol 650 mg tid × 20 d or diloxanide furoate 500 mg tid × 10 d or paromomycin 25–35 mg/kg/d in 3 divided doses × 7–10 d
Malaria (*Plasmodium falciparum, P. malariae, P. vivax, P. ovale, P. knowlesi*)	Africa, Asia, South America	Blood transfusion, IV drug use	Sporozoite clearance by hepatocytes; exoerythrocytic replication in the liver	Tender hepatomegaly, splenomegaly, rarely hepatic failure (*P. falciparum*)	Identification of the parasite on a blood smear	*P. falciparum:* Chloroquine (chloroquine-sensitive); mefloquine; or quinine and either doxycycline or clindamycin; or pyrimethamine-sulfadoxine (Fansidar); or atovaquone/proguanil (chloroquine-resistant); or artemisinins. *P. malariae:* Chloroquine *P. vivax, P. ovale, P. knowlesi.* Chloroquine and primaquine (chloroquine-sensitive) or mefloquine and primaquine (chloroquine-resistant) (eliminate exoerythrocytic forms)[b]

Continued

TABLE 31.1 ■ Parasitic Infections of the Liver and Biliary Tract—cont'd

Disease	Endemic Areas	Predisposing Factors	Pathophysiology	Manifestations	Diagnosis	Treatment[a]
Babesiosis (*Babesia* spp.)	United States	Exposure to deer tick	Hemolysis with multiorgan involvement	Fever, anemia, hepatosplenomegaly, abnormal liver test results, hemoglobinuria	Identification of the parasite on a blood smear, PCR	Azithromycin 500 mg on day 1, then 250 mg qd and atovaquone 750 mg bid × 7–10 d or clindamycin 300–600 mg IV q6h or 600 mg PO q8h and quinine 650 mg q8h × 7–10 d
Visceral leishmaniasis (*Leishmania donovani*)	Eurasia, Central America, South America	Immunosuppression (AIDS, organ transplantation)	Infection of RE cells	Fever, weight loss, hepatosplenomegaly, secondary bacterial infection, skin hyperpigmentation (kala-azar)	Amastigotes seen in the spleen, liver, or bone marrow	Pentavalent antimonial (stibogluconate sodium and meglumine antimoniate) 20 mg/kg/d × 28 d; or liposomal amphotericin B [IV] 3 mg/kg/d on days 1–5, 14, and 21; or paromomycin (aminosidine) 16–20 mg/kg/d × 21 days or miltefosine, 2.5 mg/kg/d × 28 d
Toxoplasmosis (*Toxoplasma gondii*)	Worldwide	Congenital infection, immunosuppression (AIDS, organ transplantation)	Replication in the liver leading to inflammation, necrosis	Fever, lymphadenopathy, occasionally hepatosplenomegaly, atypical lymphocytosis	Serology (IF, ELISA), isolation of the organism in the tissue	Pyrimethamine, 100 mg loading dose followed by 25–50 mg/d; plus sulfadiazine, 2–4 g/d in 4 divided doses; or clindamycin, 300 mg 4 times daily, plus folinic acid, 10–25 mg daily for 2–4 wk

TABLE 31.1 ■ **Parasitic Infections of the Liver and Biliary Tract—cont'd**

Disease	Endemic Areas	Predisposing Factors	Pathophysiology	Manifestations	Diagnosis	Treatment[a]
Nematodes						
Toxocariasis (*Toxocara canis, T. cati*)	Worldwide	Exposure to dogs or cats, especially with children younger than 5 years of age	Migration of larvae to the liver (visceral larva migrans)	Granuloma formation with eosinophilia	Larvae in tissue, serology (ELISA)	Albendazole 10 mg/kg/d × 5 d or mebendazole, 100–200 mg bid × 5 d
Hepatic capillariasis (*Capillaria hepatica*)	Worldwide	Exposure to rodents	Migration of larvae to the liver; inflammatory reaction to eggs	Acute, subacute hepatitis, tender hepatomegaly, occasionally splenomegaly, eosinophilia	Adult worms or eggs in a liver biopsy specimen	Supportive; possibly dithiazine iodide, sodium stibogluconate, albendazole, or thiabendazole
Ascariasis (*Ascaris lumbricoides*)	Tropical climates	Ingestion of raw vegetables	Migration of larvae to the liver; invasion of the bile ducts by adult worms	Abdominal pain, fever, jaundice, biliary obstruction, perioval granulomas	Ova or adult in stool or contrast study	Albendazole 400 mg × 1 dose; or mebendazole 100 mg bid × 3 d; or pyrantel pamoate 11 mg/kg up to 1 g; or ivermectin 200 µg/kg × 1 dose
Strongyloidiasis (*Strongyloides stercoralis*)	Asia, Africa, South America, Southern Europe, United States	Immunosuppression (AIDS, chemotherapy, organ transplantation) predisposes to hyperinfection	Larval penetration from the intestine to the liver	Hepatomegaly, occasionally jaundice, larvae in the portal tract or lobule	Larvae in the stool or duodenal aspirate	Ivermectin 200 µg/kg/d × 2 d; or albendazole 400 mg/d × 3 d
Trichinosis (*Trichinella spiralis*)	Temperate climates	Ingestion of undercooked pork	Hematogenous dissemination to the liver	Occasionally jaundice, biliary obstruction, larvae in hepatic sinusoids	History, eosinophilia, fever, muscle biopsy	Glucocorticoids for allergic symptoms; albendazole 400 mg bid × 10–15 d; or mebendazole 200 mg/d × 10–15 d

Continued

TABLE 31.1 ■ Parasitic Infections of the Liver and Biliary Tract—cont'd

Disease	Endemic Areas	Predisposing Factors	Pathophysiology	Manifestations	Diagnosis	Treatment[a]
Trematodes						
Schistoso-miasis (Schistosoma mansoni, S. japonicum)	Asia, Africa, South America, Caribbean	Travelers exposed to bodies of fresh water	Fibrogenic host immune response to eggs in the portal vein	*Acute:* Eosinophilic infiltrate; *chronic:* Hepatosplenomegaly, presinusoidal portal hypertension, perioval granuloma formation	Ova in the stool, rectal or liver biopsy	Praziquantel 40–60 mg/kg in 2 to 3 divided doses × 1 d; or oxamniquine (not available in United States). Acute toxemic schistosomiasis: Praziquantel 40–60 mg/kg in 2 to 3 divided doses × 1 d + glucocorticoids
Fascioliasis (Fasciola hepatica)	Worldwide	Cattle or sheep raising; ingestion of contaminated watercress	Migration of larvae through the liver; penetration of the bile ducts or surgery	*Acute:* Fever, abdominal pain, jaundice, hemobilia; *chronic:* Hepatomegaly	Ova in the stool, flukes in the bile ducts at ERC	Triclabendazole 10 mg/kg × 1 dose
Clonorchiasis and opisthorchiasis (Clonorchis sinensis, Opisthorchis viverrini, O. felineus)	Southeast Asia, China, Japan, Korea, Eastern Europe	Ingestion of raw freshwater fish	Migration through the ampulla; egg deposition in the bile ducts	Biliary hyperplasia, obstruction, sclerosing cholangitis, stone formation, cholangiocarcinoma	Ova in the stool, flukes in the bile ducts at ERC or surgery	Praziquantel 75 mg/kg in 3 divided doses × 1 d
Cestodes						
Echinococcosis (Echinococcus granulosus, E. multilocularis)	Worldwide	Cattle and sheep raising (E. granulosus)	Migration of larvae to the liver; encystment (hydatid cyst)	Tender hepatomegaly, fever, eosinophilia, cyst rupture, biliary obstruction	Serology (ELISA, IHA), hepatic imaging	Surgical resection or percutaneous drainage. Perioperative albendazole 400 mg bid continuing × 8 wk

AIDS, Acquired immunodeficiency syndrome; *CDC,* Centers for Disease Control and Prevention; *CIE,* counterimmunoelectrophoresis; *d,* day; *ELISA,* enzyme-linked immunosorbent assay; *ERC,* endoscopic retrograde cholangiography; *IF,* immunofluorescence; *IHA,* indirect hemagglutination assay; *IV,* intravenously; *PO,* by mouth; *PCR,* polymerase chain reaction assay; *RE,* reticuloendothelial; *RUQ,* right upper quadrant; *wk,* week.

[a]All drugs are given orally unless otherwise specified.

[b]For dosing guidelines for malaria, please refer to http://www.cdc.gov/malaria/pdf/treatmenttable.pdf.

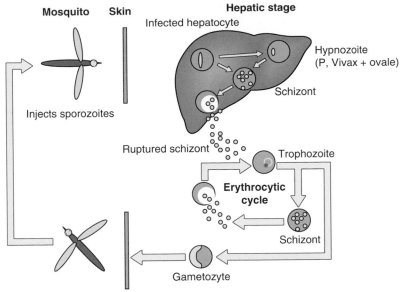

Mosquito   **Skin**   **Hepatic stage**
                        Infected hepatocyte

Injects sporozoites

Hypnozoite
(P, Vivax + ovale)

Schizont

Ruptured schizont

Trophozoite

**Erythrocytic
cycle**

Schizont

Gametozyte

Fig. 31.1 Life cycle of *Plasmodium* spp.

a. Life cycle (Fig. 31.1)
- The liver is affected during two stages of the malarial life cycle: The preerythrocytic phase and the erythrocytic phase, during which symptoms are noted.
- Malarial sporozoites injected by an infected female Anopheles mosquito circulate to the liver, enter hepatocytes, and mature to schizonts. When the schizont ruptures, merozoites are released into the bloodstream and invade erythrocytes. The four major species of Plasmodium responsible for malaria differ with respect to the number of merozoites released and the maturation times.
- Infection by ***Plasmodium falciparum*** or *P. malariae* is not associated with a residual liver stage after release of merozoites, whereas infection by *P. vivax* or *P. ovale* has an exoerythrocytic stage, the hypnozoite, which persists in the liver and can divide and mature into schizont forms again.
- The extent of hepatic injury varies with malarial species (most severe with *P. falciparum*) and severity of infection. Unconjugated hyperbilirubinemia is most commonly seen as a result of hemolysis, but occasional hepatocyte dysfunction can be seen, leading to conjugated hyperbilirubinemia as well as a prolonged prothrombin time.
- Reversible reductions of portal venous blood flow during the acute phase of falciparum malaria may be a consequence of micro-occlusion of portal venous branches by parasitized erythrocytes.

b. Histopathology
- In an acute attack of falciparum malaria, large quantities of malarial pigment, hemozoin (an iron porphyrin protein complex resulting from hemoglobin degradation by the parasite) accumulates in Kupffer cells, which hypertrophy and phagocytose erythrocytes. Sinusoidal dilatation also occurs.
- Later, a mild portal infiltrate and portal pigment deposition is often seen. All abnormalities reverse with successful treatment.

c. Clinical features

- Only the erythrocytic stage of malaria is associated with clinical illness. Symptoms develop 30 to 60 days after exposure to an infected mosquito and include cyclical fever, malaise, anorexia, nausea, vomiting, diarrhea, and myalgias. Tender hepatomegaly and splenomegaly, as well as jaundice caused by hemolysis, are common in adults, especially with heavy infection by *P. falciparum*.
- Hepatic failure is generally seen only in association with concomitant viral hepatitis or with severe *P. falciparum* infection.

d. Diagnosis

- The differential diagnosis includes hepatotropic and nonhepatotropic viral hepatitis, gastroenteritis, amebic liver abscess, yellow fever, typhoid fever, tuberculosis, leptospirosis, and brucellosis.
- The diagnosis of acute malaria rests on clinical history, physical examination, and identification of parasites on **peripheral thick or thin blood smears.** Because the number of parasites in the blood may be small, repeated smear examinations should be performed when the index of suspicion is high.
- Several rapid antigen detection assays now exist with sufficient sensitivity and specificity to be clinically useful in endemic regions.

e. Treatment

- Treatment depends on the species and the pattern of chloroquine resistance for falciparum infection. **In general, chloroquine is effective for *P. malariae*, *P. vivax*, *P. ovale*, and *P. falciparum* in areas endemic for chloroquine-sensitive species. Resistant falciparum infections can be treated with artemisinin combination therapies (ACTs), atovaquone-proguanil, quinine in combination with doxycycline or clindamycin, or mefloquine in combination with doxycycline or artemisinin derivative.**
- **For *P. vivax* and *P. ovale* infections, treatment with primaquine** (in persons who have tested negative for glucose-6-phosphate dehydrogenase deficiency) is indicated to eliminate the exoerythrocytic hypnozoites in the liver.

f. **Hyperreactive malarial splenomegaly** (tropical splenomegaly syndrome)

- Repeated exposure to malaria may lead to an aberrant immunologic response with overproduction of immunoglobulin M (IgM) malarial antibody and high levels of IgM aggregates, dense hepatic sinusoidal lymphocytosis (similar to that seen in Felty syndrome), hyperplasia of Kupffer cells, and massive splenomegaly.
- Severe anemia resulting from hypersplenism, especially in women of childbearing age, can result; variceal bleeding is uncommon.
- Treatment consists of lifelong antimalarial therapy and supportive care of anemia with blood transfusions.

3. **Babesiosis**

Babesiosis is caused by *Babesia* species and transmitted by the deer tick *Ixodes scapularis* (also known as *I. dammini*). It is a malaria-like illness endemic to the Northeast and Midwest of the United States, most often between May and September.

- Patients present with fever, anemia, hepatosplenomegaly, and abnormal liver biochemical test levels. The diagnosis can be made with polymerase chain reaction (PCR) testing, serology, or blood smear evaluation.
- Immunocompromised or asplenic patients are affected more severely.
- Combination therapy with **atovaquone** 750 mg twice daily and **azithromycin** 500 mg followed by 250 mg once daily or with **clindamycin** 600 mg three times daily and **quinine** 650 mg three to four times daily for 7 days is recommended.

4. **Leishmaniasis**

Visceral leishmaniasis is caused by *Leishmania* species, mostly *L. donovani*, and is endemic in the Mediterranean, the Middle East, Asia, Africa, and Latin America.

a. Life cycle
   - The parasite multiplies in the gut of the female sandfly as a flagellated promastigote and migrates to the pharynx. Following injection into the human host, promastigotes are phagocytosed by macrophages in the reticuloendothelial system, where they multiply as amastigotes and are taken up with the next blood meal of the sandfly.

b. Clinical features
   - Among early infections, 60% to 95% are subclinical.
   - Visceral infection begins with a papular or ulcerative skin lesion at the site of the sandfly bite (similar to the cutaneous form of the disease). Following an incubation period of 2 to 6 months, twice daily fevers, weight loss, diarrhea (of bacillary, amebic, or leishmanial origin), and progressive painful hepatosplenomegaly develop, often accompanied by pancytopenia and a polyclonal hypergammaglobulinemia. Liver biochemical test levels are typically normal.
   - Secondary bacterial infections resulting from infiltration and suppression of reticuloendothelial cell function include pneumonia, pneumococcal infection, and tuberculosis and are important causes of mortality.
   - Physical findings include often massive hepatomegaly, soft and nontender splenomegaly, jaundice, or ascites in severe disease as well as generalized lymphadenopathy, and muscle wasting. Cutaneous gray hyperpigmentation, which prompted the name **kala-azar** ("black fever"), is characteristically seen in India. Oral and nasopharyngeal nodules resulting from granuloma formation can be seen in Africa.

c. Histopathology
   - Organisms are found in macrophages of the liver and spleen, bone marrow, and lymph nodes. Kupffer cells containing amastigotes proliferate. Occasionally, parasite-bearing cells aggregate within noncaseating granulomas.
   - Hepatocyte necrosis is mild compared with that seen in cutaneous leishmaniasis. Healing is accompanied by fibrous deposition similar to that seen in congenital syphilis, and occasionally the liver looks cirrhotic (Rogers cirrhosis); complications of cirrhosis are rare.

d. Diagnosis
   - This is based on history, physical examination, and demonstration of tissue amastigotes.
   - The demonstration of parasites or parasitic DNA in tissue is diagnostic. The highest yield comes from aspiration of the spleen, with parasites seen in 95% of cases. Liver aspiration is safer and has 70% to 85% a similar sensitivity, as does bone marrow aspiration. Lymph node aspiration has 60% sensitivity.
   - Serologic testing by ELISA or direct agglutination can be used to support a presumptive diagnosis of visceral leishmaniasis with 95% sensitivity and specificity. The leishmanin skin test (Montenegro test) is typically negative and unhelpful in acute visceral disease.

e. Treatment
   - No specific measures are necessary to treat hepatic involvement. Treatment of secondary bacterial infections is essential, and specific antileishmanial chemotherapy should be initiated promptly.
   - **Liposomal amphotericin B** administered intravenously is the treatment of choice for visceral leishmaniasis. Intravenous **sodium stibogluconate** (Pentostam) is available through the Centers for Disease Control and Prevention (CDC) under an investigational protocol for treatment of infections. Alternative agents include oral meglumine antimoniate, paromomycin, and miltefosine.

- Patients with acquired immunodeficiency syndrome (AIDS) and leishmaniasis often fail to respond or relapse following treatment with conventional regimens.

5. **Toxoplasmosis**

Infection caused by *Toxoplasma gondii* is found worldwide. In the United States, serologic surveys suggest that, over years, exposure to *T. gondii* has decreased to only 9% of persons aged 12 to 49. Toxoplasmosis causes clinical disease either when transmitted congenitally or as an opportunistic infection complicating AIDS.

   a. Life cycle
      - Cats are the definitive hosts; humans and other animals are incidental hosts that become infected by ingestion of oocysts in soil, water, or contaminated meat.
      - The oocysts mature in the intestinal tract of humans to become sporozoites, which penetrate the intestinal mucosa, become tachyzoites, and circulate systemically, thus invading a wide array of cell types. They can form tissue cysts, containing many bradyzoites, which are responsible for latent infection.
      - Hepatic involvement has been observed in severe, disseminated infection.

   b. Clinical features
      - Acquired toxoplasmosis can manifest as a mononucleosis-like illness with fever, chills, headache, and lymphadenopathy. Uncommonly, hepatomegaly, splenomegaly, and minimal elevations of serum aminotransferase levels are present.
      - Infection of immunocompromised hosts can result in encephalitis, chorioretinitis, pneumonitis, myocarditis, and, uncommonly, hepatitis.
      - Atypical lymphocytosis, an otherwise unusual feature of parasitic disease, may occur.

   c. Diagnosis
      - This is best made by detecting specific IgM or IgG antibody using indirect immunofluorescence or an enzyme immunoassay (EIA) and isolation of *T. gondii* from blood, body fluids, or tissue.

   d. Treatment
      - Antibiotic therapy with **pyrimethamine and sulfadiazine, plus folinic acid** to minimize hematologic toxicity, for 2 to 6 weeks (depending on patient characteristics), should be administered to immunocompetent persons with severe infection and immunocompromised or pregnant patients.

Helminthic Infections: Roundworms (Nematodes) (see Table 31.1)

1. **Ascariasis**

Ascaris lumbricoides is estimated to infect 819 million people worldwide, especially in tropical countries and areas with poor sanitation practices.

   a. Life cycle
      - Humans are infected by ingesting embryonated eggs, usually in raw vegetables. The larvae hatch in the duodenum and migrate to the cecum, where they penetrate the mucosa, enter the portal circulation, and reach the liver, pulmonary artery, and lungs.
      - The larvae grow in the alveolar spaces, are regurgitated and swallowed, and become mature adults in the intestine 2 to 3 months after ingestion, eventually reaching 15 to 35 cm, whereupon the cycle repeats itself.

   b. Clinical features
      - Most infected persons are asymptomatic or minimally symptomatic during larval migration. Symptoms are generally proportionate to the worm burden.

- Cough, fever, dyspnea, wheezing, and substernal chest discomfort have been reported in the first 2 weeks of infection, as has hepatomegaly, when the larvae pass through the liver.
- Chronic infection is more frequently characterized by episodic epigastric or periumbilical pain. If the worm burden is particularly heavy, small bowel obstruction, intussusception, volvulus, perforation, or appendicitis may occur.
- Fragments of disintegrating worms within the biliary tract can serve as a nidus for biliary calculus formation. Preexisting disease of the biliary tract or pancreatic duct can predispose to worm migration into the bile ducts, with resulting obstructive jaundice, cholangitis, cholecystitis, pancreatitis, or pylephlebitis and intrahepatic abscesses.

c. Diagnosis
- In the absence of a history of worm passage or regurgitation, the diagnosis is made definitively by identification of characteristic eggs in stool specimens. Larvae have also been identified in sputum and gastric washings. Liver biopsy specimens may show granulomas surrounding typical eggs. Also, an infiltrate on chest x-ray and peripheral eosinophilia may be present.
- Patients with biliary or pancreatic symptoms can be evaluated by ultrasonography or by endoscopic techniques, either endoscopic retrograde cholangiopancreatography (ERCP) or direct choledochoscopy, which may identify the parasite and permit extraction of the worm.

d. Treatment
- Infected persons may be treated with a single dose of **albendazole** 400 mg, **mebendazole** 100 mg twice daily for 3 days, or **ivermectin** 200 µg/kg × 1 dose.
- In patients with intestinal obstruction, **piperazine citrate** may be used (75 mg/kg for 2 days to a maximum of 3.5 g in adults and 2 g in children under 20 kg). This agent paralyzes the worm and facilitates excretion.
- Intestinal or biliary obstruction may require surgical or endoscopic intervention and removal of the worm. In the absence of intestinal perforation or ischemia, conservative management may be attempted first for up to 24 hours.

2. Toxocariasis
Toxocara canis and *T. cati* infect dogs and cats, respectively; in other hosts, the development of the parasite larvae is arrested. Infection occurs worldwide, especially in children.

a. Life cycle
- Infection is acquired when soil or food containing eggs is ingested. The eggs hatch in the small intestine and release larvae, which penetrate the intestinal wall, enter the portal circulation, and reach the liver and systemic circulation. The immature worms bore through the vessel walls and migrate through the tissues, thereby leading to secondary inflammatory responses. They do not return to the intestinal lumen; therefore, neither eggs nor larvae appear in the feces.
- When larvae become trapped in tissue, they provoke granuloma formation with a predominance of eosinophils. The liver, brain, and eye are the most frequently affected organs.

b. Clinical features
- Most infections are asymptomatic. Two major clinical syndromes are recognized.
  - Occult infections are associated with nonspecific symptoms, including abdominal pain, anorexia, fever, and wheezing.
  - **Visceral larva migrans** is seen most commonly in children with a history of pica. Findings include fever, hepatomegaly, urticaria, and leukocytosis with persistent eosinophilia, hypergammaglobulinemia, and elevated blood group isohemagglutinins. Pulmonary, cardiac, neurologic, and ocular manifestations are often seen.

   c. Diagnosis
      ■ The diagnosis should be considered in persons with a history of pica, exposure to dogs or cats, and persistent eosinophilia.
      ■ Stool studies are not useful because the larvae do not mature to produce eggs in humans and do not remain in the gastrointestinal tract.
      ■ A definitive diagnosis is made by identification of the larvae in affected tissues, although blind biopsies have a low yield and are not routinely recommended. Ultrasound-guided liver biopsy may be necessary to differentiate visceral larva migrans from hepatic capillariasis.
      ■ A strongly positive ELISA result using excretory-secretory larval antigens provides supportive evidence of infection.
   d. Treatment
      ■ Mild cases are usually self-limited and resolve within a few weeks. More severe cases require antihelminthic treatment with **albendazole** 400 mg twice daily for 5 days or **mebendazole** 100 to 200 mg twice daily for 5 days. Significant pulmonary, cardiac, ophthalmologic, or neurologic manifestations may warrant the use of systemic glucocorticoids. The disease is rarely fatal.

3. **Hepatic capillariasis**
   Infection with *Capillaria hepatica* is acquired by ingestion of eggs in contaminated soil, food, or water, especially by children under poor hygienic conditions. Human infection is rare.
   a. Life cycle
      ■ Larvae released in the cecum penetrate the intestinal mucosa, enter the portal venous circulation, and become lodged in the liver, where adult worms develop within 3 weeks to a size of 20 mm. As the female worm dies, it releases eggs into the hepatic parenchyma and produces an intense granulomatous and fibrosing reaction.
   b. Clinical features
      ■ The features may be similar to those of visceral larva migrans, but it manifests as acute or subacute hepatitis. Patients may have tender hepatomegaly and, occasionally, splenomegaly, prominent eosinophilia, mild elevations of serum aminotransferase, alkaline phosphatase, and bilirubin levels, anemia, and an elevated erythrocyte sedimentation rate.
   c. Diagnosis
      ■ Adult worms or eggs can be detected in liver biopsy or autopsy specimens. Associated histologic findings in the liver include necrosis, fibrosis, eosinophilic infiltrate, and granuloma formation. Finding *C. hepatica* ova in stool likely reflects passage of infected animal material and is not helpful.
   d. Treatment
      ■ Treatment is generally unsuccessful. Case studies have reported success with dithiazanine iodide, sodium stibogluconate, albendazole, and thiabendazole.

4. **Strongyloidiasis**
   Strongyloides stercoralis is prevalent in the tropics and subtropics, southern and eastern Europe, and the United States. Infection is usually asymptomatic.
   a. Life cycle
      ■ Humans are infected by the filariform larvae, which penetrate intact skin, are carried to the lungs, migrate through the alveoli, and are swallowed to reach the intestine, where maturation ensues. Worms are typically found in the duodenum and proximal jejunum.
      ■ Autoinfection can occur if the rhabditiform larvae transform into infective filariform larvae in the intestine, thereby causing persistent infection even decades after exposure; reinfection occurs by penetration of the bowel wall or perianal skin and entry into the portal circulation and then the liver.

- Symptomatic infection results from a heavy infectious burden or infection in an immunocompromised person, especially in patients infected with human T-cell lymphotrophic virus-1. A hyperinfection syndrome may result from dissemination of filariform larvae into any organ, including the liver, lung, and brain, which is not ordinarily in the life cycle of the nematode.

b. Clinical features
- As with other helminthic infections, acute infection can lead to a pruritic eruption followed by fever, cough, wheezing, abdominal pain, diarrhea, and eosinophilia.
- When the liver is affected, cholestatic liver biochemical abnormalities can be seen. Liver biopsy specimens may show periportal inflammation, and larvae may be observed in intrahepatic bile canaliculi, lymphatic vessels, and small branches of the portal vein.

c. Diagnosis
- ELISA is useful in immunocompetent patients, less so in the immunocompromised. Identification of larvae in the stool is <50% sensitive. Endoscopy and intestinal biopsy are rarely required for the diagnosis. The presence of an obstructive hepatobiliary picture in a person with established strongyloidiasis suggests possible dissemination.

d. Treatment
- For acute infection, the drug of choice is **ivermectin** 200 μg/kg daily for 2 days; alternatively **albendazole** can be used. Retreatment with a second course may be necessary in immunocompromised patients or those with disseminated disease.
- Hyperinfection syndrome requires longer courses of treatment.
- Treatment options are limited following dissemination, and mortality rates are as high as 85%.

5. Trichinosis

a. Life cycle
- Humans may be infected with *Trichinella spiralis* by consuming raw or undercooked pork bearing larvae, which are released in the upper gastrointestinal tract, enter the small intestine, penetrate the mucosa, and disseminate through the systemic circulation.
- Larvae can be found in myocardium, CSF, brain, and, less commonly, liver and gallbladder.
- In the small bowel, the larvae develop into adult worms, which release larvae that migrate to striated muscle, where they become encapsulated.

b. Clinical features
- Clinical manifestations occur when the worm burden is high and include diarrhea, fever, myalgias, periorbital and facial edema, conjunctivitis, and leukocytosis with marked eosinophilia.
- Jaundice may result from biliary obstruction.
- Severe complications include myocarditis, central nervous system involvement, and pneumonitis.

c. Diagnosis
- Suggested by fever associated with eosinophilia
- Serologic studies for antibody to *Trichinella* may not be helpful in the acute phase of infection and false positives exist.
- Muscle biopsy can confirm the diagnosis.
- Rarely, hepatic histologic examination may demonstrate invasion of hepatic sinusoids by larvae.

d. Treatment
- Glucocorticoids are used to relieve allergic symptoms, followed by antihelminthic treatment with **albendazole** 400 mg twice daily for 8 to 14 days or, alternatively, **mebendazole** 200 to 400 mg three times a day for 3 days, followed by 400 to 500 mg three times a day for 10 days.

HELMINTHIC INFECTIONS: FLATWORMS (TREMATODES) (see Table 31.1)

1. **Schistosomiasis**

    Schistosomiasis (bilharziasis) is caused by trematodes (blood flukes) of the genus Schistosoma. Approximately 200 million persons are infected worldwide, with approximately 200,000 deaths annually. An estimated 400,000 people, mostly immigrants from endemic areas, are infected in the United States. Humans and mammals are the definitive hosts (see Table 31.1).

    a. Life cycle (Fig. 31.2)
       - The infectious cycle is initiated by penetration of the skin by free-swimming cercariae released from snails to fresh water. Within 24 hours, the cercariae reach the peripheral venules and lymphatics and the pulmonary vessels. They pass through the lungs and reach the liver, where they lodge, develop into adults 1 to 2 cm long, and mate.
       - Mated adult worms then migrate to their ultimate destinations in the inferior mesenteric venules (*Schistosoma mansoni*), superior mesenteric venules (*S. japonicum*), or the veins around the bladder (*S. hematobium*). These locations correlate with the clinical complications associated with each species. The eggs are deposited in the terminal venules and eventually migrate into the lumen of the involved organ, after which they are excreted in the stool or urine.
       - Eggs remaining in the organ provoke a robust granulomatous response. Excreted eggs hatch immediately in fresh water and liberate early intermediate miracidia, which infect their snail hosts. The miracidia transform into cercariae within the snails and are then released into the water, from which they may again infect humans.

    b. Clinical features
       - The severity of clinical symptoms is related to the total worm burden in the host and possibly genetic susceptibility factors and is caused by the host reaction to the schistosomes.

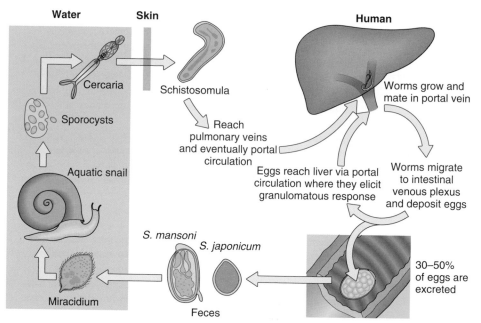

Fig. 31.2 Life cycle of *Schistosoma* spp.

- **Acute toxemic schistosomiasis (Katayama syndrome)** is believed to result from immune complex formation as a consequence of the host immunologic response to the antigenic challenge by the adult worms and eggs, occurring 4 to 8 weeks after exposure. Manifestations include headache, fever, chills, cough, diarrhea, myalgia, arthralgia, tender hepatomegaly, splenomegaly, and eosinophilia.
- Untreated acute schistosomiasis invariably progresses to chronic disease over many years. Mesenteric infection leads to hepatic complications, including periportal fibrosis, presinusoidal occlusion, and, ultimately, presinusoidal portal hypertension, as a result of the inflammatory reaction to eggs deposited in the liver. With severe schistosomal infection, portal hypertension becomes progressive, leading to ascites, gastroesophageal varices, and splenomegaly.
- Chronic schistosomal infection may be complicated by increased susceptibility to Salmonella infections. Hepatitis B and C virus infections are also common in persons living in endemic areas and may accelerate the progression of liver disease and the development of hepatocellular carcinoma.
- Laboratory findings in chronic schistosomiasis include anemia from recurrent gastrointestinal bleeding or hypersplenism, eosinophilia, an elevated erythrocyte sedimentation rate, and increased serum IgE levels. Liver biochemical test levels are generally normal until the disease is advanced.

c. Diagnosis
- The diagnosis of acute schistosomiasis should be considered in a patient with an exposure history to fresh water who has abdominal pain, diarrhea, and fever. Multiple stool examinations for ova using the Kato-Katz thick smear may be required to confirm the diagnosis, because results are frequently negative in the early phases of disease.
- Serologic testing has proved useful in facilitating earlier diagnosis. Sigmoidoscopy or colonoscopy may reveal rectosigmoid or transverse colonic involvement and may be useful in chronic disease when few eggs pass in the feces.
- Ultrasonography and liver biopsy are useful for demonstrating periportal (or "pipestem") fibrosis but not for diagnosing acute infection.

d. Treatment
- **Praziquantel** 40 mg/kg given for 1 day in two divided doses is the treatment of choice for infection caused by *S. hematobium*, *S. mansoni*, and *S. intercalatum*; cure rates are 60% to 90%. The recommended dose for *S. japonicum* and *S. mekongi* is 60 mg/kg divided into two or three doses.
- Treatment of acute toxemic schistosomiasis requires praziquantel 75 mg/kg for 1 day in three divided doses and, in some cases, prednisone for the prior 2 to 3 days to suppress immune-mediated helminthicidal or drug reactions.
- Periodic treatment of patients in endemic areas will keep the burden of infection low and will minimize chronic complications.
- Noncirrhotic, presinusoidal portal hypertension may lead to variceal bleeding requiring band ligation or sclerotherapy. Advanced chronic schistosomal liver disease can be managed with a distal splenorenal shunt with or without splenopancreatic disconnection or esophagogastric devascularization with splenectomy. Since the advent of praziquantel, complicated schistosomal liver disease has become uncommon.

2. Fascioliasis

Fascioliasis, caused by the sheep liver fluke *Fasciola hepatica*, is endemic in many areas of Europe and Latin America, North Africa, Asia, the Western Pacific, and some parts of the United States, and it causes >2 million infections worldwide.

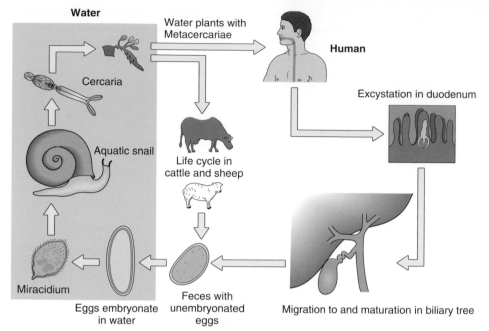

Fig. 31.3   Life cycle of *Fasciola hepatica*.

a. Life cycle (Fig. 31.3)
   ■ The life cycle is spent between herbivores and intermediate aquatic snail hosts. Eggs passed in the feces of infected mammals into fresh water give rise to miracidia that penetrate snails and emerge as cercariae, which encyst as metacercariae on aquatic plants such as watercress. Hosts become infected when they consume plants bearing the encysted organisms, which bore into the intestinal wall, enter the abdominal cavity, penetrate the hepatic capsule, and settle in the bile ducts, where they develop into adults within 3 to 4 months and reach a length of 20 to 30 mm.
b. Clinical features
   ■ Fascioliasis is divided into three phases corresponding to three syndromes.
      – **Acute:** Migration of young flukes through the liver. This phase is marked by fever, right upper quadrant pain, and eosinophilia. Urticaria with dermatographia and non-specific gastrointestinal symptoms are common. Physical examination often reveals fever and a tender, enlarged liver. Splenomegaly is reported in up to 25% of cases, but jaundice is rare. Eosinophilia can be profound (occasionally more than 80%). Abnormalities of liver biochemical tests are minimal.
      – **Latent:** Corresponds to the settling of the flukes into the bile ducts and lasts months to years. Affected persons are mostly asymptomatic but may experience vague gastrointestinal symptoms. Eosinophilia persists, and fever can occur.
      – **Chronic obstructive:** Consequence of intrahepatic and extrahepatic bile ductal inflammation and hyperplasia evoked by the presence of adult flukes. This phase may be marked by recurrent biliary pain, cholangitis, cholelithiasis, and biliary obstruction. Blood loss may result from epithelial injury, and rare cases of overt hemobilia have been described. Liver biochemical testing commonly demonstrates a cholestatic pattern. Long-term infection may lead to biliary cirrhosis and secondary sclerosing cholangitis, but no convincing association with malignancies of the liver or biliary tract exists.

   c. Diagnosis
- This diagnosis should be considered in patients with prolonged fever, abdominal pain, diarrhea, tender hepatomegaly, and eosinophilia. Because eggs are not passed during the acute phase, the diagnosis depends on a variety of serologic tests, including ELISA of genus-specific antigens and EIA of fluke excretory-secretory proteins. In the latent and chronic phases, the diagnosis is made definitively by detection of eggs in stool, duodenal aspirates, or bile. Occasionally, ultrasonography or ERCP demonstrates the flukes in the gallbladder and bile duct.
- Hepatic histologic findings include necrosis and granuloma formation with eosinophilic infiltrates and Charcot-Leyden crystals. Eosinophilic abscesses, epithelial hyperplasia of the bile ducts, and periportal fibrosis may also be seen.

   d. Treatment
- Unlike other liver fluke infections, praziquantel is not effective for fascioliasis.
- Treatment is a single dose of **triclabendazole** 10 mg/kg once or twice; alternatively, **nitazoxanide or bithionol** may be effective.

3. **Clonorchiasis and opisthorchiasis**

Clonorchis sinensis, Opisthorchis viverrini, and *O. felineus* are trematodes (liver flukes) of the family Opisthorchiidae. *C. sinensis* and *O. viverrini* are widespread in East and Southeast Asia, affecting millions of people, mostly of lower socioeconomic status. *O. felineus* infects humans and domestic animals in Eastern Europe. All three trematodes have similar life cycles and clinical features.

   a. Life cycle
- All species require two intermediate hosts—an aquatic snail and freshwater fish. Eggs are passed in the feces into fresh water, are consumed by snails, and hatch as free-swimming cercariae, which seek and penetrate fish or crayfish and encyst in skin or muscle as metacercariae. The mammalian host is infected when it consumes raw or undercooked fish. The metacercariae excyst in the small bowel and migrate into the ampulla of Vater and bile ducts, where they mature into 10- to 20-mm adult flukes. Infection can be maintained for two decades or longer.

   b. Clinical features
- Infection is clinically silent or associated with nonspecific features, with fever, abdominal pain, and diarrhea.
- Chronic manifestations correlate with the fluke burden and are dominated by fever, right upper quadrant pain, tender hepatomegaly, and eosinophilia. With a heavy worm burden in the bile ducts, chronic or intermittent biliary obstruction can ensue, with frequent development of cholelithiasis, cholecystitis, jaundice, and, ultimately, recurrent pyogenic cholangitis (see Chapter 35).
- Serum alkaline phosphatase and bilirubin levels are elevated, and mild to moderate elevations of serum aminotransferase levels are also seen. Long-standing untreated infection leads to exuberant inflammation resulting in periportal fibrosis, marked biliary epithelial hyperplasia and dysplasia, and a substantially increased risk of cholangiocarcinoma.
- **Cholangiocarcinoma** resulting from clonorchiasis or opisthorchiasis tends to be multicentric and arises in the secondary biliary radicles of the hilum of the liver. The diagnosis should be suspected in infected persons with weight loss, jaundice, epigastric pain, or an abdominal mass.

   c. Diagnosis
- The diagnosis is based on detection of characteristic fluke eggs in the stool. Stool examination is usually positive except late in the disease, when biliary obstruction supervenes. In these cases, the diagnosis is made by identifying flukes in the bile ducts or gallbladder at surgery or in bile obtained by postoperative drainage or percutaneous aspiration.

- Endoscopic or intraoperative cholangiography reveals slender, uniform filling defects within intrahepatic ducts that are alternately dilated and strictured and that may mimic sclerosing cholangitis.
- Serologic testing is generally not helpful.

  d. Treatment
- All patients with clonorchiasis or opisthorchiasis should be treated with **praziquantel,** which is uniformly effective in a dose of 75 mg/kg in three divided doses for 2 days. Side effects are uncommon and include headache, dizziness, and nausea. Alternatively, **albendazole** 10 mg/kg for 7 days can be used. After treatment, dead flukes may be seen in the stool or biliary drainage.
- When the burden of infecting organisms is high, the dead flukes and surrounding debris or stones may cause biliary obstruction necessitating endoscopic or surgical drainage.

HELMINTHIC INFECTIONS: CESTODES (TAPEWORMS)

Echinococcosis (see Chapter 30 and Table 31.1)

Fungal Liver Disease

CANDIDIASIS

Candida species are found worldwide and are common commensal organisms. They may cause invasive systemic infection in persons who are severely immunocompromised. The liver can become infected by *C. albicans* in the setting of disseminated, multiorgan disease.

1. Conditions that can predispose to disseminated candidiasis include pregnancy, immunologic defects, human immunodeficiency virus infection, diabetes mellitus, and severe zinc or iron deficiency.
2. Most cases of disseminated infections occur in leukemic patients undergoing high dose chemotherapy and become manifest during the period of recovery from severe neutropenia. In leukemic patients with disseminated candidiasis, the frequency of hepatic candidiasis is as high as 51% to 91%. The disease is often overwhelming, with a high mortality rate.
   - A less frequent presentation in the compromised host is isolated or focal hepatic candidiasis, thought to result from colonization of the gastrointestinal tract by *Candida*, which disseminates locally following the onset of neutropenia and mucosal injury caused by high dose chemotherapy.
   - Resulting fungemia of the portal vein seeds the liver and leads to hepatic micro- and macroabscesses.
3. Clinical features
   - In either focal or disseminated candidiasis involving the liver, clinical features include high fever, right upper quadrant abdominal pain and distention, nausea, vomiting, diarrhea, anorexia, and tender hepatomegaly.
   - Serum alkaline phosphatase level is nearly invariably elevated, with variable elevations in serum aminotransferase and bilirubin levels.
4. Diagnosis
   - Computed tomography of the abdomen is the most sensitive test to detect hepatic or splenic granulomas or abscesses, which are often multicentric.
   - In most cases, liver biopsy specimens reveal macroscopic nodules, portal and periportal necrosis with microabscesses, and granulomas surrounding neutrophilic abscesses, as well as characteristic yeast and hyphal forms of *Candida*. Cultures of biopsy material are negative in most cases.

- PCR testing has been used for diagnosis.
- Laparoscopy may also be used to confirm the diagnosis.

5. Treatment
   - If hepatic candidiasis is diagnosed in its focal form, response rates to therapy with **intravenous amphotericin** B 3 to 5 mg/kg/day are better (nearly 60%) than in disseminated disease. **Liposomal amphotericin** can be used to reduce the frequency of side effects, especially nephrotoxicity.
   - Other options include a **combination of amphotericin B with flucytosine, itraconazole, or fluconazole. Caspofungin, micafungin, or anidulafungin followed by fluconazole** has been shown to be effective in patients with hepatosplenic candidiasis resistant to amphotericin B.
   - Occasionally, surgical resection (e.g., splenomegaly in focal disease) may be attempted. Despite all efforts, mortality rates remain high.

HISTOPLASMOSIS

Infection with *Histoplasma capsulatum* is acquired through inhalation in an endemic area. Most patients are asymptomatic. Most symptomatic patients have disease confined to the lungs. Severely immunocompromised persons (e.g., those with AIDS) in endemic regions are predisposed to disseminated histoplasmosis, affecting mainly those organs rich in macrophages.

1. Clinical features
   - The liver can be invaded in both the acute and chronic forms of progressive disseminated histoplasmosis. Fever, weight loss, oropharyngeal ulcers, hepatomegaly, and splenomegaly may be present in chronic disease.
   - In children with acute hepatic disease, marked hepatosplenomegaly is universal and is associated with high fever and lymphadenopathy.
   - Hepatosplenomegaly is present in 30% of adults with acute disease (often the AIDS-defining illness). Serum aminotransferase and alkaline phosphatase levels are often elevated.

2. Diagnosis
   - Yeast forms are small (3 to 4 μm) but can be identified in sections of liver biopsies on standard hematoxylin and eosin staining and are best seen with a Grocott silver stain either diffusely infiltrating the sinusoids or in granulomas. The organism is difficult to culture and hardly ever grows from biopsy specimens.
   - Serologic testing for complement-fixing antibodies is helpful in confirming the diagnosis. Detection of *H. capsulatum* antigens in urine, serum, or bronchoalveolar lavage is rapid and fairly sensitive; it is particularly useful in immunocompromised persons who may not be capable of mounting a significant antibody response. The histoplasmin skin test indicates prior sensitization and has no diagnostic value.

3. Treatment
   - Disseminated histoplasmosis should be treated with **intravenous amphotericin B.**
   - **Itraconazole** is used in mild to moderate infections or to complete therapy after successful response to amphotericin.

Acknowledgment

The authors gratefully acknowledge the contributions of Wolfram Goessling, MD, PhD, to this chapter in prior editions of the book.

FURTHER READING

Albrecht H. Bacterial and miscellaneous infections of the liver. In: Zakim DS, Boyer TD, eds. *Hepatology.* Philadelphia: Saunders; 2003:1109–1124.

Bryan RT, Michelson MK. Parasitic infections of the liver and biliary tree. In: Surawicz C, Owen RL, eds. *Gastrointestinal and Hepatic Infections.* Philadelphia: Saunders; 1995:405–454.

Canto MIF, Diehl AM. Bacterial infections of the liver and biliary system. In: Surawicz C, Owen RL, eds. *Gastrointestinal and Hepatic Infections.* Philadelphia: Saunders; 1995:355–389.

Diaz-Granados CA, Duffus WA, Albrecht H. Parasitic diseases of the liver. In: Zakim DS, Boyer TD, eds. *Hepatology.* Philadelphia: Saunders; 2003:1073–1107.

Drugs for parasitic infections. *Med Lett.* 2007;5:e1–e15.

Hay RJ. Fungal infections affecting the liver. In: Bircher J, Benhamou JP, McIntyre N, eds. *Oxford Textbook of Clinical Hepatology.* Oxford: Oxford University Press; 1999:1025–1032.

Kibbler CC, Sanchez-Tapias JM. Bacterial infection and the liver. In: Bircher J, Benhamou JP, McIntyre N, eds. *Oxford Textbook of Clinical Hepatology. Oxford.* Oxford University Press; 1999:989–1016.

Kim AY, Chung RT. Bacterial, parasitic, and fungal infections of the liver, including liver abscesses. In: Feldman M, Friedman LS, Brandt LJ, eds. *Gastrointestinal and Liver Disease: Pathophysiology/Diagnosis/Management.* 10th ed. Philadelphia: Saunders Elsevier; 2016:1374–1392.

Low DE. Toxic shock syndrome: major advances in pathogenesis, but not treatment. *Crit Care Clin.* 2013;29:651–675.

Lucas SB. Other viral and infectious diseases and HIV-related liver disease. In: MacSween RNM, Burt AD, Portmann BC, eds. *Pathology of the Liver.* London: Churchill Livingstone; 2002:363–414.

Maguire JH. Disease due to helminths. In: Mandell GL, Bennet JE, Dolin R, eds. *Mandell, Douglas, and Bennett's Principles and Practice of Infectious Diseases.* 7th ed. Philadelphia: Churchill Livingstone Elsevier; 2009:3573–3575.

Palomo AM, Warell DA, Francis N, et al. Protozoal infections. In: Bircher J, Benhamou JP, McIntyre N, et al., eds. *Oxford Textbook of Clinical Hepatology.* Oxford: Oxford University Press; 1999:1033–1058.

Warren KS, Bresson-Hadni S, Miguet JP, et al. Helminthiasis. In: Bircher J, Benhamou JP, McIntyre N, et al., eds. *Oxford Textbook of Clinical Hepatology.* Oxford: Oxford University Press; 1999:1059–1086.

White NJ, Pukrittayakamee S, Hien TT, et al. Malaria. *Lancet.* 2014;383:723–735.

WHO Malaria Policy Advisory Committee and Secretariat. Malaria. Policy Advisory Committee to the WHO: conclusions and recommendations of sixth biannual meeting (September 2014). *Malar J.* 2015;(14):107.

CHAPTER 32

Surgery in the Patient With Liver Disease and Postoperative Jaundice

Andrew S. deLemos, MD ■ Lawrence S. Friedman, MD

KEY POINTS

1 Minor liver biochemical test abnormalities are common after surgery; overt liver dysfunction is uncommon but more likely if the patient has preexisting liver disease.

2 Hepatic blood flow is reduced by anesthesia, blood loss, and other hemodynamic derangements.

3 Operative mortality is increased in patients with acute hepatitis, alcoholic hepatitis, severe chronic hepatitis, and Child-Pugh class B and C cirrhosis; additional risk factors include emergency surgery, biliary surgery, cardiac surgery, liver resection, ascites, and hypoxemia.

4 The Model for End-stage Liver Disease (MELD) score predicts operative mortality with greater accuracy than the Child-Pugh classification, and the increase in risk is remarkably linear for MELD scores >8. American Society of Anesthesiologists (ASA) class IV adds an additional 5.5 MELD points, and age older than 70 years adds an additional 3 MELD points.

5 Postoperative jaundice may result from an increased pigment load as a result of transfusion or hemolysis, hepatocellular dysfunction as a result of reduced hepatic blood flow, drug toxicity, infection, or, rarely, biliary obstruction.

Effects of Anesthesia and Surgery on the Liver

OVERVIEW

1. Surgical procedures, whether performed using general or local (i.e., spinal or epidural) anesthesia, are often followed by changes in liver biochemical test results.

2. Postoperative elevations of serum aminotransferase, alkaline phosphatase, or bilirubin levels are generally minor and transient, and in patients without underlying cirrhosis, these changes are not clinically important.

3. Clinically significant hepatic dysfunction can occur in patients with preexisting acute liver disease or cirrhosis and is more common in patients with compromised hepatic synthetic function.

EFFECTS OF ANESTHETIC AGENTS ON THE CIRRHOTIC LIVER

1. At baseline, hepatic arterial and venous perfusion of the cirrhotic liver is decreased because of the following:
   ■ Portal hypertension that decreases portal blood flow
   ■ Impaired autoregulation that decreases arterial blood flow

- Arteriovenous shunting around the liver
- Reduced splanchnic inflow

2. Decreased hepatic perfusion at baseline makes the cirrhotic liver more susceptible to hypoxemia and hypotension in the operating room; induction causes a reduction in hepatic blood flow by 30% to 50%.

OTHER INTRAOPERATIVE FACTORS

Intraoperative factors that may decrease hepatic oxygenation by further decreasing hepatic blood flow or increasing splanchnic vascular resistance are as follows:

- Hypotension caused by hepatorenal syndrome or shock
- Hemorrhage
- Hypoxemia caused by ascites, hepatic hydrothorax, hepatopulmonary syndrome, portopulmonary hypertension, or aspiration
- Hypercapnia
- Heart failure
- Vasoactive drugs
- Intermittent positive pressure ventilation
- Pneumoperitoneum during laparoscopic surgery
- Traction on abdominal viscera with reflex dilatation of splanchnic capacitance vessels

HEPATIC METABOLISM OF ANESTHETIC AGENTS

1. Inhalational anesthetic agents are lipid-soluble compounds that require hepatic transformation to more water-soluble compounds for biliary excretion.
2. Consequences of hepatic metabolism
   a. Prolonged anesthetic action in patients with liver disease (also caused by hypoalbuminemia and impaired biliary excretion)
   b. Formation of toxic intermediates or reactive oxygen species, especially in the presence of hypoxia or reduced hepatic blood flow
      - Halothane → hepatitis (uncommon)
      - Enflurane → hepatitis (even less common)
3. **Isoflurane, desflurane, sevoflurane, and nitrous oxide** are preferable in patients with liver disease because these agents undergo the least hepatic metabolism and hepatic arterial blood flow alterations, and resulting hepatitis is rare.
4. **Propofol** is an excellent anesthetic choice in patients with liver disease; although it is metabolized by hepatic glucuronidation, its serum half-life remains short even in patients with cirrhosis, it increases hepatic blood flow, and it does not precipitate hepatic encephalopathy.
5. Of the induction agents, etomidate and thiopental decrease hepatic blood flow, but **ketamine** does not.

OTHER AGENTS IN LIVER DISEASE

1. Narcotics and sedatives are generally well tolerated in patients with compensated liver disease.
   a. These drugs have a prolonged duration of action in decompensated liver disease.
      - **Narcotics** have high first-pass extraction by the liver.
        - Blood levels increase as hepatic blood flow decreases.
        - Bioavailability is increased because of portosystemic shunting.
        - Preferred agents are **fentanyl and sufentanil**, which have similar durations of action in healthy persons and in patients with cirrhosis.

- ■ **Benzodiazepines** have low first-pass extraction by the liver.
  - – Those eliminated by glucuronidation (**oxazepam, lorazepam**) are not affected by liver disease.
  - – Those not glucuronidated (diazepam, chlordiazepoxide) have enhanced sedative effects in liver disease and should be avoided.
  - b. They may precipitate hepatic encephalopathy in patients with severe liver disease.
  - c. Smaller than standard doses are indicated for those drugs whose metabolism is affected by liver disease.
2. Muscle relaxants
  - a. Succinylcholine should be avoided. Resistance occurs in patients with liver disease in part because of decreased hepatic pseudocholinesterase production. The large doses required in patients with liver disease may cause difficulty in reversing their effect postoperatively.
  - b. The volume of distribution for nondepolarizing muscle relaxants is increased, and larger doses than usual may be required. **Atracurium and cisatracurium** are preferred because neither the liver nor the kidney is required for elimination.

EFFECT OF SURGERY

1. **The nature and extent of surgery may be more important determinants of postoperative hepatic dysfunction than anesthesia.**
2. Perioperative risk is increased with biliary tract and open abdominal surgery and is greatest with cardiac surgery and liver resection.
  - a. In patients with cholecystitis, laparoscopic cholecystectomy is permissible in patients in Child-Pugh class A and selected patients in Child-Pugh class B without portal hypertension; however, in patients with more advanced cirrhosis with portal hypertension, cholecystostomy is preferable.
  - b. Risk factors for hepatic decompensation after cardiac surgery include total time on cardiopulmonary bypass, use of pulsatile as opposed to nonpulsatile bypass, and need for perioperative vasopressor support; cardiopulmonary bypass may exacerbate coagulopathy.
  - c. Less invasive cardiovascular procedures (e.g., angioplasty, valvuloplasty, endovascular aneurysm repair) are preferred to open surgery in patients with advanced cirrhosis. Occasionally, however, major cardiac surgery (including heart transplantation) may be performed at the same time as liver transplantation in selected cases.

Estimation of Operative Risk in Patients With Liver Disease

Absolute contraindications to surgery (other than liver transplantation) are listed in Box 32.1.

BOX 32.1 ■ Contraindications to Elective Surgery in Patients With Liver Disease

Acute liver failure
Acute viral hepatitis
Alcoholic hepatitis
Acute renal failure
Severe cardiomyopathy
Hypoxemia
Severe coagulopathy (despite treatment)
American Society of Anesthesiologists class V

PROBLEMS IN ESTIMATING OPERATIVE RISK

- Large prospective studies and randomized controlled trials are lacking.
- Data on acute and chronic hepatitis are limited.
- The effects of comorbid conditions on surgical risk are difficult to quantitate.

ACUTE HEPATITIS (see Chapters 3, 4, and 5)

1. Acute hepatitis of any cause increases operative risk.
2. Elective surgery should be avoided in patients with acute hepatitis. In the past, exploratory laparotomy was often performed to differentiate viral hepatitis from cholestatic disorders. Currently, such a distinction is made by a combination of serologic testing, radiologic imaging, cholangiography, and/or percutaneous liver biopsy.
3. Acute hepatitis is almost always self-limited or treatable. It is best to postpone elective surgery until liver dysfunction is investigated and the course of the disease is observed. Surgery can be undertaken after the patient improves.

CHRONIC HEPATITIS (see Chapters 4 and 5)

1. Surgical risk appears to correlate with the clinical, biochemical, and histologic severity of chronic hepatitis.
   - Elective surgery is contraindicated in active, symptomatic disease, particularly when synthetic or excretory function is impaired or portal hypertension is present.
   - Patients with autoimmune hepatitis who undergo surgery and are receiving glucocorticoid therapy require "stress" doses.
2. Inactive hepatitis B or C virus carriers
   a. These patients have no increased surgical risk.
   b. In general, antiviral therapy should not be interrupted in the perioperative period.
   c. A risk exists that the patient may infect medical and surgical personnel (the higher the viral load, the higher the risk). Control measures include the following:
      - Universal precautions should be used when contacting any bodily fluid.
      - All personnel at risk should have received the hepatitis B vaccine.
      - Immediate hepatitis B immune globulin and the vaccine series should be given to unvaccinated personnel who sustain an exposure to hepatitis B.
      - No postexposure prophylaxis is recommended for hepatitis C, but personnel may be monitored for subsequent evidence of infection.

ALCOHOLIC LIVER DISEASE AND NONALCOHOLIC FATTY LIVER DISEASE (see Chapters 8 and 9)

1. Alcoholic fatty liver disease
   - Elective surgery is not contraindicated in the presence of normal liver function.
   - It may be desirable to postpone surgery until nutritional deficiencies are corrected or the acute effects of alcohol have resolved.
2. Alcoholic hepatitis
   - A spectrum of severity exists, and surgical risk is increased.
   - Acute alcoholic hepatitis is a contraindication to elective surgery.
   - Abstinence from alcohol and supportive therapy for at least 12 weeks are generally required before elective surgery.

3. Alcoholism is associated with additional perioperative risks independent of liver disease.
   - Drug metabolism is altered (e.g., acetaminophen toxicity may occur after standard doses in alcoholic patients).
   - Patients should be observed for symptoms and signs of withdrawal.
4. Nonalcoholic fatty liver disease (NAFLD)
   - NAFLD has increased in frequency as the prevalence of obesity has increased in the population.
   - At the time of bariatric surgery, approximately 3% of patients are found incidentally to have cirrhosis.
   - Hepatic steatosis of more than 30% may increase morbidity and mortality after major hepatic resection.
   - Bariatric surgery is not contraindicated in patients with compensated cirrhosis; however, clinically significant portal hypertension increases surgical risk.
   - Combined sleeve gastrectomy with liver transplantation has been studied in a small group of cirrhotic patients with a body mass index >35, with good outcomes.
   - NAFLD improves after bariatric surgery in more than 90% of cases. One year postoperatively, 34% of patients who underwent bariatric surgery experienced regression of fibrosis.

CIRRHOSIS (see Chapter 11)

1. Cirrhosis may be undiagnosed before surgery. Considerations include the following:
   - Multiple causes
   - Wide spectrum of severity
   - Lack of correlation between the presence of cirrhosis and biochemical tests of liver function
   - Importance of careful history taking and physical examination (e.g., cutaneous spider telangiectasias, palmar erythema, splenomegaly) in identifying persons with cirrhosis
2. Important consequences of cirrhosis in the postoperative period
   - Fluid and electrolyte disturbances, renal failure
   - Hypoxemia (right-to-left intrapulmonary shunts)
   - Altered drug metabolism
   - Increased susceptibility to infection (e.g., abdominal abscess, sepsis)
   - Nutritional wasting
   - Portal hypertension (ascites, variceal hemorrhage)
   - Hepatic encephalopathy

Use of the Child-Pugh Classification to Assess Surgical Risk (Table 32.1)

1. Various **risk factors** for surgical morbidity and mortality have been identified in several relatively small retrospective studies of nonportosystemic shunt surgery: Emergency surgery, upper abdominal (especially biliary) surgery, low serum albumin, prolonged prothrombin time (PT) or partial thromboplastin time (PTT), elevated serum bilirubin, anemia, ascites, encephalopathy, malnutrition, postoperative bleeding, portal hypertension, hypoxemia, infection, and Child-Pugh class (Table 32.2).
2. Difficulties in interpreting individual studies
   - Small numbers of patients in most studies
   - Nearly all are retrospective: Potential for selection bias
   - Arbitrary choices of parameters examined
3. Child-Pugh classification (see Table 32.1) reliably predicted operative mortality in independent studies over a 27-year span (Garrison et al [1984]; Mansour et al [1997]; Neff et al [2011]).

TABLE 32.1 ■ Child-Turcotte-Pugh Scoring System and Child-Pugh Classification

	1	2	3
Ascites	None	Easily controlled	Poorly controlled
Encephalopathy	None	Mild	Advanced
Albumin (g/dL)	>3.5	2.8–3.5	<2.8
Bilirubin (mg/dL)	<2	2–3	>3
Prothrombin time (seconds prolonged)	≤4	4–6	>6
Child-Turcotte-Pugh score	**5–6**	**7–9**	**10–15**
Child-Pugh Class	**A**	**B**	**C**

TABLE 32.2 ■ Risk Factors for Surgery in Patients With Cirrhosis

Patient Characteristics	Anemia
	Ascites
	Child-Pugh class B and C
	Encephalopathy
	Hypoalbuminemia
	Hypoxemia
	Infection
	Malnutrition
	Higher MELD score
	Portal hypertension
	Prolonged INR >1.5 that does not correct with vitamin K
	Higher American Society of Anesthesiologist class
Type of Surgery	Cardiac surgery
	Emergency surgery
	Hepatic resection
	Open abdominal (especially biliary and colonic) surgery

INR, International normalized ratio; *MELD,* Model for End-stage Liver Disease.

- ■ Child-Pugh class A: Mortality rate 10%
- ■ Child-Pugh class B: Mortality rate 17% to 30%
- ■ Child-Pugh class C: Mortality rate 63% to 82%
4. Experience with laparoscopic surgery in the 2000s suggests that in patients with Child-Pugh class C cirrhosis, mortality rates may be as low as 8% to 14%.
5. Limitations of the Child-Pugh classification
    - ■ Definition of terms (e.g., does "no ascites" mean clinically or sonographically absent?)
    - ■ Subjective parameters (e.g., encephalopathy: What is "mild" versus "advanced"?)
    - ■ Assignment of overall class based on components in different classes (Child-Turcotte-Pugh score uses a point system to add greater precision; see Table 32.1)

6. **The Child-Pugh class has been the most widely used predictor of surgical risk.** Its useful-
    ness has been demonstrated in retrospective, but not prospective, studies. It correlates with
    postoperative mortality and morbidity (liver failure, encephalopathy, bleeding, sepsis, ascites,
    renal failure, and pulmonary failure).
7. In addition to the Child-Pugh class, risk factors predictive of perioperative mortality include
    the following:
    - Emergency surgery
    - Biliary tract surgery: Marked vascularity of the gallbladder bed in patients with portal
      hypertension
    - Colorectal surgery
    - Hepatic resection: Generally contraindicated in decompensated cirrhosis but feasible in
      Child-Pugh class A cirrhosis (risk of morbidity and mortality correlates with preoperative
      portal hypertension and the amount of liver resected). Additional risk factors for morbidity
      and mortality in patients undergoing hepatic resection include active hepatitis, thoracot-
      omy, pulmonary disease, diabetes mellitus, malignancy, and steatohepatitis (see discussion
      later in chapter).
    - Cardiac surgery (70% mortality rate in patients with a Child-Turcotte-Pugh score ≥8)
    - Hypoxemia (Po_2 <60 mm Hg): For example, as a result of hepatopulmonary syndrome or
      portopulmonary hypertension
    - Surgery on the respiratory tract: Risk increased in patients with chronic obstructive pul-
      monary disease
    - Ascites: Risk of abdominal wall herniation and wound dehiscence

Use of the MELD Score to Assess Surgical Risk

1. **The MELD score was developed to predict outcomes following insertion of a transjugular
    intrahepatic portosystemic shunt (TIPS). It is used to prioritize candidates for liver trans-
    plantation and is increasingly used to predict surgical risk in patients with cirrhosis.** The
    MELD score is a linear regression model based on serum bilirubin, international normalized
    ratio (INR), and serum creatinine. Modifications of the traditional MELD score incorporate
    the serum sodium level and presence of ascites.
2. Advantages of the MELD score over the Child-Pugh classification
    - Objective
    - Weights the variables
    - Does not rely on arbitrary cutoff values
    The result is increased precision in predicting postoperative mortality.
3. Results of a large retrospective study of MELD as a predictor of perioperative mortality (Teh
    et al [2007]) are as follows:
    a. MELD score up to 7: Mortality rate 5.7%
    b. MELD score of 8 to 11: Mortality rate 10.3%
    c. MELD score of 12 to 15: Mortality rate 25.4%
    d. The increase in risk of death was nearly linear for MELD scores >8 (Fig. 32.1).
    e. Limitations
        - Median MELD score was 8; few patients had a MELD score >15.
        - Most patients had a platelet count >60,000/mm^3 or an INR <1.5.
4. In addition to the MELD score, risk factors predictive of perioperative mortality include the
    following:
    a. **ASA class** (Table 32.3)
        - ASA class IV: Add 5.5 MELD points.
        - ASA class V is a contraindication to surgery, except liver transplantation; 100% mortal-
          ity is expected.

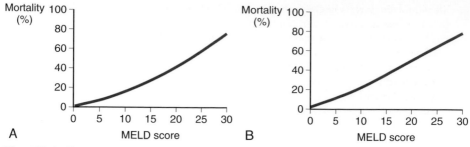

Fig. 32.1 The association between operative mortality and Model for End-stage Liver Disease (MELD) score in patients with cirrhosis undergoing surgery. A, 30-day mortality. B, 90-day mortality. (From Teh SH, Nagorney DM, Stevens SR, et al. Risk factors for mortality after surgery in 772 patients with cirrhosis. *Gastroenterology*. 2007;132:1261–1269.)

TABLE 32.3 ■ American Society of Anesthesiologists Classification

Class	
I	Healthy patient
II	Patient with mild systemic disease without functional limitation
III	Patient with severe systemic disease with functional limitation
IV	Patient with severe systemic disease that is a constant threat to life
V	Moribund patient not expected to survive >24 hr with or without surgery
E	Emergency nature of surgery (added to classification I–V above)

    b. Age: In patients whose age is >70 years, add 3 MELD points.
5. To calculate 7-day, 30-day, 90-day, and 1-year surgical mortality based on the MELD score, ASA class, and age, use the algorithm at http://www.mayoclinic.org/meld/mayomodel9.html.
6. In patients with a MELD score ≥15, a serum albumin level ≤2.5 mg/dL has been shown to be associated with a much higher postoperative mortality rate (60%) than that associated with a serum albumin level >2.5 mg/dL (14%).

Obstructive Jaundice (see Chapters 35 and 36)

SURGICAL RISK

1. Mortality rate: 8% to 28%
2. Risk factors identified in patients undergoing surgery for relief of biliary obstruction
   a. Initial hematocrit value <30%
   b. Initial serum bilirubin level >11 mg/dL
   c. Malignant cause of obstruction
      ■ All three present: Mortality rate 60%
      ■ All three absent: Mortality rate <5%
   d. Azotemia
   e. Hypoalbuminemia
   f. Cholangitis

3. Risk factors for surgery of bile duct stones
   - Serum bilirubin level
   - Other medical illnesses (however, not a risk factor for endoscopic sphincterotomy)
   - Preoperative endoscopic sphincterotomy
4. Situations in which endoscopic sphincterotomy for bile duct stones is preferable to surgery
   - Patients at high operative risk
   - Retained stones after cholecystectomy
   - Severe acute cholangitis

PERIOPERATIVE COMPLICATIONS IN PATIENTS WITH OBSTRUCTIVE JAUNDICE

Complications are presumed to result from increased circulating levels of endotoxin caused by impaired bile salt delivery to bowel and decreased hepatic reticuloendothelial function.

1. Renal failure
   - Decreased glomerular filtration rate in 60% to 75% (versus <1% of anicteric surgical patients)
   - Frank renal failure in 8% with a mortality rate >50%
2. Disseminated intravascular coagulation
3. Gastric stress ulcers and bleeding
4. Delayed wound healing, wound dehiscence, and incisional hernias

STRATEGIES TO REDUCE POTENTIAL COMPLICATIONS

1. Reduction or prevention of endotoxemia: Experimental—oral bile salts, oral antibiotics, or lactulose
2. Preoperative intravenous antibiotic administration to prevent wound infection
3. Adequate perioperative hydration: Possibly a critical factor
4. Avoidance of aminoglycosides and nonsteroidal antiinflammatory drugs because they are potentially nephrotoxic

PREOPERATIVE BILIARY DECOMPRESSION

1. Endoscopic or percutaneous biliary drainage is preferable to surgery for benign conditions in patients with cirrhosis.
   - In a large multicenter, retrospective study of 538 endoscopic retrograde cholangiopancreatographies (ERCPs) in 328 patients, the adverse event rate was 6% in Child-Pugh class A patients and 11% in Child-Pugh class B and C patients. Sphincterotomy was not associated with an increased risk of bleeding in patients with coagulopathy or thrombocytopenia.
   - EUS-guided biliary drainage is an emerging modality under investigation in cases in which ERCP is unsuccessful.
2. **Routine biliary decompression before surgery for malignant obstruction does not reduce subsequent operative mortality, but increases morbidity.**
   - No decrease in mortality occurs.
   - Complications of transhepatic biliary drainage include cholangitis, sepsis, dehydration, and catheter displacement.
   - Routine preoperative endoscopic internal biliary drainage increases the rate of morbidity, but does not decrease the rate of mortality in patients undergoing pancreatic cancer resection; therefore, it is not recommended unless surgery is delayed or the patient has cholangitis or pruritus.

3. Endoscopic biliary decompression is a useful alternative to surgery for palliation of patients with inoperable malignancy or poor surgical risk; however, it does not generally prolong survival. Endoprosthesis insertion may also be a reasonable alternative to operative bypass in selected patients; endoscopic stenting is associated with fewer early complications than surgery, with fewer late complications.

Hepatic Resection (see Chapter 29)

1. Hepatocellular carcinoma (HCC) is a common complication of cirrhosis with a frequency of 1% to 5% per year depending in part on the cause of cirrhosis.
2. The MELD score is the best available predictor of morbidity and mortality in patients with cirrhosis who undergo liver resection.
   - In a large study of 1,017 patients, a MELD score >8 was associated with a mortality rate of 4% and a morbidity rate of 16%, although most patients underwent small resections and had a mean MELD score of 6.
   - In another study, the postoperative mortality rate for patients with a MELD score ≥9 was 29% versus 0% for those with a MELD score <9. Clinically significant portal hypertension defined as a hepatic venous pressure gradient ≥10 mm Hg or the presence of gastroesophageal varices and a platelet count <100,000/mm^3 with splenomegaly is associated with clinical decompensation after surgery and possibly increased 3- and 5-year mortality rates.
3. An alternative to hepatic resection in some patients with HCC is radiofrequency or microwave ablation. A retrospective review of 837 patients with HCC and cirrhosis found a significant reduction in mortality and morbidity with ablation compared with major and minor hepatectomy.
4. **Postresection liver failure** is defined by the 50-50 rule.
   - The PT index (patient's PT relative to control PT) is <50% (i.e., INR >1.7).
   - The serum bilirubin level is >50 μmol/L (2.9 mg/dL).
   - The mortality rate is 59% when these adverse criteria are present versus 1.2% when they are absent.

Preoperative Evaluation and Preparation

GENERAL MEASURES

1. History and physical examination
   - **All patients should be screened for unrecognized liver disease preoperatively by history, physical examination, and, if there are risk factors or evidence of liver disease, biochemical testing.**
   - Patients with cirrhosis can have normal routine laboratory test results; screening laboratory testing cannot replace a thorough history and physical examination.
   - The severity of liver disease should be assessed (determine Child-Pugh class, MELD score, ASA class).
   - A careful medication and alcohol history should be included.
   - Physical examination findings in cirrhosis may include palmar erythema, spider telangiectasias, abnormal hepatic size or contour, splenomegaly, hepatic encephalopathy, ascites, testicular atrophy, and gynecomastia.
2. Liver biochemical tests: Aspartate aminotransferase (AST), alanine aminotransferase (ALT), alkaline phosphatase, bilirubin, and albumin
   a. Of unclear cost effectiveness in healthy, asymptomatic patients although often part of routine preoperative evaluation

    b. Indicated in patients who drink alcohol regularly and those with a remote history of hepatitis or risk factors for hepatitis (e.g., injection drug use); check hepatitis B surface antigen and antibody to hepatitis C virus

    c. Further investigation of any patient with clinical or biochemical evidence of liver disease (see Chapter 1):

        ■ Hepatocellular dysfunction: Biochemical and serologic testing for viral hepatitis, autoimmune liver disease, and metabolic disorders; possible liver biopsy

        ■ Cholestasis: Radiologic or endoscopic imaging (abdominal ultrasonography, possibly magnetic resonance, endoscopic, or transhepatic cholangiography), with or without liver biopsy

TREATMENT OF COAGULOPATHY

1. Impaired hemostasis in liver disease

    a. Vitamin K deficiency: Decreased levels of factors II, VII, IX, and X

    b. Decreased hepatic protein synthesis: Decrease in levels of all factors except VIII, which may be increased

    c. Low-grade disseminated intravascular coagulation causing increased fibrinolysis

    d. Pattern of hemostatic abnormalities

        ■ Prolonged PT

        ■ Normal or increased PTT

        ■ Prolonged thrombin time

        ■ Low plasma fibrinogen level

        ■ Decreased plasma levels of antithrombin, protein C, and protein S

    e. Thrombocytopenia: Result of hypersplenism or alcohol-induced bone marrow suppression

    f. The degree of prolongation of the PT does not correlate with the patient's risk of bleeding because of changes in levels of both procoagulant and anticoagulant factors in the plasma of patients with cirrhosis.

    g. Thromboelastography-guided blood product use in patients with cirrhosis before invasive procedures may reduce the need for products without increasing bleeding risk.

2. Preoperative preparation

    ■ Vitamin K 10 mg intravenously (one to three doses): Corrects hypoprothrombinemia related to malnutrition or intestinal bile salt deficiency, not hepatocellular disease

    ■ Fresh frozen plasma in patients with hepatocellular dysfunction: Aim for an INR <1.5 (the large volumes required and short half-life limit efficacy.)

    ■ Platelet transfusions: 8 to 10 U when count is <50,000/mm^3

    ■ Surgical risk and bleeding risk in patients with INR >1.5 or platelets <50,000/mm^3 are unknown because they have not been studied.

    ■ Adjunctive therapy considered only when active bleeding does not respond to standard measures: 1-deamino-8-d-arginine vasopressin (DDAVP, a factor VIII stimulant, shortens bleeding time; clinical usefulness uncertain), antifibrinolytic agents (ε-aminocaproic acid, tranexamic acid; value uncertain), recombinant factor VIIa (expensive, short half-life; of unproven benefit)

TREATMENT OF ASCITES (see Chapter 13)

1. Diagnostic paracentesis is indicated in patients with new or worsening ascites: To exclude infection or malignancy and to differentiate spontaneous from secondary (surgical) bacterial peritonitis.

2. Ascites should be controlled before abdominal surgery to reduce the risk of postoperative wound dehiscence or herniation.

    ■ Salt restriction (2-g sodium diet)

    ■ Combination diuretics: Spironolactone 100 → 400 mg/day + furosemide 40 → 160 mg/day, as necessary

- Preoperative TIPS: May lower surgical risk in patients with a low MELD score, no encephalopathy, and refractory ascites or large varices who require intraabdominal surgery
- Monitoring of patient's weight, intake and output, urinary sodium concentration (>25 mEq/L if diuretics are effective); if necessary, central venous pressure monitoring
- 1 L/day fluid restriction if hyponatremia (sodium <125 mEq/L)

3. When intraoperative volume expansion is needed, blood products, intravenous 25% salt-poor albumin, and (in the absence of hyponatremia) 5% dextrose in water (D5W) can be administered; crystalloids should be avoided if possible.

TREATMENT OF RENAL DYSFUNCTION (see Chapter 14)

1. Serum creatinine and blood urea nitrogen (BUN) should be monitored perioperatively; however, serum creatinine may underestimate renal dysfunction because of muscle wasting and decreased urea synthesis.
2. The following nephrotoxic drugs should be avoided:
   - Aminoglycosides
   - Nonsteroidal antiinflammatory drugs
   - Intravenous contrast agents
3. The differential diagnosis of acute kidney injury in patients with cirrhosis includes the following:
   - Volume depletion
   - Drug nephrotoxicity
   - Acute tubular necrosis
   - Hepatorenal syndrome
4. **Hepatorenal syndrome** is characterized by a rise in serum creatinine of ≥0.3 mg/dL compared with baseline that persists despite diuretic withdrawal and volume expansion with intravenous salt-poor albumin in the setting of cirrhosis and ascites and the absence of parenchymal kidney disease and nephrotoxic drug use (see Chapter 14).
   a. It may be precipitated by sudden volume loss (e.g., bleeding, rapid diuresis, paracentesis), infection (e.g., spontaneous bacterial peritonitis), or a decrease in cardiac output.
   b. Potential treatments are as follows:
      - Intravenous terlipressin (under study but not available in the United States) and intravenous salt-poor albumin; may be most effective approach
      - Oral midodrine (an alpha agonist), subcutaneous octreotide, and intravenous albumin (not approved by the U.S. Food and Drug Administration [FDA] for this indication)
      - Intravenous norepinephrine (titrated to increase mean arterial pressure 10 mm Hg) and intravenous albumin (not approved by the FDA for this indication)
      - Liver transplantation

TREATMENT OF HEPATIC ENCEPHALOPATHY (see Chapter 15)

1. **Importance** of preoperative recognition of encephalopathy: High frequency in the postoperative period of precipitating or exacerbating factors
   - Gastrointestinal bleeding
   - Constipation
   - Azotemia
   - Hypokalemic alkalosis
   - Sepsis
   - Hypoxia
   - Use of central nervous system depressant drugs (e.g., narcotics or benzodiazepines)

2. Treatment
   a. Control of clinically overt encephalopathy preoperatively (preemptive therapy is of unproven benefit)
   b. Correction of precipitating factors
   c. Lactulose: Oral unabsorbable disaccharide in dose needed to achieve three bowel movements per day
      ■ Converts intestinal ammonia (NH_3) to unabsorbable ammonium (NH_4^+)
      ■ Enhances growth of nonammoniagenic intestinal bacteria
   d. Oral antibiotic should be added when lactulose has not achieved adequate control (e.g., rifaximin 550 mg twice daily).

MISCELLANEOUS ISSUES

1. Risk of **hypoglycemia** in acute hepatic failure and to a lesser extent in decompensated cirrhosis: In patients at risk, an intravenous infusion of 10% dextrose in water (D10W) should be administered.
2. **Gastroesophageal varices:** Primary prophylaxis with nonselective beta blockers or endoscopic band ligation to prevent variceal bleeding is indicated.
3. All cirrhotic patients are at risk of **protein-energy malnutrition;** mortality is increased after surgery in malnourished patients.
   ■ When time permits, preoperative enteral nutritional supplementation improves immunocompetence and short-term prognosis.
   ■ Percutaneous gastrostomy is contraindicated in patients with ascites or coagulopathy.
4. There is no clear evidence that preoperative TIPS placement improves outcome in patients with cirrhosis undergoing abdominal surgery.

POSTOPERATIVE MONITORING FOR SIGNS OF HEPATIC DECOMPENSATION

■ Onset of jaundice, encephalopathy, ascites
■ Rise in serum bilirubin, prolongation of PT, worsening renal function, hypoglycemia

Postoperative Jaundice

Postoperative jaundice can occur in patients with or without underlying liver disease. Pathophysiologic mechanisms in the postoperative period are often multiple (Box 32.2).

1. **Increased pigment load** (predominantly indirect hyperbilirubinemia)
   ■ Resorption of hematoma or hemoperitoneum
   ■ Transfusion: 10% of erythrocytes in a unit of 14-day-old bank blood undergo hemolysis within 24 hours of transfusion.
   ■ Hemolysis (rare): Usually in setting of congenital erythrocyte defect, such as glucose-6-phosphate dehydrogenase (G6PD) deficiency or sickle cell disease
   ■ Postcardiac surgery status: Risk factors include preoperative elevations of serum bilirubin level and right atrial pressure, valve replacement (and number of valves replaced), and use of intraaortic balloon counterpulsation; in this setting, hyperbilirubinemia is a marker of increased mortality.
   ■ Inherited disorder of bilirubin metabolism (e.g., Gilbert syndrome): May be coincidentally diagnosed after a surgical procedure
2. **Impaired hepatocellular function**
   a. **Benign postoperative intrahepatic cholestasis:** Hepatocyte dysfunction from various stresses, such as hypoxemia, anesthesia, hemorrhage, sepsis, extensive transfusions;

BOX 32.2 ■ Causes of Postoperative Jaundice

Increased Bilirubin Load

Hemolysis after transfusion
Hematoma resorption
Underlying hemolytic anemia
Gilbert syndrome[a]

Impaired Hepatocellular Function

Anesthetic agents: Halothane, enflurane, rarely isoflurane, desflurane, sevoflurane
Antibiotics: Tetracycline, chloramphenicol, erythromycins, sulfonamides, nitrofurantoin
Other drugs: Phenothiazines, isoniazid, methyldopa, androgens, estrogens
Total parenteral nutrition
Viral hepatitis
Ischemic hepatitis
Sepsis
Benign postoperative intrahepatic cholestasis

Extrahepatic Obstruction

Bile duct stone
Cholecystitis, cholangitis, abscess
Biliary stricture, leak, tumor
Pancreatitis

---

[a]Unconjugated hyperbilirubinemia resulting from congenital defect in the hepatocyte uptake of bilirubin.

---

often occurs in the setting of prolonged, difficult surgery with postoperative multiorgan failure

- Peak serum bilirubin of up to 40 mg/dL on postoperative day 2 to 10 with variable elevation of alkaline phosphatase and no more than mild elevation of aminotransferases
- May mimic extrahepatic obstruction
- Prognosis depends on the overall condition of the patient, not liver status; liver function returns to normal if and when the patient recovers.

   b. Hyperbilirubinemia of sepsis triggered by bacterial infections, especially gram-negative sepsis and pneumococcal pneumonia

   c. Viral hepatitis
- Hepatitis C: The major cause of posttransfusion hepatitis in the past; now rare; acute hepatitis occurs 6 to 7 weeks after transfusion.
- Hepatitis B: Also uncommon with contemporary serologic screening of donated blood; incubation period 12 to 14 weeks
- Rarely Epstein-Barr virus, cytomegalovirus, or hepatitis D (with B)

   d. Drug-related hepatitis
- Halothane: Rare, with frequency of 1 in 35,000 exposures; onset of fever within 2 to 10 days of exposure; pathophysiologic mechanism involves immune sensitization to trifluoroacetylated liver proteins formed by oxidative metabolism of halothane by cytochrome P-450 2E1 in persons with a possible genetic predisposition.
- Enflurane: Less common cause of hepatitis than halothane
- Other drugs (e.g., erythromycin, sulfonamides, phenytoin, isoniazid, amoxicillin-clavulanic acid); some drugs may cause intrahepatic cholestasis (e.g., chlorpromazine, anabolic steroids). A single dose of cefazolin was implicated in 19 cases of drug-induced liver injury with a latency of 20 days, cholestatic symptoms, and a self-limited course.

   e. Ischemic hepatitis (hypoxic hepatitis, shock liver): In setting of trauma, shock, hyperthermia; typically associated with marked elevations of serum aminotransferase levels (often to >5000 U/L), as well as lactate dehydrogenase levels, that fall abruptly with stabilization of the patient; delayed rise in bilirubin up to 20 mg/dL may be seen

   f. Total parenteral nutrition: May be associated with hepatomegaly, minor elevations of serum aminotransferase levels, fatty infiltration (presumably from high glucose load or possibly carnitine or choline deficiency), or intrahepatic cholestasis and nonspecific periportal inflammation (presumably from intravenous amino acids or fat emulsions and possibly toxic bile salts such as lithocholic acid); fatty liver may be reversible with a decrease in the percentage of glucose or lecithin or choline supplementation.

3. **Extrahepatic obstruction** (uncommon cause of jaundice in postoperative period)

- Unrecognized bile duct injury with biloma formation, usually during cholecystectomy
- Cholangitis, subphrenic or subhepatic abscesses secondary to biliary obstruction
- Choledocholithiasis, biliary or pancreatic tumor
- If biliary obstruction is suspected, evaluation with ultrasonography or computed tomography and cholangiography (magnetic resonance cholangiopancreatography or ERCP) may be required.

FURTHER READING

Adler DG, Haseeb A, Francis G, et al. Efficacy and safety of therapeutic ERCP in patients with cirrhosis: a large multicenter study. *Gastrointest Endosc.* 2016;83:353–359.

Berzigotti A, Reig M, Abraldes JG, et al. Portal hypertension and the outcome of surgery for hepatocellular carcinoma in compensated cirrhosis: a systematic review and meta-analysis. *Hepatology.* 2015;61:526–536.

Cucchetti A, Cescon M, Golfieri R, et al. Hepatic venous pressure gradient in the preoperative assessment of patients with resectable hepatocellular carcinoma. *J Hepatol.* 2016;64:79–86.

De Pietri L, Bianchini M, Montalti R, et al. Thromboclastography-guided blood product use before invasive procedures in cirrhosis with severe coagulopathy: a randomized, controlled trial. *Hepatology.* 2016;63:566–573.

Heimbach JK, Watt KD, Poterucha JJ, et al. Combined liver transplantation and gastric sleeve resection for patients with medically complicated obesity and end-stage liver disease. *Am J Transplant.* 2013;13:363–368.

Im GY, Lubezky N, Facciuto ME, et al. Surgery in patients with portal hypertension: a preoperative checklist and strategies for attenuating risk. *Clin Liver Dis.* 2014;18:477–505.

Khan MA, Akbar A, Baron TH, et al. Endoscopic ultrasound-guided biliary drainage: a systematic review and meta-analysis. *Dig Dis Sci.* 2016;61:684–703.

Lassailly G, Caiazzo R, Buob D, et al. Bariatric surgery reduces features of nonalcoholic steatohepatitis in morbidly obese patients. *Gastroenterology.* 2015;149:379–388.

Li GZ, Speicher PJ, Lidsky ME, et al. Hepatic resection for hepatocellular carcinoma: do contemporary morbidity and mortality rates demand a transition to ablation as first-line treatment? *J Am Coll Surg.* 2014;218:827–834.

Montomoli J, Erichsen R, Strate LL, et al. Coexisting liver disease is associated with increased mortality after surgery for diverticular disease. *Dig Dis Sci.* 2015;60:1832–1840.

O'Leary JG, Yachimski PS, Friedman LS. Surgery in the patient with liver disease. *Clin Liver Dis.* 2009;13:211–231.

Reddy SK, Marsh JW, Varley PR, et al. Underlying steatohepatitis, but not simple hepatic steatosis, increases morbidity after liver resection: a case-control study. *Hepatology.* 2012;56:2221–2230.

Teh SH, Nagorney DM, Stevens SR, et al. Risk factors for mortality after surgery in patients with cirrhosis. *Gastroenterology.* 2007;132:1261–1269.

Telem DA, Schiano T, Goldstone R, et al. Factors that predict outcome of abdominal operations in patients with advanced cirrhosis. *Clin Gastroenterol Hepatol.* 2010;8:451–457.

van der Gaag NA, Rauws EA, van Eijck CH, et al. Preoperative biliary drainage for cancer of the head of the pancreas. *N Engl J Med.* 2010;362:129–137.

CHAPTER 33

Liver Transplantation

Andres F. Carrion, MD ■ Kalyan Ram Bhamidimarri, MD, MPH

KEY POINTS

1 Liver transplantation (LT) is a life-saving intervention for patients with acute liver failure, end-stage liver disease (ESLD), some inherited and metabolic liver diseases, and a subset of hepatic malignancies such as hepatocellular carcinoma (HCC), cholangiocarcinoma (CC), and neuroendocrine tumors.

2 Advances in surgical techniques, perioperative management, and immunosuppressive regimens have led to improved outcomes in liver transplant recipients.

3 Selection of appropriate candidates for LT remains a critical step and entails a multidisciplinary approach to identify comorbid conditions and other potential issues that may impair posttransplant outcomes.

4 Live-donor and split LT, as well as the use of extended criteria grafts, have emerged as alternatives because of the ongoing shortage for donor organs and the growing number of patients awaiting LT.

5 Long-term comprehensive care of liver transplant recipients remains critical to improving graft and patient outcomes and entails early identification and treatment of complications as well as continuous implementation of strategies to diminish complications associated with immunosuppressive drugs.

Overview

1. **LT remains the only definitive treatment for ESLD and acute liver failure (ALF), regardless of the etiology.**

2. Current post-LT survival rates of 80% to 90% at 1 year and 60% to 75% at 5 years reflect major advances in surgical technique, perioperative intensive care, immunosuppression, and selection of candidates.

3. Data from the United Network for Organ Sharing (UNOS) show that 14,753 patients were listed for LT in 2015 in the United States, but only 7127 patients actually underwent LT (48.3%).

4. Living donor liver transplantation (LDLT) has emerged as an alternative to increase the number of donor organs.

   ■ The risk of morbidity and mortality for the donor, as well as regional and center-specific differences, limits its widespread applicability.

   ■ Only 5.3% of liver transplants performed in 2015 in the United States were live-donor transplants.

5. Appropriate selection of LT candidates requires a multidisciplinary approach and remains a critical step during the pre-LT evaluation process, as it has major implications for post-LT outcomes.

6. Organ allocation within the United States and many other countries is determined by disease severity as reflected by the **Model for End-stage Liver Disease (MELD) and Pediatric End-stage Liver Disease (PELD) scores,** which predict the probability of death within a 3-month period.

- The MELD and PELD scores were implemented in 2002 to reduce waitlist mortality among liver transplant candidates.
- The **MELD** score includes the international normalized ratio (INR) for prothrombin time, serum bilirubin, and serum creatinine. This score is used for liver transplant candidates ≥12 years of age.
- **MELD-Na:** Hyponatremia is an independent predictor of mortality in patients with cirrhosis; therefore, a new policy has been in effect since January 2016 to use the MELD-Na score. Incorporation of the MELD-Na score for organ allocation is projected to prevent 50 to 60 deaths per year.
- Adult waitlisted candidates are assigned to one of the following categories: (a) Status 1A, (b) calculated or "biological" MELD score, (c) exception MELD score, or (d) inactive status.
- Adult liver transplant candidates listed as status 1A are required to be >18 years of age with one of the following conditions: ALF with life expectancy <7 days without LT, acute decompensated Wilson disease, anhepatic state, primary graft nonfunction (PNF) of whole or split liver, or graft failure due to hepatic artery thrombosis within 7 days post-LT.
- The **PELD** score includes the INR, bilirubin, albumin, and growth failure but does not include serum creatinine. The score is used for liver transplant candidates ≤11 years of age.
- Among pediatric patients, waitlisted candidates are assigned to any one category similar to adults (see earlier) but can also be ascribed an additional category, pediatric status 1B, which includes patients with nonmetastatic hepatoblastoma, organic acidemia, or urea cycle defects.

Indications

Leading indications for LT vary across different countries and regions of the world and largely reflect the incidence and prevalence of specific disorders; data for the United States are summarized in Fig. 33.1.

- The most common indications for LT due to ESLD in Western countries are hepatitis C and alcohol-induced cirrhosis, whereas cirrhosis caused by hepatitis B predominates in Asia.

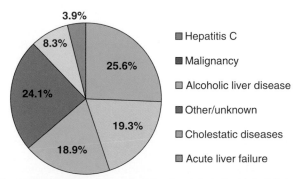

Fig. 33.1 Leading indications for liver transplantation in adults in the United States. (Data from OPTN/SRTR 2014 Annual Data Report, http://srtr.transplant.hrsa.gov.)

- ALF requiring LT is caused primarily by drug-induced liver injury in Western countries and by acute viral hepatitis in Eastern countries.

CIRRHOSIS AND ESLD (see also Chapters 11 through 15)

1. **LT is the only definitive therapy associated with markedly improved long-term survival for patients with decompensated cirrhosis and ESLD, regardless of etiology.**
2. Cirrhosis per se is not an indication for LT. Patients should be referred for liver transplant evaluation once a complication of chronic liver disease occurs (Table 33.1).
3. A substantial survival benefit is achieved through LT for patients with a MELD score ≥15.
4. Treatment of the underlying etiology of liver disease can stabilize or improve hepatic function, and such interventions should be actively pursued (e.g., administration of effective antiviral therapy against hepatitis B or C, immunosuppressive therapy for autoimmune hepatitis, complete cessation of alcohol or offending medications in alcohol- or drug-induced liver diseases).

ACUTE LIVER FAILURE (see also Chapter 2)

1. The clinical course of ALF is often rapid, and outcomes can be unpredictable, with some patients recovering spontaneously or with targeted therapy and others requiring LT or dying during evaluation.
2. Early referral of patients with ALF to an LT center is recommended.
3. Patients with ALF have the highest priority for organ allocation and are listed as status 1A according to current UNOS policies (see earlier). Criteria for UNOS status 1A designation are summarized in Table 33.2.

PRIMARY HEPATIC MALIGNANT TUMORS (see also Chapter 29)

1. **HCC** is the most common primary hepatic malignancy in adults.
   - The majority of patients with HCC in Western populations (95%) have underlying cirrhosis, thereby limiting the applicability of surgical resection. By contrast, only 60% of patients with HCC in Eastern populations have underlying cirrhosis, largely reflecting the high prevalence of hepatitis B viral infection and its oncogenic potential.
   - The **Milan criteria** are the benchmark for LT candidacy for patients with HCC: **A single tumor ≤5 cm in diameter or no more than three tumors with the largest ≤3 cm in diameter, and the absence of portal vein invasion and extrahepatic metastasis.**

TABLE 33.1 ■ **Clinical Stages of Cirrhosis, Complications, and Mortality Rate**

Stage	Complications	1-Year Mortality Rate
1	Neither varices nor ascites	1%
2	Varices	3.4%
3	Ascites	20%
4	Variceal hemorrhage	54%

Adapted from D'Amico G, Garcia-Tsao G, Pagliaro L. Natural history and prognostic indicators of survival in cirrhosis: a systematic review of 118 studies. *J Hepatol.* 2006;44:217–231.

- Criteria for prioritizing liver transplant candidates with HCC have evolved over time, and there have been several changes to listing policies.
- As per the current policy, patients with HCC remain with their "biologic" MELD score at listing and at first appeal at 3 months but accrue exception points after the second appeal at 6 months, when they are upgraded to a MELD score of 28; thereafter, patients continue to accrue 10% increments until attaining a score of 34, at which the exception score is capped.
- In order to balance the oncologic criteria and nononcologic criteria for waitlisted patients and to reduce false-positive radiologic features, a policy went into effect in October 2015 that required LT centers to follow stringent radiologic criteria for the diagnosis of HCC. The Liver Imaging Reporting Data System (LI-RADS) for HCC uses consistent terminology and permits standardized reporting by categorizing lesions according to the probability of being benign or malignant (Tables 33.3 and 33.4).
- Nodules found on imaging should be categorized in accordance with the Organ Procurement and Transplantation Network (OPTN)/UNOS classification. Only OPTN class 5 nodules (LI-RADS-5) are considered HCC (Table 33.5). OPTN class 5 nodules are further divided into subcategories: 5A (T1 lesions), 5A-g (T1 lesions with 50% interval

TABLE 33.2 ■ **Criteria for United Network for Organ Sharing Status 1A Designation in Acute Liver Failure**

Age >18 years

Life expectancy <7 days without liver transplantation

Onset of encephalopathy within 8 weeks of first symptom of liver disease

Absence of preexisting liver disease

Admission to an intensive care unit, and one of the following:
    Ventilator dependence
    Requirement for renal replacement therapy
    INR >2

Fulminant Wilson disease

Primary graft nonfunction

Hepatic artery thrombosis

INR, International normalized ratio.

TABLE 33.3 ■ **Liver Imaging Reporting Data System Categories and Definitions**

Category	Definition
LR-1	Definitely benign
LR-2	Probably benign
LR-3	Intermediate probability for HCC
LR-4	Probably HCC
LR-5 (OPTN class 5)	Definitely HCC
LR-5V	Definitely HCC with tumor in vein
LR-M	Probably malignancy, not specific for HCC

HCC, Hepatocellular carcinoma; *OPTN,* Organ Procurement and Transplantation Network.

TABLE 33.4 ■ **Liver Imaging Reporting Data System Criteria for Hepatocellular Carcinoma**

	Arterial Phase Hypoehancement or Isoenhancement		Arterial Phase Hyperenhancement		
Diameter (mm)	<20	≥20	<10	10–19	≥20
Number of features[a]:					
0	LR-3	LR-3	LR-3	LR-3	LR-4
1	LR-3	LR-4	LR-4	LR-4/LR-5[b]	LR-5
≥2	LR-4	LR-4	LR-4	LR-5	LR-5

See Table 33.3 for definitions of LR categories.

[a]Features include "washout" of tumor on imaging, presence of a capsule, and interval tumor growth.

[b]Lesions in this cell are categorized LR-4 except if there is ≥50% interval growth in ≤6 months or if washout and discrete nodules were observed on antecedent ultrasonography.

Modified from LI-RADS v2014, American College of Radiology, https://nrdr.acr.org/lirads/.

TABLE 33.5 ■ **Categorization of Organ Procurement and Transplantation Network (OPTN) Class 5 Nodules**

Category	Characteristics	Automatic Priority
5A (T1)	Single nodule 1–2 cm	No
5B (T2)	Single nodule 2–5 cm	Yes
5-g (growth)	Single nodule 1–2 cm with 50% interval growth on cross-sectional imaging within 6 months (does not apply to treated lesions)	Yes, only after the lesion grows to T2
5T (treated)	Class 5 nodule after locoregional therapy (persistent or recurrent HCC)	Yes (as per original appeal)
5X (>T2)	Lesions outside Milan criteria/>T2 lesions	No (candidates can still be listed with calculated MELD score; RRB approval is needed for priority)

HCC, Hepatocellular carcinoma; *MELD,* Model for End-stage Liver Disease; *RRB,* regional review board.

growth), 5B (T2 lesions), 5T (treated class 5 lesions), and 5X (lesions larger than T2), of which only 5B nodules are eligible for standard MELD exception points (see later).

■ OPTN 5A lesions are not eligible for standard MELD exception points unless there is more than one 5A nodule, or one or more synchronous 5B lesions are identified.

■ Approximately one third of patients with HCC are outside Milan criteria (OPTN 5X lesions) at the time of diagnosis and are not eligible for MELD exception points, even if downstaged. An individual transplant center may consider such a patient for LT, but the listing will be done as per the calculated MELD/PELD score unless the regional review board (RRB) approves exception points.

■ The use of extended criteria for HCC beyond Milan criteria (e.g., University of California, San Francisco criteria, "rule of 7") is currently not recommended.

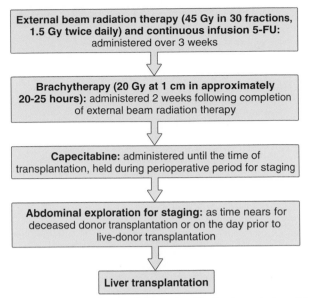

Fig. 33.2 Mayo Clinic neoadjuvant chemoradiation protocol for liver transplant candidates with hilar cholangiocarcinoma. *5-FU,* 5-fluorouracil. (Adapted from Rosen CB, Heimbach JK, Gores GJ. Liver transplantation for cholangiocarcinoma. *Transpl Int.* 2010;23:692–697.)

- Post-LT survival for patients with HCC within the Milan criteria is comparable to that of patients undergoing LT for indications other than HCC.
- Locoregional therapies (e.g., radiofrequency ablation, transarterial chemoembolization) are recommended to prevent progression of the tumors and to diminish "drop out" from the waiting list.
2. **Intrahepatic CC** is the second most common primary hepatic malignancy in adults. LT is not standard therapy for this tumor because LT for CC is associated with poor outcomes.
   - At some transplant centers use of strict protocols that incorporate neoadjuvant chemoradiation for selected patients with perihilar CC stage I or II has resulted in improved post-LT outcomes (Fig. 33.2).
3. **Hepatoblastoma** is the most common primary hepatic malignancy in children and is often treated with neoadjuvant chemotherapy and surgical resection; it commonly occurs in the absence of significant hepatic fibrosis.
4. **Fibrolamellar HCC** is an uncommon tumor variant that occurs in young adults without underlying cirrhosis; extensive surgical resection can often be performed with curative intent.
5. Although LT is currently not a standard therapeutic option for unresectable **hepatic metastases from neuroendocrine tumors,** data from the UNOS database show that 137 liver transplants were performed for this indication between 1988 and 2009, with 81% and 49% 1- and 5-year survival rates, respectively. Similar results were reported from Europe: 213 patients underwent LT between 1982 and 2009, with 81% and 52% 1- and 5-year survival rates, respectively.

METABOLIC DISORDERS

1. Metabolic disorders primarily affecting the liver are more common in pediatric than adult patients.

2. LT can be an effective therapeutic intervention for patients with liver-based metabolic disorders, resulting in cure of the underlying disease.
   - Alpha-1 antitrypsin deficiency (see also Chapter 20)
   - Hereditary hemochromatosis (see also Chapter 18)
   - Wilson disease (see also Chapter 19)
   - Familial amyloid polyneuropathy (see also Chapter 24)
   - Primary hyperoxaluria (see also Chapter 20)
   - Cystic fibrosis (see also Chapter 20)
   - Glycogen storage diseases type I and IV (see also Chapter 25)
   - Tyrosinemia (see also Chapter 25)
   - Acute intermittent porphyria (see also Chapter 20)

Contraindications

1. Absolute and relative contraindications to LT continue to evolve over time.
   - Absolute contraindications imply that successful post-LT outcomes are unlikely and thus LT should not be considered (Table 33.6).
   - Patients with relative contraindications are at high risk for experiencing suboptimal outcomes; however, LT may still be considered in selected patients.
2. Patients initially considered to be appropriate candidates for LT may develop absolute or relative contraindications after being listed; therefore, ongoing evaluation is required after listing.

Comorbid Conditions That Influence Selection

CARDIOVASCULAR DISEASE

1. The prevalence of cardiovascular diseases in patients with ESLD is at least equal to or greater compared to that of the general population.
2. Noninvasive cardiovascular evaluation with dobutamine stress echocardiography is recommended for liver transplant candidates without overt cardiovascular diseases when three or more risk factors are present: Age >60 years, systemic hypertension, diabetes mellitus, dyslipidemia, personal history of cardiovascular disease, left ventricular hypertrophy, or history of smoking.
3. Coronary angiography may be required in liver transplant candidates in whom noninvasive testing does not confidently exclude cardiovascular disease.

TABLE 33.6 ■ Absolute Contraindications to Liver Transplantation

Uncontrolled sepsis
Acquired immunodeficiency syndrome
Active alcohol or substance abuse
Advanced cardiac or pulmonary disease
Intrahepatic cholangiocarcinoma
Hemangiosarcoma
Hepatocellular carcinoma with metastasis
Extrahepatic malignancy
Anatomic abnormalities that preclude liver transplantation
Lack of social support
Persistent nonadherence to medical care

PULMONARY DISEASE

1. In addition to pulmonary disorders prevalent in the general population, such as chronic obstructive pulmonary disease, asthma, and obstructive sleep apnea, specific pulmonary conditions may develop in patients with ESLD: Hepatic hydrothorax, portopulmonary hypertension (POPH), and hepatopulmonary syndrome (HPS).
2. Insertion of indwelling catheters should be avoided in the treatment of hepatic hydrothorax in liver transplant candidates, as infections may occur and jeopardize transplant candidacy.
3. POPH must be confirmed by right heart catheterization. Moderate POPH (mean pulmonary arterial pressure [mPAP] ≥35 mm Hg) increases mortality beyond the estimates predicted by the MELD score and, if not responsive to medical therapy, is a contraindication to LT because it is associated with poor outcomes.
   - Patients with POPH who qualify for LT should have an mPAP <35 mm Hg and pulmonary vascular resistance (PVR) <400 dynes/sec/cm^{-5} with treatment.
   - Such patients accrue 22 MELD exception points, with 10% increments every 3 months if the mPAP remains <35 mm Hg.
4. All liver transplant candidates should be screened for HPS by means of pulse oximetry. In HPS, the arterial oxygen saturation (SpO$_2$) is <96% at sea level by arterial blood gas analysis; if the PaO$_2$ is <60 mm Hg or the Alveolar-arterial (A-a) gradient is ≥15 mm Hg at ambient air, imaging (beginning with contrast-enhanced echocardiography, followed by technetium-labeled macroaggregated albumin scanning if necessary) is advised for detection of intrapulmonary vascular shunts.
   - Patients with HPS qualify for MELD exception points and accrue 22 points with 10% increments every 3 months if their PaO$_2$ remains <60 mm Hg.

INFECTION

1. Active uncontrolled systemic infection is a contraindication to LT.
2. Immunizations should be updated before LT, ideally before the patient develops ESLD. The use of live-attenuated (i.e., measles, mumps, rubella, varicella, herpes zoster, oral polio, rotavirus, nasal influenza, yellow fever) vaccines is contraindicated 4 weeks before LT or any time after LT in patients on therapeutic immunosuppression.
3. Human immunodeficiency virus (HIV) infection
   - LT is performed in HIV-infected patients only in selected transplant centers.
   - The HIV viral load must be undetectable.
   - The CD4+ T cell count should be >100/μL in liver transplant candidates who have never had an opportunistic infection and >200/μL in those with a history of an opportunistic infection.
4. Hepatitis B virus (HBV) infection (see also Chapter 4)
   - Viral suppression with antiviral therapy in liver transplant candidates may improve hepatic function and obviate the need for LT in some patients.
   - Strategies to reduce the risk of recurrent HBV infection post-LT include the use of potent nucleos(t)ide analogs pre- and post-LT as well as administration of hepatitis B immunoglobulin (HBIG) at the time of LT and continued during the early post-LT period.
5. Hepatitis C virus (HCV) infection (see also Chapter 5)
   - Treatment of HCV infection has been revolutionized with licensing of direct-acting antivirals (DAAs) and continues to evolve as newer agents are approved.
   - Unlike interferon-based regimens, several antiviral regimens with combinations of DAAs are safe and effective in patients with decompensated cirrhosis.

- Effective antiviral therapy against HCV that results in a sustained virologic response (SVR) may stabilize or improve hepatic function even in patients with ESLD; however, patients may not experience significant improvement in quality of life or functional status.
- Some patients with severe hepatic decompensation may not benefit from HCV treatment pre-LT because they may not tolerate some DAAs, require a prolonged duration of therapy, achieve low rates of SVR, or lose the opportunity to shorten their waitlist time by accepting organs from an HCV-positive donor.
- In the absence of an SVR before LT, recurrence of HCV infection is universal post-LT and is associated with poor outcomes if not treated. Antiviral therapy with DAAs is indicated promptly for all liver transplant recipients with recurrent HCV infection.
- Several regimens that contain DAAs are well tolerated and highly effective in treating HCV infection in liver transplant recipients.
- Transplant teams should, therefore, be actively involved in decision making about the most appropriate timing of HCV treatment (pre- or post-LT) in a waitlisted patient.

RENAL DYSFUNCTION

1. The significance of renal dysfunction as a predictor of poor transplant-free survival in patients with ESLD is reflected by inclusion of the serum creatinine in the MELD score.
2. Acute kidney injury is common in hospitalized patients with ESLD (20%).
3. Hepatorenal syndrome (HRS) (see also Chapter 14)
   - Type 1 HRS is characterized by acute and rapidly progressive kidney injury associated with extremely poor survival in the absence of LT.
   - Type 2 HRS is more protracted and associated with less severe renal dysfunction and typically with diuretic-resistant ascites.
4. Moderate-to-severe renal dysfunction pre-LT (glomerular filtration rate [GFR] <40 mL/min/1.73 m^2) is associated with an increased frequency of primary liver graft nonfunction post-LT.
5. Simultaneous liver-kidney transplantation should be considered in the following scenarios:
   - Cirrhosis and chronic kidney disease with a GFR <30 mL/min/1.73 m^2
   - Patients with HRS who have a serum creatinine >2 mg/dL and become dialysis dependent for more than 8 weeks
   - Liver failure and chronic kidney disease with evidence of glomerulosclerosis or glomerular fibrosis in >30% of glomeruli on a renal biopsy specimen
   - End-stage renal disease (GFR <15 mL/min/1.73 m^2) and cirrhosis with symptomatic portal hypertension and a wedged hepatic vein pressure gradient ≥10 mm Hg (see Chapter 11)

SUBSTANCE ABUSE AND BEHAVIORAL DISORDERS

1. Detailed assessment of substance abuse disorders is mandatory for all patients undergoing evaluation for LT.
2. Alcohol abuse
   - At least 6 months of complete abstinence from alcohol is required by most transplant centers.
   - Predictors of recidivism for alcohol abuse post-LT include shorter length of abstinence pre-LT, family history of alcohol abuse disorders, documented episodes of past alcohol withdrawal, past failed alcohol rehabilitation, poor social support, and history of polysubstance abuse.

- Up to 25% of patients with alcoholic cirrhosis listed for LT and thought to be abstinent continue to drink alcohol.
- An important survival benefit of LT has been demonstrated for patients with severe acute alcoholic hepatitis that is unresponsive to medical therapy; these patients may undergo LT as allowed by center-specific policies or, preferably, by enrollment in clinical trials.

3. Previous active illicit drug use must be carefully assessed and is prohibited in all candidates undergoing LT evaluation.
4. Marijuana use has been under scrutiny since the mid-2000s, but no specific guidelines regarding its use and liver transplant candidacy exist.
   - Data support worsening fibrosis in marijuana users with HCV infection, and there are emerging reports of pulmonary aspergillosis post-LT.
   - Current policies are center specific and involve stringent evaluation by psychiatrists and substance abuse counselors.
5. Cigarette use should be forbidden in all liver transplant candidates because it increases the incidence of vascular complications and malignancies post-LT; however, smoking is not an absolute contraindication to LT.
6. Mental health professionals should manage psychiatric disorders pre- and post-LT.

NONHEPATIC MALIGNANCIES

1. Age-appropriate screening must be up to date for all liver transplant candidates.
2. Liver transplant candidates with primary sclerosing cholangitis (PSC) should undergo screening colonoscopy, regardless of age.
3. In liver transplant candidates with a history of a nonhepatic malignancy, the malignancy must have been cured without recurrence for at least 2 to 5 years.

Evaluation and Listing

1. Confirmation of the irreversible nature of the acute or chronic underlying liver disease is recommended.
2. Approval for LT should be obtained from the patient's insurance carrier before starting an extensive and costly pre-LT evaluation.
3. A thorough and multidisciplinary evaluation is performed over multiple encounters with members of the LT team to identify additional medical, surgical, behavioral, social, and economic issues that may affect LT candidacy and outcomes.
4. Abdominal imaging studies should be performed to screen for HCC or other hepatic and extrahepatic tumors and to evaluate the anatomy of the bile duct as well as hepatic and intraabdominal vascular structures.
5. LT candidacy should be discussed formally and in detail at an LT selection meeting at each individual transplant center.
6. Formal listing for LT is undertaken by UNOS.
   - Blood type (ABO) is the major determinant of organ compatibility.
   - MELD score determines priority for organ allocation.
   - The use of the MELD-Na score for liver transplant candidates is currently in effect as per UNOS policies (see earlier).
   - MELD exception points can be granted either automatically if the patient has a specific condition for which UNOS awards additional points or on a case-by-case basis upon request to the RRB (see discussion later in chapter).

MELD EXCEPTIONS

1. Some causes of chronic liver disease may result in diminished survival not accurately predicted by the MELD score and may be associated with extremely poor quality of life; therefore, MELD exceptions exist.
2. There are certain conditions for which standardized MELD exception criteria exist and a full RRB evaluation is not required (Table 33.7).
3. For patients with a complicating medical condition related to their liver disease (not qualifying for standard MELD exceptions) and associated with increased morbidity and mortality not adequately reflected by the calculated or biologic MELD score, additional points may be petitioned by the transplant center to the RRB. Examples of conditions that may be granted additional MELD points by the RRB include, but are not limited to, the following:
   - Recurrent bacterial cholangitis in patients with PSC
   - Intractable and debilitating pruritus in patients with primary biliary cholangitis (PBC)
   - Ascites refractory to maximum tolerated doses of diuretics
   - Hepatic encephalopathy refractory to medical therapy
   - Recurrent variceal hemorrhage despite adequate therapy

Surgical Aspects

1. The local organ procurement organization is responsible for harvesting organs once a donor is identified.
   - Warm ischemia time: Interval from cardiovascular collapse to retrieval of the organ from the donor
   - Cold ischemia time: Interval from retrieval of the organ from the donor to reinstitution of its blood supply in the recipient
2. Macroscopic evaluation of the donor liver is performed at the time of harvesting, and a rapid histologic assessment (frozen biopsy) may be obtained for further evaluation of the organ.
3. Donor-recipient matching is based primarily on ABO compatibility and the recipient's weight; human leukocyte antigen (HLA)–based compatibility is not necessary for LT.

TABLE 33.7 ■ **Medical Conditions That Qualify for Standard MELD Score Exception Points**

Condition	Comment
Hepatocellular carcinoma	T2 lesions within Milan criteria
Hepatopulmonary syndrome	PaO_2 <60 mm Hg on ambient air
Portopulmonary hypertension	Mean pulmonary arterial pressure <35 mm Hg with treatment
Familial amyloid polyneuropathy	Confirmed by DNA analysis and histology
Primary hyperoxaluria	Need for simultaneous liver-kidney transplantation
Cystic fibrosis	Forced expiratory volume in 1 sec (FEV1) <40%
Hilar cholangiocarcinoma	Stage I or II; liver transplantation center must have a UNOS approved protocol (see Fig. 33.2)
Hepatic artery thrombosis	Within 14 days of liver transplantation, not meeting criteria for status 1A

MELD, Model for End-stage Liver Disease; *UNOS,* United Network for Organ Sharing.

4. Vascular reconstruction
   ▪ Venous outflow reconstruction can be performed by either anastomosing the donor's vena cava and recipient's vena cava above and below the graft or by a "piggyback" technique that entails a suprahepatic anastomosis of the vena cava.
   ▪ The portal veins of the donor and recipient are typically anastomosed end to end.
   ▪ The hepatic arteries of the donor and recipient are anastomosed end to end without causing tension or leaving a long vessel that may kink. This is the most important vascular anastomosis, and technical problems result in increased morbidity and poor outcomes after LT.
5. Types of biliary anastomosis
   ▪ Choledococholedocostomy (duct to duct): Preferred type of anastomosis because it resembles the normal biliary anatomy and permits easy endoscopic access to the bile ducts post-LT
   ▪ Hepaticojejunostomy or choledocojejunostomy (Roux-en-Y): Traditionally performed in recipients with intrinsic bile duct disease such as PSC or when there is a significant discrepancy in the diameters of the donor and recipient bile ducts; however, there is evidence that a duct-to-duct anastomosis is safe in selected patients with PSC without extrahepatic bile duct involvement and permits continued surveillance post-LT.

APPROACHES TO EXPANDING THE DONOR ORGAN SUPPLY

1. LDLT
   ▪ The success of LDLT in pediatric patients, along with the ongoing scarcity of donor organs, has motivated many transplant centers to perform this procedure in adults as well.
   ▪ Advantages and disadvantages of LDLT are presented in Table 33.8.
2. Donation after cardiac death results in increased warm ischemia times and a higher frequency of biliary complications post-LT.
3. Hepatic grafts from hepatitis B core antibody-positive donors may be used for hepatitis B surface antigen (HBsAg)–positive recipients or even HBsAg-negative recipients, provided that effective prophylactic measures for HBV are administered post-LT (see also Chapter 4).
4. The availability of effective and safe antiviral regimens with DAAs for treatment of HCV infection has resulted in the use of grafts from HCV-positive donors, particularly for HCV-positive recipients, provided that no significant fibrosis is present in the graft.
5. Splitting suitable organs into extended right and left lateral grafts to be used in an adult recipient and pediatric recipient, respectively, may help address the ongoing donor organ shortage.

Immunosuppression

1. The primary goal of therapeutic immunosuppression in LT is to prevent graft rejection and, at the same time, minimize adverse reactions.

TABLE 33.8 ▪ **Advantages and Disadvantages of Live-Donor Liver Transplantation**

Advantages	Disadvantages
Thorough donor screening process	Only offered in selected liver transplantation centers
Elective timing of liver transplantation permitting optimization of therapies	Donor morbidity and mortality
Diminished wait time with consequent reduction in "dropouts"	Higher risk for biliary complications in the donor and recipient
Minimal cold ischemia time	

2. Currently used immunosuppressive regimens are associated with a 35% to 40% rejection rate, but graft loss due to rejection is uncommon (<5%).
3. Protocols for immunosuppression vary among LT centers.
4. Immune tolerance may develop in selected patients, thereby allowing withdrawal of immunosuppression without graft loss.

GLUCOCORTICOIDS

1. Commonly used for induction immunosuppression
2. Mainstay treatment of acute cellular rejection (ACR): Methylprednisolone 500 to 1000 mg intravenously every other day for a total of three doses
   - Approximately 90% of episodes of ACR respond to high dose glucocorticoids.
   - Associated with higher HCV RNA levels and more severe recurrence of hepatitis C, thereby resulting in diminished survival
3. Adverse effects: Diabetes mellitus, hypertension, infections, osteoporosis, hyperlipidemia, and neuropsychiatric symptoms

CALCINEURIN INHIBITORS (CNIs)

1. Strong inhibitors of the T-cell response through blockade of interleukin-2 (IL-2) production
2. **Cyclosporine** metabolism is highly dependent on cytochrome P-450 3A4 (CYP3A4) activity, which can have important genetic variations and may be significantly influenced (induced or inhibited) by drug-drug interactions and graft function.
   - Cyclosporine levels need to be monitored closely by experienced transplant providers.
   - Target therapeutic trough levels of 200 to 300 ng/mL are desirable during the first 3 months post-LT and 80 to 125 ng/mL after that.
3. **Tacrolimus** is 100 times more potent than cyclosporine, and it is also extensively metabolized by CYP3A4.
   - **First-line immunosuppressant used by most LT centers**
   - Early post-LT trough levels should be between 7 and 10 ng/mL.
   - Trough levels around 6 ng/mL are satisfactory after the first 6 months, and 4 to 6 ng/mL is typically accepted as the target level for maintenance after the first year post-LT.
4. Most common adverse effects: Nephrotoxicity, hypertension, neurotoxicity, diabetes mellitus, hyperlipidemia, and hyperkalemia
5. Tacrolimus versus cyclosporine
   - **Tacrolimus is associated with improved patient and graft survival and fewer episodes of ACR.**
   - De novo diabetes mellitus is more common with tacrolimus.
   - Neurologic adverse events are more common with tacrolimus.
   - Hirsutism and gingival hyperplasia are adverse events specific to cyclosporine.
   - The frequency of posttransplant lymphoproliferative disorders (PTLD) is comparable for both agents.

MYCOPHENOLATE MOFETIL AND MYCOPHENOLIC ACID

1. **Mycophenolate mofetil** is converted into the active compound mycophenolic acid during first-pass hepatic metabolism.

2. **Mycophenolic acid** blocks lymphocyte proliferation through inhibition of synthesis of guanine nucleotides.
3. These agents are not associated with renal toxicity and permit using lower doses of a CNI.
4. Monotherapy with mycophenolate mofetil or mycophenolic acid is not recommended for liver transplant recipients because it has been associated with high incidence of ACR.
5. Therapeutic drug monitoring is not required.
6. Most common adverse effects: Gastrointestinal symptoms and bone marrow suppression
   - Diarrhea is the most common dose-limiting adverse effect, but abdominal pain, nausea and vomiting are also common.
   - An enteric-coated formulation of mycophenolic acid is available and has improved gastrointestinal tolerability.

INHIBITORS OF THE MAMMALIAN TARGET OF RAPAMYCIN (mTOR)

1. **Sirolimus** and **everolimus** inhibit T- and B-cell proliferation through blockade of the transduction signal from the IL-2 receptor.
2. Sirolimus is licensed by the U.S. Food and Drug Administration for use in renal transplant recipients; its use in liver transplant recipients is off label. Everolimus is licensed for use in both renal and liver transplant recipients.
3. Both agents can be used as part of a renal-sparing immunosuppressive regimen in liver transplant recipients with CNI-induced nephrotoxicity.
4. Both agents have antiproliferative properties and potentially, although not yet proven, may confer recurrence-free advantage in liver transplant recipients who had HCC.
5. Adverse effects: Bone marrow suppression, hepatic artery thrombosis, delayed wound healing, hyperlipidemia, peripheral edema, and gastrointestinal symptoms

ANTIBODY THERAPY

1. **Antithymocyte globulin** is a polyclonal depleting antibody used as an induction agent or for treatment of glucocorticoid-resistant rejection.
2. **Muromonab-CD3 (OKT3)** is a murine monoclonal antibody used for induction of immunosuppression and treatment of glucocorticoid-resistant rejection.
   - Cytokine release syndrome typically occurs with the first doses; pretreatment with a glucocorticoid, acetaminophen, and antihistamine is advised.
   - Early and severe recurrence of HCV infection may occur.
   - Potentially associated with an increased incidence of PTLD
3. **Basiliximab** is a chimeric monoclonal antibody that blocks the IL-2 receptor (CD25) and inhibits T-cell proliferation.
   - Licensed for prevention of rejection in renal transplantation
   - Has been used off label as an induction agent in liver transplant recipients with renal impairment or as part of glucocorticoid-free protocols
4. **Alemtuzumab** is humanized recombinant anti-CD52 monoclonal antibody that profoundly depletes lymphocytes through antibody-dependent cellular-mediated cell lysis following binding to T and B lymphocytes.
   - Licensed for treatment of chronic B cell lymphocytic leukemia but not for use in liver transplant recipients
   - Initially proposed as an alternative agent that may permit reduction of glucocorticoid and CNI use in liver transplant recipients (off-label use), but profound immunosuppression, high risk of infections and PTLD, and lack of strong evidence supporting a benefit have reduced enthusiasm for this agent.

Complications

PRIMARY GRAFT NONFUNCTION

1. Initial graft function is a critical determinant of the long-term success of LT.
2. An extreme form of preservation injury occurs in approximately 3% to 6% of grafts.
3. Clinically manifests as ALF
   - Hepatic encephalopathy
   - Coagulopathy
   - Jaundice
   - Elevated serum aminotransferase levels
4. Risk factors for PNF
   - Donor age >50 years
   - Graft steatosis >30% of liver volume
   - Donation after cardiac death
   - Reduced-size graft
   - Severe donor hypernatremia
   - Prolonged cold ischemia time
5. **Retransplantation** is the only therapeutic option for PNF.

HYPERACUTE REJECTION

1. Graft rejection manifesting within hours of LT
2. Caused by preformed recipient antibodies against the graft endothelial cells
3. Clinical manifestations are indistinguishable from those of PNF; therefore, urgent liver biopsy is required for diagnosis: Congestive and hemorrhagic necrosis within the graft sinusoids.
4. Similar to PNF; **retransplantation** is the only therapeutic option.

ACUTE CELLULAR REJECTION

1. Typically manifests as abnormalities in liver biochemical tests
2. Liver biopsy remains the gold standard for diagnosis. Histologic features include the following:
   - Mixed inflammatory infiltrate in portal triads
   - Endotheliitis (venulitis)
   - Nonsuppurative cholangitis involving interlobular bile ducts
3. The cornerstone of treatment is **high-dose glucocorticoids:** Methylprednisolone 500 to 1000 mg every other day for three doses followed (or not) by a short prednisone taper. Glucocorticoid-resistant ACR may require treatment with thymoglobulin.

CHRONIC REJECTION

1. Histologically characterized by ductopenia and foam cell clusters or obliterative arteriopathy
2. Early chronic rejection may be reversible if diagnosed and managed appropriately, but late chronic rejection is commonly irreversible. **Retransplantation** may be needed if chronic rejection leads to graft failure.

ANTIBODY-MEDIATED REJECTION

1. Pure antibody-mediated rejection (AMR) is rare in ABO-compatible grafts.
2. Characterized by donor-specific HLA alloantibodies, microvascular endothelial injury, and linear C4d immunohistochemical staining pattern in the hepatic sinusoids

3. Antibody-depleting therapies such as **plasmapheresis and/or rituximab** are used for treatment of AMR; intravenous gamma globulin infusions have also been used.

VASCULAR COMPLICATIONS

1. Hepatic artery thrombosis (HAT)
   - Most common vascular complication post-LT (reported in 4% to 15% of liver transplant recipients; low-dose aspirin is used for primary prevention)
   - Typically occurs at the anastomosis of the native and donor hepatic arteries
   - Clinical presentation depends on the timing: Early HAT may result in acute graft failure; late HAT may result in ischemic cholangiopathy.
   - Doppler ultrasonography is the initial diagnostic test, but angiography is commonly required to confirm the diagnosis.
   - Interventional endovascular techniques may obviate the need for surgical revisions; retransplantation may be needed for untreatable cases.
2. Venous outflow obstruction
   - Clinically manifests as refractory ascites, edema, and evolving hepatic dysfunction
   - No difference in incidence between standard caval replacement and piggy-back reconstruction
   - Endovascular intervention is the treatment of choice.

BILIARY COMPLICATIONS

1. Important cause of morbidity and mortality occurring in 5% to 25% of liver transplant recipients and adversely affecting patient and graft survival
2. Biliary complications include strictures, bile leaks, filling defects within the bile ducts, and sphincter of Oddi dysfunction.
3. LDLT is associated with a higher risk of biliary complications than is deceased-donor LT.
4. Imaging studies including transabdominal ultrasonography and magnetic resonance cholangiography are important tools for diagnosis. Endoscopic ultrasonography may also be useful for diagnosis in selected cases. Endoscopic retrograde cholangiography is used for therapeutic interventions.
5. **Biliary strictures** are the most common biliary complication and can be categorized as anastomotic or nonanastomotic and differ in etiology, timing of diagnosis, number, radiologic appearance, and success of endoscopic therapy.

INFECTIONS

1. Bacterial infections typically occur early post-LT and are related to surgical complications.
2. *Pneumocystis jiroveci* pneumonia may occur because of immunosuppression; pharmacoprophylaxis is indicated during the first 6 to 12 months post-LT.
   - Trimethoprim-sulfamethoxazole is the first-line agent.
   - Pentamidine or atovaquone may be used in liver transplant recipients who are allergic to sulfonamides.
3. Invasive fungal infections pose a major threat to liver transplant recipients; antifungal prophylaxis is commonly used during the immediate post-LT period.
4. The risk for cytomegalovirus (CMV) infection is related to the recipient and donor CMV status.
   - Highest risk for recipient-negative/donor-positive pairs
   - Other risk factors include use of thymoglobulin and retransplantation.

■ Antiviral prophylaxis is standard practice, and the duration depends on risk stratification: 6 months for donor-positive/recipient-negative pairs, 3 months for all others.

5. Antiviral agents such as valganciclovir used to prevent CMV infection usually have activity against Epstein-Barr virus (EBV) as well (see later).

Long-Term Care of Liver Transplant Recipients

1. General medical care for comorbid conditions should be carried out in collaboration with the transplant center.

2. **Systemic hypertension** is common in patients treated with CNI; calcium channel blockers are the agents of choice.

3. **Hyperlipidemia** may be treated safely with statins.

4. **De novo diabetes mellitus** is often secondary to glucocorticoid or long-term CNI use.

5. **Renal dysfunction** is common in liver transplant recipients; although a CNI poses an important risk, metabolic risk factors are the most common etiologies.
   ■ Adequate glycemic control and treatment of hypertension are essential to reducing the risk of renal dysfunction.
   ■ Tailoring CNI regimens or using additional immunosuppressive agents may allow substantial reductions in the dose of CNI without jeopardizing the health of the graft.
   ■ Early identification of risk factors and implementation of strategies to prevent renal dysfunction improve long-term outcomes.

6. **Bone demineralization** is a common problem in liver transplant recipients.
   ■ Calcium and vitamin D supplementation is often required.
   ■ Dual-energy x-ray absorptiometry (DEXA) testing is indicated at regular intervals to identify progression of bone demineralization.
   ■ Bisphosphonates may be indicated to treat osteoporosis.

7. Long-term immunosuppression is associated with increased risk for **extrahepatic malignant neoplasms.**
   ■ Age-appropriate screening for colon cancer, breast cancer, cervical cancer, and prostate cancer must be continued.
   ■ Patients should avoid excessive and unnecessary direct sunlight exposure. Use of protective clothing and sunscreen and yearly dermatologic examinations are recommended because of the increased risk for skin cancers.
   ■ **PTLD** is a rare but ominous complication in liver transplant recipients that can be mediated by primary EBV infection or its reactivation. A reduction in immunosuppression is usually the initial management strategy, and some cases require chemotherapy.

8. The frequency of **recurrence of the primary hepatic disease** in liver transplant recipients is variable and largely determined by the original etiology.
   ■ Recurrence of HCV infection is universal in the absence of an SVR pre-LT.
   ■ Protocols consisting of antiviral agents and/or HBIG markedly diminish recurrence of HBV infection.
   ■ Autoimmune liver diseases have a relative high rate of recurrence post-LT; active surveillance is advised.
   ■ Surveillance for HCC should be continued in liver transplant recipients if HCC was the indication for LT or if it was discovered incidentally in the explant.
   ■ Metabolic comorbidities such as obesity, diabetes mellitus, hyperlipidemia, and hypertension are common in liver transplant recipients and result in increased risk for cardiovascular diseases. Recurrent or de novo nonalcoholic steatohepatitis is also reported with variable frequency and is related to the presence of metabolic risk factors. Lifestyle modifications and appropriate tailoring of immunosuppression are necessary steps in management.

9. Alcohol and tobacco use must be carefully monitored.
10. Pregnancy should be delayed for at least 1 year following LT, and management by a high-risk obstetrician is advised.
- Tacrolimus, cyclosporine, sirolimus, and everolimus are pregnancy category C drugs.
- Mycophenolate mofetil and mycophenolic acid are pregnancy category D drugs.
11. Weight control through dietary modifications and physical activity should be encouraged in all liver transplant recipients.

FURTHER READING

Clavien PA, Lesurtel M, Bossuyt PM, et al. Recommendations for liver transplantation for hepatocellular carcinoma: an international consensus conference report. *Lancet Oncol.* 2012;13:e11–e22.

D'Amico G, Garcia-Tsao G, Pagliaro L. Natural history and prognostic indicators of survival in cirrhosis: a systematic review of 118 studies. *J Hepatol.* 2006;44:217–231.

Darwish Murad S, Kim WR, Harnois DM, et al. Efficacy of neoadjuvant chemoradiation, followed by liver transplantation, for perihilar cholangiocarcinoma at 12 US centers. *Gastroenterology.* 2012;143:88–98.

Eason JD, Gonwa TA, Davis CL, et al. Proceedings of Consensus Conference on Simultaneous Liver Kidney Transplantation (SLK). *Am J Transplant.* 2008;8:2243–2251.

Gedaly R, Daily MF, Davenport D, et al. Liver transplantation for the treatment of liver metastases from neuroendocrine tumors: an analysis of the UNOS database. *Arch Surg.* 2011;146:953–958.

Lentine KL, Costa SP, Weir MR, et al. Cardiac disease evaluation and management among kidney and liver transplantation candidates: a scientific statement from the American Heart Association and the American College of Cardiology Foundation. *J Am Coll Cardiol.* 2012;60:434–480.

Lucey MR, Terrault N, Ojo L, et al. Long-term management of the successful adult liver transplant: 2012 practice guideline by the American Association for the Study of Liver Diseases and the American Society of Transplantation. *Liver Transpl.* 2013;19:3–26.

Martin P, DiMartini A, Feng S, et al. Evaluation for liver transplantation in adults: 2013 practice guideline by the American Association for the Study of Liver Diseases and the American Society of Transplantation. *Hepatology.* 2014;59:1144–1165.

Muzaale AD, Dagher NN, Montgomery RA, et al. Estimates of early death, acute liver failure, and long-term mortality among live liver donors. *Gastroenterology.* 2012;142:273–280.

Porrett PM, Hashmi SK, Shaked A. Immunosuppression: trends and tolerance? *Clin Liver Dis.* 2014;18:687–716.

Sharr WW, Chan SC, Lo CM. Current status of downstaging of hepatocellular carcinoma before liver transplantation. *Transplantation.* 2014;97:S10–S17.

Terrault NA, Roland ME, Schiano T, et al. Outcomes of liver transplant recipients with hepatitis C and human immunodeficiency virus coinfection. *Liver Transpl.* 2012;18:716–726.

Tiukinhoy-Laing SD, Rossi JS, Bayram M, et al. Cardiac hemodynamic and coronary angiographic characteristics of patients being evaluated for liver transplantation. *Am J Cardiol.* 2006;98:178–181.

Wells MM, Croome KP, Boyce E, et al. Roux-en-Y choledochojejunostomy versus duct-to-duct biliary anastomosis in liver transplantation for primary sclerosing cholangitis: a meta-analysis. *Transplant Proc.* 2013;45:2263–2271.

CHAPTER 34

Cholelithiasis and Cholecystitis

Ji Young Bang, MBBS, MPH ■ Stuart Sherman, MD

KEY POINTS

1 Gallstones are common and generally asymptomatic.

2 Gallstones can result in various clinical sequelae, including biliary pain and acute cholecystitis.

3 Cholecystectomy is the first-line treatment for symptomatic gallstones and acute cholecystitis.

4 In patients who are poor surgical candidates, alternative therapeutic options include percutaneous gallbladder drainage, transpapillary gallbladder drainage, or endoscopic ultrasound (EUS)–guided gallbladder drainage.

Cholelithiasis (Gallstones)

1. Gallstone disease is common and affects 20 to 25 million persons in the United States. About 20% of women and 10% of men have gallstones by 60 years of age.
2. Gallstone disease is costly, with an estimated annual direct cost of $15 billion. Approximately 750,000 cholecystectomies are performed annually.
3. Gallstones are asymptomatic in 80% of persons who have them; however, the stones can cause significant abdominal pain in up to 20% and carry a mortality rate of up to 0.6%.
4. Gallstones can be broadly divided into cholesterol, black pigment, and brown pigment.
5. Cholecystectomy, the first-line therapy for symptomatic gallstones, is the most commonly performed nonemergent gastrointestinal surgical procedure in the United States.

TYPES OF GALLSTONES

1. **Cholesterol stones**
   a. **In the American population, 70% to 80% of gallstones are cholesterol stones.**
   b. Cholesterol stones are composed of 50% to 100% cholesterol, in combination with mucin and calcium salts. The stones are generally yellow-brown in color.
   c. Cholesterol stones form primarily in the gallbladder as a result of increased secretion of cholesterol by the liver, supersaturation of bile with cholesterol, and an increase in gallbladder mucin and calcium. A stone nidus is formed by aggregation of calcium salts and mucin, following precipitation of cholesterol monohydrate crystals.
   d. **Risk factors** for cholesterol stone formation
      ■ Older age: Prevalence rises with increasing age in men and women.

- Female gender: Risk of gallstone formation in women is twice that of men.
- Diet: Cholesterol gallstone formation is associated with a diet high in saturated fat and low in fiber. Cholesterol stones are more frequent in North America and Europe compared with Asia and Africa.
- Obesity
- Rapid weight loss
- Pregnancy
- Genetics
- Ethnicity: High prevalence among North American Indians, Mapuche Indians
- Medications: Estrogens

2. **Pigment stones**
   a. **Black pigment stones** account for about 20% to 30% of gallstones in Americans.
      - They form primarily in the gallbladder.
      - Main composition: Calcium bilirubinate, calcium phosphate, and calcium carbonate
      - They are black, hard, and radiopaque.
      - Risk factors for formation
        - Chronic hemolysis
        - Cirrhosis
        - Cystic fibrosis
        - Crohn disease
   b. **Brown pigment stones** form primarily in the bile duct.
      - They are composed of calcium bilirubinate, calcium palmitate, calcium stearate, cholesterol, and mucin.
      - Risk factors for formation
        - Stagnation of bile in combination with bacterial and parasite infection of the bile duct, including *Escherichia coli*, *Bacteroides* spp, *Clostridium* spp, *Opisthorchis viverrini*, and *Ascaris lumbricoides*.

DIAGNOSIS

1. **Ultrasonography (US) is the primary modality for the diagnosis of cholelithiasis;** it is both noninvasive and sensitive for the detection of cholelithiasis, with a sensitivity of 95% for gallstones >2 mm in size.
2. The sensitivity of computed tomography (CT) for the detection of cholelithiasis is 79%—lower than that of US—because of insufficient calcium content in some stones.
3. Magnetic resonance imaging (MRI) is also not recommended as a first-line imaging modality for detection of cholelithiasis; however, MRI has a role in the diagnosis of bile duct stones, with a sensitivity of 93%.
4. EUS is at least as sensitive as abdominal US for the detection of cholelithiasis, including very small stones <2 mm in size and sludge (Fig. 34.1); however, use of EUS is limited by the invasive nature of this technique.
5. Although CT, MRI, and EUS can be used for diagnosing cholelithiasis, these imaging modalities should be reserved for detecting complications that can arise from gallstones, such as acute cholecystitis, acute pancreatitis, or choledocholithiasis, rather than as the primary modality for uncomplicated cholelithiasis.
6. Occasionally, other diseases of the gallbladder, such as cholesterolosis ("strawberry gallbladder") and adenomyomatosis, are identified on imaging studies, including oral cholecystography (Table 34.1).

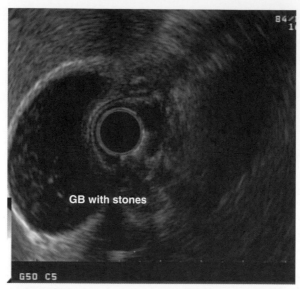

Fig. 34.1 Endoscopic ultrasonographic image of a gallbladder (GB) filled with gallstones. (Courtesy David M. Freidel, MD)

TABLE 34.1 ■ **Diseases of the Gallbladder**

	Clinical Features	Laboratory Features	Initial Diagnostic Test(s)	Treatment
Asymptomatic gallstones	Asymptomatic	Normal	Ultrasonography	None
Symptomatic gallstones	Biliary pain	Normal	Ultrasonography	Laparoscopic cholecystectomy
Acute cholecystitis	Epigastric or right upper quadrant pain, nausea, vomiting, fever, Murphy sign	Leukocytosis	Ultrasonography, HIDA scan	Antibiotics, laparoscopic cholecystectomy
Chronic cholecystitis	Biliary pain, constant epigastric or right upper quadrant pain, nausea	Normal	Ultrasonography (stones), oral cholecystography (nonfunctioning gallbladder)	Laparoscopic cholecystectomy
Cholesterolosis	Usually asymptomatic	Normal	Oral cholecystography	None
Adenomyomatosis	May cause biliary pain	Normal	Oral cholecystography	Laparoscopic cholecystectomy if symptomatic
Porcelain gallbladder	Usually asymptomatic, high risk of gallbladder cancer	Normal	Radiograph or CT	Laparoscopic cholecystectomy

CT, Computed tomography; *HIDA,* hepatic iminodiacetic acid.

COMMON CONSEQUENCES (see also Chapter 35)

1. **Asymptomatic gallstones**
   a. Gallstones are discovered incidentally in 80% of affected persons; they are therefore asymptomatic and remain so for several decades in the majority of cases.
   b. Biliary pain develops in 2% to 3% in persons with gallstones each year, and in 10% by 5 years.
   c. Complications from gallstones are observed in only 1% to 2% persons with gallstones each year.
   d. Persons with asymptomatic gallstones do not require prophylactic cholecystectomy, which should only be considered in the following special circumstances:
      ■ Persons with an increased risk of gallbladder cancer, including those with porcelain gallbladder (calcification of the gallbladder wall), anomalous pancreaticobiliary duct junction, and large gallstones >3 cm
      ■ Persons who undergo solid organ transplantation, due to high morbidity associated with complications arising from gallstones in these patients
      ■ Persons who undergo abdominal surgery for other indications, especially bariatric surgery; these patients are predisposed to gallstone formation because of rapid weight loss
2. **Biliary pain**
   a. Biliary pain ("colic") is characterized by intermittent right upper quadrant abdominal pain, typically with radiation to the right shoulder, lasting 30 minutes to 4 hours and occurring with variable frequency.
   b. The pain commonly follows a large or fatty meal because of contraction of the gallbladder in the presence of an obstructed cystic duct.
   c. The diagnosis is confirmed by visualization of gallstones on US, with exclusion of other etiologies of abdominal pain, such as acute pancreatitis, choledocholithiasis, peptic ulcer disease, and nephrolithiasis.

TREATMENT

1. **Ursodeoxycholic acid (UDCA)**
   a. UDCA, a secondary bile acid given in a dose of 8 to 10 mg/kg body weight/day, is suitable in only a select group of patients with gallstones: Those with uncomplicated biliary pain from small cholesterol stones (<5 mm in size), a nonoccluded cystic duct, and normal gallbladder contraction to allow passage of stones from the gallbladder.
   b. UDCA should be reserved for patients who are unable or unwilling to undergo cholecystectomy. The treatment success rate is only 37%, and recurrence of stones occurs in up to 50% of patients by 5 years after therapy.
2. **Extracorporeal shock wave lithotripsy (ESWL)**
   a. ESWL involves the breakdown of gallstones with external application of sound waves to increase the efficacy of UDCA.
   b. As with oral dissolution therapy, ESWL is reserved for patients with small cholesterol stones and uncomplicated gallstones disease and requires an open cystic duct and normally contracting gallbladder to encourage passage of stone fragments into the duodenum.
   c. ESWL is also reserved for patients who are unable or unwilling to undergo cholecystectomy, with reasonable treatment success rates of 68% to 84%; however, recurrence rates are 54% at 10 years when ESWL is used in conjunction with UCDA.
3. **Cholecystectomy**
   a. 750,000 cholecystectomies are performed annually in the United States for symptomatic gallstones via either an open or laparoscopic approach.
   b. Cholecystectomy results in resolution of abdominal pain in patients with symptomatic gallstones, with treatment success rate of around 90%; it is the **treatment of choice for patients with biliary pain.**

c. Mortality rates for open cholecystectomy range from 0.02% to 1.5%, with complication rates of 4% to 5%, including bile duct injury, acute pancreatitis, and wound infections.

d. **Laparoscopic cholecystectomy is preferred** over the open approach because of a shorter length of hospitalization, more rapid resumption of daily activities, and lower analgesic requirement. Complication rates range from 4.3% to 14.6% (including bile duct injury in 0.14% to 0.86%), with mortality rates of up to 0.3%.

e. Intraoperative cholangiography is often performed during laparoscopic cholecystectomy to delineate the biliary system in case of aberrant anatomy, and hence minimize the risk of bile duct injury, and detect bile duct stones, which can be present in 8% to 16% of patients with cholelithiasis.

Acute Cholecystitis

ACUTE CALCULOUS CHOLECYSTITIS

1. Acute cholecystitis most commonly complicates gallstone disease.
2. It occurs in 1% to 3% patients with cholelithiasis when a stone becomes lodged at the junction of the gallbladder and cystic duct, with resulting local inflammation, ischemia, and secondary bacterial infection with gram-negative and/or gram-positive bacteria.

ACUTE ACALCULOUS CHOLECYSTITIS

1. Comprises 5% of cases of acute cholecystitis
2. Most frequently seen in critically ill patients
3. Risk factors include burn injury, trauma, bone marrow transplantation, chemotherapy, administration of total parenteral nutrition, and chronic medical conditions that result in vascular insufficiency, such as vasculitis.
4. The main differences between calculous and acalculous acute cholecystitis are the association with gallstones only in the former and the need for more urgent gallbladder decompression in the latter, either with cholecystectomy, if possible, or cholecystostomy tube placement followed by cholecystectomy when clinical stability is achieved. The urgent need for decompression is due to mortality rates of up to 50% and a high risk of complications that include perforation, gangrene, and empyema associated with acute acalculous cholecystitis.

CLINICAL FEATURES

1. According to the **Tokyo guidelines,** the diagnosis of **acute cholecystitis** requires fulfillment of clinical, laboratory, and imaging criteria indicating the presence of a local and systemic inflammatory process.
2. Patients present with **right upper quadrant pain that is usually unremitting; tenderness and guarding; a positive Murphy sign; and fever, leukocytosis, and/or C-reactive protein level of ≥3 mg/dL.**
3. Mild jaundice may also be present.
4. The severity of acute cholecystitis can be classified as mild (grade I), moderate (grade II), and severe (grade III). These distinctions impact clinical management, surgical risk, and the urgency of intervention.
   - **Mild** acute cholecystitis is defined by the absence of organ failure and severe local inflammation.
   - **Moderate** acute cholecystitis is defined by symptoms persisting for >72 hours, significant leukocytosis, and features of local complications such as an abscess or peritonitis.
   - **Severe** acute cholecystitis requires the presence of dysfunction of at least one organ system: Cardiovascular, respiratory, renal, hepatic, hematologic, or neurologic.

5. Unlike acute calculous cholecystitis, acute acalculous cholecystitis may present in an atypical fashion, commonly without abdominal pain in up to 75% of patients and associated with fever, systemic inflammatory response, and shock.

6. **Chronic cholecystitis** may occasionally result from repeated episodes of acute cholecystitis. Other complications include **hydrops of the gallbladder** (when acute cholecystitis subsides but cystic duct obstruction persists) and **xanthogranulomatous cholecystitis**, a rare variant of chronic cholecystitis.

DIAGNOSIS

1. Various imaging modalities can be used to verify the diagnosis.

2. **Cholescintigraphy** involves injection of radiolabeled hepatic 2,6-dimethyliminodiacetic acid (HIDA) or diisopropyl iminodiacetic acid (DISIDA), which under normal circumstances is taken up by the liver, is excreted in the bile, enters the gallbladder, and is excreted into the duodenum in 1 to 2 hours. The test is highly sensitive (95%) and specific (95%) for the diagnosis of acute cholecystitis, with a positive scan characterized by nonvisualization of the gallbladder 1 hour after injection of the radioisotope, in association with filling of the bile duct and duodenum.

3. **US, CT, and MRI** of the abdomen show an enlarged gallbladder, thickening of the gallbladder wall (>4 mm), and presence of pericholecystic fluid.

4. Murphy sign can also be elicited during US ("sonographic Murphy sign").

5. In patients with acute acalculous cholecystitis, US is commonly performed because of its high sensitivity (up to 92%), high specificity (around 90%), rapid availability, and the convenience of being able to do the study at the bedside in critically ill patients. Moreover, scintigraphy has lower specificity in patients with acute acalculous cholecystitis because of the risk of false-positive results in fasting patients and false-negative results due to an unobstructed cystic duct.

TREATMENT

1. **Cholecystectomy**
   a. Following administration of broad-spectrum antibiotics with coverage of gram-negative bacteria, making the patient nil per os, and intravenous fluid resuscitation, cholecystectomy is performed as the **first-line treatment** for acute cholecystitis.
   b. Cholecystectomy can be conducted via an open or laparoscopic approach, usually within 72 hours of presentation (or as soon as possible in patients with acute acalculous cholecystitis).
   c. The number of laparoscopic cholecystectomies has been increasing, and that of open cholecystectomies has been decreasing; the rate of conversion during surgery for a laparoscopic to an open approach ranges from 5% to 10%.
   d. In a national population study comprising 1.39 million patients who underwent a cholecystectomy for acute cholecystitis between 1998 and 2005 in the United States, better outcomes were observed in the laparoscopic group, with significantly greater rates of discharge to home (91% vs. 69%, $P < 0.0001$), short hospitalization of 2 days or less (37% vs. 6%, $P < 0.0001$), and lower mortality rates, even when taking into account the patient's clinical status (1.7% vs. 6.4% for the sickest patients, $P < 0.0001$). Laparoscopy was also less costly by nearly $15,000 ($21,743 vs. $36,335, $P < 0.0001$).

2. **Cholecystostomy tube**
   a. Percutaneous insertion of a tube to achieve successful gallbladder drainage is an effective, minimally invasive option in patients with acute cholecystitis who are not suitable surgical candidates.

b. The tube can be left in place indefinitely or until the patient becomes more stable for cholecystectomy.

c. In a study of 185 patients with comorbidities, including chronic obstructive pulmonary disease (COPD), coronary artery disease, and cirrhosis, who underwent placement of either a percutaneous or surgical cholecystostomy tube, cholecystectomy was subsequently performed in 56.8% of patients, with a laparoscopic approach used in >80% of the cases. Adverse events such as pain, leakage, and tube dislodgement occurred at a rate of around 11%.

d. In a study comparing percutaneous cholecystostomy tube placement with emergency cholecystectomy, there was no significant difference in morbidity, but there was a significant difference in the mortality rate between the two groups, with higher mortality observed in the cholecystostomy group (17.2% vs. 0%, $P = 0.02$). Therefore, **cholecystectomy should be performed whenever possible, and the placement of a cholecystostomy tube should be reserved for patients who are unable to undergo surgery for acute cholecystitis.**

3. **Endoscopic therapy**

a. Endoscopic therapy can be performed in poor surgical candidates with significant comorbidities or those with contraindications to percutaneous gallbladder drainage such as ascites and absence of a safe window for catheter insertion.

b. Endoscopic therapy should be avoided in patients with gallbladder perforation.

c. **Endoscopic retrograde cholangiopancreatography (ERCP) with transpapillary gallbladder drainage**

   ■ Has been reported since the 1980s

   ■ Decompresses the gallbladder via the cystic duct. Once the major papilla is identified with the duodenoscope in the second portion of the duodenum, the bile duct is cannulated with a catheter and a 0.025- or 0.035-inch guidewire.

   ■ Under fluoroscopic guidance, the guidewire is advanced into the cystic duct and gallbladder and allowed to coil several times within the gallbladder lumen.

   ■ A 7-10 Fr double-pigtail plastic stent or 5-7 Fr nasogallbladder drainage catheter is then inserted through the cystic duct and into the gallbladder for decompression.

   ■ Unlike a transpapillary stent, a nasogallbladder drainage catheter allows irrigation of the gallbladder with sterile normal saline.

d. The pooled technical success rate of endoscopic transpapillary stent placement is higher than that of nasogallbladder catheter insertion at 96% (95% CI, 91.1% to 98.7%) and 80.9% (95% CI, 74.7% to 86.2%), respectively, with clinical resolution in 88% (95% CI, 81.2% to 93.2%) and 75.3% (95% CI, 68.6 % to 81.2%) of patients, respectively.

   ■ The adverse events encountered during endoscopic transpapillary gallbladder drainage include perforation of the gallbladder or cystic duct, pancreatitis, and cholangitis, with pooled adverse event rates of 0% to 16%.

e. **EUS-guided gallbladder drainage**

   ■ EUS can be used to decompress the gallbladder by creating a fistulous tract between the gallbladder and gastroduodenal lumen.

   ■ A therapeutic linear array echoendoscope is advanced into the stomach or duodenum to visualize the gallbladder and identify the optimal site of gallbladder access. A 19-gauge fine aspiration needle is used to puncture the gallbladder wall from the enteral lumen under EUS guidance (Fig. 34.2A).

   ■ A 0.035-inch guidewire is inserted through the needle into the gallbladder and allowed to coil several times within the gallbladder lumen. The needle is then removed, and a catheter or needle knife is inserted over the guidewire to create a fistula between the gallbladder wall and the stomach or duodenal lumen.

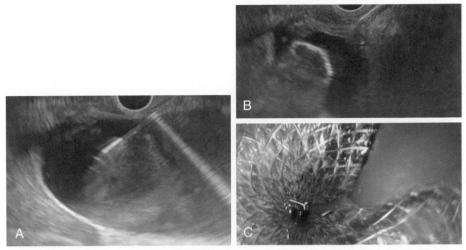

Fig 34.2 Endoscopic ultrasonography (EUS)–guided drainage of the gallbladder. A, The gallbladder is punctured from the duodenal lumen with a 19-gauge needle under EUS-guidance. B, A lumen-apposing metal stent is first deployed in the gallbladder under EUS-guidance. C, The proximal end of the metal stent is then deployed in the duodenal lumen under direct endoscopic guidance.

- The fistulous tract is then dilated with a dilating balloon or catheter up to maximum of 6 mm to allow insertion of a double-pigtail plastic stent, fully covered metal stent, or nasogallbladder catheter into the gallbladder from the lumen (Fig. 34.2B–C).
- Studies investigating EUS-guided gallbladder drainage are small because of the relative novelty of this technique; however, the technical and treatment success rates with both plastic and metal stents have been encouraging. Adverse events have included pneumoperitoneum and bile peritonitis.
- In a randomized trial of 59 patients, EUS-guided gallbladder drainage was compared with percutaneous gallbladder drainage. When a noninferiority margin was set at 15%, technical (97% for both modalities) and clinical (100% for EUS-guided gallbladder drainage vs. 96% for percutaneous gallbladder drainage) success rates were comparable. There was also no significant difference in adverse event rates.

Emphysematous Cholecystitis

1. Emphysematous cholecystitis is thought to result from vascular insufficiency of the gallbladder and subsequent gallbladder infection with gas-forming bacteria such as *Clostridium* spp. and *E. coli.*
2. Risk factors include diabetes mellitus and elderly age.
3. Treatment involves administration of broad-spectrum antibiotics and cholecystectomy.

Uncommon Consequences of Gallstones

MIRIZZI SYNDROME

1. Definition: External impingement of the common hepatic duct by gallstones located in the cystic duct or gallbladder neck
2. Can lead to obstructive jaundice
3. Managed by biliary stent placement during ERCP, cholangioscopic-guided electrohydraulic or laser lithotripsy, and/or cholecystectomy

CHOLECYSTOENTERIC FISTULA

1. Rare condition
2. Characterized by formation of a fistula between the gallbladder and the small bowel, proximal colon, or stomach because of direct passage of the gallstone through the gallbladder and enteral wall and into the enteral lumen.
3. The fistula can then lead to obstruction of the enteral lumen, usually by gallstones >25 mm in size, resulting in **gallstone ileus** (obstruction in small bowel) or **Bouveret syndrome** (obstruction in the duodenum).
4. The diagnosis can be confirmed by visualization of pneumobilia on a plain abdominal film or with a small bowel series and/or barium enema to visualize the fistula. The fistula can seal spontaneously; however, cholecystectomy with fistula closure is the definitive treatment.
5. Laparotomy is always required for gallstone ileus; the mortality rate is 20% with delayed treatment.

FURTHER READING

Andersson KL, Friedman LS. Acalculous biliary pain, acute acalculous cholecystitis, cholesterolosis, adenomyomatosis and gallbladder polyps. In: Feldman M, Friedman LS, Brandt LJ, eds. *Sleisenger and Fordtran's Gastrointestinal and Liver Disease: Pathophysiology/Diagnosis/Management*. Philadelphia: Saunders Elsevier; 2016:1152–1165.

Cherng N, Witkowski ET, Sneider EB, et al. Use of cholecystostomy tubes in the management of patients with primary diagnosis of acute cholecystitis. *J Am Coll Surg*. 2012;214:196–201.

Csikesz NG, Tseng JF, Shah SA. Trends in surgical management for acute cholecystitis. *Surgery*. 2008;144:283–289.

Fogel E, Sherman S. Diseases of the gallbladder and bile ducts. In: Goldman L, Schafer AI, eds. *Goldman's Cecil Medicine*. Philadelphia: Saunders Elsevier; 2016:1038–1048.

Glasgow RE, Mulvihill SJ. Treatment of gallstone disease. In: Feldman M, Friedman LS, Brandt LJ, eds. *Sleisenger and Fordtran's Gastrointestinal and Liver Disease: Pathophysiology/Diagnosis/Management*. Philadelphia: Saunders Elsevier; 2016:1134–1151.

Hirota M, Takada T, Kawarada Y, et al. Diagnostic criteria and severity assessment of acute cholecystitis: Tokyo guidelines. *J Hepatobiliary Pancreat Surg*. 2007;14:78–82.

Itoi T, Coelho-Prabhu N, Baron TH. Endoscopic gallbladder drainage for management of acute cholecystitis. *Gastrointest Endosc*. 2010;71:1038–1045.

Jang JW, Lee SS, Park do H, et al. Feasibility and safety of EUS-guided transgastric/transduodenal gallbladder drainage with single-step placement of a modified covered self-expandable metal stent in patients unsuitable for cholecystectomy. *Gastrointest Endosc*. 2011;74:176–181.

Jang JW, Lee SS, Song TJ, et al. Endoscopic ultrasound-guided transmural and percutaneous transhepatic gallbladder drainage are comparable for acute cholecystitis. *Gastroenterology*. 2012;142:805–811.

Rodríguez-Sanjuán JC, Arruabarrena A, Sánchez-Moreno L, et al. Acute cholecystitis in high surgical risk patients: percutaneous cholecystostomy or emergency cholecystectomy? *Am J Surg*. 2012;204:54–59.

Song TJ, Park do H, Eum JB, et al. EUS-guided cholecystoenterostomy with single-step placement of a 7F double-pigtail plastic stent in patients who are unsuitable for cholecystectomy: a pilot study (with video). *Gastrointest Endosc*. 2010;71:634–640.

Stinton LM, Myers RP, Shaffer EA. Epidemiology of gallstones. *Gastroenterol Clin North Am*. 2010;39:157–169.

Stinton LM, Shaffer EA. Epidemiology of gallbladder disease: cholelithiasis and cancer. *Gut Liver*. 2012; 6:172–187.

Venneman NG, van Erpecum KJ. Pathogenesis of gallstones. *Gastroenterol Clin North Am*. 2010;39:171–183.

Wang DQ-H, Afdhal NH. Gallstone disease. In: Feldman M, Friedman LS, Brandt LJ, eds. *Sleisenger and Fordtran's Gastrointestinal and Liver Disease: Pathophysiology/Diagnosis/Management*. Philadelphia: Saunders Elsevier; 2016:1100–1133.

Diseases of the Bile Ducts

Petros C. Benias, MD ■ Douglas M. Weine, MD ■ Ira M. Jacobson, MD

KEY POINTS

1 Diseases of the bile ducts (BDs) usually manifest with symptoms and signs related to BD obstruction, including pain, jaundice, pruritus, fever, and elevated serum levels of liver biochemical tests.

2 Choledocholithiasis, the most common benign disorder of the biliary tract, may manifest in patients with an intact gallbladder, soon after cholecystectomy, or up to many years after cholecystectomy. Predictors of BD stones in patients with a compatible history include elevated liver biochemical test levels, BD dilatation, stones visualized in the duct on imaging studies, and an initial presentation of biliary-type pain or cholangitis.

3 In the diagnosis and management of BD stones before laparoscopic cholecystectomy, endoscopic retrograde cholangiopancreatography (ERCP) should be restricted to patients in whom BD stones are strongly suspected and in whom therapeutic intervention is likely. Magnetic resonance cholangiopancreatography (MRCP) is used commonly for noninvasive diagnosis. Endoscopic ultrasonography (EUS), while operator dependent, can be highly sensitive for even small bile duct stones.

4 Endoscopic sphincterotomy is the most common technique used for removal of BD stones, either before or after cholecystectomy. Laparoscopic extraction of BD stones during cholecystectomy is an alternative approach when ERCP by an expert has failed and surgical expertise is available.

5 Endoscopic intervention plays an important role in the diagnosis and treatment of complications of cholecystectomy, such as biliary leaks and strictures.

6 Anatomic and congenital anomalies, such as choledochal cysts, can lead to jaundice, pancreatitis, secondary cirrhosis, and biliary carcinoma if these anomalies are not recognized and treated.

7 Premalignant lesions of the biliary system mimic their pancreatic counterparts in histology and premalignant potential and may be encountered with increased frequency as the quality of cross-sectional imaging and cholangioscopy improves. They can result in cholangitis, strictures, secondary cirrhosis, and, most importantly, cholangiocarcinoma.

8 Biliary strictures remain a diagnostic challenge because many benign entities can mimic malignancy. In addition to pancreatic cancer or cholangiocarcinoma, benign entities such as immunoglobulin (Ig)G4 cholangiopathy and primary sclerosing cholangitis (PSC) are diagnostic considerations.

Bile Duct Stones

RISK FACTORS

1. **In Western countries, most cases of choledocholithiasis are secondary to the passage of gallstones from the gallbladder into the bile duct.**
   - Most of these stones are cholesterol rich and have formed in the gallbladder.
   - Black pigment stones are also formed in the gallbladder and are associated with hemolytic disorders such as sickle cell disease and occasionally cirrhosis.
2. Certain groups of patients are at risk of forming primary duct stones, including the following:
   - Older adults with large bile ducts and periampullary diverticula
   - Patients with recurrent pyogenic cholangitis (RPC)
   - Patients with chronic biliary strictures
   - Patients at risk for biliary stasis (e.g., with cystic fibrosis)

CLINICAL FEATURES

1. Symptomatic BD stones may present as follows:
   - Pain
   - Cholangitis
   - Pancreatitis
   - Jaundice
2. Asymptomatic incidentally found stones
   - Typically, the patient is afebrile with normal complete blood count and pancreatic enzyme levels.
   - Serum alkaline phosphatase or gamma-glutamyltranspeptidase (GGTP) levels may be mildly elevated.
   - Stones may be found incidentally on routine imaging or intraoperative cholangiography during cholecystectomy.
   - In older patients, anorexia may be an overlooked sign.
3. Pain from BD stones resembles pain of gallbladder origin.
   - The pain is typically located in the epigastrium or right upper quadrant and is often prolonged but resolves within 6 hours.
   - Abdominal tenderness is greater with cholecystitis than with BD stones.
   - Obstructive jaundice from BD stones is usually accompanied by pain and may be accompanied by evidence of infection, including fever and chills; the latter may predominate as the presenting feature.
   - The pain from choledocholithiasis resolves when the stone either passes spontaneously or is removed. Occasionally, some patients have intermittent pain due to transient blockage of the BD termed a "ball valve" effect.
   - Jaundice associated with malignancy is more likely to be painless.
4. **Features of cholangitis** include the following:
   - **Charcot's triad,** consisting of **abdominal pain, fever, and jaundice:** Each feature may not be present in all patients with cholangitis.
   - **Reynolds pentad** consists of **Charcot triad plus hypotension and altered mental status.**
   - Fever may be accompanied by severe rigors.
   - Cholangitis is more frequent with BD stones than with malignant BD obstruction.
   - **Severe cholangitis must be considered life threatening and requires urgent intervention.**
5. The timing of clinical presentation with BD stones is variable.
   - Before cholecystectomy
   - During intraoperative cholangiography (IOC)
   - Shortly after cholecystectomy
   - Months to years or decades after cholecystectomy

6. Gallstone pancreatitis (see discussion later in chapter)
   ■ Small gallstones pose a greater risk of pancreatitis than do large stones; they migrate more easily through the cystic duct.

LABORATORY FEATURES

1. Elevations in serum liver biochemical test levels, including alanine aminotransferase (ALT), aspartate aminotransferase (AST), alkaline phosphatase (ALP), GGTP, and bilirubin
   ■ Marked elevations in serum ALT and AST levels may occur, even levels >1000 U/L transiently, especially with cholangitis.
   ■ A high level of suspicion is required. No single blood test accurately predicts the presence of stones. In the appropriate clinical setting, an elevation in serum bilirubin has a sensitivity of 69% and a specificity of 88% for diagnosing a BD stone. For elevations in serum ALP, the values are 57% and 86%, respectively.
   ■ On the other hand, the negative predictive value of normal liver biochemical test levels is high.
   ■ Aminotransferase levels typically fall rapidly, even as the ALP level rises if stone impaction persists.
   ■ This condition can be confused with hepatitis.
2. Elevations in serum amylase and lipase levels suggest concomitant acute pancreatitis.
3. Elevations in the white blood cell (WBC) count occur with cholangitis or pancreatitis.
4. Positive blood cultures can be found with cholangitis.
5. Distention of the liver capsule from hepatitis can cause right upper quadrant discomfort often confused with biliary pain in the setting of abnormal liver enzyme levels.

IMAGING STUDIES

1. Ultrasonography
   ■ Excellent for detecting gallbladder stones; less sensitive for BD stones
   ■ May be limited by obesity and gas in the intestine
   ■ Sensitive for detecting BD dilatation
   ■ More sensitive for BD stones when the duct is dilated
   ■ Absence of BD dilatation or detectable stones does not exclude BD stones.
2. Computed tomography (CT)
   ■ Sensitivity <50% for BD stones
   ■ Detection depends on the presence of calcifications in stones
   ■ Sensitivity similar to that of ultrasonography for detecting a dilated BD
   ■ Oral contrast agents should be avoided on initial images (can obscure BD stones).
3. MRCP (Fig. 35.1)
   ■ Detection of BD stones depends on T2-weighted images
   ■ Contrast provided by fluid in the ducts
   ■ Sensitivity and specificity >90%
   ■ Sensitivity lower for small stones
   ■ Limited availability and high cost; contraindications include a pacemaker, defibrillator, or certain other metallic implants. The feasibility of an MRCP in a patient with an orthopedic implant should be discussed with the radiologist.
4. EUS (Fig. 35.2)
   ■ Sensitivity and specificity rival those of ERCP.
   ■ Less risk than ERCP but still requires sedation
   ■ Most suitable for choledocholithiasis when EUS and ERCP can be performed at the same session

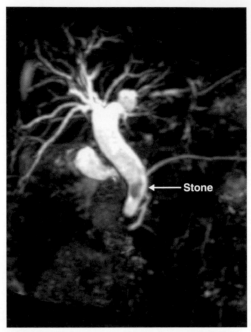

Fig. 35.1   Magnetic resonance cholangiographic image showing a large stone (*arrow*) in the distal bile duct.

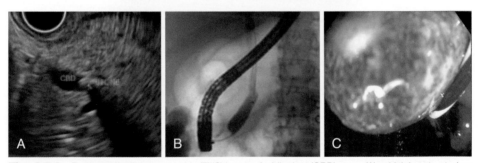

Fig. 35.2   Endoscopic ultrasonographic (EUS) image of a bile duct (CBD) stone (A), which is not noted on a subsequent cholangiogram (B), and finally extracted after a formal sweep of the bile duct is performed (C), thereby demonstrating the sensitivity of EUS for BD stones.

5. ERCP (Fig. 35.3)
    ■ Has been the gold standard for detecting BD stones
    ■ Can miss small stones, especially in a dilated duct
    ■ Sweeping the duct with a balloon catheter increases the chance of finding and removing small stones.
    ■ Most often done when therapeutic intervention is anticipated
    ■ Risks include pancreatitis, bleeding (usually from a sphincterotomy), retroperitoneal perforation, and anesthesia-related complications.
6. Percutaneous transhepatic cholangiography (THC)
    ■ Seldom used for evaluation or treatment of BD stones, except in patients with acute cholangitis when ERCP is unavailable or fails or is anatomically impossible because of prior surgery

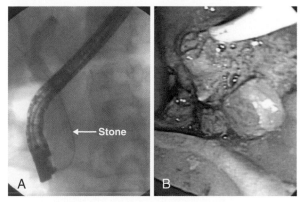

Fig. 35.3   A, Endoscopic retrograde cholangiogram showing a distal bile duct stone *(arrow)* before stone extraction. B, Stone adjacent to the sphincterotomy site after balloon extraction.

- Occasionally used to facilitate a "rendezvous procedure" (combined THC and ERCP) when ERCP alone fails

7. Overall approach
- Patients at high risk for a BD stone should proceed to ERCP with stone removal, followed by elective cholecystectomy.
- Patients at intermediate risk for a BD stone should undergo preoperative EUS or MRCP or laparoscopic cholecystectomy with intraoperative cholangiography or ultrasonography. If a stone is found preoperatively, patients should undergo ERCP with stone removal, followed by elective cholecystectomy if gallbladder stones or sludge were seen on preoperative imaging.
- Patients at low risk for a BD stone should undergo cholecystectomy without additional testing, provided gallstones or sludge were seen on preoperative imaging.
- In the setting of acute cholecystitis a dilated BD on transabdominal ultrasonography may be suggestive of, but not specific for, choledocholithiasis. In a nondilated duct (<6 mm) the risk of having a stone is <10%. At 6 mm, the risk of having a stone is up to 20%, and when the duct is >10 mm, the risk is at least 50%.

TREATMENT

1. ERCP with endoscopic sphincterotomy
- **Treatment of choice at most centers**
- Successful clearance of BD in more than 90% of patients
- Definitive treatment of BD stones in postcholecystectomy patients
- Most common treatment of BD stones when laparoscopic cholecystectomy is planned and BD stones are documented or strongly suspected
- Permits the gallbladder to be left intact after ERCP in patients at high risk for surgery; need for subsequent cholecystectomy is 10% to 20% within 5 to 10 years.

2. Preoperative versus postoperative ERCP
- ERCP has no routine role before cholecystectomy.
- Factors that may predict the presence of BD stones are as follows:
  - Elevated liver biochemical test levels
  - BD dilatation on imaging
  - Initial presentation with cholangitis

- **Preoperative ERCP is appropriate when the suspicion for BD stones is high.**
- **Postoperative ERCP is effective therapy if BD stones are confirmed on IOC.**
- If preoperative ERCP fails in the setting of known BD stones, alternatives include a repeat ERCP at a tertiary referral center, where a variety of methods for cannulation and stone extraction may be used, surgically assisted ERCP, or laparoscopic exploration and stone extraction when the bile duct is large.
  - High success rates (80% to 90%) have been reported by expert surgeons when IOC results are positive for BD stones.
  - The usual approach is the transcystic duct route.
  - Laparoscopic choledochotomy is also possible.
  - Surgical expertise is generally only available at expert centers.
  - Many surgeons still prefer preoperative or postoperative ERCP.
3. Surgical exploration and open choledochotomy
   - Standard of care before ERCP in the 1970s; currently seldom performed except for large retained stones not extractable by other methods
   - If the gallbladder contains stones, laparoscopic cholecystectomy after ERCP extraction of BD stones is usually performed, but leaving the gallbladder intact is an option in high-risk patients.
4. ERCP techniques for the treatment of choledocholithiasis include the following:
   - Guidewire cannulation of BD with a sphincterotome is a common technique; the sphincterotome is advanced over a guidewire into the BD.
   - Needle-knife-access sphincterotomy is performed when cannulation of the BD is difficult.
   - Similarly, needle-knife fistulotomy can be performed in the setting of a large impacted stone at the level of the ampulla.
5. Large stones: May require one or more of the following advanced ERCP techniques:
   - Mechanical lithotripsy with a large basket
   - Laser lithotripsy through choledochoscopy: "Baby scope" inserted into the BD through the channel of a side-viewing endoscope
   - Electrohydraulic lithotripsy through a "baby scope"
   - Extracorporeal shock wave lithotripsy (rarely used in the United States because of the lack of availability)
6. **Complications of ERCP and sphincterotomy**
   - **Pancreatitis** occurs in 5% of patients. It may result either from the diagnostic portion of the procedure or from cautery-induced injury to the pancreatic duct orifice.
     - Symptoms of pancreatitis may not occur until 6 to 12 hours following the procedure.
     - Management of post-ERCP pancreatitis is similar to that for other forms of pancreatitis.
     - Rectal indomethacin may decrease the risk and severity of post-ERCP pancreatitis. It has proven efficacy in combination with a pancreatic stent and as stand-alone therapy.
     - Pancreatitis is more common in patients with a difficult cannulation requiring more cannulation attempts, suspected or proven sphincter of Oddi dysfunction (SOD), and small-caliber ducts.
     - Early evidence suggested that techniques such as needle-knife precut sphincterotomy or transseptal sphincterotomy have a greater risk for pancreatitis; however, when they are used early in the procedure by an expert, the risks of pancreatitis, bleeding, or perforation are equivalent to those for standard ERCP.
     - Temporary placement of a stent in the pancreatic duct appears to reduce the risk, as well as the severity, of post-ERCP pancreatitis.
   - **Bleeding** occurs in 2% to 3% and is usually self-limited.
     - It may occasionally require blood transfusions and even angiographic embolization or surgery.

- Epinephrine injection, endoscopic hemostatic clip placement, deployment of a large fully covered self-expandable metal stent, balloon tamponade, or electrocautery at the time of ERCP may stop bleeding.
- **Perforation** (usually retroperitoneal) occurs in 1%.
  - Post-ERCP imaging may identify benign retroperitoneal air. A small amount of retroperitoneal air can be demonstrated in up to 30% of asymptomatic patients on postprocedural CT. This must be distinguished from a true perforation or even microperforation.
  - Initial symptoms after ERCP that should cause concern for perforation are chills, rigors, and back pain.
  - Perforation often responds to nonsurgical management with nasogastric decompression, nasobiliary drainage (if the complication has been recognized during ERCP), and intravenous broad-spectrum antibiotics.
  - Surgery may be required if signs of infection cannot be controlled with antibiotics.
  - Radiologic drainage may be required if a collection forms.
- **Infection** may occur when adequate drainage is not provided following ERCP.
  - An endoprosthesis can be placed to provide drainage until the BD can be cleared.
7. Long-term stent placement
   - Reserved for patients in whom stone extraction is not accomplished or who have a stricture
   - May be appropriate for frail or elderly patients
   - Cholangitis occurs in 10% to 40% in ensuing years.
   - Treatment with ursodeoxycholic acid, in combination with biliary stenting, may help facilitate subsequent stone extraction.

Gallstone Pancreatitis

Related to impaction of a stone in the ampulla of Vater with occlusion of the pancreatic duct orifice. This may be transient, and the stone may ultimately pass despite having caused pancreatitis.

CLINICAL FEATURES

- Epigastric pain radiating through to the back bilaterally
- Nausea and vomiting
- Low-grade fever or chills
- Tachycardia
- Hypotension, if sequestration ("third-spacing") of fluid is significant

LABORATORY FEATURES

- Leukocytosis
- Elevated liver biochemical test levels (usually to a greater degree than in alcoholic and other causes of pancreatitis)
- Elevated serum amylase and lipase levels
- Elevated blood urea nitrogen and creatinine levels if third-spacing is sufficient to compromise renal blood flow
- Hypocalcemia in moderate to severe cases
- Hyperglycemia
- Hypoxemia, in severe cases, resulting from pulmonary capillary leak, which may result in acute respiratory distress syndrome

  Ranson criteria: The most commonly used of the many classification systems to predict the severity of an episode of acute pancreatitis.

At time of admission:
- Age >55 years
- Blood glucose level >200 mg/dL
- WBC count >16,000/mm^3
- Serum lactate dehydrogenase (LDH) level >350 U/L
- Serum AST level >250 U/L

At 48 hours, the following are noted:
- Decrease in hematocrit value by more than 10%
- Serum calcium level <8 mg/dL
- Base deficit >4 mmol/L
- Blood urea nitrogen level increase >5 mg/dL
- Estimated fluid sequestration >6 L
- Arterial oxygen tension <60 mm Hg
  - The presence of fewer than three criteria indicates mild pancreatitis.
  - **Three or more criteria are associated with more severe pancreatitis and higher mortality rates.**
  - A simpler scoring system (**BISAP** [Bedside Index of Severity of Acute Pancreatitis: blood urea nitrogen >25 mg/dL, impaired mental status, systemic inflammatory response, age >60 years, pleural effusion]) can be used.

TREATMENT

- Similar to that for other forms of pancreatitis
- Strictly nothing by mouth initially; trend in the 2010s has been toward earlier enteral feeding during recovery
- Intravenous hydration
- Careful recording of intake and output
- No role for antibiotics to prevent infection in severe acute pancreatitis or sterile necrosis in the absence of cholangitis
- Monitoring of laboratory data, including blood counts and electrolytes
- Serial contrast-enhanced CTs to monitor patients with moderate or severe pancreatitis for the development of pancreatic necrosis, pseudocysts, or abscesses
- **Role of ERCP in gallstone pancreatitis**
  - ERCP has no benefit in mild gallstone pancreatitis unless clear evidence of a retained BD stone exists.
  - One study demonstrated a reduced risk of local and systemic complications and shorter durations of hospitalization in severe pancreatitis.
  - Meta-analyses have shown no benefit to urgent ERCP.
  - The greatest benefit of ERCP is in the setting of concomitant cholangitis or pancreatic duct disruption (often presenting as severe pancreatitis).

Postcholecystectomy Syndrome

DEFINITION

Postcholecystectomy syndrome is a term used for the **persistence of gastrointestinal symptoms, usually biliary-type pain, in a patient who has undergone a cholecystectomy**.
1. Causes are numerous and are often unrelated to cholecystectomy or the biliary tract.
2. Soon after cholecystectomy, postsurgical complications such as a bile leak must be excluded.

DIFFERENTIAL DIAGNOSIS

In addition to BD stones, the following nonbiliary entities should be considered:
- Irritable bowel syndrome
- Gastroesophageal reflux disease
- Esophageal spasm
- Peptic ulcer
- Chronic pancreatitis
- Musculoskeletal or neurologic pain

SPHINCTER OF ODDI DYSFUNCTION

1. A possible cause of postcholecystectomy syndrome
2. Clinical criteria for diagnosis
   - Biliary- or pancreatic-type pain
   - BD and/or pancreatic duct dilatation (bile duct >10 mm)
   - Elevated serum aminotransferase or ALP levels or elevated pancreatic enzyme levels (more than two times the upper limit of normal) on repeated occasions during episodes of pain
3. Diagnosis (SOD should be considered as a diagnosis only after cholecystecomy.)
   - The gold standard for the diagnosis of SOD is an elevated sphincter of Oddi (SO) pressure (>40 mm Hg) at SO manometry during ERCP.
   - SO manometry is not available at all centers that perform ERCP.
   - SO manometry may add to the risk of pancreatitis during ERCP.
   - For SOD type 1 (sphincter stenosis, see later), there is little benefit to performing manometry as opposed to proceeding with an ERCP sphincterotomy.
   - Noninvasive imaging such as MRCP with secretin may help raise clinical suspicion of SOD when fewer than three criteria are met (accuracy relative to manometry is approximately 75% for SOD type 2 [sphincter disorder]).
   - Provocative testing with cholecystokinin before ultrasonography or EUS can be helpful; an increase of 2 mm or more in BD diameter is abnormal (sensitivity is <25%, specificity >90%).
   - The sensitivity of a hepatobiliary iminodiacetic acid (HIDA) scan for delayed biliary transit is about 50%.
   - Long-term durable response to sphincterotomy is greatest (>70%) for SOD type 1.
4. Traditional classification
   - **Type 1 (sphincter stenosis)**
     - All three clinical criteria are met.
     - SOD is almost always present, and SO manometry is not required.
   - **Type 2 (sphincter disorder)**
     - The patient meets one or two clinical criteria.
     - This type accounts for about one half of patients with SOD.
     - Only patients with abnormal SO manometry results have a good long-term response to sphincterotomy.
   - **"Type 3" (functional pain)**
     - Patients have biliary- or pancreatic-type pain alone.
     - None of the other clinical criteria are present.
     - SO manometry may be abnormal in up to one half of patients.
     - The response to sphincterotomy is low regardless of SO manometry results.
     - Most cases are thought to be unrelated to SOD; therefore, the designation "type 3" SOD has been abandoned.
     - Treatment decisions should be individualized.

Postoperative Bile Duct Injuries and Leaks

OVERVIEW

1. BD injuries occur in about 0.5% of laparoscopic cholecystectomies.
2. The most common biliary injury is a complete transection of the BD, which accounts for approximately 61% of cases and is the most difficult to manage.
3. Bile leaks can result from direct biliary injury or failure to occlude a transected duct and cause acute illness resulting from intraperitoneal bile collections.
4. Bile leaks can occur from a simple cholecystectomy and as a complication of liver transplantation (see Chapter 33) or other pancreaticobiliary surgeries such as a pancreaticoduodenectomy.
5. Other resulting complications include a chronic BD stricture with recurrent cholangitis, liver atrophy, and secondary biliary cirrhosis.

CLASSIFICATION

1. Types of biliary tract injuries during cholecystectomy
   - Bile leak without interruption of ductal continuity
   - Injury to one or more ducts with impairment or complete interruption of bile flow but without a bile leak
   - Combined bile leak and damage to a duct resulting in interrupted flow
2. Classification system proposed by Strasberg et al (1995):
   - **Type A:** Bile leak from a minor duct with preservation of continuity between the liver and duodenum. Examples of type A leaks include injury to the cystic duct remnant or the duct of Luschka, a series of small biliary conduits connecting the gallbladder to the liver bed. Another example is transection of an aberrant accessory right hepatic duct.
   - **Type B:** Occlusion of the right hepatic duct or one of its branches (occurs because the right hepatic duct is mistaken for the cystic duct during cholecystectomy as a result of an anatomic variant in which the cystic duct joins the right hepatic duct rather than the BD)
   - **Type C:** Transaction, rather than occlusion, of an aberrant right hepatic duct
   - **Type D:** Lateral injury to an extrahepatic duct with preserved communication between the biliary tract and duodenum and a resulting stricture
   - **Type E:** Occlusive injury of the BD at any level from the hepatic bifurcation to the duodenum

CAUSES

- Failure to occlude the cystic duct
- Injury to the liver bed caused by entry into a plane deep to the fascial plate of the gallbladder
- Direct thermal injury to a duct at the time of gallbladder dissection
- Forcible pulling on the gallbladder with a resulting injury at the junction of the BD and hepatic duct

DIAGNOSIS

1. A bile leak or injury may be recognized intraoperatively, or the diagnosis may be delayed for years.
2. Presenting symptoms and signs of bile leaks
   - Pain
   - Low-grade fever
   - Abdominal tenderness
   - Leukocytosis
   - Minor liver biochemical test elevations

3. Presenting symptoms and signs of major occlusive injuries to BDs
   - Jaundice
   - Pruritus
   - Elevated liver biochemical test levels
   - Cholangitis
4. Standard imaging studies
   - A nuclear HIDA scan is useful for the diagnosis of a bile leak.
   - Ultrasonography or CT may detect an intraperitoneal bile collection.
   - Benign BD strictures may not result in ductal dilatation on imaging.
   - MRCP can delineate ductal injury; it is the best initial test for identifying proximal biliary injuries and excluded segments. A bile-secreted contrast agent such as gadolinium can also be used to identify a bile leak.
   - ERCP is the preferred modality for the diagnosis of major BD injuries.
5. THC may be necessary in certain situations.
   - Involvement of the biliary tract above the bifurcation, in which THC can localize the proximal extent and access the injured duct better than ERCP
   - Suspicion of an excluded segment of the biliary tract with absent communication between the liver and the distal BD
6. IOC may significantly reduce the risk of biliary injury in complex cholecystectomies (2.2% vs. 16.9%).

TREATMENT

1. The goal of therapy for a bile leak is to reduce outflow resistance in the duodenum.
   - **The procedure of choice is ERCP with stent placement, with or without sphincterotomy.**
   - The stent does not need to bridge the site of the leak.
2. Percutaneous or operative drainage may be needed for large bile collections.
3. Antibiotics should be administered until the leak is controlled or drained.
4. Surgical treatment
   - For major injuries, ligation of the BD and creation of a Roux-en-Y connection between the proximal biliary tract and the jejunum are indicated.
   - Smaller injuries may be repaired by suturing the BD over a T tube.
   - Treatment of a complete transection of the BD during surgery by suturing over a T tube is rarely successful in the long term.
5. Endoscopic therapy of postoperative biliary strictures
   - Biliary dilatation and stent placement (multiple plastic stents are preferred) are followed by stent exchanges every 3 to 6 months for at least 1 year; a covered self-expandable metal stent can be used in selected cases.
   - Published series differ on the need for balloon dilatation of a stricture before stent placement.
   - Good long-term results are achieved in 50% to 80% of patients.
   - Endoscopic and surgical treatment have led to similar results in retrospective comparison studies.

Recurrent Pyogenic Cholangitis

OVERVIEW

1. RPC is characterized by primary intrahepatic stones associated with strictures of the intrahepatic ducts.

2. **It is found almost exclusively in people who live or have lived in Southeast Asia.**
3. Stones are composed mainly of calcium bilirubinate.
4. The syndrome was known previously as Oriental cholangiohepatitis.
5. Patients typically present with recurrent bouts of cholangitis.

PATHOGENESIS

1. RPC is associated with bacterial infection of bile.
   - Bacterial beta glucuronidases hydrolyze conjugated bilirubin.
   - Unconjugated bilirubin binds with calcium and precipitates as calcium bilirubinate, the major constituent of intrahepatic stones.
   - Infection with parasites, such as *Ascaris lumbricoides* or *Clonorchis sinensis,* may play a role.
2. RPC is seen in rural rather than urban areas in endemic countries.
   - The low-protein diet prevalent in rural areas decreases biliary glucuronolactone, an inhibitor of beta glucuronidase.
   - Endogenous beta glucuronidase activity is enhanced, with further deconjugation of bile that leads to precipitation of calcium bilirubinate.

CLINICAL AND LABORATORY FEATURES

1. RPC occurs at a younger age than Western gallstone disease.
   - It may occur in young adults and children.
2. Clinical features
   - Abdominal pain
   - Jaundice
   - Infection
   - Patients may be asymptomatic for many years.
3. Laboratory features
   - Leukocytosis
   - Elevated serum ALP and bilirubin levels
4. Potential consequences
   - Liver abscesses (see Chapter 30)
   - Approximately 30% chance of stone recurrence even if all of the stones are initially removed
   - Atrophy of affected liver segments
   - Cirrhosis and portal hypertension
   - Cholangiocarcinoma in approximately 10% of these cases at time of surgery; lifelong risk is unknown but elevated.

DIAGNOSIS

1. Ultrasonography or CT may reveal focal segmental dilatation of BDs, gross dilatation of ducts within an entire segment or lobe with intrahepatic stones, abrupt tapering intrahepatic duct, and/or strictures. The most common location for disease is the left lobe of the liver.
2. Definitive diagnosis requires ERCP or THC. MRCP is helpful in providing a "roadmap." Cholangioscopy should be considered for evaluation of the ductal mucosa as well as for therapy of stones.

TREATMENT

1. Broad-spectrum antibiotics are administered intravenously to treat episodes of acute cholangitis (see discussion earlier in chapter).
   - Short courses of antibiotics have no proven role to prevent stone formation or episodes of cholangitis.
   - Ursodeoxycholic acid has been used frequently, but there is no evidence that it can provide prophylaxis against stone recurrence.
2. Long-term relief includes surgical options tailored to the individual patient.
   - Resection of atrophic hepatic segments (possibly even lobectomy) and diseased ducts draining the affected liver portion
   - Anastomosis of jejunum to intrahepatic segments proximal to sites of obstruction
   - Creation of permanent access to the BD via the skin through which subsequent therapeutic maneuvers may be performed
   - Creation of a T tube tract or loop of jejunum brought to a subcutaneous site to which the BD has been anastomosed
3. Endoscopic therapy
   - The proximal location of strictures and stones makes the endoscopic approach difficult.
   - ERCP is the first choice for therapeutic intervention, but THC may be necessary because removal of intrahepatic stones by ERCP can be difficult.
   - Cholangioscopy can be useful in assessing duct strictures and treating stone disease (Fig. 35.4).

Biliary Cysts

OVERVIEW

1. Biliary cysts are anomalies of the biliary tract characterized by cystic dilatation of variable portions of the intrahepatic and/or extrahepatic ducts.
2. They are associated with significant complications such as ductal strictures, stone formation, cholangitis, rupture, and secondary biliary cirrhosis.

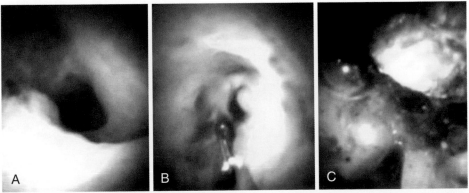

Fig. 35.4 Digital cholangioscopy showing a benign-appearing right intrahepatic stricture (A) in a patient with recurrent pyogenic cholangitis and subsequent biopsy (B). The segment of duct containing multiple stones (C) was then treated with electrohydraulic lithotripsy.

3. The incidence in Western populations is estimated to be 1 in 100,000 and up to 1 in 1000 in Japan, with a female to male ratio of 3 to 1.
4. They primarily affect children and young adults, but reported age ranges vary greatly.
5. Certain types of biliary cysts have a high risk of malignancy.

PATHOGENESIS

1. A cyst may result from an abnormality in biliary epithelial proliferation when fetal ducts are solid that leads to an abnormally dilated proximal portion and a normal or stenotic distal portion.
2. A distal BD stenosis may induce proximal cystic dilatation.
3. Intrinsic autonomic dysfunction may lead to cyst formation.
   - This theory is based on finding a paucity of postcholinergic neurons in portions of the cyst wall.
4. Abnormal pancreaticobiliary junction (APBJ)
   - APBJ is characterized by junction of the BD and pancreatic duct outside the duodenal wall with a long common ductal channel (at least 8 mm, and often >20 mm, in length) leading to the duodenal lumen (Fig. 35.5).
   - APBJ is considered a rare congenital anomaly among the general population but is found in up to 50% of patients with a biliary cyst.
   - APBJ may result in lack of normal SO function and reflux of pancreatic enzymes into BDs, thereby inducing progressive ductal damage and dilatation.
   - APBJ elevates the risk of cancer formation within a cyst.
   - It is common in type I cysts, but not in types II, III, and V cysts (see discussion later in chapter).
   - The observation that the ampulla of Vater is diminutive or flat in patients with APBJ supports this hypothesis.

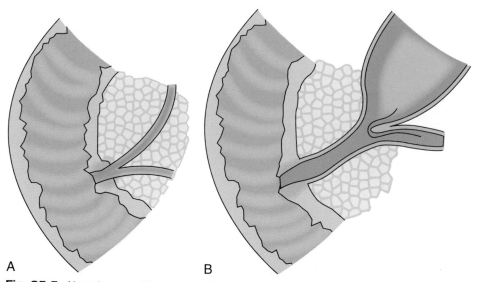

A   B

Fig. 35.5 Normal anatomy (A) contrasted with an anomalous pancreaticobiliary junction (B) thought to be responsible for free reflux of pancreatic enzymes and choledochal cyst formation. (Adapted from O'Neill JA. Choledochal cysts. *Curr Probl Surg.* 1992;29:365–410.)

Classification by Todani et al (1977) (Fig. 35.6)

- Type I: Dilatation of the extrahepatic duct alone; the most common type
- Type II: Diverticulum of the extrahepatic BD
- Type III: Choledochocele, involving only the intraduodenal duct
- Type IVA: Multiple extrahepatic and intrahepatic cysts
- Type IVB: Multiple extrahepatic cysts only
- Type V: Single or multiple intrahepatic cysts (Caroli disease)

CLINICAL FEATURES

1. Right upper quadrant pain
2. Jaundice
   - Often the sole symptom in infants
3. Palpable abdominal mass
4. Fever
5. Epigastric or diffuse abdominal pain if pancreatitis is present

DIAGNOSIS

1. Ultrasonography or CT may reveal or suggest the diagnosis; MRCP is also a diagnostic modality.

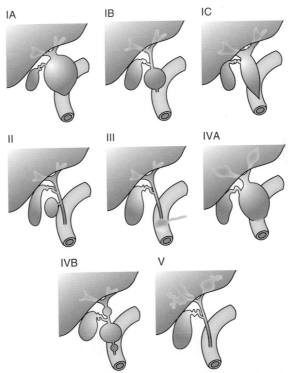

Fig. 35.6 Classification scheme of choledochal cysts suggested by Todani et al. in 1977 (see text). (From Crittenden SL, McKinley MJ. Choledochal cyst-clinical features and classification. *Am J Gastroenterol.* 1985;80:643–647.)

2. ERCP or THC is usually diagnostic.
   - It is also important for classification and planning therapy.
3. THC is best for delineating and potentially draining the proximal biliary ducts.
4. ERCP enables evaluation of the pancreatic duct and the pancreatic-biliary junction.
   - It often reveals an anomalous junction, especially in patients with a type I cyst.
5. MRCP obviates the need for ERCP in many cases.

COMPLICATIONS

1. Stone formation within cysts
2. Cholangitis and liver abscesses
3. Acute pancreatitis, with or without stones
   - This is most common with a choledochocele (type III cyst).
4. Secondary biliary cirrhosis
5. Carcinoma (see also Chapter 36)
   - It usually occurs within cysts and is often multifocal.
   - Carcinomas in cysts are frequently associated with metaplasia and biliary intraepithelial neoplasia formation (see discussion later in chapter).
   - A significant risk exists after nonresectional surgery.
   - Primary cyst excision reduces the cancer risk markedly but not completely.
   - A preoperative diagnosis of cancer is rare.
   - It has a poor prognosis because of extensive spread.
6. Portal hypertension
7. Cyst rupture with bile peritonitis

TREATMENT

1. Type I and type II cysts
   - Excision is followed by reconstruction of the biliary tract with a Roux-en-Y hepaticojejunostomy.
   - Reports have noted success with a laparoscopic approach.
2. Type III cysts (choledochoceles)
   - Endoscopic sphincterotomy may be definitive therapy.
3. Type IV cysts
   - Excision of the extrahepatic cyst, partial resection of intrahepatic cysts when present, and hepaticojejunostomy are performed.
   - Predominant involvement of the left lobe in type IVA disease may necessitate left hepatic lobectomy.
4. Type V cysts (Caroli disease)
   - Partial hepatectomy is performed for localized disease.
   - Roux-en-Y hepaticojejunostomy with placement of transhepatic stents is performed for diffuse disease.
   - Recurrent stones and strictures are treated with percutaneous techniques.
   - Liver transplantation may be required for severe diffuse disease.

Premalignant Lesions of the Bile Duct (see Chapter 36)

- Two early lesions of the BD that may occur de novo or in conjunction with other underlying biliary disease are recognized.

- While most patients will frequently have a predominance of just one of these lesions, both types of epithelial change can be seen in the same specimen as part of a spectrum.
- The lesions are speculated to be part of a multistep sequence of carcinogenesis.

1. **Biliary intraepithelial neoplasia (BilIN)**
   - Subcategorized as BilIN 1-3: BilIN-1 has mild atypia, whereas BilIN-3 has severe atypia and carcinoma in situ.
   - Considered the biliary counterpart of pancreatic intraepithelial neoplasia (PanIN)
   - In the past, it was often called biliary dysplasia, biliary adenoma, and/or biliary epithelium with atypia.
   - Often microscopic and not visible with current cholangioscopic technology
   - BilIN manifests microscopically as flat pseudopapillary (loss of cellular polarity and pseudostratification) and micropapillary (papillary growth with/without indistinct fibrovascular cores) lesions.
   - BilIN and PanIN exhibit similar expression patterns of mucin core proteins (MUC1 and MUC2), suggesting identical phenotypic changes.
   - Commonly associated with PSC, hepatolithiasis, and biliary cysts
   - Also noted as a multifocal lesion in transplant resection specimens from patients with chronic hepatitis B and C and alcoholic cirrhosis
   - Early *KRAS* mutation with later overexpression of *TP53* is similar to that seen in cholangiocarcinoma.

2. **Intraductal papillary neoplasia of the biliary system (IPN-B)**
   - Subcategorized similarly to intraductal pancreatic mucinous neoplasm
     - Gastric (rare in BD)
     - Intestinal (most common type in Asian patients with history of hepatolithiasis and/or clonorchiasis)
     - Oncocytic
     - Pancreaticobiliary (most common type found in BD especially in Western patients)
   - Previously referred to as biliary papillomatosis or biliary papilloma
   - Macroscopically visible and often symptomatic resulting in biliary obstruction either due to the lesion itself or the production of mucin (Fig. 35.7)
   - Gross morphology of the liver shows dilated fusiform and cystic BDs with soft papillary intraductal lesions with the appearance of fish eggs.
   - Most prominent in Asia
   - Often segmental, but 25% of cases are multifocal and best recognized on MRCP.

DIAGNOSIS

1. BilINs are often asymptomatic and frequently identified postresection in the pathologic specimen.
2. MRI and MRCP can identify intraductal polypoid lesions with segmental dilatation of ducts. The use of gadolinium can often help identify mucin as a filling defect on MRI.
3. ERCP with or without cholangioscopy can aid in diagnosis by identifying lesions and intraductal mucin.
   - BilINs can be identified as flat erythematous or nodular areas during cholangioscopy with targeted biopsy.
   - IPN-B can be identified as papillary projections and can have a "fish-egg" appearance. Suspicion is raised when mucin is observed flowing from or in the duct. Mucin may also present as a filling defect on a cholangiogram.

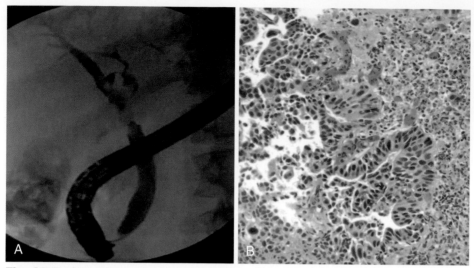

Fig. 35.7 Cholangiogram showing a polypoid lesion (A) causing partial bile duct obstruction. Biopsy of the lesion revealed intraductal papillary neoplasia of the biliary system with areas of high-grade dysplasia (B) (hematoxylin and eosin).

- "Mother-daughter" cholangioscopy is used less frequently because of fragility but offers narrow-band imaging capability and superior optics.
4. Other imaging studies are not helpful for detecting BilIN.

TREATMENT

1. Often associated with underlying biliary pathology and a likely pathway to carcinoma
2. Surgical resection of the underlying lesion needs to be considered, keeping in mind that lesions can be multifocal.
3. Multifocal IPN-B may require liver transplantation because of the risk of cancer and development of secondary biliary cirrhosis.

Bile Duct Strictures

Determining the etiology of a biliary stricture can be challenging, with up to 20% of strictures categorized as indeterminate after initial evaluation. A variety of benign diseases frequently mimic malignancy; the approach needs to be multimodal and multidisciplinary from the beginning.

1. **Benign strictures**
   - Even benign biliary strictures can result in liver abscess, cholangitis, and secondary cirrhosis.
   - Chronic strictures are associated with hepatic lobe atrophy and may result in hypertrophy of unaffected segments along with secondary biliary cirrhosis and portal hypertension.
   - Usually form as a response to acute or chronic injury
     - Chronic inflammation with collagen deposition, fibrosis, and narrowing
     - Acute injury, resulting in segmental ischemia, inflammatory infiltration, fibrosis, and narrowing

■ Causes include bile duct injury (80% of all cases), PSC, choledocholithiasis, hepatolithiasis (RPC), chronic pancreatitis, IgG4 disease with cholangiopathy, human immunodeficiency virus infection, liver transplantation, Mirizzi syndrome (compression of the common hepatic duct by a stone in the neck of the gallbladder), radiation, and benign tumors.

   a. **PSC** (see Chapter 17)

■ 60% of patients develop a dominant stricture in the intrahepatic or extrahepatic biliary tract. This is defined as a stenosis with a ductal diameter of ≤1.5 mm in the BD and ≤1 mm in the hepatic ducts.

■ Generally not responsive to glucocorticoids

■ Affected patients have a 10% to 15% lifetime risk of developing cholangiocarcinoma with an annual incidence of 1.5%.

   b. **IgG4 cholangiopathy** (see Chapter 24)

■ IgG4-related sclerosing cholangitis is the most frequent extrapancreatic manifestation of type 1 autoimmune pancreatitis and is present in over 70% of patients.

■ Tissue biopsy reveals infiltrates of IgG4+ plasma cells, severe interstitial fibrosis, elevated IgG4 serum levels (usually >135 mg/dL). Tissue can also be obtained from the papilla and/or stomach.

■ EUS findings include segmental thickening of the BD wall without an intraductal component. Intraductal masses are more consistent with cholangiocarcinoma.

■ Suspicion should remain high to exclude malignancy especially before placing a patient on immunosuppressive therapy.

■ Usually responsive to glucocorticoids; other immunosuppressive medications (azathioprine, mycophenolate) may be used adjunctively.

2. **Malignant strictures** (see Chapter 36)

■ Pancreatic cancer is the most common cause of malignant extrahepatic BD strictures. Cholangiocarcinoma is the second most common cause and should be suspected especially when there is no mass seen on cross-sectional imaging of the pancreas.

■ Tissue acquisition and cytology are helpful in establishing a diagnosis but are not crucial in patients with potentially resectable disease and a stricture suspicious for carcinoma.

■ The following sampling methods are used:
   – Intraductal fluoroscopically guided biopsies (60% to 80% sensitivity)
   – Cholangioscopy with directed microforceps biopsies (60% sensitivity)
   – Brush cytology (30% to 60% sensitivity)
   – A combination multimodal approach (>85% sensitivity)
   – EUS with fine-needle aspiration or fine-needle biopsy should be avoided in extrahepatic cholangiocarcinoma because of the risk of tumor seeding.

■ Serologic tests such as CA19-9 have a limited sensitivity (50% to 90%).

■ Serum carcinoembryonic antigen (CEA) combined with CA19-9 testing has been proposed as a method to survey PSC for malignancy.

■ IgG4-related cholangiopathy should be excluded.

■ MRI with MRCP and/or ERCP are indicated for preoperative imaging of hilar tumors to determine extent and accurately determine Bismuth classification (see Chapter 36).

■ If there is no evidence of metastatic disease or lymph node involvement and a positron emission tomography (PET) scan is negative, patients should undergo laparoscopy and possible resection. Biliary epithelium is considered extremely 18F-fludeoxyglucose (FDG) avid, and FDG-PET/CT can detect lesions as small as 1 cm.

FURTHER READING

Bowlus CL, Olson KA, Gershwin ME. Evaluation of indeterminate biliary strictures. *Nat Rev Gastroenterol Hepatol*. 2016;13:28–37.

Du S, Liu G, Cheng X, et al. Differential diagnosis of immunoglobulin G4-associated cholangitis from cholangiocarcinoma. *J Clin Gastroenterol*. 2016;50:501–505.

Fan ST, Lai EC, Mok FP, et al. Early treatment of acute biliary pancreatitis by endoscopic papillotomy. *N Engl J Med*. 1993;328:228–232.

Filip M, Saftoiu A, Popescu C, et al. Postcholecystectomy syndrome: an algorithmic approach. *J Gastrointestin Liver Dis*. 2009;18:67–71.

Folsch UR, Nitsche R, Ludtke R, et al. Early ERCP and papillotomy compared with conservative treatment for acute biliary pancreatitis: the German Study Group on Acute Biliary Pancreatitis. *N Engl J Med*. 1997;336:237–242.

Freeman ML. Pancreatic stents for prevention of post-endoscopic retrograde cholangiopancreatography pancreatitis. *Clin Gastroenterol Hepatol*. 2007;5:1354–1365.

Jablonska B, Lampe P. Iatrogenic bile duct injuries: etiology, diagnosis and management. *World J Gastroenterol*. 2009;15:4097–4104.

Neoptolemos JP, Carr-Locke DL, London NJ, et al. Controlled trial of urgent endoscopic retrograde cholangiopancreatography and endoscopic sphincterotomy versus conservative treatment for acute pancreatitis due to gallstones. *Lancet*. 1988;2:979–983.

Nguyen T, Powell A, Daugherty T. Recurrent pyogenic cholangitis. *Dig Dis Sci*. 2009;55:8–10.

Petrov MS, Savides TJ. Systematic review of endoscopic ultrasonography versus endoscopic retrograde cholangiopancreatography for suspected choledocholithiasis. *Br J Surg*. 2009;96:967–974.

Petrov MS, van Santvoort HC, Besselink MG, et al. Early endoscopic retrograde cholangiopancreatography versus conservative management in acute biliary pancreatitis without cholangitis: a meta-analysis of randomized trials. *Ann Surg*. 2008;247:250–257.

Soreide K, Korner H, Havnen J, et al. Bile duct cysts in adults. *Br J Surg*. 2004;91:1538–1548.

Strasberg SM, Hertl M, Soper NJ. An analysis of the problem of biliary injury during laparoscopic cholecystectomy. *J Am Coll Surg*. 1995;180:101–125.

Toouli J. Sphincter of Oddi: function, dysfunction, and its management. *J Gastroenterol Hepatol*. 2009;24:S57–S62.

Williams EJ, Green J, Beckingham I, et al. Guidelines on the management of common bile duct stones (CBDS). *Gut*. 2008;57:1004–1021.

CHAPTER 36

Tumors of the Biliary Tract

Michael G. House, MD, FACS ■ Keith D. Lillemoe, MD, FACS

KEY POINTS

1 Cancers of the biliary tract are categorized into four groups: Gallbladder cancer, intrahepatic cholangiocarcinoma, perihilar cholangiocarcinoma, and distal cholangiocarcinoma.

2 Disregarding cases discovered incidentally at cholecystectomy, carcinoma of the gallbladder, because of its late stage of clinical presentation, has an overall 5-year survival rate <20%.

3 Surgical resection that leads to negative margins may be curative for patients with localized cancers limited to the gallbladder wall.

4 Cholangiocarcinoma is strongly associated with cystic disease of the biliary tract (choledochal cysts, Caroli disease), parasitic infection (*Clonorchis sinensis* or *Opisthorchis viverrini*), primary sclerosing cholangitis, and hepatolithiasis.

5 Patients with perihilar cholangiocarcinomas have poor overall survival, although aggressive resection that includes hepatectomy to achieve negative margins may provide cure.

6 Distal bile duct tumors, which manifest similarly to other periampullary malignant tumors, are associated with a higher rate of resectability and better long-term survival than more proximal (hilar and intrahepatic) cholangiocarcinomas.

Benign Tumors of the Gallbladder

PSEUDOPOLYPS (CHOLESTEROL POLYPS)

1. The most commonly observed polypoid lesion of the gallbladder; accounts for approximately 50% of such lesions
2. Not true neoplasms, but rather cholesterol-filled projections of gallbladder mucosa protruding into the lumen
3. Usually <1 cm in size; visualized on gallbladder imaging studies (ultrasonography, oral cholecystography) as nonmobile filling defects
4. Usually asymptomatic unless associated with gallstones or chronic cholecystitis (e.g., porcelain gallbladder [see later and Chapter 35])
5. No malignant potential

ADENOMYOMATOSIS

1. Consists of a thickened gallbladder muscular layer with Rokitansky-Aschoff sinuses
2. **Three types: Fundal** (most common), appearing as a hemispheric lesion with a central dimple; **segmental,** consisting of an annular stricture; or **diffuse,** involving the entire gallbladder

499

3. May manifest as muscular hypertrophy secondary to gallbladder dysmotility; therefore, symptoms are relieved by cholecystectomy
4. May be associated with carcinoma of the gallbladder

ADENOMAS

1. True neoplastic epithelial tumors of the gallbladder mucosa
2. Usually manifest as solitary, nonmobile filling defects seen on gallbladder ultrasonography
3. Premalignant, with carcinoma in situ found in larger polyps
4. Unlikely to play a major role in the pathogenesis of most gallbladder cancers

TREATMENT

1. Because the histology of polypoid lesions of the gallbladder cannot be determined nonoperatively by current methods, even high-quality ultrasonography, patients with polyps >8 mm should undergo cholecystectomy.
2. Polyps up to 8 mm in size, regardless of total number, should be followed by repeat imaging studies every 3 to 6 months. Changes in ultrasonographic size or features (e.g., involvement of the gallbladder wall) are indications for cholecystectomy.
3. Any patient with biliary symptoms and a gallbladder polyp should undergo cholecystectomy.

Benign Tumors of the Bile Duct (see also Chapter 35)

1. Much less common than benign gallbladder tumors
2. Histologic types
   - Papillomas
   - Adenomas
   - Cystadenomas: Tumors with inner layers of mucin-secreting epithelium, mesenchymal stroma, and an outer layer of hyalinized fibrous tissue
   - Other lesions that may mimic a malignancy
     - Benign tumors: Soft tissue sarcoma, neuroendocrine tumors, and neuromas
     - Inflammatory conditions: Viral hepatitis infection, cholangiopathy due to immunoglobulin (Ig)G4–related disease, biliary sclerosis, radiation-induced cholangiopathy, human immunodeficiency virus (HIV)–associated cholangiopathy (see Chapter 27), and iatrogenic injuries postcholecystectomy of the extrahepatic biliary tract
3. They may be solitary or multiple.
4. Symptoms are usually caused by bile duct obstruction, which results in intermittent jaundice or cholangitis.
5. The diagnosis can usually be made by magnetic resonance, endoscopic retrograde, or percutaneous transhepatic cholangiography.
6. Treatment consists of surgical resection of the bile duct, most commonly with reconstruction by hepaticojejunostomy.
7. Both benign cystadenomas and multiple papillomatosis of the bile duct can be associated with a high rate of local recurrence if complete resection is not accomplished.

Carcinoma of the Gallbladder

EPIDEMIOLOGY

1. **Carcinoma of the gallbladder is the most common biliary tract malignancy and the fifth most common gastrointestinal cancer (3% to 4% of gastrointestinal tumors).**

> **BOX 36.1 ■ Risk Factors for Gallbladder Carcinoma**
>
> Gallstones
> Chronic cholecystitis
> Choledochal cysts
> Anomalous pancreatobiliary duct junction
> Carcinogens
> Estrogens
> Chronic typhoid infection
> Porcelain gallbladder
> Gallbladder polyps

2. The incidence has increased as the population has aged. Approximately 7000 new cases are diagnosed each year (three cases per 100,000 population).
3. The female to male ratio is 3 to 1 due to the greater prevalence of cholelithiasis in women.
4. The usual age of onset is the sixth or seventh decade of life.
5. An increased incidence is seen in southwestern Native Americans, Native Alaskans, Mexicans, and Hispanics living in the United States and in residents of northern Japan, Israel, and Chile.
6. A much lower incidence is seen in African Americans and residents of India, Nigeria, and Singapore.

RISK FACTORS (Box 36.1)

1. **Gallstones and chronic cholecystitis**
   - **Gallstones are present in >90% of patients with gallbladder carcinoma; conversely, only 1% of patients with gallstones have gallbladder carcinoma.**
   - Larger stones (>3 cm) are associated with a 10-fold higher risk of gallbladder cancer compared with smaller stones.
   - The role of gallstones in the development of gallbladder cancer is likely related to chronic inflammation.
   - Gallstone composition does not seem to affect pathogenesis.
2. **Choledochal cysts** (see also Chapter 35)
   - Choledochal cysts are associated with carcinomas throughout the biliary tract, including the gallbladder.
   - The risk of biliary carcinoma increases with age.
   - The risk may be related to an association with an anomalous pancreaticobiliary duct junction, which is frequently seen with choledochal cysts.
   - Surgical removal of choledochal cysts (and the gallbladder) is recommended to prevent further reflux of bile and stasis and to eliminate the cancer risk.
3. **Anomalous pancreaticobiliary duct junction** (see also Chapter 35)
   - The long common channel of the pancreatic and common bile duct (type 3B anomaly) appears to be associated with a significantly increased risk of gallbladder cancer.
   - Reflux of pancreatic juice into the biliary tract with bile stasis is the proposed mechanism.
4. **Carcinogens**
   - Industrial exposure: Rubber industry
   - Thorotrast agent: Used in medical imaging until 1960; long latency for development of cancer of 20 to 40 years
   - Animal studies: Azotoluene, nitrosamines
5. **Estrogens**: This epidemiologic association may simply be related to the associated increased incidence of gallstones.

6. ***Salmonella typhi* infection**: This is likely related to chronic irritation and inflammation of the gallbladder.
7. **Gallbladder wall calcification**: Diffuse calcification of the gallbladder wall (porcelain gallbladder) was formerly an indication for cholecystectomy because of the risk of cancer even in asymptomatic patients. Subsequent studies have suggested that this risk had been overestimated and is likely <5%. Calcification of the gallbladder mucosa is typically a marker of chronic cholecystitis and is associated with an increased frequency of gallbladder cancer.
8. **Gallbladder polyps**
   - Adenomas and adenomyomatosis have clear premalignant potential.
   - Cholecystectomy is indicated for any polyp >8 mm (see discussion earlier in chapter).

PATHOLOGY

1. Histologic type
   a. Adenocarcinoma: 90%
      - Infiltrative (90%): Sclerosing and desmoplastic, obliterating the gallbladder lumen and invading the liver; early lymphovascular and perineural invasion
      - Papillary (5%): Polypoid, slow growing; late metastasis and adjacent organ invasion
      - Colloid (5%): Soft, gelatinous, mucinous tumors that fill the gallbladder
   b. Anaplastic: 5%
   c. Squamous or adenosquamous: 2%
   d. Miscellaneous types (sarcomas, neuroendocrine carcinoma): 3%
2. Routes of spread
   a. Local extension into adjacent organs (i.e., liver, omentum, colon, duodenum), typically for fundus-based tumors. Direct invasion of adjacent structures including the common hepatic duct and duodenum occurs, especially for cancers involving the gallbladder infundibulum.
   b. Lymphatic drainage is to adjacent lymph node basins first: Cystic duct, pericholedochal, and hepatoduodenal lymph nodes (N1). Secondary basins include the retropancreatic, celiac axis, aortocaval, and periaortic nodes (N2).
   c. The veins of the gallbladder drain directly into the liver parenchyma and to branches of the portal vein of segments V and IVB of the liver leading to hepatic metastasis.
   d. Widespread dissemination occurs to the peritoneal surfaces of the hollow and solid viscera of the abdomen.

CLINICAL FEATURES

1. Symptoms (frequency)
   - Abdominal pain (80%): Usually <1-month duration and difficult to distinguish from symptoms of acute cholecystitis or biliary pain
   - Nausea and vomiting (50%)
   - Weight loss (40%)
   - Jaundice (30% to 40%): Usually a poor prognostic finding for fundus-based cancers
   - Incidental finding at cholecystectomy for gallstones (10% to 20% of all gallbladder cancers are discovered incidentally; incidental cancers are found in 1% of cholecystectomies for symptomatic gallstones)
2. Physical findings: Usually indicate advanced disease
   - Right upper quadrant mass
   - Hepatomegaly
   - Jaundice
   - Ascites

DIAGNOSIS

1. Laboratory tests
   - Abnormal liver biochemical test levels when tumor or periportal lymphadenopathy is associated with biliary obstruction
   - No reliable tumor marker, including carcinoembryonic antigen (CEA) and carbohydrate antigen 19-9 (CA19-9)
2. Imaging
   - a. Ultrasonography
     - Sensitivity of 75% to 80%
     - Findings
       - Complex mass filling the gallbladder lumen
       - Asymmetric gallbladder wall thickening
       - Polypoid gallbladder mass
       - Gallbladder wall invasion
       - Gallstones
       - Normal in up to 10% of patients
   - b. Computed tomography (CT)
     - Findings are similar to those of ultrasonography with respect to gallbladder wall thickening or mass.
     - CT defines the extent of disease better than ultrasonography; it demonstrates liver or adjacent organ invasion, liver metastases, lymph node involvement, vascular invasion, and biliary obstruction.
   - c. Magnetic resonance imaging (MRI)
     - Magnetic resonance cholangiopancreatography (MRCP) provides a single noninvasive imaging modality that allows complete assessment of the hepatic parenchyma, biliary tract, vasculature, and lymph nodes.
   - d. Endoscopic ultrasonography (EUS) aids in determining the extent of local invasion and nodal involvement.
   - e. Cholangiography
     - Endoscopic retrograde cholangiopancreatography (ERCP) or percutaneous transhepatic cholangiography (THC) is indicated in patients with clinical evidence of biliary obstruction.
     - The typical cholangiographic appearance is a long stricture of the midportion of the bile duct usually below the hepatic duct bifurcation.
     - Endoscopic or percutaneous stents can be placed for preoperative biliary decompression, to aid in surgical management, or to provide long-term palliation.
   - f. Positron emission tomography (PET) lacks sensitivity and is not part of the routine evaluation for gallbladder cancer. PET may be useful for assessing adenopathy suspected at N2 basins (celiac, retroperitoneum).
3. Preoperative biopsy and cytologic findings
   - No indication exists to pursue a preoperative tissue diagnosis in patients who are considered candidates for surgical resection.
   - Percutaneous or EUS-guided fine-needle biopsy for histologic or cytologic analysis should be avoided. Biopsy for tissue diagnosis should only be performed in patients with unresectable or metastatic gallbladder cancer.
   - Bile duct or bile cytologic specimens or brushings, even with a cytogenetics assay (e.g., fluorescence in situ hybridization [FISH]), have a low diagnostic yield.

STAGING

Please refer to the Table 36.1 for the carcinoma staging of the gallbladder.

TABLE 36.1 ■ American Joint Commission on Cancer (Tumor, Node, Metastasis) Staging for Carcinoma of the Gallbladder

Stage	Definition
0	Carcinoma in situ (T0)
I (T1N0M0)	Tumor invades lamina propria (T1a) or muscular layer (T1b)
II (T2N0M0)	Tumor invades perimuscular connective tissue on the peritoneal side (T2a) or hepatic side (T2b)
IIIA (T3N0M0)	Tumor perforates the serosa (visceral peritoneum) and/or directly invades the liver and/or one other adjacent organ, such as stomach, duodenum, colon, pancreas, or extrahepatic bile ducts (T3); no lymph node involvement
IIIB (T1-3N1M0)	T1-3 with positive nodes confined to the hepatic hilus including nodes along the bile duct, hepatic artery, portal vein, and cystic duct (N1)
IVA (T4N0M0)	Tumor invades main portal vein or hepatic artery or invades two or more extrahepatic organs (T4); no lymph node involvement
IVB (any T, any N, M1 or any T, N2M0, or T4N1M0)	Any T with distant metastases (M1); any T with lymph node metastases to celiac, periduodenal, peripancreatic, and/or superior mesenteric lymph nodes (N2); T4 with N1 nodes

Adapted from Zhu AX, Pawlik TM, Kooby DA, et al. Gallbladder. In: Amin MB, Edge SB, Greene FL, et al, eds. *AJCC Cancer Staging Manual,* 8th ed. New York: Springer Nature; 2017:303–309.

TREATMENT

1. Nonoperative palliation
   - Nonoperative palliation is indicated in patients in whom preoperative evaluation reveals extensive local or metastatic disease that precludes resection (stage IVA or IVB disease).
   - Obstructive jaundice can be palliated with either a Silastic or metallic endoprosthesis or internal-external transhepatic Silastic stent; internal or internal-external Silastic stents must be changed at 2- to 3-month intervals.
   - Pain, if significant, can be managed with oral narcotics or a percutaneous or EUS-guided celiac axis block.
   - Palliative systemic chemotherapy (gemcitabine plus cisplatin) can be considered for patients with preserved performance status and a life expectancy >6 months.
2. Surgical management
   a. Incidental discovery of gallbladder carcinoma at laparoscopic cholecystectomy
      - With the widespread use of laparoscopic cholecystectomy for symptomatic gallstones, many gallbladder cancers are first encountered in this setting.
      - **Laparoscopic cholecystectomy is contraindicated if gallbladder carcinoma is suspected preoperatively.**
      - **If gallbladder carcinoma is recognized at the time of laparoscopic cholecystectomy, the operation should be converted to an open resection.**
      - If gallbladder carcinoma is recognized pathologically after laparoscopic cholecystectomy, management is dictated by the histologic findings.
        - If the carcinoma is limited to the lamina propria of the gallbladder wall and has a negative cystic duct margin (pathologic stage T1a), cholecystectomy is adequate.
        - If the carcinoma penetrates into the muscular layer (pathologic stage T1b), an extended cholecystectomy (similar to that for pathologic stage T2) should be considered.
        - If the carcinoma penetrates into the perimuscular connective tissue (pathologic stage T2), the patient should undergo repeat exploration and partial central hepatectomy,

TABLE 36.2 ■ Morbidity and Mortality Rates for Resection of Gallbladder Carcinoma

Resection	Overall Morbidity Rate (%)	30-Day Mortality Rate (%)
Cholecystectomy	10	1
Extended cholecystectomy with central hepatectomy	25	2
Major hepatectomy	40	5
Hepatectomy and pancreatoduodenectomy	50–70	15

including liver segments IVB and V, plus regional periportal lymph node dissection (for adequate staging) and excision of the cystic duct stump.
  - Laparoscopic port site excision is no longer advocated because port site disease typically indicates diffuse peritoneal seeding.
  b. Surgical management of suspected gallbladder carcinoma based on clinical or imaging findings
   ■ The resectability rates for gallbladder carcinoma range from 15% to 30%.
   ■ If the tumor is confined to the lamina propria or muscular layer (pathologic stage T1), simple cholecystectomy is adequate resection in most cases.
   ■ If the tumor penetrates the gallbladder wall, resection includes the gallbladder, segment V, and the anterior portion of segment IV of the liver with a lymph node dissection, including hepatoduodenal, choledochal, and retropancreatic nodes.
   ■ Japanese investigators have advocated more aggressive resection, including combined hepatic resection and pancreatoduodenectomy.
   ■ Postoperative morbidity and mortality rates are directly related to the extent of resection (Table 36.2).
3. Adjuvant chemotherapy following resection
   ■ A high frequency of distant recurrence supports the need for systemic adjuvant therapy.
   ■ The number of relevant randomized prospective trials is limited.
   ■ One prospective randomized phase III trial of adjuvant chemotherapy with 5-fluorouracil and mitomycin C versus surgery alone found that 5-year survival was significantly better in the adjuvant therapy group (26%) than in the control group (14%). The 5-year disease-free survival rates were 20.3% and 11.6%, respectively.
4. Treatment of unresectable disease
   ■ Modern chemotherapy (gemcitabine and platinum-based agents) is associated with response rates of approximately 20% and improves progression-free survival by 8 weeks.
   ■ Radiation therapy, including external beam and intraoperative radiation therapy and brachytherapy, has not been shown consistently to improve survival and does not play a major role in palliation.

PROGNOSIS

1. Because of the late stage of presentation, **the overall 5-year survival rate is <10%, with a median survival of 6 months**.
2. Survival depends on the stage of tumor (see Table 36.1).
   ■ Patients with stage I tumors have a 5-year survival rate approaching 100% following simple or extended cholecystectomy.

TABLE 36.3 ■ **Frequency of Cholangiocarcinoma at Various Locations (%)**

Intrahepatic bile duct	25
Perihilar bile duct (superior to cystic duct orifice)	40
Distal bile duct (inferior to cystic duct orifice)	25
Diffuse/multifocal	10

- Patients with stage II tumors treated with extended cholecystectomy may have a 60% to 80% 5-year survival rate.
- Patients with stage IIIa tumors treated with extended resection have 3- and 5-year survival rates of 60% and 25%, respectively. Stage IIIb gallbladder cancer is associated with a 5-year survival rate of <20%.
- The median survival for patients with unresectable stage IV disease is only 3 to 4 months.
- Long-term survival after curative resection as a second procedure (following an inadequate first operation) is no different from that after a single procedure.

Carcinoma of the Bile Duct (Cholangiocarcinoma)

THREE TYPES (Table 36.3)

- Intrahepatic cholangiocarcinoma
- Perihilar cholangiocarcinoma
- Distal cholangiocarcinoma

EPIDEMIOLOGY

- Distinct from that of gallbladder cancer
- The incidence of bile duct cancer in the United States is 0.8 per 100,000 population per year.
- 3000 to 4000 new cases per year in the United States
- Male to female ratio of 1.3 to 1
- Age range of 50 to 70 years

RISK FACTORS (Table 36.4)

1. **Caroli disease and choledochal cysts** (see also Chapter 35)
   a. The reported frequency of cholangiocarcinoma in patients with cystic abnormalities of the biliary tract ranges from 6% to 30%.
   b. Patients with cystic lesions of the bile duct tend to develop cholangiocarcinoma at an age two to three decades earlier than patients with sporadic cholangiocarcinoma.
   c. In more than 75% of patients with cholangiocarcinomas associated with choledochal cysts, symptoms first appear in adulthood.
   d. Factors that may account for the development of cholangiocarcinoma in patients with cystic disease of the biliary tract include the following:
      - Reflux of pancreatic exocrine secretions as a result of an anomalous pancreatobiliary duct junction

TABLE 36.4 ■ Risk Factors for Cholangiocarcinoma

Strong Association

Caroli disease
Choledochal cyst
Clonorchis sinensis
Opisthorchis viverrini
Hepatolithiasis
Primary sclerosing cholangitis
Ulcerative colitis
Thorotrast exposure

Possible Association

Chronic hepatitis B or C viral infection with or without cirrhosis (intrahepatic cholangiocarcinoma)
Asbestos
Dioxin (Agent Orange)
Isoniazid
Methyldopa
Oral contraceptives (mixed hepatocellular cholangiocarcinoma)
Polychlorinated biphenyls
Radionucleotides

- Bile stasis
- Chronic inflammation and bacterial infection within the cyst
- Stone formation within the cyst

2. **Parasitic infection** (see also Chapter 31)
   - *C. sinensis* is common in Asia, particularly China, Hong Kong, and Korea, and is associated with the ingestion of raw fish.
   - The adult trematode resides in the intrahepatic and, less commonly, extrahepatic bile ducts, can obstruct biliary flow, and can cause periductal fibrosis, hyperplasia, stricture, and stone formation.
   - *O. viverrini* is another liver fluke associated with cholangiocarcinoma and is found mostly in Thailand. Metacercariae are present in flesh and skin of freshwater fish.

3. **Hepatolithiasis** (recurrent pyogenic cholangitis) (see also Chapter 35)
   - Cholangiocarcinoma develops in 5% to 10% of patients with hepatolithiasis.
   - Bile stasis, bactibilia, and cystic dilatation may all be associated with this increased risk.
   - Cholelithiasis is seen in up to one third of patients with and without cholangiocarcinoma; therefore, gallbladder stones are not considered a risk factor for cholangiocarcinoma in this setting.

4. **Primary sclerosing cholangitis** (see also Chapter 17)
   - Average age at diagnosis: 45 to 50 years
   - Unrecognized cholangiocarcinoma is found in up to 25% of autopsies in patients dying with, and 15% of patients undergoing liver transplantation for, primary sclerosing cholangitis.
   - Patients with primary sclerosing cholangitis have a lifetime risk of cholangiocarcinoma of 6% to 36%.
   - Cholangiocarcinoma in patients with primary sclerosing cholangitis often presents with rapid clinical deterioration and progressive jaundice.
   - Controversy exists regarding the relation between the duration of primary sclerosing cholangitis and the risk of cholangiocarcinoma.

- Cohort studies report the diagnosis of cholangiocarcinoma within 1 to 2 years of the diagnosis of primary sclerosing cholangitis.
- Most studies do not show an association between the presence or duration of inflammatory bowel disease and primary sclerosing cholangitis–associated cholangiocarcinoma.
- The prognosis in patients with clinically detected cholangiocarcinoma and primary sclerosing cholangitis is poor, with a median survival of <1 year.

5. **Ulcerative colitis**
   - The frequency of cholangiocarcinoma in patients with ulcerative colitis ranges from 0.14% to 0.9%, >100 times that of the general population.
   - Cholangiocarcinoma develops 20 years earlier in patients with ulcerative colitis than in others.
   - Patients with cholangiocarcinoma and ulcerative colitis tend to have pancolonic involvement and a long duration of disease.
   - The risk of cholangiocarcinoma does not appear to be affected by proctocolectomy.

6. **Thorotrast** (thorium dioxide)
   - This radiocontrast agent used before 1960 emits alpha particles and, when injected intravenously, is retained in the reticuloendothelial system for life.
   - Cholangiocarcinoma may develop after a mean latent period of 35 years.

PATHOLOGY

1. Histologic type
   - Adenocarcinoma accounts for more than 95% of cases.
   - Rare histologic types include squamous and mucoepidermoid carcinomas, cystadenocarcinomas, carcinoid tumors, and leiomyosarcomas.
   - Histologic types of adenocarcinoma include sclerosing (most common), scirrhous, diffusely infiltrating, and papillary (unifocal or multifocal).
2. Location (see Table 36.3)
3. Route of spread
   - Spread occurs most commonly (70%) by direct invasion of the adjacent liver, portal vein, hepatic artery, pancreas, or duodenum.
   - Liver and peritoneal metastases occur in up to 25% of patients, with an even higher frequency in patients with intrahepatic cholangiocarcinoma.
   - Regional lymph nodes are involved in 60% to 75% of patients.

CLINICAL FEATURES

1. Symptoms
   - Jaundice: The most common presenting symptom; present in >90% of patients
   - Pruritus
   - Weight loss
   - Abdominal pain: Vague, nonspecific, and mild; sometimes the only symptom in patients with a proximal tumor located above the hepatic bifurcation
   - Cholangitis (uncommon)
2. Physical findings
   - Jaundice
   - Hepatomegaly
   - Palpable gallbladder: Only with distal tumors
   - Ascites

DIAGNOSIS

1. Laboratory tests
   - Serum bilirubin and alkaline phosphatase levels are increased.
   - The prothrombin time is prolonged in patients with long-standing biliary obstruction.
2. Tumor markers
   - Serum CA19-9 levels are usually elevated, particularly in patients with jaundice.
3. Imaging
   a. Ultrasonography and CT
      - Findings in patients with a hilar tumor are a dilated intrahepatic biliary tract, contracted gallbladder, and normal-caliber extrahepatic biliary tract and pancreas.
      - Findings in patients with a distal tumor are a dilated intrahepatic and extrahepatic biliary tract and a distended gallbladder.
      - Hilar adenopathy and portal vein patency should be assessed.
      - Involvement of hepatic artery branches is assessed most accurately with CT angiography or careful ultrasonography.
      - Celiac, aortocaval, and retroperitoneal lymph nodes (all indicating N2 disease) should be assessed.
   b. MRI and MRCP
      - These techniques can usually identify the primary tumor, level of biliary sectoral or segmental involvement, patency of hilar vascular structures, nodal or distal metastases, and sectoral liver atrophy.
      - MRI with MRCP is more valuable than invasive cholangiography for revealing obstructed and isolated ducts and avoids early biliary instrumentation with a risk of cholangitis.
   c. Cholangiography
      - **Either ERCP or percutaneous THC should be performed to define the location and extent of the tumor.**
      - THC is preferred at some centers because of its greater accuracy in defining the proximal extent of the tumor (i.e., segmental duct involvement).
      - The cholangiographic appearance can predict resectability (with regard to ductal involvement) in perihilar cholangiocarcinoma (positive predictive value of 60%).
      - Percutaneous or endoscopic placement of biliary catheters should be planned to permit adequate drainage of the future liver remnant following operative resection of a perihilar cancer.
      - ERCP is most appropriate for distal bile duct cancers.
   d. PET may detect small tumors (e.g., intrahepatic cholangiocarcinoma in patients with primary sclerosing cholangitis), advanced regional lymph node involvement, or distant metastases.
   e. Preoperative biopsy and cytologic findings
      - A tissue diagnosis to rule out malignancy is necessary in patients being considered for nonoperative management of a presumably benign stricture or in those with primary sclerosing cholangitis who are being evaluated for liver transplantation.
      - Bile cytology demonstrates malignant cells in only 30% of cases of cholangiocarcinoma.
      - Cytologic brushings performed either percutaneously or endoscopically yield positive results in <50% of patients; results improve with multiple attempts; cytogenetic molecular markers (e.g., FISH analysis) may increase detection rates.
      - **EUS-guided fine-needle aspiration or ERCP-directed cholangioscopic biopsies for perihilar tumors may increase the diagnostic yield to 60%.**

TABLE 36.5 ■ **American Joint Commission on Cancer (Tumor, Node, Metastasis [TMN]) Staging for Extrahepatic (Perihilar) Cholangiocarcinoma**

Stage	Definition
0	Carcinoma in situ or high-grade dysplasia
I (T1N0M0)	Tumor confined to the bile duct wall up to the muscle layer or fibrous tissue (T1)
II (T2a or 2b N0M0)	Tumor invades beyond the bile duct wall to the surrounding adipose tissue (T2a) or the adjacent liver parenchyma (T2b)
IIIA (T3N0M0)	Tumor invades unilateral branches of the portal vein or hepatic artery (T3); no lymph node involvement
IIIB (T1-3N1M0)	T1-3 with regional lymph node metastases
IVA (T4N0-1M0)	Tumor invades the main portal vein or branches bilaterally or common hepatic artery; or second-order biliary radicles bilaterally; or second-order biliary radicles with contralateral portal vein or hepatic artery involvement
IVB (any T, N2M0 or any T, any NM1)	Any T with periaortic, pericaval, superior mesenteric, or celiac lymph node metastases (N2) or with distant metastasis (M1)

Adapted from Nagorney DM, Pawlik TM, Chun YS, et al. Perihilar bile ducts. In: Amin MB, Edge SB, Greene FL, et al, eds. *AJCC Cancer Staging Manual,* 8th ed. New York: Springer Nature; 2017:311–316.

STAGING

Please refer to Table 36.5 for the staging for extrahepatic (perihilar) choangiocarcinoma.

TREATMENT

1. Nonoperative palliation
   - This is indicated in patients with extensive local or metastatic disease that precludes resection (if determined preoperatively).
   - Obstructive jaundice can be palliated with either Silastic or metallic endoprostheses or internal-external Silastic stents; Silastic stents must be changed at 3-month intervals.
   - In patients with perihilar cholangiocarcinoma, percutaneous bilateral access may be necessary if endostenting cannot be accomplished with ERCP.
   - Death is usually the result of recurrent biliary sepsis and liver failure.
2. Surgical palliation
   a. Only indicated for patients who undergo operative exploration with the potential for cure (i.e., good-risk patients not determined to have unresectable or metastatic disease by preoperative staging)
   b. The surgical approach to palliation of a locally unresectable cholangiocarcinoma is determined at exploration.
      - For perihilar tumors: Cholecystectomy with placement of Silastic stents and a Roux-en-Y choledochojejunostomy or hepaticojejunostomy or a segment III biliary bypass to the left hepatic duct using a Roux-en-Y limb of jejunum
3. Surgical resection
   a. The approach to intrahepatic cholangiocarcinoma is similar to that for hepatocellular carcinoma, with a standard hepatic resection to accomplish complete removal of the tumor.
   b. **Perihilar cholangiocarcinomas** require local resection of the hepatic duct cephalad to the level of the hepatic duct bifurcation to achieve a microscopically negative margin, including hepatic resection as indicated, with reconstruction to a Roux-en-Y jejunal limb; hepatoduodenal lymphadenectomy should be performed.

TABLE 36.6 ■ **Morbidity and Mortality Rates for Resection of Cholangiocarcinoma**

	Overall morbidity rate (%)	30-day mortality rate (%)
Hepatic bifurcation resection and hepaticojejunostomy	40	<5
Hepatectomy without bile duct resection	25	2
Hepatic bifurcation resection, reconstruction, and hepatectomy	65	15

- Many surgeons advocate routine resection of the caudate lobe (segment I) of the liver for cancers involving the bile duct bifurcation or left hepatic duct.
- The addition of a major hepatic resection significantly increases perioperative morbidity and mortality (Table 36.6).
- **Liver transplantation** offers the advantage of resection of all structures potentially involved by tumor even in locally advanced disease. Liver transplantation should only be performed at centers with careful selection protocols that include neoadjuvant therapy after meticulous staging.
  c. **Distal cholangiocarcinomas** require pancreatoduodenectomy, with a perioperative mortality rate <4% and morbidity rate of 30% to 40%.
4. Adjuvant therapy following resection
   - No relevant randomized, prospective trials have been reported.
   - To date, no single chemotherapeutic agent or combination of agents, with or without radiation, has been shown to be of clear benefit in reducing locoregional recurrence.
   - In the absence of prospective data, most groups advocate adjuvant chemotherapy and/or radiation therapy for resected distal cholangiocarcinomas based on the results of prospective trials for resectable pancreatic carcinoma.
5. Treatment of unresectable disease: Randomized controlled trials have shown an overall survival benefit of 2 to 4 months with combination chemotherapy (gemcitabine plus cisplatin).

PROGNOSIS

1. Intrahepatic cholangiocarcinoma
   - Intrahepatic cholangiocarcinoma usually manifests at an advanced stage (only 25% resectability rate).
     a. Resectable: 3-year survival rate of 45%; median survival of 18 to 30 months
     b. Unresectable: Median survival of 9 months
     c. Metastatic: Median survival of 3 to 6 months
2. Perihilar cholangiocarcinoma (Table 36.7)
   - Factors adversely influencing survival include positive surgical margin, low preoperative serum albumin level, and postoperative sepsis.
     a. Unresectable (determined at surgery)
        - Median survival of 9 months
        - 1-year survival rate of 27%
        - 2-year survival rate of 6%
     b. Unresectable (determined preoperatively)
        - Median survival of 6 months
        - 1-year survival rate of 25%
        - 2-year survival rate of 5%

TABLE 36.7 ■ **Management of Perihilar Cholangiocarcinoma and Outcomes**

Management or Outcome	Frequency (%)
Liver resection required	75–100
Margin of resection negative (R0) after surgery	50–80
5-yr survival:	
R0 resection	40
R1 resection	10

3. Distal cholangiocarcinoma
   a. Resectable
      ■ Median survival of 24 months
      ■ Overall survival rates at 1, 3, and 5 years of 70%, 40%, and 25%, respectively
      ■ Factors adversely influencing survival following resection are positive lymph node status and poor tumor differentiation.
   b. Unresectable: Median survival of 15 months

FURTHER READING

Aljiffry M, Walsh M, Molinari M, et al. Advances in diagnosis, treatment and palliation of cholangiocarcinoma: 1990-2009. *World J Gastroenterol.* 2009;15:4240–4262.

Burke ED, Jarnigan WR, Hochwald SN, et al. Hilar cholangiocarcinoma: patterns of spread, the importance of hepatic resection for curative operation, and a presurgical clinical staging system. *Ann Surg.* 1998;228:385–394.

Cho C, Ito F, Rikkers L, et al. Hilar cholangiocarcinoma: current management. *Ann Surg.* 2009;250:210–218.

Endo I, House MG, Endo I, et al. Clinical significance of intraoperative bile duct margin assessment for hilar cholangiocarcinoma. *Ann Surg Onc.* 2008;15:2104–2112.

Fong Y, Jarnigan W, Blumgart L. Gallbladder cancer: comparison of patients presenting initially for definitive operation with those presenting after prior noncurative intervention. *Ann Surg.* 2000;232:557–569.

House MG, Chauhan A, Nakeeb A, et al. Postoperative morbidity results in decreased survival after resection for hilar cholangiocarcinoma. *HPB.* 2011;13:139–147.

Ito F, Agni R, Rettammel RJ, et al. Resection of hilar cholangiocarcinoma: concomitant liver resection decreases hepatic recurrence. *Ann Surg.* 2008;248:273–279.

Jarnigan WR, Fong Y, DeMatteo RP, et al. Staging, respectability, and outcome in 225 patients with hilar cholangiocarcinoma. *Ann Surg.* 2001;234:239–251.

Loehrer AP, House MG, Nakeeb A, et al. Cholangiocarcinoma: are North American outcomes optimal? *J Am Coll Surgeons.* 2013;216:192–200.

Mohamadnejad M, Dewitt JM, Sherman S, et al. Role of EUS for preoperative evaluation of cholangiocarcinoma: a large single-center experience. *Gastrointest Endosc.* 2011;73:71–78.

Rea DJ, Heimbach JK, Rosen CB, et al. Liver transplantation with neoadjuvant chemoradiation is more effective than resection for hilar cholangiocarcinoma. *Ann Surg.* 2005;242:451–458.

Rea DJ, Munoz-Juarez M, Farnell MB, et al. Major hepatic resection for hilar cholangiocarcinoma: analysis of 46 patients. *Arch Surg.* 2004;139:514–523.

Shih SP, Schulick RD, Cameron JL, et al. Gallbladder cancer: the role of laparoscopy and radical resection. *Ann Surg.* 2007;245:893–901.

Takada T, Amano H, Yasuda H, et al. Is postoperative adjuvant chemotherapy useful for gallbladder carcinoma? A phase III multicenter prospective randomized controlled trial in patients with resected pancreaticobiliary carcinoma. *Cancer.* 2002;95:1685–1695.

Vauthey JN, Pawlik TM, Abdalla EK, et al. Is extended hepatectomy for hepatobiliary malignancy justified? *Ann Surg.* 2004;239:722–730.

INDEX

Page numbers followed by *f* indicate figures; *t*, tables, *b*, boxes.